FORENSIC NURSING

A HANDBOOK FOR PRACTICE

EDITED BY

RITA M. HAMMER, PhD, RN, BC
Professor of Forensic Nursing
Quinnipiac University
Hamden, CT

BARBARA MOYNIHAN, PhD, APRN, BC
Associate Professor of Nursing
Coordinator MSN, Forensic Nursing Track
Quinnipiac University
Hamden, CT

ELAINE M. PAGLIARO, JD, MS
Assistant Director
CT Forensic Science Laboratory
Meriden, CT

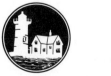

JONES AND BARTLETT PUBLISHERS
Sudbury, Massachusetts
BOSTON   TORONTO   LONDON   SINGAPORE

World Headquarters
Jones and Bartlett Publishers
40 Tall Pine Drive
Sudbury, MA 01776
978-443-5000
info@jbpub.com
www.jbpub.com

Jones and Bartlett Publishers Canada
6339 Ormindale Way
Mississauga, ON L5V 1J2
CANADA

Jones and Bartlett Publishers International
Barb House, Barb Mews
London W6 7PA
UK

Jones and Bartlett's books and products are available through most bookstores and online booksellers. To contact Jones and Bartlett Publishers directly, call 800-832-0034, fax 978-443-8000, or visit our website www.jbpub.com.

Substantial discounts on bulk quantities of Jones and Bartlett's publications are available to corporations, professional associations, and other qualified organizations. For details and specific discount information, contact the special sales department at Jones and Bartlett via the above contact information or send an email to specialsales@jbpub.com.

Library of Congress Cataloging-in-Publication Data

Forensic nursing : a handbook for practice / [edited by] Rita M. Hammer,
   Barbara Moynihan, Elaine M. Pagliaro.
    p. ; cm.
   ISBN 0-7637-2610-9
   1. Forensic nursing. I. Hammer, Rita M. II. Moynihan, Barbara.
   III. Pagliaro, Elaine M.
   [DNLM: 1. Nursing Care—methods. 2. Forensic Medicine—methods.
   3. Specialties, Nursing—methods. WY 100 F715 2006]

RA1155.F63 2006
614'.1—dc22

                                         2005018287

Production Credits
Acquisitions Editor: Kevin Sullivan
Associate Editor: Amy Sibley
Production Director: Amy Rose
Production Editor: Renée Sekerak
Production Assistant: Rachel Rossi
Marketing Manager: Emily Ekle
Manufacturing Buyer: Amy Bacus
Composition: Graphic World, Inc.
Cover Design: Kristin E. Ohlin
Printing and Binding: Malloy Incorporated
Cover Printing: Malloy Incorporated

Printed in the United States of America
09 08 07 06 05   10 9 8 7 6 5 4 3 2 1

Contents

APPENDICES

Foreword

Almost ten years ago, I authored federal legislation for the Violence Against Women Act that provides millions of dollars each year to state and local authorities and victim service providers for the investigation, prosecution, treatment, and prevention of domestic violence, sexual assault, and stalking. I also overhauled our nation's federal criminal laws to better prosecute these crimes. Significantly, the Violence Against Women Act mandated the Attorney General to evaluate and recommend standards for training and practice for licensed health care professionals performing sexual assault forensic exams.

In the course of drafting the Violence Against Women Act, I became aware of the critical work sexual assault forensic nurses do in our country's hospitals. I learned that these nurses are particularly sensitive to the trauma of sexual assault and try to ensure that the patient is not revictimized after reporting the crime. When forensic nurses are involved in the treatment of a sexual assault victim, there is typically better collaboration with law enforcement, higher reporting rates, better documentation of the crime, accurate forensic evidence collection, and more successful prosecutions of the assailants. Forensic nurses play an integral role in bridging the gap between law and medicine. They should be in each and every emergency room.

Ten years ago, DNA analysis cost thousands of dollars and took months to get results, today it can be done for $40 in a matter of days. Ten years ago, it took a bottle cap of blood for forensic scientists to do the tests. Now, testing can be done with a sample the size of a pinhead. Today, DNA testing is 99.9 percent accurate. The changes in DNA technology are remarkable and mark a sea of change in how forensic science can help us fight crime, particularly sexual assault crimes. But DNA matching is only effective if the evidence is collected and maintained appropriately. It is clear that if we are going to capitalize on the power of DNA, forensic nurses must be key players. Arming our forensic nurses with resources and tools will help us bring to justice thousands of criminals who are only one DNA test away from conviction.

The examples of what can be done are clear. Just last year, Alabama authorities charged a man in the rape of an 85-year-old woman almost 10 years after the assault because he was linked to the case by a DNA sample he was compelled to submit while in prison on unrelated charges. In Colorado, prosecutors brought to trial a case against a man accused of at least 14 rapes and sexual assaults. Due to the national DNA database, prosecutors were able to trace the defendant to rapes and assaults that occurred in Colorado, California, Arizona, Nevada, and Oklahoma between 1999 and 2002.

Undoubtedly, DNA matching by comparing evidence gathered at the crime scene with offender samples entered on the national DNA database has proven to be *the* deciding factor in solving stranger sexual assault cases—it has revolutionized the criminal justice system and brought closure and justice for victims. Federal, state, and local lawmakers have begun to focus attention on DNA evidence and ensure that our crime-fighting professionals, including forensic nurses, have adequate tools to harness the power of DNA.

Most recently, Congress proposed new federal legislation (the Advancing Justice through DNA Technology Act of 2003), passed legislation such as the DNA Analysis Backlog Elimination Act of 2000, and held several hearings that focused on DNA and sexual assault crimes and oversight of the forensic sciences. The current Administration also launched a DNA initiative last year calling for $232.6 million in federal funding in fiscal year 2004 and continuing this level of funding for five years—a total commitment of over $1 billion.

Forensic nurses are foot soldiers in the response to and treatment of violence against women. Therefore, I am pleased that this groundbreaking textbook will help educate and prepare tomorrow's forensic nurses. Recognizing the complexity of forensic nursing, this textbook covers a wide variety of issues, such as forensic photography, offender profiling, and court testimony. It also devotes an entire chapter to disaster management.

Forensic Nursing: A Handbook for Practice brings together in one volume many of the field's most accomplished experts. I am certain that this textbook will serve as an invaluable resource for the entire forensic examiner community and help shape a new generation of forensic nurses.

Joseph R. Biden, Jr.
United States Senator

Preface

Forensic nursing is an area of clinical expertise that is an evolving phenomenon on the verge of maturing into a significant new nursing specialty. Its development reflects a response designed to fulfill a societal need: The growing public health problem of societal violence. A few enthusiastic and dedicated individuals with a vision recognized not only the need for forensic nurses and forensic nursing, but also the fact that nurses have been practicing in forensic roles for many years. This role was informally recognized among nurses themselves, but never formally acknowledged. A pioneer among those visionary nurses was Virginia Lynch, the founding president of the International Association of Forensic Nurses and a contributing author of this text. This handbook was developed in recognition of the need for a resource that could enhance the ability of the forensic nurse to function effectively in this new and evolving role. Thus, it is a book intended for use by both practicing forensic nurses as well as those just beginning the study of forensic nursing.

Current global conditions have our attention riveted on violence as an international concern. Although war and acts of terrorism are indeed a real and omnipresent threat, no less demanding of our attention is the issue of violence within our own borders. Until recently, the death and disability caused by violence was viewed as a social problem that came under the purview of the criminal justice system. Recognizing violence as a public health problem mandates that successful interventions must encompass a collaborative effort among health care professionals, scientists, and professionals within the criminal justice system. A coalition of these professionals gives rise to the hope that strategies will be created and tested that address the problem of violence from the standpoint of both prevention and intervention. To develop interventions to prevent violent behavior and to protect at risk populations, professionals are needed who understand the dynamics of both victimization and criminal behavior. Forensic nurses are uniquely positioned to fulfill this role and to form the necessary collaborative relationships and coalition of resources that need to exist among the health care system, forensic science, and the criminal justice system.

These disciplines have come together with the common goal of meeting the needs of individuals and groups who have been affected by violence. In addition, there are forensic situations that are not associated with interpersonal violence, such as natural disaster, organ procurement, Internet safety and others. Holistic forensic nursing practice recognizes the uniqueness of each situation and draws upon the expertise of the nurse in all three purviews—nursing, science, and the law.

This handbook is organized around what the authors consider to be significant concepts that support forensic nursing practice, as well as what they consider to be challenges to that practice in the 21st century. Basic foundations of forensic nursing are explored, as are some significant roles of the forensic nurse and the skills required to meet the challenges of those roles. In this handbook, individuals with diverse expertise have been brought together to share their knowledge, experience, and insights. The editors hope that the reader will benefit from the broad scope of content and the depth of knowledge presented by these experts, who are highly renowned in their respective fields.

Acknowledgments

Many people generously gave their time to provide insight and assistance during the writing of this book. Among those who deserve particular thanks are Patricia Esposito, Secretary for the Graduate Nursing Program, Quinnipiac University, for her valiant efforts to keep us organized, and the editorial and production staffs of Jones & Bartlett Publishers. In addition, we would like to thank the contributing authors for their time, expertise, and dedication to this ground-breaking project.

We would also like to thank our students, co-workers, and other professional colleagues, especially those at Quinnipiac University and the Connecticut Department of Public Safety Division of Scientific Services, who provided ideas, comments, and encouragement throughout this endeavor.

Finally, a special thank you is extended to our families and friends for their patience, understanding, and support throughout the entire project.

Contributors

Ellen Russell Beatty, PhD, RN
Associate Professor, Department of
  Nursing
Southern Connecticut State
  University
New Haven, CT

Frederick Berrien, MD
St. Francis Medical Center
Hartford, CT

**Edwin "Ted" Brandhurst,
  PhD, CCFC**
Therapist
Center for the Treatment of
  Problem Sexual Behavior
Middletown, CT

**Nancy B. Cabelus,
  BS, RN, DABFN**
CT State Police
  Department of Public Safety
Middletown, CT

**Jacquelyn C. Campbell,
  PhD, RN, FAAN**
Associate Dean
Johns Hopkins University School
  of Nursing
Baltimore, MD

Bonnie R. Bentley Cewe, JD
Office of the State's Attorney
Danielson, CT

**Paul T. Clements, PhD,
  APRN-BC, DF-IAFN**
Assistant Professor
College of Nursing
Albuquerque, NM

**David A. D'Amora,
  MS, LPC, CFC**
Director–CQI-TCI
Director
Center for the Treatment of
  Problem Sexual Behavior
Middletown, CT

Linda C. Degutis, DPH, MSN
Associate Professor of Emergency
  Medicine and Public Health
Associate Clinical Professor of
  Nursing
Yale University
New Haven, CT

**Joseph T. DeRanieri, PhD,
  RN, CAN, BCECR**
Assistant Professor
Thomas Jefferson University
Philadelphia, PA

David Duff, MPA
Hamden, CT

Mary M. Galvin, JD
State's Attorney
Judicial District Ansonia/Milford
Milford, CT

Maryann Glendon, PhD, RN
Associate Professor, Department
  of Nursing
Southern Connecticut State
  University
New Haven, CT

Rita M. Hammer, PhD, RN, BC
Professor of Forensic Nursing
Quinnipiac University
Hamden, CT

Shadonna L. Hawkins, BSN, RN
Johns Hopkins University School
of Nursing
Baltimore, MD

Anita G. Hufft, PhD, RN
Dean of College of Nursing
Valdosta State University
Valdosta, GA

**Arlene Kent-Wilkinson,
RN, MN**
Forensic Nurse
Educator/Consultant
Calgary AB, Canada

Anne Klein, APR, Fellow PRSA
President
Anne Klein & Associates
Marlton, NJ

Carll Ladd, PhD
Supervising Criminalist
CT Forensic Science Laboratory
Meriden, CT

Patricia LaMonica, MSN, SANE
Director
Emergency Department
MidState Medical Center
Meriden, CT

Henry C. Lee, PhD
Chief Emeritus
CT Forensic Science Laboratory
Meriden, CT

Nathan Light, PhD
Visiting Assistant Professor
Department of Sociology
and Anthropology
University of Toledo
Toledo, OH

Virginia A. Lynch, MS, RN
Director of Forensic Health Science
University of Colorado
Colorado Springs, CO

Jennifer L. Makely, BSN, RN
Johns Hopkins University School
of Nursing
Baltimore, MD

Monique Mattei Ferraro, JD
Associate Professor
Post University
Waterbury, CT

Edward T. McDonough, MD
Office of the Chief Medical
Examiner
Farmington, CT

**Barbara Moynihan, PhD,
APRN, BC**
Associate Professor of Nursing
Coordinator MSN, Forensic
Nursing Track
Quinnipiac University
Hamden, CT

Michael E. Moynihan, MSW
President and CEO
United Way of Camden County
Camden, NJ

Catherine R. Nash, MSN, RN
Johns Hopkins University School
of Nursing
Baltimore, MD

Douglas Olsen, PhD, RN
Yale School of Nursing
New Haven, CT

Elaine M. Pagliaro, JD, MS
Assistant Director
CT Forensic Science Laboratory
Meriden, CT

Paul Penders, CFPEI
CT Forensic Science Laboratory
Meriden, CT

Edwin F. Renaud, LCSW, PhD
Department of Social Work
VA Connecticut Healthcare System
West Haven, CT
Youth Continuum Incorporated
New Haven, CT

Joseph V. Saitta, EdD
Director, Public Safety Institute
Fredericksburg, VA

**Daniel J. Sheridan,
PhD, RN, FAAN**
Assistant Professor
Johns Hopkins University School
of Nursing
Baltimore, MD

Katherine Spangler, MS, RN
Forensic Nurse Consultant
Jupiter, FL

Evan Stark, PhD, MSW
Woodbridge, CT

Tracy A. Swan, MPA
Rutgers, The State University
of New Jersey
Camden, NJ

Randall Wallace, PsyD
Licensed Psychologist
Juvenile Coordinator–CTPSB
Middletown, CT

Dian Williams, PhD, RN
Center for Arson Research, Inc.
Lafayette Hill, PA

**Mary Jane M. Williams,
PhD, RN**
Professor Emeritus
Central Connecticut State
University
Associate Professor, Department
of Nursing
University of Hartford
West Hartford, CT

Kenneth B. Zercie, MS
Assistant Director
CT Forensic Science Laboratory
Meriden, CT

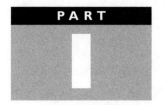

FOUNDATIONS

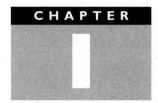

CHAPTER

Forensic Nursing Science

Virginia A. Lynch

This chapter introduces an innovative framework for forensic health care and identifies the opportunities and challenges inherent in the development of forensic nursing practice.

CHAPTER FOCUS_____

History and Development
Advent of Forensic Nursing
The Forensic Nurse
Forensic Case Management
The Investigation of Death
Vicarious Trauma
Forensic Nursing, Present and Future

KEY TERMS_____

clinical forensic practice
forensic case management
forensic gerontology
forensic health care
forensic nursing
forensic patient/client
International Association of Forensic Nurses
multidisciplinary collaboration
vicarious traumatization

INTRODUCTION

Forensic nursing is an innovative and evolving nursing specialty that seeks to address healthcare issues that have a medicolegal component. Although forensic nursing has been practiced informally by nurses in various sectors for many years, it has only recently been recognized formally in response to an increasing level of sophistication in identifying its unique body of knowledge.

Crime and violence bring together two of the most powerful systems that impact the daily lives of citizens throughout the world: health and justice. Violent crime and its associated trauma is an issue that concerns physicians, nurses, attorneys, judges, sociologists, psychologists, social workers, forensic and political scientists, advocates, and activists, as well as criminal justice agencies. None of these disciplines can continue to work in isolation. Effective management of forensic cases has been hampered by lack of sufficient policy and legislation to ensure protection of patients' legal, civil, and human rights. Reducing and preventing human violence requires a multidisciplinary, multidirectional approach.

As we move into the 21st century, a new nursing specialty is emerging in response to the healthcare issues presented by criminal violence. This chapter will introduce an innovative framework for forensic health care and for the nurse's role in processing victims, perpetrators, and families through the health and justice systems. In partnership with the forensic medical sciences and the criminal justice system, the emerging discipline of forensic nursing science is assuming responsibility for those affected by human violence and liability-related accidents.

The forensic nurse examiner as clinical investigator represents one member of an alliance of healthcare providers, law enforcement officials, and forensic scientists joined in a holistic approach to the study and intervention of physical, psychological, and sexual violence. While the role of a forensic nurse specialist augments and enhances traditional nursing with exciting and intellectually stimulating responsibilities, it also brings with it a new identity, new language, new terms, and new definitions. It expands the traditional concept of holistic practice—*body, mind, spirit*—to include *the law* (Lynch, 2006).

It is important to emphasize that the forensic nurse does not serve as a criminal investigator; this function remains outside the boundaries of nursing practice. Forensic nurses do not compete with, replace, or supplant other practitioners—rather, they fill voids by performing select forensic tasks in cooperation with other health and justice professionals. This new specialty brings to forensic medicine a perspective that historically has been absent, providing the practice with a uniquely qualified clinician who blends biomedical knowledge with an understanding of the basic principles of law and human behavior.

The advancement of forensic nursing practice in the last decade has brought a new image and higher profile to nursing as a profession and has redefined forensic services for both the living and the deceased. The conceptual framework for the forensic nursing specialty has evolved from society's need to reduce and prevent interpersonal violence and criminal behavior. Benefits derived from clinical forensic intervention, collection, and preservation of forensic evidence, effective sexual assault examinations, identification and reporting of abuse, investigation of suspicious deaths, court-ordered mental health evaluations, and expert testimony by forensically skilled experts in nursing are clearly recognized. These forensic services have been historically absent or insufficient as a result of the failure to integrate the practice of clinical forensic medicine or the principles of forensic pathology into traditional clinical medicine and nursing curricula.

BACKGROUND PERSPECTIVES

Daily, nurses are faced with the extremes of human behavior: child abuse, domestic violence, crimes against the elderly, catastrophic accidents, self-inflicted injuries, blatant neglect, and maltreatment. These incidents must be reported to a law enforcement agency and investigated. Special skills are also required of nurses who provide treatment to or court-ordered assessments of patients in legal custody. As trends in crime and violence change, new legislation is implemented as a means of anti-violence strategies; new resources are required in order to meet the needs of a society at war against crime. Nurses have been challenged to conjoin patient care with the legal system in order to augment resources available to patients with liability-related injuries, mentally disordered offenders, crime victims, and suspects or offenders in police custody.

Forensic nursing represents a new perspective on the holistic approach to legal issues surrounding patient care in clinical or community-based settings. The application of forensic science to contemporary nursing practice allows practitioners a wider role in the clinical investigation of crime and the legal process that contributes to public health and safety (Lynch, 1995). It is not surprising that there is strong support for nurse specialists who possess the combination of knowledge and skills required to go beyond the traditional treatment of forensic patients to fulfill today's requirements for forensic expertise in health care.

Because the majority of forensic patients first present to the emergency department, trauma care providers must be aware of the indicators of liability-related injuries, abuse of children and the elderly, sexual assault, interpersonal violence, and unnatural deaths. Other forensic patients will present in different departments of the hospital, private or public clinics, law offices, jails, penal institutions, hospital forensic wards, disaster sites, and the morgue or mortuary.

All trauma is classified as a forensic case until proven otherwise. These cases require a clinical and criminal investigation in order to confirm or rule out use of force and criminal intent. Failure to meet forensic requirements in the clinical setting can compromise the investigation. A nurse's ignorance of forensic issues could leave unanswered questions related to trauma that later may be of relevance in a court of law.

Forensic Nursing Defined

Forensic nursing is defined as the application of the nursing process to public or legal proceedings, and the application of forensic health care in the scientific investigation of trauma and/or death related to abuse, violence, criminal activity, liability, and accidents (Lynch, 1990, 1993a, 1995, 2004). Forensic science is defined as the application of science to the just resolution of legal issues (AAFS, 2000). The American Academy of Forensic Sciences (AAFS) remains the oldest and most prestigious organization of forensic specialists worldwide. The Academy, established in 1948, was the first formal association to recognize forensic nursing as a scientific discipline and give credence to this new specialty (Lynch, 1991a). Forensic medicine, one of many specialties within the forensic sciences, applies the standards and principles of medical practice to questions of law. This specialty includes both forensic pathology, and clinical forensic medicine.

Other specialties within the boundaries of the forensic sciences include psychiatry and behavioral science, anthropology, odontology, criminalistics, questioned document examination, radiology, biology, jurisprudence, engineering, toxicology, and others. The newest specialties in forensic science comprise unique, emerging areas of expertise, specialties represented by professionals who practice in such innovative areas as forensic accounting, voice analysis, forensic wildlife, and forensic botany; however, these growing specialties will remain uncategorized until a sufficient number of experienced experts in each group are identified. At this point in time, forensic nurses represent one of these emerging disciplines and their membership in the AAFS is expanding annually. With the acceptance of forensic nursing science by the AAFS, greater credibility has been established.

Traditionally, in the United States, the term *forensic science* carries connotations of crime, death, and murder. This association exists because we have, until recently, only practiced one kind of forensic medicine in North America: forensic pathology, which is the scientific investigation of death. Survivors of trauma requiring investigation of their injuries are the concern of the clinician, not the pathologist. Forensic nursing focuses on those areas where medicine, nursing, and individuals impacted by violence interface with the law.

In order to understand the concept of a forensic nurse specialist, we must first accurately define the term *forensic.* Healthcare and justice professionals in the United Stated often misinterpret and misuse this term. According to Taber's Cyclopedic Medical Dictionary (2001), *forensic* means "pertaining to the law," specifically, that which is related to public debate (Latin: *forensis*: a forum) in a court of law, implying the debate between the prosecution and defense to determine the innocence or guilt of the accused.

The original application for recognition as a scientific discipline within the AAFS described forensic nursing as "the application of the forensic aspects of health care combined with the bio/psycho/social/spiritual education of the registered nurse in the scientific investigation and treatment of trauma and/or death" (Lynch, 1990). The forensic nurse provides direct services to individual clients, consultation services to nursing, medical and law-related agencies, as well as providing expert court testimony in areas dealing with questioned death investigative processes, adequacy of services delivery and specialized diagnoses of specific conditions as related to nursing." (Lynch, 1991b, p. 1). This description was derived from original research at the University of Texas in Arlington, which was published in 1990. Since that time, this description has remained the standard, while at the same time expanding and evolving into broader definitions and emerging subspecialties.

A theoretical framework evolved from the 1990 study and continues to evolve as the practice of forensic nursing expands to address society's needs for forensic intervention in health care. The consequences of criminal and interpersonal violence have been recognized as a primary healthcare and human rights concern. As a public service profession, nursing has a responsibility to maintain standards of practice in forensic-related cases. Because of the legal issues involved in caring for victims of human violence, the risk of using forensically unskilled personnel to provide healthcare intervention has become antiquated. Today, enlightened healthcare institutions, death investigation systems, government agencies, and institutes of higher learning have recognized the benefits of the forensic nurse.

HISTORY AND DEVELOPMENT

The concept of forensic nursing emerged from the practice of clinical forensic medicine. A subspecialty of forensic medicine defined as the application of forensic medical knowledge and techniques to living patients has existed in Europe and Great Britain as well as Asia, South America, Australia, Africa, and many other countries for more than two centuries (McLay, 1990). Medical professionals in this field go by various titles but most often are referred to as police surgeons, forensic medical officers, and most recently, forensic medical examiners (FME). The role of the police surgeon or FME in the United Kingdom served as the conceptual model for the development of the clinical forensic nurse.

Clinical forensic medicine is defined as a medical specialty that applies the principles and practices of clinical medicine to the elucidation of questions in judicial proceedings for the protection of the individual's legal rights prior to death (Eckert et al., 1986). Historically, this healthcare role had been viewed worldwide as a medical specialty and had been restricted to physicians alone. Until recently, practitioners of clinical medicine and nursing in the United States have largely ignored forensic issues in the care of the living patient (Smock, 1998, 2004). Medical examiners or coroners (ME/C), or combined coroner–medical examiner systems (which are responsible for the investigation of unnatural and suspicious deaths), traditionally have not been assigned the responsibility of dealing with living forensic patients. Yet forensic pathologists strongly believe that if vital legal questions are not addressed during the care of the living patient, justice will suffer, criminals will go free, and innocent persons could be convicted of crimes they did not commit. The practice of clinical forensic medicine is often either unrecognized as such or is consciously or subconsciously evaded by practicing clinical physicians. If clinical physicians and forensic pathologists do not consider themselves responsible for the forensic issues surrounding living patients, who does?

By the 1980s, U.S. physicians and forensic pathologists were beginning to recognize the inadequacies of the medicolegal structure and the need to establish a more effective partnership between the health and justice systems. The first article to appear in American emergency medicine literature regarding clinical forensic medicine was published in the *Emergency Medicine Clinics of North America* (Smialek, 1983). Smialek stated that "medical care of the critically ill in the emergency department has a significant impact on the practice of forensic medicine. Many victims of homicide or accidents receive some degree of medical or surgical treatment prior to expiration" (p. 699). Smialek recognized that the evidence necessary to accurately reconstruct the event, prove guilt, or establish innocence was disappearing or being destroyed, either by commission or omission, during trauma treatment. That same year, the *American Journal of Nursing* published the article "Preserving Evidence in the Emergency Department" by Roger Mittleman, a forensic pathologist, Hollace Goldberg, an emergency nurse, and David Waksman, a state attorney in Florida (Mittleman et al., 1983). This article emphasized the importance of recognizing and preserving the evidence found on patients presenting to the emergency department: In order to avoid unnecessary negative consequences for both individuals and the system.

In 1988, Dr. C. Everett Koop, then U.S. Surgeon General, criticized our social and legal systems' responses to victims as late and inadequate. He also pointed out that the resources available to help law enforcement and the courts—resources from community and social service organizations—should include those of medicine and health care. Yet none of these institutions are up to the task in light of the dimensions of the problem. Koop stated that it is the responsibility of healthcare professionals—doctors, nurses, physician assistants, paramedics, emergency medical technicians (EMTs), hospital administrators, and other executives with the power to influence change—to maintain a high index of suspicion in the protection of the victim's rights (Koop, 1988).

As medical professionals began to weigh risk and liability issues involved in the medicolegal management of forensic patients they were required by law to treat, a concerted effort by Dr. William Smock and Dr. George Nichols II of the University of Louisville, Kentucky, established the first clinical forensic medicine program in 1993 (Smock et al., 1993). As often happens with an idea whose time has come, nursing was not far behind. The University of Texas at Arlington implemented the first formal degree in forensic nursing in 1986.

With the exception of some academic emergency medical centers and progressive ME/C programs, clinical forensic medicine has not enjoyed the same success as forensic nursing (Smock, from Lynch, 2006). In 2000, the American College of Emergency Physicians (ACEP) still had no position or statement regarding the role of clinical forensic physicians (police surgeons) in emergency departments in America. The College's only training guidelines related to the collection of evidence are those for recognizing, assessing, and intervening in case of child abuse. On the other hand, ACEP has recognized the benefits of sexual assault nurse examiners and strongly supports their presence in the emergency department (ACEP, 1999, 2000). In spite of some initial resistance from the medical and legal communities, forensic nursing has become the moving force in clinical forensic practice in the United States and Canada. In countries where clinical forensic medicine is already established, current restructuring of forensic services will no doubt result in a greater emphasis on forensic nursing science.

Clinical Forensic Practice

The combined energies of medicine, nursing, and the law have developed into a mutually beneficial, collaborative practice in which knowledge and responsibility are shared in order to reach common goals. The evolution of forensic nursing science has revolutionized the medicolegal management of forensic patients and has reduced the risk of liability due to violation of patients' legal rights for clinical and community facilities in the United States.

Clinical forensic practice is now defined as the application of medical and nursing sciences to the care of living victims of crime or liability-related accidents, as opposed to forensic pathology, which focuses upon the deceased. Clinical forensic practice also applies the principles and philosophies of forensic science to the investigation of trauma in living patients, with the aim of the just resolution of legal issues. Forensic scientists and police have long recognized that there are intervals between the forensic patient's trauma, emergency care, admission to the clinical setting, and initiation of the investigation. During these periods of time, a series of events occur that may compromise the recovery, preservation, and security of forensically significant trace and physical evidence. Biological evidence, which is highly perishable and fragile, is often the most essential evidence that links the perpetrator to the victim or the crime scene. When the clinical staff handling the case lacks forensic education and skills, the loss and destruction of such evidence is predictable.

ADVENT OF FORENSIC NURSING

As a medicolegal death investigator member of the American Academy of Forensic Sciences (AAFS) and the National Association of Medical Examiners (NAME), Lynch recognized the value of forensic education and forensic roles for nurses, Lynch proposed the development of a forensic nursing specialty in 1986. The concept became a reality when the University of Texas at Arlington School of Nursing's department of graduate studies accepted the proposed curriculum and implemented the first master's degree for forensic clinical nurse specialists (FCNS). Although the original proposal focused on preparing the forensic nurse to assist forensic pathologists in death investigations, Lynch rapidly expanded this focus to include the practice of clinical forensic nursing. The first articles on the subject of forensic nursing were incorporated into the introduction of CFM presented at the 1988 annual meeting of the AAFS. These articles, influenced by Lynch's association with the forensic pathologists in NAME, combined with the mandate from Dr. C. Everett Koop, became the impetus to define forensic nursing as a scientific discipline.

Lynch identified all areas of nursing in which nurses were currently providing a *nursing* service within a forensic environment to forensic patients, or were providing a *forensic* service within a healthcare environment to forensic patients. At that time, these nurses had no specialty practice recognition, yet they were highly aware that they were filling a unique role. Their jobs included providing death scene investigations, sexual assault examinations, psychiatric evaluations, and treatment of offenders. There were nurses practicing in various venues including law offices, penal institutions, and other areas where they interfaced with the law.

The initial intent of the forensic nursing curriculum was to combine instruction in nursing science, forensic science, and the law, expanding existing nursing education to address critical healthcare and legal issues surrounding patient care. Traditional nursing education was conspicuously lacking in forensic knowledge and skills, yet nurses were expected daily to provide forensic services. By 1995, however, forensic nursing had been recognized as one of the four major areas for nursing development in the 21st century (Marullo, 1995). The framework for the specialty is now poised to meet legal requirements and to ensure that the Joint Commission on Accreditation for Healthcare Organizations (JCAHO) guidelines are fulfilled with reasonable certainty (JCAHO, 1995).

An Integrated Practice Model

As a graduate student at the University of Texas at Arlington, Lynch finalized research, titled "Clinical Forensic Nursing: A Descriptive Study in Role Development," in 1990 (Lynch, 1990). The purpose of this descriptive study was to identify forensic role behaviors and to clarify role expectations of the emergency department nurses working with trauma victims. It further sought to identify and examine the differences between the frequency and perceived importance of selected forensic role behaviors performed by emergency department nurses. This study promoted the need for a multidisciplinary team approach to the identification of forensic trauma and the recovery and preservation of evidence. Research results defined the appropriate application of selected forensic concepts to professional nursing practice and education and described the potential for a forensic clinical nurse specialist. Since that time, replications of this study have assessed trauma centers and first responders, as opposed to emergency departments, further validating the significance of forensic health care (Rooms, 2004, Drake, 2002).

Progressive trauma centers that include forensic nurses assign a high value to the services provided. The American College of Surgeons encourages establishment of comprehensive systems to assure that standards of trauma care are being met in the form of trauma centers that provide state-of-the-art care to patients with life-threatening injuries (ACS, 1999). While recognizing the overwhelming importance of the physiological need of the patient, the clinician must also acknowledge the patient's psychological trauma and the priority of legal requirements (Rooms, 2004). The application of forensic science to contemporary nursing practice reveals a wider role for the nurse in the clinical investigation of crime and the legal process that contributes to public health and safety (Lynch, 1995).

The integrated practice model for forensic nursing science incorporates a synthesis of shared theory from a variety of disciplines, including social science, nursing science, and forensic sciences. It presents a global perspective on the interrelated disciplines and knowledge bases that affect forensic nursing practice and social justice. An integrated practice model is especially relevant to the applied health sciences.

Theoretical Foundations

Forensic nursing derives its theoretical foundations from several mainstream nursing theories, which are integrated with theories from sociology and philosophy. Like every nursing specialty, forensic nursing offers specific strategies and considerations for addressing the biological, psychological, social, and spiritual dimensions of patient care—with the important addition of the legal dimension. The connection that brings the philosophies of nursing science together with the law that define forensic nursing's body of knowledge (Lynch, 1990, 2006).

Forensic nursing theory incorporates the various human dimensions pertinent to all nursing theories of care, yet projects beyond the bio-psycho-social-spiritual and cultural aspects to incorporate the dimension of law. Forensic nursing is holistic in nature, addressing these concepts individually and collectively, and has been recognized by the professional bodies of nursing that direct the development of nursing education, research, and practice (Lynch, 1990, 2006).

Truth as a Central Paradigm

The forensic nursing practice model integrates sociology (sociopolitical impact), criminology (crime, violence, criminal justice, social sanctions, and human rights), clinical and criminal investigation (forensic science), and education (nursing and medicolegal knowledge, education of staff and patient/clients). The cyclic nature of the model speaks to continuance, perpetuation, and balance. The scales of justice are balanced when justice is served to those who have been victimized, to those accused of a crime, and to society as a whole. Justice is served when truth is identified, verified, and demonstrated. Thus, the forensic nurse becomes an advocate for justice and an advocate for truth. Truth and justice perpetuate holistic health in its biological, psychological, sociological, spiritual, and cultural dimensions (Lynch, 1990, 2006).

The dynamics of the interlocking circles are omnidirectional (see Figure 1–1). The outer circle, framing and encompassing these components, is symbolic of the environment: society, education, and other social systems. At the center of the internal triangle, the symbol of forensic nursing is displayed. This symbol, reflecting the legal sciences, forensic medical, physical, psychosocial, and nursing sciences, is composed of the scales of justice, the bundle of public service, the caduceus, and the eternal flame of nursing. The flame illustrates enlightenment of humanity and the challenge in nursing to continually evolve and expand into new roles as societal trends demand.

This enlightenment reflects awareness of the connectedness that the healthcare system has to other social systems. A caduceus represents medical science and, enmeshed in this symbol, the interdisciplinary collaboration that integrates nursing into the multitude of highly specialized scientific psychocultural arenas. The bundle of public service represents the complexity and weight of public service obligations, which all modern systems in our society bear. Finally, the scales of justice emphasize the necessary balance to determine the truth and the notion that patient care must now require the consideration of legal as well as human rights.

THE FORENSIC NURSE

Roles and Relevance

Nurses who apply concepts and strategies of forensic science in their specialty practice include the following:

Clinical Forensic Nurse: Provides care for the survivors of crime-related injury and deaths that occur within the healthcare institution. This specialist has a duty to defend the patient's legal rights through the proper collection and documentation of evidence.

Forensic Nurse Investigators: Employed in an ME/C's jurisdiction and represents the decedent's right to social justice through scientific investigation of the scene and circumstances of death. This role may also include the investigation of criminal behavior in long-term care facilities, institutionalized care, insurance fraud and abuse, or other aspects of investigative exigency.

Forensic Nurse Examiner: Provides an incisive analysis of physical and psychological trauma, questioned deaths, and/or psychopathology evaluations related to forensic cases and interpersonal violence; i.e., child

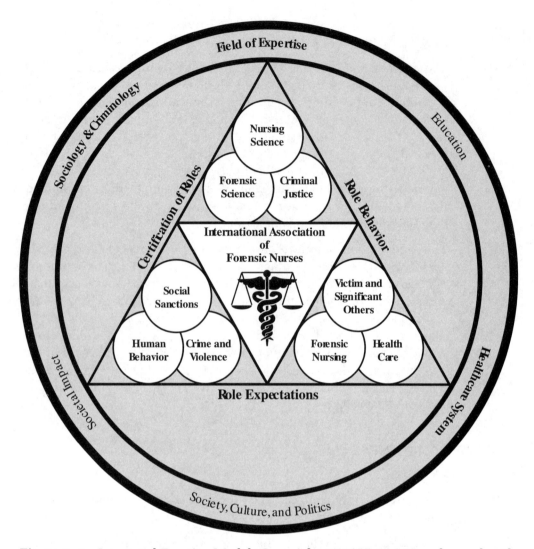

Figure 1–1   Integrated Practice Model. Copyright 1990 Virginia Lynch, used with permission.

abuse, domestic violence, elder abuse, sexual assault, or injury resulting from lethal weapons, torture, police brutality, etc.; is cross trained in several subspecialties and serves a wider population of forensic patients.

Sexual Assault Nurse Examiner: A registered nurse specially trained to provide the forensic/medical examination and evaluation of sexual trauma while maximizing the collection of biological, trace, and physical evidence and minimizing the patient's emotional trauma.

Forensic Psychiatric Nurse: Specializes in the assessment and intervention of criminal defendants and patients in legal custody who have been accused of a crime or have been court mandated for psychiatric evaluation.

Forensic Correctional, Institutional, or Custodial Nurse: Specializes in the care, treatment, and rehabilitation of persons who have been sentenced to prisons or jails for violation of criminal statutes and require medical assessment and intervention.

Legal Nurse Consultant: Provides consultation and education to judicial, criminal justice, and healthcare professionals in areas such as personal injury, product liability, and malpractice, among other legal issues related to civil and criminal cases.

Nurse Attorney: A registered nurse with a Juris Doctorate degree who practices as an attorney-at-law, generally specializing in civil or criminal cases involving healthcare-related issues.

Nurse Coroner: A registered nurse serving as an elected officiator of death duly authorized by state and jurisdictional statutes to provide the investigation and certification of questioned deaths; to determine the cause and manner of death, as well as the circumstances pertaining to the decedent's identification and notification of next of kin.

Each of these forensic nursing roles is investigative in nature, requiring specific knowledge of the law and the skill of expert witness testimony. The prevalence of criminal and liability-related trauma indicates a growing need for healthcare providers to intercede on behalf of social justice; to recognize and reported crime-related injury and death; to ensure accurate documentation and security of evidence; and to evaluate, assess, and treat offenders.

The Forensic Nurse Examiner

A registered nurse specifically trained to provide comprehensive care in the medicolegal management of forensic patients, with demonstrated competency in the performance of the forensic examination and the ability to testify as an expert witness in a court of law, can assume the title forensic nurse examiner (FNE). Documented nursing and forensic education, certification, clinical performance, and other pertinent credentials determine the nurse's competency.

Forensic nurse examiners will encounter individuals of all ages who present with suspected criminal or liability-related trauma. Physical, psychological, or sexual trauma in both living and deceased patients mandate a forensic evaluation.

Forensic nurse examiners enhance patient care through their expertise, patient education, referrals, and crisis intervention. Forensic nursing services address perceived physical and/or emotional symptoms associated with criminal violence, abuse, and neglect, which are often undiagnosed and may require prompt intervention as well as ongoing investigation of causative factors. The forensic nurse examiner is also responsible for the forensic care of the criminal suspect or offender, providing unbiased, objective assessment and treatment in the clinical or correctional setting.

Forensic nursing care is often episodic, primary, and acute in nature. It is frequently unscheduled, most commonly occurring as the need arises in a specific care setting, such as an emergency department, a mobile unit, a suicide prevention center, the crime scene, the scene of death, or the forensic pathology laboratory. Forensic nurse examiners share a common interest with medicine and law, where scientific knowledge and human caring is applied to the administration of social justice.

Education for the forensic nurse examiner should encompass study of the following:

- Forensic photography
- Nursing and emergency medical technician responsibilities
- Bite mark interpretation and analysis
- Death investigation
- Psychological abuse
- Deviant behavior and psychopathology assessment
- Interpretation of blunt, sharp, or fast (e.g., gunshot) trauma
- Sexual abuse and rape
- Jurisprudence
- Injuries to individuals held in legal custody
- Elder abuse
- Child abuse and neglect
- Drug abuse
- Psychological and physical abuse from occult or "religious" practices
- Tissue and organ donation

The Forensic Clinical Nurse Specialist

The forensic clinical nurse specialist was the first formal role to incorporate forensic science into nursing practice. The forensic clinical nurse specialist is defined as a nurse educated at the graduate level (master of science in nursing) in a clinical specialist program in forensic nursing at a regionally accredited institution of higher learning. Texas was the first state to address the issue of the FCNS as an advanced practice role through the State Board of Nurse Examiners. Advanced practice, credentialed by the state, is still premature without a greater number of practicing forensic nurses with advanced degrees. However, the majority of nurses who first applied forensic science to patient care were registered nurses without advanced education in nursing or forensic science. These nurses were the collective force that established the forensic nursing specialty, showing the commitment and dedication that is the strength of forensic nursing today.

Times change, as science and technology continue to advance and challenge the knowledge and skills of nurses. No physicians, lawyers, scientists, or judges practice their profession without advanced education. Yet these are the colleagues with whom we interface, collaborate, and consult on forensic issues as well as debate within courts of law. Ideally, FCNS candidates would hold a BSN or MSN and have 3–5 years of clinical experience plus a forensic specialization background. As forensic nurses become the standard by which forensic health care is measured, we must step up to the witness stand qualified, certified, and credentialed in our specialty area.

Flexibility is critical in the development of a role that remains in constant evolution based on the needs and demands of society. The role of the forensic nurse will remain flexible and continue to evolve as changing trends in crime and criminality present new challenges.

Expertise in Court

As in any forensic discipline, forensic nurses must be prepared to give testimony in court—the natural resolution of a forensic case. Nurses have long been subpoenaed to recite facts of a case in which they were involved. Until the advent of forensic nursing, few nurses were called as experts to give their professional opinion of the case at hand. It is now more common for forensic nurses to be qualified to give court testimony as nurse expert witnesses. Contemporary advances and reform in judicial procedures have brought greater numbers of nurses into the courtroom than ever before. Prosecutors and defense attorneys alike recognize forensic nurses as formidable witnesses.

The nurse expert witness is defined as a nurse qualified by education, experience, present position, and professional organization membership to give an opinion as to whether the nursing care administered in a particular case met the acceptable standard of care.

Novice forensic nurses who not have yet fulfilled these criteria would do well to take special courses or educational programs in forensic nursing and obtain membership in both forensic and nursing organizations. They can also establish their credibility by earning additional degrees, securing employment positions with "forensic" in their job titles, taking leadership positions, and publishing.

With these requirements in mind, nurse educators, schools of nursing, and practicing forensic nurses sought to expand informal forensic courses, primarily offered by nonnursing professionals, into formal academic programs, which would qualify forensic nursing professionals for the roles they were destined to fill. Simultaneously, this same group of pioneering nurses began to establish a forensic organization specifically to meet the objectives of forensic nursing as a professional entity. The International Association of Forensic Nurses was founded as an organization that would speak with one voice to the development of new concepts, new roles, and new responsibilities.

Forensic Health Care

As holistic approaches to clinical forensic health care are explored and developed, it becomes apparent that this field is expanding. Although forensic health care also addresses the dying and the dead, it is important to consider there are more living forensic patients at any given time than those who die, and thus the importance of clinical forensic practice. In a rather comprehensive article that concentrated upon "enhanced involvement in assisting the living," several well-known forensic scientists explored new roles for the emerging clinical forensic medical specialist (Eckert et al., 1986, pp. 182–5). According to Eckert, these roles require new responsibilities, which include the following:

- Determination of trauma (physical, sexual, and emotional abuse; assault; rape; drug abuse)
- Identification of human rights violations (physical and emotional torture as well as neglect while in the custody of foreign governments, law enforcement agencies, jails, correctional institutions, detoxification centers, juvenile homes, foster and nursing homes, institutions for the mentally challenged, public and private psychiatric institutions, or in private homes)
- Determination of unsafe conditions and products (analysis of injuries and illnesses resulting from electrical burns; fires; toy-related accidents; food and foreign body asphyxiation; ingestion of toxic agents; including lead poisoning; hyperthermia; and hypothermia; environmental hazards in the workplace, as well as in the general environment) (Eckert et al., 1986)

Healthcare professionals are among the most effective advocates for social justice. The nurse or EMT may be the first to suspect that the patient he or she is treating is, in fact, a victim or a perpetrator of a crime. With the identification of a medicolegal case comes the responsibility of notifying the proper authorities. Because of the unique position of the healthcare professional—often the first to see the patient after the perpetration of the crime—it is essential that the nurse or EMT be knowledgeable of the state reporting statutes, the hospital policy for reporting, and the procedures associated with local or state law enforcement agencies, as well as with the Department of Human Services.

State reporting statutes specifically mandate that healthcare profession-als who have cause to believe that an individual is being abused or neglected must report that suspicion to the proper authorities. Depending on the size and location of the hospital, emergency department practi-tioners may frequently treat a high percentage of medicolegal patients, and will routinely have to report to the appropriate agencies.

Reporting laws vary from state to state as to what must be reported, who should receive the report, and what degree of protection from lia-bility the law offers to the person making the report. Emergency department staff and EMTs must maintain familiarity with current fed-eral, state, and local laws and regulations that may apply when they make a report. It is essential that forensic policies and procedure man-uals are current, complete, and unambiguous pertaining to reporting responsibilities.

Reporting is a request for investigation. The healthcare professional does not need to confirm that the suspicion is valid. The Department of Human Services (or its equivalent), ME/C, or law enforcement agency will conduct the investigation, determine the extent of the problem, evaluate the circumstances of the incident, and take the appropriate action to protect the patient. Incidents that healthcare personnel are required to report include:

- Injuries caused by any lethal weapon (gunshot wounds, stab wounds, etc.)
- Self-inflicted injuries
- Drug overdoses
- Poisonings
- Animal bites
- Automobile accidents (if laws classify automobiles as lethal weapons)
- Child and elder abuse (physical or psychological neglect or inflicted injury by other than accidental means)
- Sexual assault
- Dead on arrival (or death occurring in the emergency department)
- Medical aid, treatment, or hospitalization for any person suffering from any wound that could have been inflicted as a result of violence
- Death due to blood transfusion (federal laws mandate reporting such deaths to the U.S. Food and Drug Administration)

Making a report can be the beginning of a process that ends the cycle of violence and protects the victim's legal and human rights. Offenders are likely to continue their behavior unless intervention occurs. If a family member or guardian is a suspected abuser, there may be reason not to contact that person until after the Department of Human Services or law enforcement agency has responded and conducted an investigative interview. With the forensic practitioner's legal responsibilities also comes the moral responsibility of patient advocacy. This includes respect for the rights of families.

Forensic Nursing Process

In 1995, the American Nurses Association Congress of Nursing Practice granted specialty status to forensic nursing based on its demonstrated use of the nursing process. The forensic nursing process is client centered, and establishes a feedback loop that ensures a dynamic mechanism for the reevaluation and revision of care plans. Collaboration is vital to the forensic nursing process (Lynch, 2006).

The following concepts are among the variables that influence the forensic nursing process:

- Assessment: Identification of trauma
- Planning: Investigation
- Intervention: Documentation pertaining to the incident, collection of evidence (specimens), reporting to appropriate legal agency
- Evaluation: Post-investigation review

The forensic nurse also provides traditional nursing interventions such as crisis care for traumatized victims and their families (Lynch, 1990, 2006).

FORENSIC CASE MANAGEMENT

Forensic cases require the management of a multitude of details outside of medical or nursing intervention. Various trauma cases require immediate, crucial intervention by physicians, nurses, technicians, and other specialists. Yet, a number of forensic cases require only one professional to perform an examination, assessment, or evaluation. Depending on the size of a hospital or trauma center and the number of forensic cases, how many forensic healthcare professionals does a facility need at any given time?

The American Hospital Association reports that two Pennsylvania legislators have introduced a bill that would set minimum nurse–patient ratios for hospitals in that state. The law would require that operating rooms and trauma units have at lease one registered nurse per patient, while emergency departments and pediatric departments would have to have at least one nurse per three patients. Other departments would have varying requirements. Is one nurse per three patients enough when one case may require many nurses' attention? Considering the chaos that generally erupts when life-threatening cases take precedence in the trauma room, it is best to have one nurse who is not a member of the trauma team to provide the medicolegal management of forensic cases.

Who, then, is prepared to photograph, diagram, and document injury; collect clothing, trace, and physical evidence; interview family or friends; or liaison with police and notify the ME/C if necessary? With the employment of forensic nurse examiners, who are qualified to provide a forensic consult on each trauma patient, liability or crime-related investigations would become one central aspect of patient care. The FNE documents the circumstances of injury or death, tracking patient progress from intake to outcome, leaving the trauma team to manage life-saving intervention.

The Forensic Patient

Forensic patients are classified as those whose injury or death within the clinical setting is required by law to be reported to a legal agency. Also included among forensic patients is the suspected offender, whose care requires collection and documentation of injury and evidence. Categories of forensic cases include:

- Victims of violent crime
- Sexual assault (rape, incest, child molestation)
- Domestic violence (child, spouse, and elder abuse)
- Substance abuse (drug and alcohol addiction, fetal alcohol syndrome, drug-dependent newborns, driving while intoxicated)
- Non-fatal assaults
- Automobile or/ pedestrian trauma
- Suicide attempts
- Occupation-related injuries (worker's compensation cases)
- Disputed paternity (DNA testing)
- Medical/nursing malpractice (and resulting injuries)
- Police and corrections custody abuse
- Drug and food tampering
- Product liability, manufacture of unsafe products (e.g., toys, contraceptive devices, tools, foods)
- Physiological and psychological abuse (occult, spousal, religious)
- Anatomical gifts (near-death tissue or organ donation)
- Environmental hazards (radon gas, dioxin, chlordane)
- Nursing home injuries (abuse, neglect, inappropriate administration of medication)
- Epidemiological issues (communicable diseases posing threat to public safety)
- Suspicious, unrecognized, or unidentified trauma and death

Nurses are cautioned to resist lapsing into personal detachment when dealing with victims, perpetrators, and families. It is important not to treat crime-related tragedies as mere cases or statistics. Essential intervention includes understanding that any feelings the victim is experiencing are normal for that individual. A nurse should express regret for the terrible crime that has happened and reassure the patient that she or he did nothing wrong. Tell the patient what will happen next—interviews, hospital procedures, and detective interviews—and explain the roles of the nurse, the physician, and the detective. Assure patients that they are safe now. The nurse must remain aware that her or his manner of approaching the patient, tone of voice, eye contact, and body language all send a subliminal message.

Forensic Pediatrics

As the nature of abuse and family violence continues to change, clinical forensic nursing and death investigation changes also. A major component of forensic practice in the emergency department is the diagnosis and reporting of child abuse. Emergency department nurses are urged to become cognizant of signs and symptoms of child abuse and to develop and adhere to standardized care plans. A multidisciplinary network approach to child protection that includes the forensic nurse examiner should be proposed and included in an interdisciplinary forensic protocol. As with other liability issues, threats of legal retaliation by parents or guardians demand that the emergency department nurse comply with laws to accurately document and report suspected child abuse.

An effective multidisciplinary approach to identifying, confirming, and confronting crimes against children requires a planned, objective, and coordinated response with defined policies and procedures that can be put into effect the moment that abuse becomes a possible diagnosis (Pasqualone & Fitzgerald, 1999). The pediatric forensic nurse examiner (PFNE) is an ideal clinician for validating suspicion and developing a plan in which hard evidence can be provided for diagnosis, treatment, and referral to the department of social services (Volz, 1995).

The foundation to any trauma investigation is *to determine whether the physical injuries and the evidence are consistent with the patient's history or statement of how the injury or illness occurred.* If what the nurse sees does not match what the nurse hears, he or she should document the disparities for further evaluation and report the case to a legal agency. Familiarization with the warning signs and objectivity during the collection of evidence are important aspects of the clinical forensic investigation of child abuse. Recognition of abuse involves an in-depth assessment of patient history, including physical conditions, lab results, and family functioning over time.

Forensic Gerontology

Elder abuse is the most recent form of societal violence to be noted and elicit concern. The U.S. Senate Special Committee on Elder Abuse reported that an estimated 500,000 to 2.5 million cases of elder abuse occur each year in the United States, but only one in six cases is reported. Underreporting has been attributed to the lack of a definition of elder abuse, fear of retribution, and fear of institutionalization. Community agencies most likely to encounter elder abuse or neglect include social service agencies, police departments, and hospital emergency departments.

The role of the forensic geriatric nurse examiner parallels that of the forensic pediatric specialist. Because both geriatric and pediatric patients depend on caretakers for activities of daily living, the forensic nurse working with these populations must remain aware of the warning signs of abuse.

Intimate and Interpersonal Violence

Intimate partner violence (IPV) involves acts of violence occurring between two people that are in an intimate relationship with each other. Once called domestic violence or spousal abuse, IPV can occur between heterosexual or homosexual couples or former couples, married or unmarried, and can include relationships with elderly people or children (USDHHS, 2003).

IPV should be differentiated from interpersonal violence, as IPV is specifically between two people in an intimate relationship. Conversely, interpersonal violence is violence involving one or more person(s), regardless of relationship. This includes but is not limited to IPV, physical and/or sexual assault or abuse, child abuse, elder abuse, firearm violence, physical battery, and homicide. Interpersonal violence also includes self-mutilation, suicide, or attempted suicide.

Emergency personnel have often failed not only to identify battering in women, but have frequently compounded the abuse by making the victim wait several hours to be examined while other emergency patients were treated. Derogative labeling in medical records projects blame the abuse on the victim. Campbell, Pliska, Taylor, and Sheridan (1994) contend that emergency department nurses are changing the medical system's traditional treatment of battered women. Nurses are encouraged to study and learn the signs and symptoms of IPV against women and to respond to victims' needs. Any trauma in a female patient must be considered IPV until battering is ruled out.

If the emergency department staff provides care that is perceived as negative or victim blaming, it may result in the development of what is termed "battering syndrome," characterized by unsuccessful help seeking, general medical complaints, and serious psychosocial problems such as substance abuse. The characteristic pattern of injuries to the following areas: head, neck, face, breasts, abdomen, and genitalia, should be regarded with suspicion and are indicative of battering. Also suspicious are multiple injuries to various parts of the body, as well as injury during pregnancy. Emergency care practitioners examining a female trauma victim need to be aware that the victim's partner, if responsible for her injuries, poses a threat not only to the victim but also to the staff, and should be kept in the waiting area until battering has been eliminated as cause of injury.

These women are also at risk for committing suicide or homicide and for becoming abusers themselves. A battered woman in the emergency department should be viewed as appropriately reaching out to the healthcare system for help for a situation that will result in, if left untreated, further injury and possible death to her, her partner, and/or her children. Never hesitate to question a patient concerning the possibility of abuse. Conduct questions in a non-judgmental and non-assuming tone. Forensic documentation is crucial in all cases of known or suspected abuse. Often of vital need are the following:

- History pertaining to the nature, frequency, and severity of the battering
- Names and addresses of witnesses, if beating has been witnessed
- Subjective and objective data regarding observation and evaluation of the patient
- Photographs and body maps

Battery is a crime that should be reported to the police, even if such reporting is not mandated. It is the nurse's responsibility to inform the survivor that he or she is a crime victim and has a right to pursue criminal charges. This may be the only help a victim will receive that can prevent future abuse. Medical records may be valuable evidence in future criminal or civil litigation, and may also be the only evidence the patient has.

Forensic Gynecology

The sexual assault nurse examiner (SANE) fulfills a crucial role in providing comprehensive care for victims of sexual crimes, collecting evidence from suspects, and conducting postmortem examinations in cases of rape homicide. A SANE is a registered nurse specially trained to provide comprehensive care to the sexual assault patient, with demon-

strated competency in the performance of the medical/forensic examination and the ability to testify as an expert witness in a court of law.
The SANE provides care for victims of sexual assault or abuse. However,
as this role expands to include care for victims of intimate partner and
interpersonal violence, as well as for a wider range of forensically significant injuries and public health concerns, such as liability-related
issues and communicable diseases (HIV/AIDS, STDs), the SANE is
evolving into the more encompassing role of the FNE.

The sexual assault patient is categorized as a trauma case. Each case is
approached as any other medical problem, requiring a history of the
event. The SANE provides appropriate physical examination, collects
essential laboratory specimens and trace and physical evidence, refers
the patient for therapy as needed, and writes a report outlining the findings and interpretation of results. This approach utilizes state-of-the-art
medicolegal technique and technology, facilitates the examination and
initial treatment of the sexual assault patient, and fulfills an investigative
protocol based on IAFN Standards and Scope of Practice (IAFN, 1997).

All information is pertinent to the investigation of the current case and
may lend itself to correlation with past rape cases. A rapist may be a
recidivistic individual who tends to utilize the same or very similar procedures in each of his attacks. Therefore, if a pattern has been established, it may facilitate the institution of preventative measures in the
community, and also form a basis for multijurisdictional cooperation in
the search for and eventual apprehension of the criminal. It is imperative that the SANE handling rape cases has a working knowledge of the
law enforcement investigator's needs and responsibilities.

The hospital emergency department sexual assault liaison or the SANE
must be aware that in most areas the investigation of a sexual assault is initiated by a uniformed police officer. The primary function of the police is
to determine whether the victim is seriously injured, arrange immediate
transportation to a hospital as necessary, ascertain the proper jurisdiction,
secure the area, and make an arrest if possible. The case is then turned over
to an experienced investigator from the sex crimes division. Although
statutes may vary in different states or jurisdictions, it is not uncommon for
the sex crimes investigator, in coordination with the prosecutor's office, to
request a medical–forensic examination to be performed at one of the local
hospital emergency departments. Other systems provide a sexual assault
examination upon request. A detailed history of the reported attack
obtained by the police investigator should include the following:

- Date and time of the attack
- Description of how the attack was initiated and the environment in
  which it occurred (home, shopping center, car, wooded area)

- How many people were involved in the attack
- Physical characteristics of the suspect including estimated age, race, estimated height and weight, scars, tattoos, and any physical defects
- Description of physical force used to restrain the victim (use of hands, arms)
- Restraints used—belts, ligatures
- Weapons used to threaten or to inflict wounds
- Dildoes or other objects placed in body orifices
- Lubricants, powders, or other chemical substances used
- What the rapist said and whether there were any distinguishing voice characteristics
- What, if anything, was stolen (money, pictures, undergarments)

Gathering this information may become a shared responsibility as it is accumulated throughout the interviews and examination. The SANE can significantly aid law enforcement efforts by retaining evidence, maintaining the chain of custody, preventing changes in the physical condition of the evidence, and assuring that evidence-collecting procedures are adequately witnessed. These responsibilities bring the SANE's role in line with that of a clinical investigator. The common goal is the identification and apprehension of the perpetrator and the physical and emotional treatment of the victim. To this end, the SANE avoids using the term "alleged" to describe or document a sexual assault. This term may imply to the victim that they are believed to be untruthful, and therefore have a negative impact to their psychological state.

Similarly, the SANE must never describe or document that the victim has been "raped." Such language constitutes a conclusion, which is legally up to the court to decide. The victim of sexual violence should be referred to as a "trauma patient." All documentation should note the attack as "patient reported sexual assault," and should always be in quotation marks in order to be admissible in court.

Physical Examination

The physical examination of any forensic patient is referred to as a medical–forensic or nursing–forensic examination to differentiate between the assessment by physicians and nurses in a healthcare facility and that of the *criminalist* who examines the clothing, projectiles, weapons, and other evidence in the crime laboratory. Any evidence of trauma, no matter how minimal, involving any part of the body, is documented and outlined on a body map (wound chart) and also photographed. This includes contusions (bruises), abrasions (scratches), incised wounds (cuts), and lacerations (puncture wounds and tears).

Wound characteristics should be described as to the anatomic area, quantity, size, color, age, and so on, with individual photographs taken of each wound next to a measuring scale. The descriptions should state whether the trauma is consistent with a pattern-type injury (such as a bite or a wound inflicted by fingernails or a weapon). Finger-tip bruises on the neck are consistent with attempted strangulation; superficial lacerations of the mucosal surface of the mouth suggest oral penetration. Linear superficial abrasions are consistent with ligature marks made by belts or ropes. The SANE should not use the term "choking" in describing or documenting external pressure caused by a ligature or manual strangulation, as "choking" refers to an obstruction inside the throat and pressure by ligature or manual strangulation is considered attempted murder in assault cases.

Evidence on Trial

Evidence is defined as any species of proof, in the form of witness testimony, records, documents, concrete objects, etc., presented at a trial by either party for the purpose of inducing belief in the minds of the court or jury as to the party's contention (Black's Law Dictionary, 2002). Simply said, evidence is proof of conduct or lack thereof. Far too often it is the evidence that is on trial rather than the defendant.

Historically, a gap has existed between clinical practitioners, the justice system, and forensic scientists. This gap arises from inadequate communication, disorganization, lack of structure, lack of cooperation, and failure to understand the consequences of inaction. Misinterpretation, omission, or loss of valuable forensic evidence has resulted in miscarriage of justice. Failure to address forensic issues continues to confound effective processing of incidents of trauma. This systemic weakness creates serious outcomes in the lives of affected citizens. Failure to accommodate change threatens all individuals' legal rights, including those of the victims, witnesses, relatives, defendants, and professionals who investigate trauma.

The forensic psychiatric nurse, who may view the collection of evidence as contrary to the nurse–patient relationship, must consider that the evidence could exonerate the client as well as reinforce guilt, based on the corroboration of circumstances individual to each case (Lynch, 1990).

When ambulance or emergency department personnel treat victims of crime, valuable forensic evidence may be lost because these personnel are not aware of its presence or potential value. The problem of gathering evidence in the emergency department is not restricted to the failure to recognize or collect forensic evidence, but also reflects the failure to properly preserve fragile or perishable evidence. The accurate documentation of medicolegal evidence is essential. It is not only appropriate, but often legally required that evidence be identified, collected, and preserved. Studies show the causes of this critical failure are poor communication between medical, nursing, and law enforcement personnel, and lack of forensic education (Rooms & Shapiro, 2005).

In the absence of a specially educated forensic physician or forensic nurse, the emergency department staff is potentially liable. It is recommended that the staff seek legal counsel or information about forensic procedures when questions concerning the legality of evidence collection arise. Once medical personnel are taught the value of physical evidence and the proper procedures for handling it, they generally support police requests for assistance.

Prior to the advent of the forensic nurse examiner within the clinical setting, the justice system had little confidence in the healthcare system to prevent the discarding of clothing, projectiles, particles of broken glass, paint chips, hairs, fibers, body fluids, and other valuable clues that could determine if a crime had been committed or identify the offender.

Patient Advocacy

In trauma care, most forensic patients are victims, although when the patient may be the suspect or offender, patient advocacy remains the same. In other categories of forensic cases, such as patients in custody and forensic mental health cases, the patients are most often suspects or offenders. Forensic nurses must not forget that their role is not that of a victim advocate, but rather that of a patient advocate, one who remains unbiased and scientifically objective when providing forensic services to this patient population.

As nursing professionals, we must be sensitive to the needs of the victims in our society, understand a victim's reaction to crisis, and be able to provide psychological first aid. A new focus on victims' rights and needs has emerged and has compelled health professionals to participate in the movement to improve services to forensic patients. Victims' rights includes the rights of those who have been accused of crimes they did not commit. With the advent of DNA evidence and programs such as the Innocence Project, individuals falsely prosecuted and incarcerated are being identified and pardoned. We help prevent the prosecution of innocent individuals through:

- Sharing responsibility for victim care
- Detecting abuse and neglect
- Improving response to victims' needs

- Calling for outside intervention
- Providing tangible support
- Protecting victims' human rights
- Supporting greater legal rights for victims

With this care, the victim will feel safe, secure, and supported, and is likely to cooperate with law enforcement. Although crime is not always violent, a sense of violation remains. The victim may be blaming herself or himself for the crime, feeling that her or his behavior provoked the attack. Explain to the victim that she or he is not to blame. The fault always lies with the offender.

Victim management should reflect sincerity as well as expert patient care. Every victim deserves to be treated with dignity and respect, regardless of the crime, and her or his appearance, race, or class. Clinicians must also consider the care of the patient in police custody. The young, male first-time offender often presents with significant anxiety, guilt, shame, and depression. It is recognized that this category of prisoners are at extremely high risk for suicide. The FNE may provide psychosocial intervention and suicide assessment during the intake examination and collection of forensic evidence. Prevention of suicide is a responsibility of all healthcare professionals.

Survivors of Suicide

Emergency department nurses frequently encounter suicidal patients. Although many suicide attempts should be obvious, they frequently go unrecognized. Wound characteristics, patterned injuries, or type and amount of drugs or chemicals, as well as the patient's medical history, differentiate the suicide attempt from the accidental injury or harm inflicted by an assailant. Forensic nursing emphasizes methods for detecting potentially self-destructive behavior prior to a fatal event. If subtle signs and indicators of suicide are ignored or misjudged, victims may go on without help, only to repeat the behavior with tragic results. Caring confrontation in a therapeutic environment may provide the necessary impetus to initiate psychiatric intervention and a resolution of the problem.

Suicide ranks higher than homicides among causes of death in the United States. Physical findings supported by behavioral clues are often the only evidence of suicidal intent. Because motor vehicle trauma is a common event in the emergency department, nurses may not consider that 10–15% of single vehicle crashes may represent suicide attempts. Such attempts may be misreported as accidents because of lack of evidence. Emergency department nurses and first responders need to be able to recognize suicidal gestures in patients who survive attempted vehicular suicide and other violent events resulting in near-death trauma. However, it is difficult to differentiate a lifestyle that incorporates frequent risk-taking activities from an active attempt to end a life. Those who attempt suicide and survive are at high risk for repeating self-inflicted assaults. Without medication and therapy, it is most likely they will eventually succeed. Deaths as a result of trauma require a forensic evaluation by the clinician that will help confirm or rule out suicide as the manner of death.

THE INVESTIGATION OF DEATH

The role of the forensic nurse examiner in a death scene investigation was another first to prove beneficial to the forensic medical community and law enforcement officers. In Canada, as early as 1975, nurses were designated death investigators representing the ME/C's office at the scene of death, working with homicide detectives, and the Royal Canadian Mounted Police. As forensic clinicians in the scientific inquiry of death, forensic nurse death investigators and nurse coroners have demonstrated the requirements necessary to investigate trauma, medical cause of death, mechanism of injury, multi-organ system failure, and pharmacology, as well as provide psychosocial intervention in grief and bereavement management.

When all attempts to succeed with life-saving intervention cease, death is pronounced and notification of next of kin becomes the next priority. Any sudden, unexpected, or unexplained death is difficult for the victim's family. But the act of human violence that may have taken an innocent life is a complicating factor. Homicide ranks 11th among leading causes of death in the United States. It stands to reason that hospital emergency departments will experience these events frequently. The law requires the ME/C to take charge of the body. An autopsy is generally unavoidable in these cases. The ME/C has jurisdiction over the body of any person who dies as a result of violence, trauma, accident, suicide, homicide, or suspected foul play.

Although criterion may vary in different locals, the following cases are generally those within the ME/C's jurisdiction:

- Patient dies within 24 hours of admission to the hospital
- Patient dies from unnatural causes
- Circumstances of death are unknown
- Suspicion of foul play
- Suspicion of suicide
- Physician is unable to certify the cause of death

The ME/C may also be notified of patients who die with no known pertinent medical history. This category is intended to include only those for whom no medical records can be found, for instance, a traveler passing through the state who dies at the bus station. It does not include a person who is found dead under nonsuspicious circumstances whose regular attending physician or clinic doctor happens to be temporarily absent. Generally, the ME/C has no authority to assume jurisdiction over the body of a person who has died of an obviously natural cause in nonsuspicious circumstances, and should not be summoned merely because the decedent's private doctor is temporarily unavailable. This may not be the case in all jurisdictions, however.

Finally, death brings with it innocent living victims: the survivors. In this area as well forensic nurses have made pioneering inroads, often times acting out of necessity, by providing grief counseling and crisis intervention in the absence of designated professionals. The FNE on staff is responsible for organizing and delegating responsibilities concerning the notification of death, reporting to the police or ME/C, collecting evidence, and maintaining chain of custody until the body is turned over to the proper legal agency. The FNE also directs the manner in which the body is prepared for transfer to the autopsy laboratory or mortuary facility. When the death is a forensic case, routine postmortem care is no longer appropriate. The body should not be washed; clothing and treatment paraphernalia should not be removed, tied, or clamped off; and all specimens of body fluids should be sent to the ME/C with the decedent.

Death in the Emergency Department (ED)

Violent death is not an uncommon visitor to the emergency department. No single event, with the possible exception of an epidemic, brings more agencies or tension into the ED than sudden death. For example, a commercial aircraft disaster brings criminal justice agencies into the emergency department, along with ME/Cs and a host of others.

Saving lives is the obvious priority for ED nurses treating catastrophic near-death cases. Despite this priority of patient care, the importance of properly identifying, securing, and preserving items that can later be considered evidence—even if the patient dies—must not be forgotten. The ME/C and the crime laboratory rely on the attending staff to provide:

- Accurate documentation
- Detailed description of wounds

- Collection and preservation of admission (samples taken when the patient is admitted to the ED) or postmortem samples of blood and body fluids
- Recognition and recovery of trace evidence
- Gathering of documents
- Notification of appropriate authorities and/or agencies
- Notification of death
- Care of the decedent's family

Death in the Community

When a catastrophic death occurs, the first responders are usually the police, the EMTs, and the forensic nurse investigator or nurse coroner. Probably no other aspect of homicide investigation is more open to error than the preservation and protection of the crime scene. Preservation of evidence at the crime scene is crucial to a successful investigation and subsequent prosecution of perpetrators. Therefore, crime scene protection is essential. The first official acts taken at the scene will either help to bring the investigation to a successful conclusion or will negatively affect both the investigation and eventual prosecution of the case (Geberth, 1996).

According to Drake (2002), forensic pathologists indicate that most problems that occur in medicolegal death investigations are related to crime scene preservation. These problems are usually caused by emergency medical service (EMS) professionals, who are first to arrive at the crime scene, yet who have not had sufficient training or education to recognize the significance of forensic evidence or how their presence may alter the scene. Whether or not most EMS professionals have sufficient training and knowledge of Child Protective Services (CPS) related to Medicolegal Death Investigator (MDI) is largely unknown, as delivery of forensic educational content in their training is not regulated. In order to assist the first responder with evidence preservation, a 2002 study by Drake surveyed the basic training and continuing education of EMS related to CSP in a midwestern state and made recommendations to improve forensic services.

Drake identified how role behaviors as well as roles overlap, and how role confusion often led to tension when any investigating agencies requested information regarding the death scene from other agencies. Typical questions included how the crime scene presented upon arrival, what prehospital treatments were provided, what evidence was altered, and how the family and witnesses presented themselves. While it was apparent that each agency knew its role in the investigation, a coordinated knowledge of death scene investigation could have better assisted law enforcement with collecting evidence and aided the coroner in determining cause and manner of death.

Problems identified include lack of coordination leading to miscommunication, lack of mandatory education in crime scene preservation, and lack of quality review of death scene management. From this review it was clear that EMTs receiving additional education in crime scene preservation and its relevance lead to effective judicial prosecution. The medicolegal framework of investigation and outcome based upon effective preparation of each member of the team and subsequent collaborative teamwork provides effective interaction between medicine and law (Drake, 2002).

Shared responsibilities at the scene of death include interviewing survivors and documenting evidence. The task of communicating with the decedent's survivors requires tact and empathy. When the shock of the loved one's death is compounded by violence, the death scene is frequently an overwhelming scenario of despair and anguish. Whether the interaction with the next of kin or significant other is at the scene of death or in the emergency department, the alleviation of human suffering remains the objective of the empathetic health professional (Lynch, 1995).

Psychosocial Issues

Social scientists have begun to study the survivors left behind, victims by extension. These individuals display signs and symptoms of posttraumatic stress disorder (PTSD) resulting not only from the death trauma, but also from "secondary wounds" due to the circumstances surrounding the aftermath (Masters, 1988). Secondary trauma begins with the notification of death.

The task of notifying a family member of the death of a loved one is unpleasant and requires compassion and respect. Hostility is often projected toward the one making the notification, complicating an already difficult task. Although the forensic nurse examiner must not let emotions interfere with professionalism, she or he must be sensitive enough to feel the family's loss. This requires a balance of objectivity and empathy. Health professionals have a responsibility to understand the survivors' verbal and nonverbal clues and to determine how to help them. The most common defense mechanisms in reaction to the notification of a sudden and unexpected death are shock, panic, guilt, confusion, rage, and resentment.

As an immediate source of support, the forensic nurse examiner or the emergency department nurse making the notification provides the opportunity for the bereaved to vent their feelings. The primary emotional injury to the victim's survivors cannot be prevented, yet those making the notification of death have a responsibility to prevent secondary wounds caused by indifference to the survivors' pain. The staff member designated to make the notification of death should reflect on how it would feel to receive such devastating news.

Anatomical Gifts

There is probably no other area where the worlds of law and medicine collide that carries a more dramatic psychosocial impact than obtaining consent for the recovery of organs for transplant. This is a new and important role for the forensic nurse. Organ donor and transplant requests are frequently as emotionally traumatic for the nurse making the request as for the family being asked. This responsibility generally falls to the emergency department nurse or another designated staff member.

Approaching a family to ask for consent is never an easy task. Even if the potential donor has expressed a wish to donate or has signed a donor card, it is a common practice to seek family consent. Knowing that the decedent's wish is being fulfilled can make a difference to the grieving family, yet the interaction between the nurse and the relatives remains delicate.

The clinical forensic nurse, cross trained in death investigation and psychosocial intervention, can help the family understand the concept of brain death. It is the physician's responsibility to explain the medicolegal aspect of brain death, but often the nurse is left to respond to the aftermath. It is important to use clear, concise language that the family can understand. State clearly that the patient has died. Realize the family is in a state of shock and denial and may look to the nurse to identify and define reality.

Be certain the family has accepted the death, and then present the organ donation as an option. Never use the term "life support" when referring to artificial ventilation, for this can be confusing to the family who wants to believe the patient is still alive. Stress the critical need for various organs and tissues and explain that they can donate only which organs they wish. Questions about the forensic status of a deceased person may be difficult for a family to ask. It may be difficult for the nurse to answer if she or he is unfamiliar with medicolegal protocol in organ donor cases.

The family is generally informed of the manner of death if it is known or is under investigation. In the case of a suspicious death, the consent must come from the ME/C as well as the family. If there is no next of kin, consent can be obtained from the ME/C. When clearance from the ME/C is necessary, it must be obtained after death is pronounced but before the organs are removed.

Circumstances that require the medical examiner's consent for organ donation vary from state to state. The nurse designated by the hospital to offer the option for tissue donation must obtain the ME/C's clearance. Nurses should know if their state has a "must ask" law in effect. This law says that when a patient dies, and is not ruled out as a donor, the healthcare staff must ask the next of kin for permission to donate the patient's organs. There is a shortage of donors relative to those in need of transplantable organs. Two-thirds of those who need an organ will likely die before a donor can be found. The forensic nurse becomes an asset to both the donor family and the recipient of the gift of life.

Before the donation of tissues, the forensic nurse should take photographs to document the condition and appearance of the organs before any changes are made, specifically in cases of motor vehicle or crime-related trauma, or in circumstances likely to end in claims or litigation. Months or years later, the defense attorney may try to show in court that some injury did not result from the acts of her or his client. Often the photo documentation provides the critical response to these questions.

Sudden Infant Death Syndrome (SIDS)

One of the most difficult forensic cases is the death of an infant or child. Sudden infant death syndrome (SIDS) is a major cause of infant mortality and a tragedy for families. The death of an infant signifies the loss of a future life, and brings the shared joys of a baby in the family to a distressing and poignant end.

Before 1960 many infants died without an investigation into the cause of death. It was difficult to differentiate between natural and unnatural deaths without an autopsy, death scene investigation, and toxicology evaluation. Medical science and research, determined to seek answers, initiated the first inquiry into these deaths. After much deliberation, a name and official definition was given for unexplained infant deaths. SIDS was defined as: The death of an infant in apparent good health who dies suddenly and unexpectedly, and in whose case an autopsy does not reveal a commonly accepted cause of death (NIH, 1974). Unfortunately, little more is known today regarding the medical cause of infant deaths in this category. Nurses have been identified as those most likely to interface with these cases and the grieving parents, in the clinical setting or as death scene investigators. It is essential that nurses be prepared to assess and document information pertinent to the investigation as well as to intervene in the grieving process.

Emergency department nurses have complained that police and ME/C's investigators tend to complicate the investigation of SIDS with accusatory or insensitive questioning. Yet the fact remains that the cause of death must be determined. In the past, inadequate medicolegal investigation frequently resulted in an unrecognized or misdiagnosed cause of death. Often the cause of death was certified as smothering. The lack of a definite explanation and cause for these deaths has lead to many theories, the majority of which are not correct. The incidence of SIDS amounts to a few (perhaps 2 or 3) per 1,000 live births in Western urban society. The age distribution is interesting: only about 1% of infants die within the first 2 weeks of life. The peak occurs between 2 and 4 months of age; about 91% of SIDS victims die in the first 6 months of life. The incidence then declines steadily and the condition is seldom encountered after 12 months. Thus, a child dying suddenly at 18 months of age should not be considered a SIDS case. Nursing care requires an awareness of the indicators of SIDS, laws regarding the certification of SIDS deaths, and preparedness to help the family understand the necessity of an autopsy.

When the unexplained death of a child less than 1 year of age in apparent good health occurs, the death requires an intensive investigation to confirm or rule out abuse. The forensic pathologist makes every effort to provide a prompt diagnosis to help alleviate the family's grief, as well as to inform the local law enforcement agency should abuse be determined. The forensic nurse examiner should have informative literature to leave with the family after the initial investigation. Many ME/C offices provide a personal letter to help explain the facts of SIDS. Referral for counseling services, such as SIDS support groups, should also be considered by the forensic nurse, who should understand the seriousness of unresolved grief. Indeed, SIDS is a major potential cause of divorce, hesitancy to have other children, and overprotection of other offspring, to say nothing of destructive feelings of guilt and blame. The forensic nurse investigator is in a difficult position, having to be suspicious and inquiring while at the same time empathic and prepared to participate in handling grief.

VICARIOUS TRAUMA

Working with trauma victims affects the provider. It is imperative for the provider to know that this accumulated exposure to trauma and abuse will affect him or her. It is equally important to know the steps to prevent such traumatization.

Vicarious traumatization is the continued, residual effects of witnessing and assisting the victims of rape, child abuse, domestic violence, and death (Iliffe & Steed, 2000). Vicarious trauma is also referred to as "empathic strain," "secondary victimization," or "compassion fatigue." It is important that forensic nurses become knowledgeable about the insidious and inevitable nature of vicarious traumatization. Of primary importance, realize that when working with trauma, "the important part of coping with the intensity of the work is to acknowledge that it will affect you. ... Recognizing that it is normal to be affected by this type of work is the most important coping skill that you can give to yourself" (Nelson, 2004). It's normal to be shocked, horrified, outraged, saddened, scared, and vulnerable. Know that it's normal to "distance" oneself from the immediate task at hand, that it can be stressful and sometimes lead to sheer exhaustion from both the physical tasks and coping. Know that one isn't alone and that others feel the same way.

Vicarious trauma accumulates over time and across patients. It produces symptoms of post traumatic stress disorder (PTSD) and it changes a clinician's view of her- or himself and the world (McSwain et al., 1999). Signs and symptoms of PTSD may include intrusive nightmares related to trauma, addictive or compulsive behaviors, feelings of isolation, numbness, generalized anxiety, poor coping, feeling of helplessness and being overwhelmed, sleep disturbances, hyperarousal, intrusive images and thoughts, and dissociative reactions.

Not unlike the victims and victims by extension, the forensic nurse examiner experiences distress and reactions associated with victimization. Somatic complaints such as headaches, joint pain, abdominal discomfort, and diarrhea may present themselves (Clark, 1998). According to McSwain, vicarious trauma can cause a person's belief system to "feel a loss of safety and control, have a loss of trust and connection with others, be disillusioned, cynical and lose compassion, feel despair and have low self-esteem." In the workplace vicarious trauma can cause negativity, blaming, victimhood, and feelings of powerlessness (McSwain, 1999).

FORENSIC NURSING, PRESENT AND FUTURE

International Association of Forensic Nurses

Since its founding in 1992, the International Association of Forensic Nurses (IAFN) has promoted the education of forensic nurses and the implementation of forensic nursing roles worldwide. The vision of the founding group was to develop an organization that would encompass a wide and diverse body of those who practice nursing within the arena of the law. Nurses who apply concepts and strategies of forensic science while providing nursing interventions fall within this field of practice. Each year, the organization holds the Annual Scientific Assembly of Forensic Nurses for the purpose of disseminating knowledge and expertise to members and nonmembers from the United States and abroad.

With the establishment of graduate and undergraduate education programs, role development in forensic nursing in the United States and abroad is recognized as an essential component of anti-violence strategies. The IAFN recognizes membership numbers of over 2000 in 11 countries and territories. Institutions of higher learning offer formal and informal curricula in Australia, Canada, England, Scotland, Singapore, Brunei, Central America, Italy, South Africa, Sweden, Turkey, Zimbabwe, India, and Japan. South Africa has become the first country to designate forensic nursing as a national priority program. Through the media of the World Wide Web, Internet education and information connects this new frontier in forensic health care with the global community.

Advancing Humanity

One final aspect of forensic nursing science is the issue of human rights. Worldwide, forensic nurses must address the dynamics of archaic cultural traditions and religious practices that continue to pose threats to vulnerable subjects in each society—women, children, the disabled, the elderly, and the poor. An awareness of cultural and traditional practices such as female genital mutilation, honor killings, bride burning, and dowry deaths; criminal issues such as child prostitution and the incarceration of rape victims; and the effects of poverty and lack of education for women must become a part of forensic nursing education.

Within our strategic plan for nursing, we must strive to include issues that the World Health Organization has identified as having the highest priority, not limiting our concerns only to state and national agendas. In addition to basic and advanced forensic studies, a strong emphasis on human rights and international law is an integral part of the educational curricula for forensic nurses. Another critical aspect of their education is a broader focus on transcultural nursing, covering issues unique to immigrants and refugees who are survivors of war or torture, and victims of cultural practices that have maimed and crippled them, physically and emotionally (Lynch, 2006).

Our research, curricula, and practices must address prevention of HIV/AIDS and its direct connection to sexual assault. Forensic nursing must encompass the consequences of disease and death related to the lack of early detection and management of chronic conditions. The need to reduce the abuse of women and children and to curb infant mortality arising from multiple causes must be emphasized. Frank, open, culturally sensitive discussions are imperative for achieving positive responses from victims representing a vast array of social and cultural experiences (Lynch, 2006).

Interpersonal violence and its associated trauma impact all societies. Crimes against women, children, and the elderly are common. In order for forensic nurses to better assist in the management of medicolegal cases, they must be trained in transcultural nursing perspectives, the ethical and moral dimensions of health care, healthcare practices of diverse cultures, and local, national, and international laws as well as the United Nations Declaration of Human Rights.

Challenges and Opportunities

The development of a new field of practice is a challenging experience that brings together diverse professionals who recognize a mutual benefit through collaborative practice, exchange of knowledge, and shared successes in order to reach common goals. We must remain concerned with improving the health care of at-risk populations and advancing the information technologies that are revolutionizing forensic nursing research, clinical care, and education. A partnership must be nurtured between forensic nurses and professionals from all disciplines with similar interests in eliminating threats to health and justice.

Antiquated laws and social policies, restrictive family values, disregard for human equality, and inequalities in health care access and delivery must be addressed within the forensic sciences in order to reduce and prevent interpersonal violence. The health and justice challenges that arise from violent crime will not be eradicated for many generations, but it is imperative that the mission is launched within this decade.

AN AGENDA FOR THE 21ST CENTURY

Advances in the forensic and nursing sciences have brought this new discipline to the forefront as one of the four major areas for nursing development in the 21st century. Forensic nursing addresses the manner in which nursing is practiced within various countries, the unique cultures and traditions that influence crimes in each specific locale, the court system and the law, as well as the current and future application of forensic nursing science.

These are extraordinary times for personnel in the health sciences, and both challenges and opportunities abound in every sector of healthcare delivery. The sophisticated capabilities of medical and nursing sciences, rapid transportation, instant communication, and an interdependent world economy have compelled healthcare personnel to reexamine their missions and geographical boundaries of practice. A healthy world cannot be achieved merely within a vacuum of highly industrialized nations. Governments alone cannot meet the immense needs of adults and children who need preventive and restorative health care. Forensic medical and forensic nursing personnel have been among the first to step forward and become involved in the global issues of health care. This involves a broad acumen of knowledge, skills, and attention to justice concerns of the world's peoples (Lynch, 2006).

In achieving an international focus, nurses who have reached out to address human violence and its associated trauma have recognized the similarities of interpersonal crime in all societies. In order for nurses to assist in the forensic assessment and management of medicolegal cases, the incorporation of transcultural nursing perspectives, the ethical and moral dimensions of human care, healthcare practices of diverse cultures, and a review of the law—local, national, and international, as well as an in-depth knowledge of individual human rights, is required.

A strong working knowledge of the law promotes interaction with local law enforcement agencies and helps to develop an accurate approach to forensic nursing interventions. Nurses who apply concepts and strategies of forensic nursing science in their specialty practice are becoming recognized as a vital resource to the global health and justice system. To meet the healthcare needs of an increasingly diverse population of patients with forensic assessment needs, the establishment of formal and informal education programs, in addition to role development in forensic nursing in the United States and abroad, is recognized as one important component of antiviolence strategies. Individuals who have embraced the challenges of today will provide leadership and solutions for the future.

QUESTIONS FOR DISCUSSION

1. Why is there a specialty identified as forensic nursing?
2. What are the various roles inherent in forensic nursing practice?
3. What are the various roles inherent in forensic nursing?
4. How has the development of the International Association of Forensic Nurses influenced forensic nursing practice?
5. What is the historical background of forensic nursing?

REFERENCES

American Academy of Forensic Sciences. (1989). Membership information brochure. Colorado Springs: Author.

American College of Emergency Physicians. (1999). Management of the patient with the complaint of sexual assault. (ACEP Policy Statement #400130). Irving, TX: Author.

American College of Emergency Physicians. (2000). Child abuse. (ACEP Policy Statement #400279). Irving, TX: Author.

American College of Surgeons. (1999). *Resources for optimal care of the injured patient.* Chicago, IL: Author.

Black's Law Dictionary (7th ed). (2002). Frederick, MD: Aspen Publishers.

Campbell, J., Pliska, M., Taylor, W., & Sheridan, D. (1994). Battered women's experiences in the emergency department. *Journal of Emergency Nursing, 20*(4), 280–288.

Clark, M. (1998). Nurses, indirect trauma, and prevention. *Journal of Nursing Scholarship, Sigma Theta Tau International, 30*(1), 85–87.

Drake, S. (2002). Crime scene preservation and the emergency medical services. Unpublished thesis. University of Colorado at Colorado Springs.

Eckert, W.G., Bell, J.S., Stein, R.J., Tabakman, M.B., Taff, M.L., & Tedeschi, L.G. (1986). Clinical forensic medicine. *American Journal of Forensic Medical Pathology, 7*(3), 182–185.

Geberth, V. (1996). *Practical homicide investigation: Checklist and field guide.* Boca Raton, FL: CRC Press.

Iliffe, G. & Steed, L. (2000). Exploring the counselor's experience of working with perpetrators and survivors of domestic violence. *Journal of Interpersonal Violence, 15*(4), 393–412.

International Association of Forensic Nurses. (1997). *Scope and standards of forensic nursing practice.* Washington, DC: American Nurses Publishing.

Joint Commission on Accreditation of Healthcare Organizations. (1995). *Accreditation manual for hospitals.* Oakbrook Terrace, IL: Author.

Koop, C.E. (1988). President and surgeon general condemns violence against women, call for new attitudes, programs. *National Organization Victims Assistance Newsletter*, 13.

Lynch, V. (1990). *Clinical forensic nursing: A descriptive study in role development.* Unpublished master's thesis. University of Texas Health Science Center at Arlington.

Lynch, V. (1991a). Proposal for a new scientific discipline: Forensic nursing. Presentation to the general section at the Annual Meeting of the American Academy of Forensic Sciences. Anaheim, CA.

Lynch, V. (1991b). Forensic nursing in the emergency department: A new role for the 1990s. *Critical Care Nursing Quarterly, 14*(3), 69–86.

Lynch, V. (1993a). Forensic aspects of health care: New roles, new responsibilities. *Journal of Psychosocial Nursing, 31*(11), 5–6.

Lynch, V. (1993b). Forensic nursing: Diversity in education and practice. *Journal of Psychosocial Nursing, 31*(11), 7–14.

Lynch, V. (1995, September). A new perspective in the management of crime victims from trauma to trial. *Critical Care Nursing Clinics of North America.*

Lynch, V. (Ed.). (2006). *Forensic nursing.* St. Louis: Elsevier.

McLay, W.D.S. (1990). *Clinical Forensic Medicine.* London: Pinter.

McSwain, K., Robinson, R., & Panteluk, L. (1999). *Manitoba.* Retrieved January 18, 2004, from http://www.drjontry.com/handouts/vicarious.htm.

Marullo, G. (1995). Keynote address. Annual Scientific Assembly of the International Association of Forensic Nurses. Kansas City, MO.

Mittleman, R., Goldberg, H., & Waksman, D. (1983). Preserving evidence in the emergency department. *American Journal of Nursing, 83*(12), 1652–1656.

National Institute of Health. (1974). Report on National Institute of Child Health and Human Development Research Planning Workshop. *Recognition of Infants at Risk for Sudden Infant Death: An Approach to Prevention* (Pub. no. 76-1013). Bethesda, MD: Department of Health, Education and Welfare.

Nelson, T. (2004). *Vicarious trauma: Bearing witness to another's trauma.* Retrieved January 18, 2004, from http://www.isu.edu/bhstamm/ts/vt.htm.

Pasqualone, G., & Fitzgerald, S. (1999). Munchausen by proxy syndrome: The forensic challenge of recognition, diagnosis and reporting. *Critical Care Nursing Quarterly, 22*(1), 52–64.

Rooms, R. (2004). *Forensic nursing practice in United States trauma centers.* Unpublished master's thesis, University of Texas Health Science Center at Houston.

Smialek, J. (1983). Forensic medicine in the emergency department. *Emergency Medicine Clinics of North America, 1*(3), 1685.

Smock, W., Nichols, G., & Fuller, P. (1993). Development and implementation of the first clinical forensic medicine training program. *Journal of Forensic Sciences, 38*(4), 835–839.

Smock, W. (1998). Clinical forensic medicine. In *Emergency medicine: Concepts and clinical practice* [P. Rosen] (pp. 248–262). St. Louis, MO: Mosby.

Taber's Cyclopedic Medical Dictionary (19th ed.). (2001). Philadelphia: FA Davis Co.

U.S. Department of Health and Human Services. (2003). *Costs of intimate partner violence against women in the United States.* Atlanta, GA: Author.

Volz, A. (1995). Nursing interventions in Munchausen syndrome by proxy. *Journal of Psychsocial Nursing and Mental Health, 33*(9), 51–54.

Theoretical Foundations for Advanced Practice Forensic Nursing

Anita G. Hufft

This chapter proposes organizing a conceptual framework for forensic nursing to define and establish the relationships among selected concepts identified as relevant to the practice of forensic nursing and to the understanding of the domain concepts of nursing. Such a framework provides opportunities to review relationships between healthcare systems and forensic systems (judicial, correctional, legal) and establish the assumptions upon which these views are based.

CHAPTER FOCUS

Organizing forensic nursing theory
Environment/Violence
Human beings/Victimization
Nursing
Health

KEY TERMS

assumptions
caring
critical thinking
evidence-based practice
health
lived experience
manipulation
organizational framework
revictimization theory
violence

INTRODUCTION

The nursing profession is based on a specialized body of knowledge that reflects different philosophies and views about those phenomena of interest to nursing. Conceptualized as the science and technology of human caring, nursing is concerned with reality-based changing life patterns and experiences of humans (Kenney, 1996; Rodgers & Knafl, 2000). Nursing theory provides a conceptual framework for organizing and relating knowledge for nursing within what are recognized as domain concepts. Health, the environment, human beings, and nursing are the domain concepts of nursing science, and, when defined and interrelated sufficiently within a specific population or health event, have the potential to increase our understanding of human experiences within the context of their lives (Alligood & Marriner-Tomey, 1997).

A conceptual framework provides a structure by which a discipline can be understood in terms of philosophical assumptions, theoretical methods, and developmental influences. Those forces that have shaped the development of forensic nursing occur in the wider context of society and represent the point of contact between healthcare systems and legal systems. Consistent with the framework for nursing, forensic nursing can be described in terms of the domain concepts of nursing as a distinct area of education, practice, and scientific inquiry. A heuristic approach to understanding advanced practice nursing lies in the elaboration of definitions and relationships among the concepts of human beings, environment, health, and nursing.

The forum of medicine and forensic science is an unlikely environment for the development of a nursing specialty if one considers the common conception of nursing as a caring profession that emphasizes holistic understanding of the lived experience of persons (Kenney, 1996). Traditional views of nursing place caregivers at the bedside of a sick person, applying the art and science of compassion and healing to the restoration of the human body, mind, and spirit. Contemporary understandings of nursing encompass a wide variety of settings and roles, including the care of society and communities through the identification and prevention of violence and traumatic injury (Burgess, Berger, & Boersma, 2004; Sheridan, 2004). A theoretical foundation for forensic nursing establishes linkages between caring constructs and forensic principles.

Current trends in nursing include increased numbers of nurses with graduate preparation and shared experiences with forensic populations. New themes in nursing education stress critical thinking, evidence-based practice, and theoretical as well as experiential preparation of advanced nurse practitioners (Kenney, 1996; Oberle & Allen, 2001). Observation of phenomena unique and common to forensic experiences along with emerging prescriptions for nursing interventions specific to forensic populations signal the need to organize theoretical knowledge applied to forensic nursing.

The general conception of any field of inquiry ultimately determines the kind of knowledge the field develops. The patterns and images that emerge as we observe forensic clients, forensic settings, and the interactions of forensic nurses and colleagues are indicative of the basic understanding we have of our field of work. It is characterized by bias and the influence of other experiences and disciplines, reflecting the nature of existing environments in which forensic nursing takes place (McEwen & Wills, 2002; Meleis, 1997). In addition to empirical knowledge, nursing decisions are based on knowledge derived from our ethics and values, our sense of aesthetics, and our personal experience. The aim of the application of this knowledge is to organize nursing practice by comprehensively assessing clients, recognizing patterns, diagnosing problems, and using selected nursing methods and technology to care for and assist clients and their families, as well as communities, in their responses to those problems. Nurses in forensic practice are obliged to identify an organizing framework as the foundation of practice in order to systematically and reliably carry out its aims.

ORGANIZING FORENSIC NURSING THEORY

In order to understand forensic nursing practice as a distinct nursing specialty, a body of knowledge must be identified that is unique to this application of nursing, along with a set of nursing interventions aimed at using this knowledge to apply the nursing process. The value of a conceptual framework for forensic nursing is threefold: (1) It allows for the public debate of philosophical assumptions about the specialty, providing the opportunity for self-evaluation and accountability to the public and to the profession; (2) the development of a conceptual framework provides for the structure of theoretical statements and hypotheses suggesting appropriate and effective nursing interventions; and (3) hypotheses derived from a conceptual framework allow for systematic scrutiny and analysis of emerging care protocols. A conceptual framework also identifies developmental and political influences on the practice of forensic nursing, giving the profession a base from which to determine best practices and best policies for regulation within the field.

Forensic nursing is an evolving entity in search of an identity; it is in competition with and in collaboration with such other disciplines and professionals as forensic psychiatry, forensic psychology, physician assistants, forensic pathologists, emergency room physicians, and medical examiners, to name a few. Major trends in nursing education and nursing practice in the United States include advanced education for nursing practice (nurse practitioners and clinical nurse specialists) and nationally recognized certification in an area of clinical specialization. Other trends include use of specialized bodies of knowledge and skills to deliver research-based or evidence-based practice, use of nontraditional practice sites, and the growth of community-based nursing care. Building on these trends, it is reasonable and prudent for those who identify themselves as forensic nurses to systematically build a body of nursing knowledge by which to differentiate the specialty, providing a framework for basic and advanced nursing education and an agenda for research.

Because this new forensic nursing identity is just emerging, there are very different conceptualizations of it in the United States compared to the United Kingdom and other countries. In Canada and the United Kingdom, the term *forensic nurse* most commonly applies to those nurses working in secure settings with psychiatric patients. In the United States, the term *forensic nurse* is most commonly identified with nurses working in forensic medical settings such as the medical examiner's office and the coroner's office. These nurses, at first appraisal, seem to share nothing but a common term, *forensic,* and the public, along with many in nursing, are confused and at times offended by the association of this name with nursing.

Nursing practice—the science and technology of human caring—is viewed within our understanding of the domain concepts of nursing: human beings, environment, health, and nursing. The nursing profession is based on a specialized body of knowledge that reflects different philosophies and views about those phenomena of interest to nursing (Kenney, 1996; Meleis, 1997). Health, the environment, human beings, and nursing are all concepts that emerge as components of nursing science, and, when defined and interrelated sufficiently within the context of a particular population, have the potential to increase our understanding of human experiences of health and wellness. As an applied practice profession, nursing has emerged as a dominant integrator of knowledge applicable to human caring. Nursing "borrows" from fields of social and biological sciences, as well as the humanities and other applied fields, in order to understand principles explaining health and the nature of human beings. Nursing theory tells us how to apply this knowledge to activities and problems that are distinctly *nursing.*

One can look beyond the stereotype of analyzing the criminal mind or investigating the scene of a crime for a comprehensive role for nursing, which can be understood as the diagnosis and treatment of human responses to actual or potential health problems among clients (individuals, groups, families, or communities) who are victims or perpetrators of crime, violence, or trauma as they articulate against or are involved with the criminal justice system.

Forensic nursing, like so many other nursing specialties, came into being because there was a need that was not being met, in settings where nurses have access, and in which the knowledge and skill set of the nurse could be exploited (Baly, 1980; Oberle & Allen, 2001). Forensic nursing evolved from the caretaking of special populations. Inmates and those accused of crime, along with those victims of crime presenting with mental disorders and other psychological and physical wounds, have long been in the care of nurses. Addressing the needs of these individuals and their families developed as an application of general nursing skills and specialized skills from the critical care, emergency room, and women's healthcare settings, along with psychiatric and community health nursing. Over the years, nurses have recognized that the needs of these people required skills and knowledge outside usual nursing preparation. Nurses turned to forensic psychiatry and forensic medicine to acquire information and techniques appropriate to the problems they encountered. Based on disciplines such as these and others, nurses have acquired knowledge to enhance assessment and interventions appropriate to the needs presented in forensic practice (Goll-McGee, 1999; Lynch, 1995).

Nurses have always received and cared for victims of crime and trauma. From emergency rooms to schools, nurses have assessed and triaged, and planned for and intervened with victims and their families. Law enforcement officers and other representatives of the court intersect with nurses and the healthcare system when evidence collection overlaps with assessment and medical care. Nurses have, out of necessity, looked to forensic science and criminal justice codes as additional sources of knowledge from which to analyze factors affecting client care.

Models of nursing care provided to forensic populations, both perpetrators and victims of crime and their families, have been compared anecdotally and through publications, emphasizing common recurring issues and problems. Observation of phenomena unique and common to forensic experiences, along with emerging prescriptions for nursing interventions specific to forensic populations, signal the need to organize theoretical knowledge applied to forensic nursing.

ENVIRONMENT

Violence is a significant component of understanding environment, particularly in the United States, where violence is more common than in any other industrialized country that is not engaged in a civil war (Gellert, 2002). Consistent with contemporary conceptualizations, violence is viewed as a major public health problem and establishes a context for understanding factors contributing to social resource deficits, political priorities and sensitivities, and acknowledgment or recognition of mental disorders, deviancy, victimization, and trauma (American Association of Colleges of Nursing, 1999; Canadian Public Health Association, 1997; Rosenberg, 2002; Rosenberg & Fenley, 1991; Roth, 1994; Winett, 1998) The National Institutes of Health, recognizing the relationship of violence and trauma to mental health, has prioritized research studying acute reactions to trauma and risk for psychopathology, disaster mental health, and mass violence, as well as exposure to domestic and community violence (National Institutes of Health, 2004).

Environments for forensic nursing are viewed as both physical surroundings and social realities that serve as the context for analyzing and understanding the human responses to forensic phenomena of violence and abuse. Crime scenes and settings in which violence has occurred, as well as formal organizational settings such as medical examiner offices and emergency rooms, are environments for forensic nursing. Any event or location where violence or abuse occurs, or where victims or perpetrators of violence or abuse receive care, is potentially an environment for forensic nursing. The unique aspect of environment, as constructed by forensic nursing, is the potential for human suffering or trauma with accompanying interest or involvement of the criminal justice system.

Violence is defined as the intentional use of force to harm a human being; the intended outcome is physical or psychological injury, fatal or nonfatal (Rosenberg, 2002). Violence takes many forms, from verbal attacks to murder. Both short-term and long-term responses to violence affect individual and group health, including psychological and physical impairment, disintegration of family and community cohesiveness, and destruction of physical and financial bases for social sustainability (American Association of Colleges of Nursing, 1999; OPHA, 1997). Violence is part of the environment, and the experience of individuals and communities in response to violence is a phenomenon of concern to nursing. As society attempts to cope with the growing incidence of violence in individual, group, and societal acts, increased attention is being given to violence as it occurs in everyday life. A growing awareness of limited resources to deal with person-on-person violence has prompted legislators to respond to public demands for action. Violence must be understood in terms of gender, race, culture, and time (Gellert, 2002), and nurses working in forensic settings must be able to construct nursing interventions based on knowledge of violence as a complex environmental concept occurring at every level of social organization, from interpersonal violence among intimate partners to impersonal violence perpetrated as an act of global terrorism.

Growing intolerance for any sort of threat to personal safety and public peace is a stimulus for action and provides a societal need to which nursing has responded by developing forensic nursing roles. Healthcare providers have responded to the issue of violence as a major public health problem, documenting the incidence and impact of violence on the health status of communities through epidemiological research approaches. The conception of violence as a health and medical issue is evidenced by the development of concepts of post-traumatic stress disorder and interventions such as critical incident stress management (Cloitre et al., 2001). Nurses, who use these constructs to develop plans of care for patients, are now being placed in the position of developing effective nursing strategies to respond to the effects of violence and trauma on individuals, groups, and communities (Clements et al., 2003; Glaister & Kesling, 2002). In the absence of a framework for forensic nursing, nurses are challenged to consider diagnoses and interventions related to violence without acknowledgment of the criminal justice system that also intersects with these patients as a result of their involvement in violence related to criminal offense.

HUMAN BEINGS

A concept related to violence, critical to the understanding of forensic nursing, is *victimization*. The concept of victim and the field of victimology have traditionally been applied almost exclusively to crime victims who were victimized by individuals. An emerging understanding of victimization includes other forms of harmful behavior that may or may not be criminal and may or may not be perpetrated by one individual upon another. This approach broadens the definition of victimization: A victim is defined as one who is harmed or killed by another; one who is harmed by or made to suffer by an act, circumstance, agency, or condition; a person who suffers injury, loss, or death as a result of an involuntary undertaking; or a person who is tricked, swindled, or taken advantage of. A theoretical exploration of the meaning and impact of victimization relevant to advanced practice forensic nursing is based on defining *victim* as a recipient of physical and/or psychological trauma. This approach to victimization involves the analysis of the experience of recipients of harm or injury, as well as accompanying issues of guilt, powerlessness, anger, fear, and impaired problem-solving abilities, which so often characterize victims (Campbell & Humphreys, 2003; Elklit, 2002; Nettlebeck & Wilson, 2002; Price, 2001; Fishman, Mesch, & Eisikovits, 2002).

Although considerable data exist reflecting statistics on the incidence and cost of victimization, there is only beginning to be a significant body of literature identifying the process and consequences of victimization. Within a forensic nursing framework, *human beings* are distinguished as either victims or perpetrators of crime or trauma whose care is partially determined by their involvement with and resolution of criminal or justice issues. They are identified as individuals, groups, families, or communities. Relational victimization theory recognizes the commonality of loss experienced by individuals, families, and communities and stratifies victims into primary (actual victims of crime), secondary (families of perpetrators), and tertiary (law enforcement, correctional and criminal justice personnel, and the community at large) (McCarthy & Bruin, 2002). Victims can be survivors or deceased, and perpetrators may also be victims. Nurses working with forensic populations are more likely than not to be caring for a patient who is a victim of crime and abuse. How we evaluate the impact of previous traumatization of an individual or group affects the scope of care we are able to deliver and influences the attitudes we sustain in order to care for these patients. Individuals can assume the role of victim as a learned behavioral response to social and interpersonal cues present in the environment. Many traumatized people expose themselves, seemingly compulsively, to situations reminiscent of the original trauma. These behavioral reenactments are rarely consciously understood to be related to earlier victimization. Behavioral reenactment of a trauma may manifest itself as one or more of three responses, which may involve the individual as victim or victimizer.

1. *Harm to others:* Reenactment of victimization is thought to be a major cause of violence. Criminals have often been physically or sexually abused. One researcher, describing acts of self-mutilation among male inmates, concluded that "the constellation of withdrawal, depressive reaction, hyperactivity, stimulus-seeking behavior, impaired pain perception, and violent aggressive behavior may be the consequence of having been reared under conditions of maternal social deprivation."
2. *Self-destructiveness:* Self-destructiveness is seen frequently in correctional or secure settings. Often a characteristic of borderline personality disorder, self-destructiveness is common in those who have been abused. Self-destructive behaviors, including those acts that deprive an inmate of privileges or discharge from incarceration, are not primarily related to conflict, guilt, and superego pressure but are related to more primitive behavior patterns originating in painful encounters with hostile caretakers early in life or dependent relationships later in life.
3. *Revictimization:* Revictimization is a consistent finding in which rape victims and victims of abuse or violence are more likely to be abused again as adults.

Compliance with an abuser's demands legitimizes those demands, creates an accumulation of repressed anger and frustration in the victim, and creates an environment of violence, threats, degradation, and humiliation. This process deprives the victim of opportunities to build up an effective social support system, and the repressed anger can support continued victimization or lead to acts of aggression or victimization on the part of the original victim.

Information processing of trauma is a theoretical context that identifies victimization behaviors as a neuropsychiatric response (Burgess, Hartman, & Baker, 1995; Walker, Scott, & Koppersmith, 1998). This model assumes the basic constructs of information processing of a living system and that experiences are processed on a sensory, perceptual, cognitive, and interpersonal level. The individual first registers a traumatic experience through the sensory level, after which the perceptual level (within the sensory) begins to classify the event. The cognitive and interpersonal levels further classify the event and give it meaning to the individual.

Post-traumatic Stress Disorder

A general response syndrome to trauma, first described by Horowitz in 1976, occurs in two major stages: First, the disturbing psychological phenomena are presented as a cluster of intrusive and repetitive imagery associated with memory. Second, the victim develops avoidance strategies to keep associations with the trauma out of awareness. Resolution of the event occurs when there is sufficient processing for the information to be stored in distant memory; when the event is remembered, the attendant feelings are neutralized, and the anxiety generated by the event is controlled. When the victim does not resolve the event and it either remains in active memory or becomes defended by a defense mechanism (such as denial, dissociation, or splitting), the diagnosis is generally post-traumatic stress disorder (PTSD). In this case the individual experiences the trauma both unconsciously and consciously (Burgess, Hartman, & Clements, 1995).

Forensic nursing contains a structure for understanding the tensions and variability among definitions and responses to social deviance and trauma and for caring for those who experience such problems. Using the construct of victimization and the micro-theories explaining the process and impact of victimization, forensic nursing applies specific approaches to assessment and planning care specific to the conditions and imperatives determined by the criminal justice system, with whom the patient is also interacting.

Theories of oppression describe the unjust use of authority and provide explanations for deviant human behavior. Oppression is a complex, pervasive social problem emanating from and sustained by oppression of race, class, gender, and even age, as in the application of differential oppression theory to the development of delinquency. In this model, the adult oppression of children is reflected in parents' ability to force children into socially defined and controlled inferior roles. Children's reactions to this oppression are reflected in maladaptive or problem behaviors, one of which is delinquency (Hewitt & Regoli, 2003). In this model, the deviant behavior is actually conceptualized as adaptation through one of four modes: passive acceptance, exercise of illegitimate coercive power, manipulation of one's peers, and finally retaliation (Regoli & Hewitt, 1994). Advanced practice forensic nursing applies theoretical knowledge of violence and oppression in relation to social causes of violence. Analyzing health in relation to racism, sexism, classism, and ageism establishes constructs for the prevention of violence and the impetus for social change (Varcoe, 1996).

The experience of *boundary violations* is a theme for understanding victims and perpetrators of crime and abuse. Boundary violations exist when role behaviors of one person are not consistent with the societal norms or personal expectations of another. The degree of boundary violation, and therefore the impact, is determined by the symbolic meaning of the act that is considered deviant, unacceptable, or intrusive. Boundary violation results in emotional or physical discomfort and perceived threat to the person for whom the boundary violation occurs. Boundary violations can occur in terms of space, as when one person touches another or otherwise intrudes upon another's personal space (Cote, 2001; Gutheil & Simon, 2002; Radden, 2001). Boundary violations can also include verbal interruption, speaking for another, or taking away another's opportunity to speak or express ideas. Boundary violations also occur in social terms when one performs an act outside the range of expected or acceptable behaviors, as when a nurse forms a sexual relationship with a patient or when a person deprives another of their personal belongings (theft). When one member of a couple engages in adultery, he or she invades the roles of his or her spouse, enacting boundary violations on them and their families. Boundary violations also occur when a person unwittingly enters into familiar or inappropriate interaction with another, such as when tourists invade a private social hangout of local inhabitants of a small town and proceed to sit at a regular patron's favorite table, or when a victim of a crime proceeds to find the perpetrator on their own, bypassing the legal system to enact vigilante justice. Any time boundary violations take place, a sense of loss, personal threat, and anxiety occurs. People who are involved with the criminal justice system frequently exert boundary violations, due to either cognitive disorders, social pathology, anxiety, or ignorance.

Every theoretical construct used to define and explain the practice of forensic nursing is dependent upon the understanding of theories of violence and victimization and their application to the nursing process for individuals, groups, and communities, along with social systems and global agencies who are recognized as victims or perpetrators of victimization.

NURSING

Forensic nurses care for those who are victims or perpetrators of crime, violence, or abuse. The nursing process focuses on specific applications of forensic and other sciences and sociocultural sensitivities to the formal assessment, diagnosis, planning, and evaluation of interventions aimed at the resolution of human responses to violence. Forensic nurses must assess boundary violations and intervene to reorient the client to his or her expected role; apply consistent and effective strategies to support the client in recognizing their behavior as a boundary violation; recognize where physical, social, and legal boundaries are; and develop a repertoire of skills that enable them to maintain appropriate boundaries.

Essential skill sets for forensic nurses include advanced physical and psychological assessment of violence, trauma, and abuse, such as recognition and identification of patterned injury, assessment for risk of violence or self-injurious behavior, differentiation of factitious disorders and manipulation, and delineation of boundaries. Handling, processing, and documenting assessments and interventions as evidence is clearly a distinguishing feature of forensic nursing.

Ethical dilemmas are part of every nurse's role, but the blurred boundaries and conflicting role expectations of nurses working in forensic settings magnify the impact of ethical decision making on forensic nursing outcomes. The intersection of criminal justice with healthcare systems, and the balancing of rights between individuals and society, are hallmarks of forensic events. The protection of vulnerable individuals' human rights is a common issue addressed in forensic settings, in which nurses are conflicted between the rights of individuals to autonomy and care through a therapeutic and helping relationship, and nursing obligations to preserve evidence, security, and control (Fisher, 1995; Grace et al., 2003; IAFN, 2002; Peter & Morgan, 2001).

The ability to sustain objectivity and a healthy skepticism when assessing individuals and communities in a forensic context often depends on distancing oneself from a relationship with the individual or community. Mastery of the theoretical basis for establishing a trusting professional relationship must incorporate a sound knowledge of legal and ethical principles that serve as boundaries for forensic nursing practice

(Austin, 2001; Daly, 2002). Older approaches to nursing ethics—built on contracts, paternalism, and care—are being replaced by a trust approach for nursing ethics (Peter & Morgan, 2001). In this model the ethics of care and justice are integrated, with emphasis on acknowledging vulnerability and the potential for malevolence. The importance of ethical decision making is clear within the competition for power that exists in events and processes related to the criminal justice system and governments (Austin).

The process and effects of institutionalization and social isolation are factors that determine options in therapeutic interventions for those nurses working with clients in secure settings. Long-term confinements in rigid settings that dictate behaviors narrowly have a profound effect on patients and caregivers alike. Forensic nurses, especially those working in psychiatric settings, need a theoretical base from which to determine the therapeutic value of interventions, particularly when the goal of rehabilitation and wellness held by the nurse may be in conflict with the goal of punishment and retribution held by the institutional staff and the community. The social isolation that often accompanies victims of heinous crimes such as rape or incest can have the same devastating effects as incarceration or confinement in a mental institution. The revictimization that is said to occur often when a victim is processed through the criminal justice system has predictable consequences, which must be taken into account in any understanding of specialized care of these individuals.

Manipulation is a predictable adaptation strategy among clients, and necessitates prescribed, consistent, and firm responses on the part of the nurse. Dealing with manipulative individuals who may falsify information and fake signs and symptoms or deny them is challenging and exhausting. Recognizing manipulation and dealing with it in a manner that is supportive to the environment in which the client exists is critical to successful forensic nursing.

HEALTH

Defining health within a forensic nursing context is a challenging and evolving process, primarily focusing on successful resolution of the effects of traumatization or victimization. Successful applications of different nursing models allow for a pluralistic approach to understanding health, from adaptation to violence to finding meaning in survivorship. A growing body of literature on victimology distinguishes victimization from survivorship, establishing characteristics of successful response to violence, trauma, or abuse (Adkins, 2003; Clements et al., 2003; Cloitre et al., 2001; Gallop, 2002; Gellert, 2002; Lanza et al.,

2003; McCarthy & Bruin, 2002). Assessment of survivor characteristics and implementation of interventions to promote learned behaviors promoting survivorship are essential components of forensic nursing.

Health is constructed in terms of multiple views of human beings and in relation to different contexts or environments in which violence or abuse occurs. Successful resolution of conflicts related to trauma or violence; movement from victim to survivor; and healing of psychological or physical wounds sustained as a result of violence, trauma, or abuse are views of health through a forensic nursing perspective. Promotion of interpersonal or community peace, restoration of family or community integrity, and increasing the resiliency or hardiness of individuals and communities are also indicators of forensic health (National Mental Health Association, 1995; Rosenberg, 2002).

An example of the application of forensic health concepts to forensic nursing can be articulated in the nurse death investigator role. The role of death investigator is perhaps the most challenging to relate to traditional definitions of nursing and health. In this situation the patient is the deceased and/or the family or those with whom the deceased had a relationship prior to death. Any unexplained or unexpected death is accompanied by forensic data collection and additional trauma for family and significant others. The forensic nursing model applied to the death investigator role preserves the caring aspect of the nursing relationship with those connected to the deceased and the death event. Rights to nursing care extend beyond death, and this obligation is assumed by the nurse death investigator.

An awareness of the social construction of deviancy provides a foundation for understanding the relative and changing nature of diagnoses and responses to human behaviors associated with crime, trauma, and abuse. The issue of personality disorder as a mental illness is currently being scrutinized. The question of whether someone who has a personality disorder can be treated or whether that person is sick at all or just "mean" is debated among those who ultimately must either assign care or pay for it (Breeze & Repper, 1998; Gellert, 2002; Mason & Mercer, 1996; Mercer, Mason, & Richman, 1999). Nurses must understand that conditions for which we treat individuals can change over time as the nature of public sensibilities in the process of medicalizing human behavior changes. Today, most mental illnesses do not qualify as a defense of innocence for a crime, while being a spouse abuse victim or having premenstrual syndrome may or may not be taken into account as rationale for one's deviant or illegal behavior. A useful nursing framework provides a structure for understanding maladaptive human responses regardless of their standing in the medical/legal system, and provides an understanding of appropriate nursing responses. A forensic nursing framework will account for the changing nature of social contexts for care, balancing the need for culturally competent care with universal care needs. Knowledge of the social and criminal justice systems increasingly dictate the conditions under which nurses care for their clients and the resources and priorities assigned to the care of those clients. The conceptual framework for forensic nursing must stand apart from these social systems and propose the range of overlap that best serves the needs of society and the profession.

A conceptual framework for forensic nursing not only must define these considerations, but also must describe the relationships among the concepts, indicating, among other things, the relationships between the healthcare systems and forensic systems. The social and legal processes by which specific human behaviors and responses are categorized and treated as healthcare problems rather than cruel, evil, or just stupid behavior, and the differentiation between victimization and a sense of entitlement, must be accounted for as part of the environmental context in which nursing and human health occurs.

SUMMARY

A conceptual framework for forensic nursing is the foundation for education and practice not only for nurses who practice in the specialty, but also for every nurse. A careful examination of the current social and environmental conditions reveals a society that is acutely aware of the relationship between violence and health. Basic education for nursing already includes many areas of content that can be identified as forensic. The value in isolating that content, labeling it as forensic, and incorporating it into the education of the professional nurse is significant. This approach puts a value on forensic knowledge and skills and sets aside specific applications that emphasize the need to raise awareness of the overlap between healthcare systems and criminal justice/forensic systems.

Identifying forensic content in a nursing curriculum lays down the foundation for the recognition of the specialty, encouraging undergraduate experiences in forensic settings. Role socialization for the nurse working in forensic roles begins with a clear conceptualization of the role in basic nursing education. This provides for increased recruitment opportunities of forensic employers, increases the career opportunities for graduates, and supports the nurses working in those settings.

Identification and integration of forensic content into basic nursing education provides a basis for generalist nursing practice inclusive of skills necessary for the care and referral of forensic patients who are cared for in general hospital settings, schools, community settings, and private physician offices. The ability to define concepts central to forensic nursing that differentiate forensic nursing and explain the relationships among those concepts allows nurses to develop a method for organizing our thinking about specialty practice and a guide for evolving as advanced nursing practice. *Forensic nursing* is a term that is emerging in the literature and in practice. Establishing a significant body of theoretical knowledge unique to this specialty will be the challenge of the future.

QUESTIONS FOR DISCUSSION

1. Which nursing interventions impact the health of individuals and communities experiencing violence?
2. What is the process of victimization and how can nursing intervene to prevent, to treat, and to rehabilitate?
   a. What kind of support is necessary for families who participate in the trial, conviction, and execution of the murderer of a family member?
   b. Which clients benefit from reviewing an abusive or victimizing event?
   c. Which nursing interventions can be effective in managing revictimization of patients in incarceration?
3. Which boundary violations characterize perpetrators and victims of crime, trauma, and abuse? How can nurses intervene to promote healthy boundaries among patients?
   a. What is the therapeutic role boundary for a nurse working in a correctional setting?
   b. How does the therapeutic goal for the inmate differ from the patient in a nonsecure setting?
   c. What is the role of the offense in planning and delivering care for persons convicted of crimes?
4. Which processes of institutionalization can be positively impacted by nursing?
5. How does the limitation of citizenship or human rights among offenders affect nursing practice?
6. What is the role of nursing in evidence identification and collection? How does this affect the image of nursing and the public trust?

REFERENCES

Adkins, E. (2003). The first day of the rest of their lives. *Journal of Psychosocial Nursing and Mental Health Services, 41*(7), 29–32.

Alligood, M.R. & Marriner-Tomey, A. (1997). *Nursing theory: Utilization and applicaton.* St. Louis, MO: CV Mosby.

American Association of Colleges of Nursing. (1999). *Violence as a public health problem.* Washington, DC: AACN.

Austin, W. (2001). Relational ethics in forensic psychiatric nursing. *Journal of Psychosocial Nursing and Mental Health Services, 39*(9), 12–17.

Baly, M. (1980). *Nursing and social change* (3rd ed.). London: Heinemann Medical.

Breeze, J.A. & Repper, J. (1998). Struggling for control: The care experiences of "difficult" patients in mental health services. *Journal of Advanced Nursing, 28*(6), 1301–1311.

Burgess, A., Hartman, C.R., & Baker, T. (1995). Memory presentations of childhood sexual abuse. *Journal of Psychosocial Nursing & Mental Health Services, 33*(9), 9–16.

Burgess, A., Hartman, C.R., & Clements, P.T. Jr. (1995). Biology of memory and childhood trauma. *Journal of Psychosocial Nursing and Mental Health Services, 33*(3), 16–26; 52–53.

Burgess, A.W., Berger, A.D., & Boersma, R.R. (2004). Forensic nursing: Investigating the career potential in this emerging graduate specialty. *American Journal of Nursing, 104*(3), 58–64.

Campbell, J. & Humphreys, J. (2003). *Family violence and nursing practice.* Philadelphia: Lippincott, Williams and Wilkins.

Canadian Public Health Association. (1997). *Violence in society: A public health perspective.* CPHA Issue Paper.

Clements, P.T., Vigil, G.J., Henry, G.C., Kellywood, R., & Foster, W. (2003). Cultural perspectives of death, grief and bereavement. *Journal of Psychosocial Nursing and Mental Health Services, 41*(7), 18–26.

Cloitre, M., Cohen, L.R., Edelman, R.E., & Han, H. (2001). Posttraumatic stress disorder and extent of trauma exposure as correlates of medical problems and perceived health among women with childhood abuse. *Women and Health, 34*(3), 1–17.

Cote, I. (2001). A case of pain, factitious disorder and boundary violations. *Pain Research & Management, 6*(4), 197–200.

Daly, B. (2002). Moving forward: A new code of ethics. *Nursing Outlook, 50*(3), 97–99.

Elklit, A. (2002). Victimization and PTSD in a Danish national youth probability sample. *Child and Adolescent Psychiatry, 41*(2), 174–181.

Fisher, A. (1995). The ethical problems encountered in psychiatric nursing practice with dangerously mentally ill persons. *Scholarly Inquiry for Nursing Practice, 9*(2), 193–208.

Fishman, G., Mesch, G.S., & Eisikovits, Z. (2002). *Variables affecting adolescent victimization: Findings from a national youth survey.* Retrieved from http://wcr.sonoma.edu/v3n2/fishman.html.

Gallop, R. (2002). Failure of the capacity for self-soothing in women who have a history of abuse and self-harm. *Journal of the American Psychiatric Nurses Association, 8*(1), 20–26.

Gellert, G.A. (2002). *Confronting violence: Answers to questions about the epidemic destroying America's homes and communities* (2nd ed.). Washington, DC: American Public Health Association.

Glaister, J.A. & Kesling, G. (2002). A survey of practicing nurses' perspectives on interpersonal violence screening and intervention. *Nursing Outlook, 50*(4), 137–143.

Goll-McGee, B. (1999). The role of the clinical forensic nurse in critical care. *Critical Care Nursing Quarterly, 22*(1), 8–18.

Grace, P.J., Fry, S.T., & Schultz, G.S. (2003). Ethics and human rights issues experienced by psychiatric-mental health and substance abuse registered nurses. *Journal of the American Psychiatric Nurses Association, 9*(2), 17–23.

Gutheil, T.G. & Simon, R.I. (2002). Non-sexual boundary crossings and bound-ary violations: An ethical dilemma. *Psychiatric Clinics of North America, 25*(3), 585–592.

Hewitt, J.D. & Regoli, R. M. (2003). *Differential oppression theory.* Retrieved from http://www4.gvsu.edu/cj/members/hewitt/Dotheory.html.

Horowitz, M.J. (1976). *Stress response syndromes.* New York: Jason Aronson.

International Association of Forensic Nursing. (2002). *Code of ethics.* Retrieved September 15, 2002, from: http://www.forensicnurse.org/about/code.html.

Kenney, J.W. (Ed.). (1996). *Philosophical and theoretical perspectives for advanced nursing practice.* Boston: Jones & Bartlett.

Lanza, M.L., Kazis, L., & Lee, A. (2003). Using the violence prevention commu-nity meeting protocol. *Journal of the American Psychiatric Nurses Association, 9*(3), 86–89.

Lynch, V. (1995). Clinical forensic nursing: A new perspective in the manage-ment of crime victims from trauma to trial. *Critical Care Nursing Clinics of North America, 7*(3), 489–507.

Mason, T. & Mercer, D. (1996). Forensic psychiatric nursing: Visions of social control. *Australian and New Zealand Journal of Mental Health Nursing, 5,* 153–162.

McCarthy, K.J. & Bruin, M.J. (2002). *Managing community-based outcomes through the application of relational victimization theory and practice.* Retrieved on October 10, 2002, from: http://www.uic.edu/orgs/convening/managing.html.

McEwen, M. & Wills, E.M. (2002). *Theoretical basis for nursing.* Philadelphia: Lippincott, Williams and Wilkins.

Meleis, A.A. (1997). *Theoretical nursing: Development and progress* (3rd ed.). Philadelphia: Lippincott.

Mercer, D., Mason, T., & Richman, J. (1999). Good & evil in the crusade of care. Social constructions of mental disorders. *Journal of Psychosocial Nursing and Mental Health Services, 37*(9), 13–17.

National Institutes of Health. (2004). *Health consequences of violence and trauma.* PA-04-075, Department of Health and Human Services. Retrieved May 18, 2005, from http://grants.nih.gov/grants/guide/pa-files/PA-04-075.html.

National Mental Health Association. (1995). *Violence in America: A community mental health response.* Position Statement. Retrieved May 18, 2005, from http://www.nmha.org/prevention/previol.html.

Nettelbeck, T. & Wilson, C. (2002). Personal vulnerability to victimization of people with mental retardation. *Trauma Violence and Abuse, 3*(4), 289–306.

Oberle, K. & Allen, M. (2001). The nature of advanced practice nursing, *Nursing Outlook, 49*(3), 148–153.

Ontario Public Health Association. (1997). *Violence: A public health issue.* Resolution adopted at the 1997 OPHA Annual General Meeting (1997-01).

Peter, E. & Morgan, K.P. (2001). Explorations of a trust approach for nursing ethics. *Nursing Inquiry, 8,* 3–10.

Price, G.M. (2001). *Non-rational guilt in victims of trauma.* Retrieved May 18, 2005, from http://www.inpsyte.ca/priceg.html.

Radden, J. (2001). Boundary violation ethics: Some conceptual clarifications. *Journal of the American Academy of Psychiatry and the Law, 29*(3), 319–326.

Regoli, R. & Hewitt, J.D. (1994). *Delinquency in society.* New York: McGraw-Hill.

Rodgers, B.L. & Knafl, K.A. (2000). *Concept development in nursing: Foundations, techniques, and applications.* Philadelphia: WB Saunders.

Rosenberg, M.L. (2002). The problem of violence. Retrieved October 8, 2002, from http://www.annenberg.nwu.edu/pubs/violence/viol3.html.

Rosenberg, M.L. & Fenley, M.A. (1991). *Violence in America: A public health approach.* New York: Oxford University Press.

Roth, J.A. (1994). *Understanding and preventing violence.* Washington, DC: National Institute of Justice, U.S. Department of Justice.

Sheridan, D.J. (2004). Legal and forensic nursing responses to family violence. In J. Humphreys & J. C. Campbell (Eds.), *Family violence and nursing practice* (pp. 385–406). Philadelphia: Lippincott, Williams & Wilkins.

Varcoe, C. (1996). Theorizing oppression: Implications for nursing research on violence against women. *Canadian Journal of Nursing Research, 28*(1), 61–78.

Walker, G.C., Scott, P.S., & Koppersmith, G. (1998). The impact of child sexual abuse on addiction severity: An analysis of trauma processing. *Journal of Psychosocial Nursing and Mental Health Services, 36*(3), 10–18; 40–41.

Winett, L.B. (1998). Constructing violence as a public health problem. *Public Health Reports, 113*(6), 498–507.

Epidemiology of Violence

Linda C. Degutis

In order to appreciate the range of violent events that may be encountered in the practice of forensic nursing, it is important to understand the various forms of violence that result in injury, as well as the proportions of these events in the population in general, and in specific subgroups of the population. An understanding of the basic principles of epidemiology, with specific reference to injury epidemiology, is also essential.

CHAPTER FOCUS

Definition of violence
Description of types of interpersonal violence
Sources of Data
Epidemiology of violence
Risk factors for violence

KEY TERMS

epidemiology
firearms
homicide
intentional injury
intimate partner violence
National Violent Death Reporting System
suicide
surveillance
terrorism
violence
war

On any given day, it is possible to read multiple news reports that reinforce the fact that violence is a part of our everyday lives. Dramatic events such as suicide bombings and other acts of terrorism have taken over the front pages of our newspapers, and the "common" acts of violence such as homicides and assaults that occur around the country are relegated to other parts of the paper. Biases in reporting can lead one to either underestimate or overestimate the number of events that take place in any particular city or state, or in any given population subgroup. Putting together the data about all of these events is important in understanding the true nature of violence and its impact on our society.

VIOLENCE DEFINED

Violence has many forms. In this chapter, only physical violence will be discussed in detail. In addition, the standard terms to describe intent with respect to injury will be used. Unintentional injuries are injuries that result from events that have traditionally been thought of as "accidents." Some examples of such events are a motor vehicle crash that occurs when a driver fails to stop quickly enough to avoid hitting the car in front of him, an elderly woman tripping and falling over a loose rug in the bathroom, or a toddler who is walking and cuts his chin on the sharp edge of an end table. What these events have in common is that they were not intentional—neither the injured person nor another person deliberately caused the event that resulted in an injury.

Intentional injuries or injuries related to violence are the result of a deliberate act that is committed by the person who is injured, or by another person, with intent to cause harm. These events include an overdose of licit drugs, a fistfight that leads to facial injuries, and a drive-by shooting of two adolescents walking down a street. The types of violent events that occur, and the mechanisms by which they occur, can be defined further. Homicide is an intentional killing of one person by another. Suicide is the deliberate taking of one's own life. Assault is the physical attack by one person upon another, which may or may not result in physical injury. Intimate partner violence (IPV) is the occurrence of physically violent acts between persons who have an intimate relationship, regardless of their sex. Weapons include any object or body part that is used to inflict physical harm on a person. Firearms are handguns, long guns, and any other type of gun that may be used to inflict harm upon oneself or another person. Terrorism is the deliberate and planned act of a person or group of people against another person or group of people in order to achieve political or economic gain. War is a conflict that results in broad-scale violence against specific groups of

can be queried in order to identify specific rates of both fatal and non-fatal injury events due to various causes.

Rates

Rates of injuries or deaths due to violence are often reported. In general, the rate is expressed as the rate per hundred thousand of the population of interest. This provides useful information for comparing rates across age groups, sexes, racial/ethnic groups, and other population groups.

THE EPIDEMIOLOGY OF VIOLENCE

Of the approximately 150,000 injury-related deaths in the United States each year, 31 percent are due to violence. Suicide accounts for 62 percent of the intentional injury deaths, homicide accounts for approximately 37 percent, and legal interventions for less than 1 percent (WISQARS, 2004). Intentional injuries are one of the leading causes of death for several age groups, as illustrated in Table 3–1. Injuries resulting from violence are responsible for approximately 9 percent of the years of potential life lost prior to age 75. Tables 3–1, 3–2, and 3–3 illustrate the leading causes of death, injury-related death, and violence-related death across the lifespan for the year 2001.

Suicide

Each year, suicide accounts for approximately 31,000 deaths in the United States. It is important to keep in mind the appropriate terms to use when discussing suicide. A completed suicide occurs when the victim dies. A suicide attempt is an event in which the victim does not die. Suicide disproportionately affects adolescents, young adults, and the elderly. The methods by which these events occur are also important to understand. The instrument most often used in suicide is a firearm. In 2001, 16,869 firearm-related suicides occurred, with the greatest number of these (3,943) in the 65 and over age group (WISQARS, 2004). Other means of committing suicide include drug overdose, hanging, suffocation, and carbon monoxide poisoning. Table 3–4 compares some of the common mechanisms of homicides and suicides.

There are multiple risk factors for suicide that may change across the life span. One of the most important risk factors is depression. Other factors that contribute to the risk of suicide include alcohol problems, chronic illness, mental health problems, and impulsive behavior.

Table 3–1 Ten Leading Causes of Death, United States 2001, All Races, Both Sexes

Rank	<1	1–4	5–9	10–14	15–24	25–34	35–44	45–54	55–64	65+	All Ages
											Age Groups
1	Congenital Anomalies 5,513	Unintentional Injury 1,714	Unintentional Injury 1,283	Unintentional Injury 1,553	Unintentional Injury 14,411	Unintentional Injury 11,839	Malignant Neoplasms 16,569	Malignant Neoplasms 49,562	Malignant Neoplasms 90,223	Heart Disease 582,730	Heart Disease 700,142
2	Short Gestation 4,410	Congenital Anomalies 557	Malignant Neoplasms 493	Malignant Neoplasms 515	Homicide 5,297	Homicide 5,204	Unintentional Injury 15,945	Heart Disease 36,399	Heart Disease 62,486	Malignant Neoplasms 390,214	Malignant Neoplasms 553,768
3	SIDS 2,234	Malignant Neoplasms 420	Congenital Anomalies 182	Suicide 272	Suicide 3,971	Suicide 5,070	Heart Disease 13,326	Unintentional Injury 13,344	Chronic Low Respiratory Disease 11,166	Cerebrovascular 144,486	Cerebrovascular 163,538
4	Maternal Pregnancy Comp. 1,499	Homicide 415	Homicide 137	Congenital Anomalies 194	Malignant Neoplasms 1,704	Malignant Neoplasms 3,994	Suicide 6,635	Liver Disease 7,259	Cerebrovascular 9,608	Chronic Low Respiratory Disease 106,904	Chronic Low Respiratory Disease 123,013
5	Placenta Cord Membranes 1,018	Heart Disease 225	Heart Disease 98	Homicide 189	Heart Disease 999	Heart Disease 3,160	HIV 5,867	Suicide 5,942	Diabetes Mellitus 9,570	Influenza & Pneumonia 55,518	Unintentional Injury 101,537
6	Respiratory Distress 1,011	Influenza & Pneumonia 112	Benign Neoplasms 52	Heart Disease 174	Congenital Anomalies 505	HIV 2,101	Homicide 4,268	Cerebrovascular 5,910	Unintentional Injury 7,658	Diabetes Mellitus 53,707	Diabetes Mellitus 71,372
7	Unintentional Injury 976	Septicemia 108	Influenza & Pneumonia 46	Chronic Low Respiratory Disease 62	HIV 225	Cerebrovascular 601	Liver Disease 3,336	Diabetes Mellitus 5,343	Liver Disease 5,750	Alzheimer's Disease 53,245	Influenza & Pneumonia 62,034
8	Bacterial Sepsis 696	Perinatal Period 72	Chronic Low Respiratory Disease 42	Benign Neoplasms 53	Cerebrovascular 196	Diabetes Mellitus 595	Cerebrovascular 2,491	HIV 4,120	Suicide 3,317	Nephritis 33,121	Alzheimer's Disease 53,852
9	Circulatory System Disease 622	Benign Neoplasms 58	Cerebrovascular 38	Influenza & Pneumonia 46	Influenza & Pneumonia 181	Congenital Anomalies 458	Diabetes Mellitus 1,958	Chronic Low Respiratory Disease 3,324	Nephritis 3,284	Unintentional Injury 32,694	Nephritis 39,480
10	Intrauterine Hypoxia 534	Cerebrovascular 54	Septicemia 29	Cerebrovascular 42	Chronic Low Respiratory Disease 171	Liver Disease 387	Influenza & Pneumonia 983	Homicide 2,467	Septicemia 3,111	Septicemia 25,418	Septicemia 32,238

From: Centers for Disease Control, National Center for Injury Prevention and Control WISQARS: http://webappa.cdc.gov/sasweb/ncipc/leadcaus10.html. Accessed February 2004.

Table 3–2   Ten Leading Causes of Injury Deaths, United States 2001, All Races, Both Sexes

Rank	Age Groups										All Ages
	<1	1–4	5–9	10–14	15–24	25–34	35–44	45–54	55–64	65+	
1	Unintentional Suffocation 614	Unintentional MV Traffic 558	Unintentional MV Traffic 660	Unintentional MV Traffic 884	Unintentional MV Traffic 10,513	Unintentional MV Traffic 6,759	Unintentional MV Traffic 6,891	Unintentional MV Traffic 5,422	Unintentional MV Traffic 3,328	Unintentional Fall 11,623	Unintentional MV Traffic 42,443
2	Unintentional MV Traffic 139	Unintentional Drowning 458	Unintentional Drowning 168	Unintentional Drowning 165	Homicide Firearm 4,200	Homicide Firearm 3,308	Unintentional Poisoning 5,036	Unintentional Poisoning 3,547	Suicide Firearm 2,083	Unintentional MV Traffic 7,256	Suicide Firearm 16,869
3	Homicide Other Spec., classifiable 117	Unintentional Fire/Burn 230	Unintentional Fire/Burn 164	Suicide Suffocation 163	Suicide Firearm 2,130	Suicide Firearm 2,564	Suicide Firearm 3,030	Suicide Firearm 3,023	Unintentional Fall 1,004	Unintentional Unspecified 5,806	Unintentional Fall 15,019
4	Homicide Unspecified 107	Homicide Unspecified 146	Homicide Firearm 59	Homicide Firearm 121	Unintentional Poisoning 1,362	Unintentional Poisoning 2,507	Homicide Firearm 1,978	Suicide Poisoning 1,439	Unintentional Poisoning 798	Suicide Firearm 3,943	Unintentional Poisoning 14,078
5	Unintentional Drowning 68	Unintentional Suffocation 138	Unintentional Other Land Transport 48	Suicide Firearm 90	Suicide Suffocation 1,235	Suicide Suffocation 1,373	Suicide Poisoning 1,541	Unintentional Fall 1,024	Suicide Poisoning 578	Unintentional Suffocation 3,204	Homicide Firearm 11,348
6	Unintentional Fire/Burn 50	Unintentional Pedestrian, Other 81	Unintentional Suffocation 44	Unintentional Fire/Burn 88	Unintentional Drowning 596	Homicide Transportation Related 842	Suicide Suffocation 1,534	Suicide Suffocation 952	Unintentional Fire/Burn 395	Adverse Effects 1,995	Unintentional Unspecified 7,218
7	Undetermined Suffocation 47	Homicide Other Spec., classifiable 80	Unintentional Fall 33	Unintentional Other Land Transport 83	Homicide Cut/Pierce 481	Suicide Poisoning 753	Undetermined Poisoning 1,121	Homicide Firearm 934	Suicide Suffocation 392	Unintentional Fire/Burn 1,147	Suicide Suffocation 6,198
8	Homicide Suffocation 40	Homicide Firearm 55	Unintentional Pedestrian, Other 26	Unintentional Suffocation 68	Suicide Poisoning 337	Undetermined Poisoning 549	Homicide Transportation Related 1,061	Undetermined Poisoning 761	Unintentional Unspecified 385	Unintentional Poisoning 722	Unintentional Suffocation 5,555
9	Adverse Effects 26	Homicide Other Spec., NEC[N] 49	Unintentional Struck by or Against 25	Unintentional Firearm 39	Unintentional Fall 256	Homicide Cut/Pierce 472	Unintentional Fall 647	Homicide Transportation Related 644	Adverse Effects 384	Unintentional Natural/Environment 621	Suicide Poisoning 5,191
10	Unintentional Fall 23	Unintentional Natural/Environment 42	Unintentional Other Transport 22	Unintentional Pedestrian, Other 38	Unintentional Other Land Transport 250	Unintentional Drowning 374	Unintentional Drowning 462	Unintentional Suffocation 461	Unintentional Suffocation 381	Unintentional Other Spec., NEC[N] 578	Unintentional Fire/Burn 3,423

From: Centers for Disease Control, National Center for Injury Prevention and Control WISQARS: *http://webappa.cdc.gov/sasweb/ncipc/leadcaus10.html*. Accessed February 2004.
[N]Not elsewhere classified (NEC).

Table 3–3   Ten Leading Causes of Violence-Related Injury Deaths, United States 2001, All Races, Both Sexes

Rank	1–4	5–9	10–14	15–24	25–34	35–44	45–54	55–64	65+	All Ages
1	Homicide Other Spec., classifiable 117	Homicide Unspecified 146	Homicide Firearm 163	Homicide Firearm 4,200	Homicide Firearm 3,308	Suicide Firearm 3,030	Suicide Firearm 3,023	Suicide Firearm 2,083	Suicide Firearm 3,943	Suicide Firearm 16,869
2	Homicide Unspecified 107	Homicide Other Spec., classifiable 80	Homicide Unspecified 121	Suicide Firearm 2,130	Suicide Firearm 2,564	Homicide Firearm 1,978	Suicide Poisoning 1,439	Suicide Poisoning 578	Suicide Suffocation 543	Homicide Firearm 11,348
3	Homicide Suffocation 40	Homicide Firearm 55	Homicide Other Spec., classifiable 12	Suicide Suffocation 1,235	Suicide Suffocation 1,373	Suicide Poisoning 1,541	Suicide Suffocation 952	Suicide Suffocation 392	Suicide Poisoning 530	Suicide Suffocation 6,198
4	Homicide Other Spec., NEC[N] 19	Homicide Other Spec., NEC[N] 49	Homicide Suffocation 10	Homicide Cut/Pierce 481	Homicide Transportation Related 842	Suicide Suffocation 1,534	Homicide Firearm 934	Homicide Firearm 364	Homicide Firearm 307	Suicide Poisoning 5,191
5	Homicide Drowning 16	Homicide Fire/burn 24	Homicide Cut/Pierce 8	Suicide Poisoning 337	Suicide Poisoning 753	Homicide Transportation Related 1,061	Homicide Transportation Related 644	Homicide Transportation Related 250	Homicide Unspecified 173	Homicide Transportation Related 3,008
6	Homicide Firearm 11	Homicide Suffocation 18	Homicide Fire/Burn 8	Homicide Unspecified 164	Homicide Cut/Pierce 472	Homicide Cut/Pierce 458	Homicide Cut/Pierce 266	Homicide Unspecified 117	Homicide Cut/Pierce 143	Homicide Cut/Pierce 1,971
7	Homicide Poisoning 10	Homicide Drowning 14	Homicide Other Spec., NEC[N] 8	Homicide Transportation Related 139	Homicide Unspecified 204	Homicide Unspecified 298	Homicide Unspecified 250	Suicide Cut/Pierce 112	Suicide Fall 112	Homicide Unspecified 1,506
8	Homicide Struck by or Against 10	Homicide Struck by or Against 11	Suicide Suffocation 6	Homicide Suffocation 115	Homicide Other Spec., NEC[N] 156	Homicide Other Spec., NEC[N] 166	Homicide Other Spec., NEC[N] 155	Homicide Other Spec., NEC[N] 75	Suicide Cut/Pierce 91	Homicide Other Spec., NEC[N] 831
9	Homicide Cut/Pierce 2	Homicide Cut/Pierce 10	Homicide Drowning 5	Homicide Other Spec., NEC[N] 105	Homicide Suffocation 132	Homicide Suffocation 145	Suicide Fall 129	Suicide Fall 73	Homicide Other Spec., NEC[N] 89	Homicide Suffocation 690
10		Homicide Transportation Related 5	Three Tied 4	Legal Int. Firearm 87	Suicide Fall 109	Suicide Fall 139	Suicide Cut/Pierce 115	Suicide Cut/Pierce 60	Homicide Suffocation 87	Suicide Fall 651

From: Centers for Disease Control, National Center for Injury Prevention and Control WISQARS: *http://webappa.cdc.gov/sasweb/ncipc/leadcaus10.html.* Accessed February 2004.

[N] Not elsewhere classified (NEC).

Table 3–4 Injury Deaths Classified by Type of Injury

Mechanism	Suicide	Homicide
Firearm	16,869 (55.1%)	11,348 (55.9%)
Suffocation	6,198 (20.2%)	690 (3.4%)
Transportation-related	91 (0.3%)	3,008 (14.8%)
Poisoning	5,191 (17.0%)	64 (0.3%)

From WISQARS: *http://webappa.cdc.gov/sasweb/ncipc/leadcaus10.html.* Accessed February 2004.

Homicide

Homicide accounts for approximately 37 percent of intentional injury deaths and was responsible for 20,308 deaths in 2001 (WISQARS, 2004). The vast majority of homicides in the United States are committed with a firearm; other mechanisms of homicide include knives or sharp objects, assaults with a blunt instrument, fire, or use of a motor vehicle. Although there are fewer homicides than suicides each year, the primary mechanism for each is a firearm, accounting for approximately 55 percent of these events. Homicide continues to be the leading cause of death for black males between the ages of 15 and 24, as it has been for the past several years. In addition, black females between 10 and 19 experience homicide at a rate that is three times that of white females in the same age group. The homicide rate among black females aged 15 to 45 years has increased over the past several years so that it is now the leading cause of death in this group. Other groups in which homicide is one of the leading causes of death are children between ages 1 and 4, and youth between ages 15 and 19 of all racial groups. Despite this, there has been a steady decrease in the rate of homicide deaths over the past 10 years. This may be attributable to many interventions, and it is difficult to determine exactly what proportion of the decrease is due to these changes.

Intimate Partner Violence

Intimate partner violence (IPV) includes violence between two people of either sex who are currently, or have been, intimate partners. Women who experience IPV are higher utilizers of healthcare services than other women, making more emergency department visits for injuries and medical complaints, as well as more visits to primary care and mental health services (Centers for Disease Control, 2004). Women are victims of IPV far more often than men, and in the United States, women who are homicide victims are most likely to have been killed by a partner. IPV is responsible for approximately 40 percent of homicides, but only a small percentage of these deaths occur in men. Generally, homicide in an intimate relationship is not the first act of violence that occurs.

Rather, the violence within the relationship escalates over time, with injuries becoming more severe and/or violent episodes becoming more frequent. Estimates are that approximately 1.5 million women are the victims of IPV each year in the United States (Tjaden and Thoennes, 2000). Multiple risk factors contribute to IPV, as well as IPV resulting in homicide. A recent study by Campbell and associates demonstrated that unemployed abusive men were four times more likely to commit femicide than employed men who abused their partners (Campbell et al., 2003). Prior arrest for IPV decreased the risk of femicide, whereas an abuser's access to a firearm increased the risk. Women who left a highly controlling abusive partner were at greater risk of being killed, whereas women who never lived with the abusive partner had a lower risk of femicide.

Dating Violence

Physical violence in a dating relationship has been reported to occur in as many as 32 percent of relationships in high school and college women (White & Koss, 2003). Sexual assault occurs with some frequency in this age group, as half of sexual assaults against females occur to those ages 12 to 24 (Bachman & Saltzman, 1995). A recent study found a rate of dating violence against young women of 88 percent (Smith, White, & Holland, 2003). The greatest risk of victimization was in women who had been victimized in childhood and adolescence.

Terrorism

The Code of Federal Regulations defines terrorism as ". . . the unlawful use of force and violence against persons or property to intimidate or coerce a government, the civilian population, or any segment thereof, in furtherance of political or social objectives" (U.S. Regulations, 1998). Terrorism has been a problem for many years, with some of the most dramatic examples including not only the events that took place in the United States on September 11, 2001, but also events such as the bombing of the Murrah Federal Building in Oklahoma City on April 19, 1995; the intentional poisoning using contaminated food of the citizens of Dalles, Oregon, by a religious cult that sought to take over the town by winning an election; and the distribution of weaponized anthrax through the mail.

The epidemiology of terrorist events is evolving, as researchers identify methods of collecting data in multiple victim incidents and providing real-time information on the extent of injuries and illness occurring. Some of the particular challenges related to the study of terrorist events include the need to protect sensitive data that may be used in legal actions, and the sheer volume of data that may be necessary in order to include all of the victims of these acts in any analysis. As opposed to the epidemiology of violence-related injury, where there are identifiable specific causes of the incidents, the mechanism of any particular terrorist event may not be predicted, and the temporal nature of these events will be different than that of other types of violence, which focus more on individuals than large groups of people.

War

During a war or conflict, many types of violence may occur, and various population groups may be affected. Military units or civilian groups fighting against one another might be expected to suffer fatal and nonfatal injuries, but civilians who are not part of the conflict may also be injured or killed, either intentionally or unintentionally. In addition, other risks may exist during a conflict or time of little governmental control, including sexual assaults of women and young girls. Other consequences of war include those related to landmines that are placed during a conflict but left undetonated, which place the population in the area at risk for injury and long-term disability.

SUMMARY

Epidemiology serves as an investigative method that can be used to examine patterns of injury, patterns of circumstances, and patterns of behavior of humans, vehicles, and environments that contribute to violent events. Knowledge of the epidemiology of violence, as well as epidemiological methods that are used to study injury and violence, can provide a basis for determining the likelihood that specific events are the result of specific causes and circumstances. The consistent use and practice of these methods can enhance the expertise of the forensic investigator, and provide excellent tools for practice.

QUESTIONS FOR DISCUSSION

1. How can forensic nursing contribute to the collaborative investigation of violent events?
2. What is the role of forensic nursing in identifying risk factors for violence?
3. What role can forensic nursing play in preventing violence?
4. How can forensic nurses use epidemiology to assist in the investigation of violent events?

REFERENCES

Agency for Healthcare Research and Quality. HCUPnet. (n.d.). Retrieved February 20, 2004, from http://www.ahrq.gov/data/HCUPnet.ase.

Bachman, R., & Saltzman, L.E. (1995). *Violence against women: Estimates from the redesigned survey.* Washington, DC: U.S. Dept of Justice, Office of Justice Programs. Bureau of Justice Statistics Special Report NCJ-154348.

Campbell, J.C., Webster, D., Koziol-McLain, J., et al. (2003). Risk factors for femicide in abuse relationships: Results from a multisite case control study. *American Journal of Public Health, 93*(7), 1089–1097.

Centers for Disease Control and Prevention. (2004). *Web-based injury statistics query and reporting system (WISQARS).* Retrieved February 20, 2004, from http://www.cdc.gov/ncipc/wisqars/.

Centers for Disease Control and Prevention, National Center for Injury Prevention and Control. (2003). *Costs of intimate partner violence against women in the United States.* Retrieved February 20, 2004, from http://www.cdc.gov/ncipc/pub-res/ipv_cost/ipv.htm.

Haddon, W., Jr. (1968). The changing approach to the epidemiology, prevention and amelioration of trauma: The transition to approaches etiologically rather than descriptively base. *American Journal of Public Health, 58*(8), 1431–1438.

McCaig, L.F., & Burt, C.W. (2003). *National hospital ambulatory medical care survey: 2001 emergency department summary. Advance data from vital and health statistics.* Hyattsville, MD: National Center for Health Statistics.

Paulozzi, L.J., Mercy, J., Frazier, L., & Annest, J.L. (2004). CDC's National Violent Death Reporting System: Background and methodology. *Injury Prevention, 10*(1), 47–52.

Smith, P.H., White, J.W., & Holland, L.J. (2003). A longitudinal perspective on dating violence among adolescent and college-age women. *American Journal of Public Health, 93*(7), 1104–1109.

Tjaden, P. & Thoennes, N. (2000). *Full report of the prevalence, incidence, and consequences of intimate partner violence against women: Findings from the National Violence Against Women Survey.* Report for grant 93-IJ-CX-0012, funded by the National Institute of Justice and the Centers for Disease Control and Prevention. Washington, DC: National Institute of Justice.

United States Code of Federal Regulations, Title 28, Volume 1, Parts 0 to 42. (July 1, 1998). From the U.S. Government Printing Office via GPO Access. Accessed on February 20, 2004, from http://www.gpoaccess.gov/cfr.htm.

United States Federal Bureau of Investigation. Uniform Crime Report. (2004). Retrieved February 20, 2004, from http://www.fbi.gov/ucr/ucr.htm.

White, J.W., & Koss, M.P. (2003). Courtship violence: Incidence and prevalence in a national sample of higher education students. *American Journal of Public Health, 93*(7), 1104–1109.

Multidisciplinary Collaboration

Joseph V. Saitta

Given the array of people, agencies, levels of private and public sector inter-action, concepts, regulations, laws, and so forth that forensic nurses must deal with, it should be clear that practical methods for developing these necessarily interrelated processes are needed. Even a quick scan of the other chapter titles of this text will reveal that close interagency coopera-tion and coordination between agencies and individuals is needed: Forensic nurses may have to work in conjunction with law enforcement agencies, medical examiners and/or coroners, social services agencies, public health departments, hospitals, private healthcare practitioners, psychologists and other mental health professionals, the media, arson investigators, emergency management agencies, the court system, correctional facilities, and more. Thus, in framing an understanding of the word *multidisciplinary*, it will be used in its broadest, most inclusive sense: multiple career fields that impact the practice of forensic nursing.

CHAPTER FOCUS

Multidisciplinary collaboration defined
A theory of collaboration
Internal and external collaboration
Practical collaboration
Future directions in collaboration

KEY TERMS

external collaboration
internal collaboration
multidisciplinary collaboration
search for shared ground
task force concept

MULTIDISCIPLINARY COLLABORATION DEFINED

The derivation and history of collaboration is a fascinating one. The etymology of the word has a Latin base (*com* + *laborare*), which essentially means to "labor with" someone. Unfortunately, the word suffered a fall in fortunes during World War II when it took on a negative, traitorous connotation: A collaborator was viewed as an individual who provides assistance to the enemy. The acts of a collaborator were known as "collaboration." It was not until the 1981 publication of the classic conflict resolution text, *Getting to Yes: Negotiating Agreement Without Giving In*, that the word began its rehabilitation. The text's authors, Fisher and Ury, described a variety of methods that could be used to resolve conflict, from avoiding conflict entirely to the methods of accommodating, compromising, competing, and collaborating. Any of the methods could be appropriate, given the situation and the individuals involved. More importantly, collaboration was characterized as a "win/win" solution with significant advantages to the conflicting parties. For the purposes of this chapter, this more positive connotation is intended whenever the word *collaboration* is used.

Within the field of business, collaboration is often known by other names, such as networking. It may even go by the grandiose moniker of "strategic alliance," the concept of which connotes something far more structured than is being discussed in this chapter. A strategic alliance encompasses the development of joint ventures and similar legal entities. Of course, the concept of collaboration is not alien to the nursing profession. Numerous medical and public health articles point to either the need for collaboration or its use in clinical or managerial activities. This chapter seeks to address a different aspect of collaboration, with an emphasis on its practical application. Our definition, then, of "multidisciplinary collaboration" is the process of working effectively with people from multiple career fields to accomplish forensic nursing goals, while maintaining existing organizational structures. These goals could involve clinical, psychiatric, correctional/institutional, or other forensic nursing areas.

As it pertains to our definition of multidisciplinary collaboration, the phrase "working effectively with people" is worth closer examination. It implies reciprocal communication, tact, trust, and a comprehensive understanding of how all of the pieces fit together to produce a user-friendly forensic system.

A THEORY OF COLLABORATION

According to Charles McClintock (1998) the term *collaboration* also implies commitment, which usually develops over quite a long period of time. This commitment may take a variety of forms, as will be demonstrated with the "Practical Collaboration" section later in this chapter. McClintock cites Konrad (1996) and Himmelman (1994) in more fully discussing a collaboration continuum that contains five types of collaboration built on each other; the following list organizes these types from least formal (networking) to most formal (integration):

Networking requires the least commitment and is characterized by informal information sharing and support for common objectives. Thus, an act as simple—yet, as useful—as sending an e-mail about a recent forensic article to a colleague is considered a networking activity.

Coordinating maintains the informality of networking but also attempts to unify certain services to accomplish common goals. For example, a hypothetical forensic nurse works in a correctional facility. Instead of developing a sexually transmitted diseases (STD) prevention program for her clients by working independently, she coordinates with the nearby health department's STD educator to develop a cutting-edge program that combines the resources of both agencies.

Cooperating closely mirrors our definition of collaboration: People from different organizations work together to develop *and* to accomplish common goals, and share resources. However, the existing organizational structures are maintained. The development of a forensic task force is a prime example of cooperating, and will be discussed further in this chapter's "Practical Collaboration" section.

Consolidating has many of the foregoing elements, but also requires a structural change with some type of oversight committee or umbrella group being created to manage administrative tasks. Meanwhile, lower in the food chain, the functional units remain largely the same. An example of consolidating is the establishment of a joint training committee for a homicide work group composed of forensic nurses, 911 communication dispatchers, the medical examiner's staff, homicide investigators, prosecutors, and crime scene investigators. The purpose of the committee is to develop a training program for this diverse group that will address appropriate procedures for managing a homicide incident, from receipt of the 911 call through the prosecution of the perpetrator. The committee will have the authority to prepare or purchase training materials, contract with instructors, and conduct the class or classes. Each participating agency and organization has agreed to these activities, and the financial support thereof, because the training is intended to produce a cost-effective, systematic result.

Integrating is a total restructuring of organizations. The most recent national example of this is the development of the U.S. Department of Homeland Security from scores of pre-existing and newly developed agencies. The ultimate success of such a massive undertaking depends on a variety of complex factors, including the change management process itself, the smoothness of the transition from separate organizational cultures to a new one, the new agency's ability to refocus employees toward new goals and objectives, the effectiveness of the department's new leadership, and so on.

INTERNAL AND EXTERNAL COLLABORATION

Multidisciplinary collaboration can be further delineated into "internal collaboration" and "external collaboration." By internal collaboration, we mean the daily, face-to-face effective interaction that must occur *within* your primary work unit; external collaboration refers to the effective interaction that must occur *outside* of your primary work unit. The thrust of this chapter is external collaboration. But, if internal collaboration does not already exist—essentially, if you are "at war" with others in your primary work unit—you will be unable to devote much time or effort to external collaboration. In other words, a house divided cannot effectively collaborate externally. Settle these internal issues first, then build your network outward.

The first step in external collaboration is determining what *your* current job entails. This situational analysis may be as uncomplicated as reviewing your job description. Most jobs change over time, however, sometimes in subtle ways and at other times in not so subtle ways. Furthermore, people tend to mold their jobs to fit their own strengths and weaknesses. Even if you have determined what your current job entails, this is not a one-time process; your job will change as the career field of forensic nursing changes and as your local conditions change. There is a high probability that, when the job changes, the people you need to collaborate with will change as well.

The next step is to determine who—outside of your primary work unit—has similar goals, patient interaction, legal or regulatory authority, and other duties that touch on your speciality within forensic nursing. Jay Conger (1998), writing on management persuasiveness, devotes an entire chapter to the "search for shared ground." He builds a strong case that success in management is based on the outcomes of this search. According to Conger, the core elements in framing this search for shared ground are shared goals and rewards, shared values and beliefs, and shared language (p. 79).

Forensic nurses should frame their search for shared ground similarly. For example, a hypothetical forensic nurse works in a subspecialty as a nurse coroner. This role calls for dealing with an elected coroner, a hospital-based medical examiner, and law enforcement personnel. What are their shared goals and outcomes? One such goal would surely be to accurately determine the cause of death of a victim. And, just as surely, a shared value and belief would be to treat the families of said victim with empathy.

Unfortunately, shared language between agencies cannot be taken as a given. I recall a counterterrorism class I once conducted for a group on the West Coast. The audience included police and fire/rescue personnel (career fields that I knew well), and public health nurses and doctors (a field that, at that time, I did not know as well). In describing the types of detection equipment that a fire company may carry on its responding apparatus, I started by listing the equipment (flame ionization detector, combustible gas meter, etc.) but then lapsed into using an acronym: "PID." As a result, the police personnel did not know what I meant and the doctors and nurses *apparently* thought I was referring to pelvic inflammatory disease, and got a great deal of enjoyment from my confusion and chagrin. Only the firefighters knew that I was referring to a photo ionization detector. Never assume that shared language exists. When in doubt, clarify and define.

THE DRIVE TO BOND

Is the need to work collaboratively reinforced by innate human characteristics? According to Paul R. Lawrence and Nitin Nohria in their 2002 book, *Driven: How Human Nature Shapes Our Choices*, the answer is definitely "yes." Both Harvard Business School professors maintain that their extensive research indicates that " . . . bonding between humans starts with a one-on-one pairing, moves on to the nuclear family and thence to the primary face-to-face group, is extended to social networks and then to social networks that are interlocked and clustered into all kinds of collective entities, organizations, and associations" (p. 99). Given this, one is on firm ground in forming a collaborative group that nurtures this need to bond.

PRACTICAL COLLABORATION

Here are some practical tips, drawn from a variety of sources including real world experience, to get you started on multidisciplinary collaboration. Please bear in mind that, like fine wine, these practical tips may not travel well (just because these tips have worked for me and for others does not mean that they will automatically work for you). However, give them a real-world trial. Some permutation of this randomly arranged smorgasbord of ideas probably will work for you.

Task Force Concept

The incident command system (ICS) is used extensively in public safety and should already be a part of one's baseline knowledge. According to the ICS concept, a "task force" is "a group of any type or kind of resource, with common communications and a leader, temporarily assembled for a specific mission . . . " (Federal Emergency Management Agency, 1999, p. A-5). Many communities have taken this ICS task force concept and used it to form ad hoc collaborative groups. For example, there are scores of regional counterterrorism task forces, which usually include participation from the FBI's weapons of mass destruction (WMD) coordinator(s), state and local law enforcement agencies, medical examiner's office representatives, area hospital and healthcare providers, the public health department, the local chapter of the American Red Cross, the region's emergency medical services council, social service agencies, and area fire/rescue and emergency management agencies. Together these groups are working effectively to prepare for, and respond to, domestic terrorism incidents. (As an aside: You should consider membership in such a group.)

The task force concept lends itself quite well to collaborative efforts with others in the forensic field. Starting a forensic task force, which meets periodically to discuss common issues and concerns and to develop a working relationship, can really "jump-start" your collaborative efforts. Several other terms are often used for similar ad hoc teams, such as "working group." Select a group name that most accurately provides clarity of your group's intended functions.

Common Goals and Objectives

Developing Goals. Whether or not you decide to use the task force concept in developing your collaborative efforts or you select another method of getting your group together, start off the first meeting (or first few meetings) of the group you plan to develop into your collaborative network with the usual introductions. Then seek to develop common written goals and objectives. Goals are broad "targets" to be accomplished. As preferred outcomes, they should be written with an action verb or verbs (such as improve, reduce, or increase). An example of a common goal would be "to increase the effectiveness of the Forensic Task Force in preventing, investigating, and prosecuting homicides in the XYZ region." The goals that you develop should be reasonable (meaning that they are, in fact, attainable), politically astute, important, and forward-looking. Goals are not written in a vacuum; they should represent the cooperative work effort of a group of willing and knowledgable colleagues. It may take longer to write goals in this manner, but it offers two distinct advantages. First, you will end up with a better, more representative product. Second, you will have more "buy in" from the people who worked on these goals. These involved stakeholders can then go forward to persuade the rest of your group, intellectually "selling" the results of their combined work efforts. If opposition develops, set aside a time for any dissenters to provide their input. Ultimately, everyone involved must have "buy in."

Developing Objectives. As opposed to the broad-based nature of goals, objectives should be precise, written statements of what the group intends to accomplish at the end of a specified period of time. As such, objectives are designed to be more measurable than goals, use an observable action verb (such as describe, conduct, or purchase), include pertinent conditions (such as cost figures, locations, or implementation parameters), and provide an end date. An example of an objective is: "By July 1, 2004, the Forensic Task Force will develop a protocol for use by all personnel investigating suspicious death cases in the XYZ region." Dividing this objective into understandable pieces, we find that the observable action verb is "will develop." This indicates that at the end date, July 1, 2004, there will be a hard copy document prepared as a work deliverable. The pertinent conditions included in this objective include "by all personnel" and "in the XYZ region." In short, think of objectives as more specific and measurable when compared to goals.

Developing Ground Rules

Associated with developing common goals and objectives is determining your group's ground rules. These can include items such as how you will contact each other (via e-mail, fax, or perhaps by calling home telephone numbers in the event of an emergency), how often the group will meet, if the leadership function will rotate, whether meeting minutes will be taken (and who will do so), and so on. It is probably more effective to have less formal ground rules in the early development of the group. Too much formality increases the workload of someone (probably you), and causes fears that an individual or group is trying to take over or has some other devious hidden agenda. Often this fear of a turf battle is all it takes to kill the success of the collaborative effort. After the individuals in the group have had an opportunity to get to know and trust each other, formality can be interposed, if needed.

Offer Training

One surefire way to get to know your counterparts and to develop effective professional interactions is to offer them training. There's an old saying in the intelligence community to the effect that "you've got to give a little to get a little." Although this saying refers to the exchange of classified information, it can be used to understand why training is an appealing entrée to another group of forensic professionals. There is an inherent interest in continuing the learning process that has brought them to their current high level of expertise, not to mention a competitive desire to exceed that level.

Using the earlier example of providing the rest of a forensic task force with training about the "role of forensic nurses," you would be offering these group members insights into a newly emerging facet of their profession, and how it will mesh with the existing forensic field. This provides your "students" with extremely current information, but it also affords you the opportunity to further "sell" forensic nursing. Bear in mind that a reciprocal training, where you learn about their various specialties, is also in order. As a result, you may be learning about forensic epidemiology, law enforcement procedures, prehospital emergency medical services documentation, disaster operations, or hazardous materials. These are all of great value to you in understanding the entire forensic system. Most of your counterparts in the forensic task force will have some type of continuing education requirements similar to your own. If you can arrange for them to obtain continuing education credits or hours through their authorizing professional association, you provide an added incentive for their ongoing involvement in the group's training program.

Take a Field Trip

Do you recall how much you enjoyed the field trip your fifth grade class took to the museum? You can still use the concept. As long as your destination will result in accomplishing a specific learning objective, such an out-of-class experience is still useful . . . and fun. For example, would members of your forensic task force need a better understanding of how your state laboratory system works? If so, a tour of one of the state's laboratory facilities would be a worthwhile training event.

Be Willing to Work

If your collaborative work effort is going to succeed, it will require a great deal of hard work. I have often found that one committed and hardworking person can *start* the process needed to unify a group. It would be great if everyone involved would be willing to work at the development of this collaborative effort, but *you* may have to make the personal commitment to be that one person who initially invests the time and effort into this project until others can clearly see its usefulness. If your schedule does not permit that level of time commitment, then find someone whose schedule *does* permit it, or get permission to "off-load" some of your everyday work duties for a specified period.

Leadership Team

Of course, a different tack than having you initiate the bulk of the work would be to pull together a "leadership team" or cadre of motivated people—naturally, including you—from the agencies and organizations involved. Allow them (and you) to do the initial foundation work of developing the goals and objectives, contacting other interested persons, and so on. One important decision to make early on is whether to include "distinguished colleagues" in this leadership team. I am sure that you have seen the letterhead of virtually any large charitable organization: at the top left there is usually a list of the board of directors. The board is composed of the esteemed, the rich, and the famous . . . plus a few "worker bees." To the extent that the "big names" draw in funds, motivate others to contribute, and lend legitimacy to the charity, they more than earn their places. Should you include similar people in your leadership team? To some degree the answer depends on local conditions, personalities, past experiences, and other such imprecise factors. My recommendation would be to exercise care in the selection of any member of your leadership team, especially those who do not directly contribute to the work effort. However, I would not rule out anyone who could help further your group's efforts, including "distinguished colleagues." If carefully chosen, your leadership team will be in a position to initiate the development of the group and the development of the individuals in the group, so that both excel. This "transformational leadership" process is no small feat, and implies the ability to cause positive change in a group of people and in their organizational culture.

The Team Concept

While on the subject of having a leadership team, some note should be made on the usefulness of the team concept in general. There are signs at your local post office with the acronym **TEAM** boldfaced, followed by the explanation "**T**ogether **E**veryone **A**ccomplishes **M**ore." The Postal Service has definitely delineated a key element of the nature of teams. We can use this team concept whether or not we use a leadership team. In fact, an athletic team is a useful analogy for how a forensic work group should perform. Successful athletic teams have a common vision and mission, a finely developed sense of how the different roles interrelate, and a clear understanding of procedures. They are intensely focused on positive outcomes. Athletic teams also know how to deal with failure and move forward. They even have some things that your work group may not yet have: an identifying logo, a common uniform, and a slogan or motto. The closer your work group replicates these successful athletic team characteristics the more positive its outcomes may become.

Don't Neglect the Interpersonal

Strong, trusting collaborative relationships are built one step after another over a long period of time. Although we have already begun to discuss the ways you can build that relationship as a group effort, also consider ways that you can develop that relationship with each individual in the group. This can be done by engaging in activities such as making reciprocal visits to each other's offices, "breaking bread" over lunch, and conducting mutually supportive functions that, although unrelated to the development of the task force, are related to your job functions. For example, sharing how your office files are arranged (essentially, providing the titles of each file folder) with another forensic nurse may be very helpful to that individual, especially if he or she is new to the field. In return, he or she may suggest ways for you to add to or consolidate your files. Again, such little things foster better relationships.

Conduct Productive Meetings

Several points can be made concerning the process of running an effective meeting (Table 4–1). Each member of your collaborative group already has pre-existing commitments, both personal and work-related. Be respectful of the time they are sacrificing to attend a group meeting. Although meeting management is an art in itself, several simple actions increase the likelihood of holding productive meetings:

- *Start with a clear need for a meeting.* This need should be included in a written agenda that is circulated well in advance of the meeting. This agenda should spell out the purpose of the meeting, the major topics to be discussed, and who will lead or present each topic, plus it will indicate the exact meeting time and location. Be sure to include some social time in each meeting where people can have an opportunity to informally chat. Providing coffee and munchies (unfortunately, often at your own expense) may seem unimportant, but these "comfort items" represent a courtesy that people invariably appreciate.

Table 4–1 Elements of a Productive Meeting

Respect for the commitments of others
Articulation of a clear need for the meeting
Inclusion of social time
Promptness
Adherence to agenda
Clarification of decisions after each agenda item
Completion of "homework" prior to the meeting

- *Start your meeting on time.* It is rude to those already in attendance to wait for the arrival of someone else, no matter how important that person's role in the meeting. I have found that once it becomes known that you start on time, the meeting attendees tend to actually be prompt, ready to go when the stated time arrives.
- *Stick to your agenda.* If it appears that the group is falling behind in its scheduled discussions, it is often effective for the meeting's leader to survey the group members to see if they think the issue can be resolved in another 10 to 20 minutes of further discussion or if the members prefer to postpone the issue until the next meeting. Finally, move from each agenda item with a clear understanding of what decision was made. If an action is to be taken, it should be equally clear to all attendees who will be taking said action, when it will be completed, and what the work product will be. And, remember, often the real meeting has occurred *before* the actual meeting. Do your homework and confer with those who are persuasive, extremely opinionated, and/or powerful before the actual meeting begins.

Share Successes

When your collaborative group or task force accomplishes something especially noteworthy (attaining a grant, solving a crime, etc.), take that opportunity to enjoy the occasion. An informal meeting with food and soft drinks is definitely in order. These social occasions serve another purpose: to reaffirm that the group is, in fact, accomplishing worthwhile objectives. Sometimes in the hustle-and-bustle to get started on the next case or manage the next patient, our successes go unnoticed to us. With that in mind, some groups are a bit too driven. A little unstructured pleasantness to the "fun deprived" is more than merely therapeutic; it makes people want to continue to affiliate with your group. At the same time as you share successes, I would remind you to exercise care in doing so. Be especially vigilant about group members maintaining professional decorum, even as they have fun. It only takes one untoward event to embarrass an individual or the entire group, cause an injury, or result in a lawsuit.

Use the Media Effectively

The chapter on media management provides some very useful ideas on grabbing the attention of the print and electronic media. Use these tips to "toot the horn" of your collaborative group. Most agencies and individuals like to see their names referred to by the media in a positive light. Properly written press releases can attract media coverage, and can include such events as the formation of the group, the initial call for members, the completion of the goals and objectives, the establishment of a speakers' bureau, the award of a grant, or the solution of a particularly thorny problem or case. The media thrive on human interest stories, so use these opportunities as well.

Another media opportunity is to develop a media "school," wherein the media are invited to learn about the different components of your forensic task force. The "pay-off" for the media will be a succinct overview of forensics, and a chance to meet good future agency contacts or news sources. Turnabout is fair, so perhaps the media in your area will offer a reciprocal training for your task force membership that explains how the media functions, what kinds of stories the press are interested in, and what format they prefer for press releases.

Public Forensic Academy

Many law enforcement agencies and fire departments have initiated citizens' academies to familiarize the public with the organization, procedures, and operation of their respective agencies. Given the popularity of television shows addressing forensic issues, this may be the appropriate time to offer *your* public a forensic academy. Even a 1-hour program explaining how your forensic team is organized would be viewed positively by the public. Because you probably will not be able to select attendees, bear in mind that the content will have to be prepared very carefully so that it does not allow any sensitive information to be included in the presented content.

Evaluate Failures

When things do not go as well as they should, the tendency is to point fingers at another individual or agency . . . in public. Instead, hold a closed session "postincident analysis" or "lessons learned" meeting to determine what specifically needs improvement. Make sure that you end the session with an acknowledgment of the importance of all of the assembled individuals and agencies to the attainment of your common goals. The attendees should leave the meeting with a clear action plan of the steps that need to be taken to ensure that the same problem does not occur again. As warranted, agencies may have to change policies and procedures, offer more training, and/or shift individuals to other positions. Every failure, if treated as a learning opportunity, contains the seeds for a future success.

Also, remember that your group's failure *may* be related to how successful the group has been at becoming cohesive. Although this sounds counterintuitive, the phenomenon is well known in the social sciences as the concept of "groupthink." Essentially, it takes a great deal of hard work to become a cohesive group and to internalize Conger's elements of shared goals and rewards, shared values and beliefs, and shared language. As a result, the group's members tend to avoid any ideas or actions that may cause discord. This tendency to uncritically reject those things that cause discord *and* uncritically accept those things that reinforce the appearance of agreement may lead to critical errors. Meanwhile, the group continues to deny that its initial course of action is in error. Always be on the lookout for groupthink. This is especially true when the group makes a hasty, little-discussed decision on a critical issue.

Establish a Conflict Resolution Mechanism

This might seem similar to the previous tip of evaluating failures, but here I am referring to interpersonal conflicts, those little niggling things (and sometimes very big issues) that cause conflict. Most people prefer to solve a problem quickly, at the lowest level possible (meaning that you do not contact someone's supervisor until you make good faith efforts to solve the problem directly with that individual), and in a way that does not damage the future relationship you may have with the involved individual. A good starting point for brushing up on conflict resolution techniques is the *Getting to Yes* book mentioned earlier (Fisher & Ury, 1981). Additionally, the Thomas-Kilmann Conflict Mode Instrument (TKI) is a test—available at the counseling departments of most community colleges and online for a fee—that can be utilized to determine and evaluate your predominant conflict resolution style.

Stay in Touch

If your collaborative partners only meet with you on a monthly or a quarterly basis, you may need to devote extra effort to maintaining the working relationship with them. One colleague of mine goes so far as to clip business cards of his associates to his calendar. Then, each week he calls one or two of them just to "touch base." He also keeps notations of their professional interests: If an article or research report crosses his desk that he thinks will be useful to an associate, he refers it to them. I would suggest going a bit further. Learn about associates' hobbies, avocations, and so forth. Once again, if you locate something of interest to them, just let them know.

Good working relationships are built slowly, and in both big and small ways. So, do not forget to send appropriate congratulations to those who are newly promoted, recently married, or involved in other such happy events. Appropriate condolences should also be provided on occasions where there has been a death in the family of an associate or the like.

Be Polite

At the risk of stating the obvious, a little bit of courtesy goes a long way. If common courtesy was so very common, we would not boast about our rare good fortune when we encounter a polite salesclerk. Use "please" and "thank you," return telephone calls and e-mails promptly, answer letters, and so on. In short, act as you would like to be treated. If someone does something helpful for you or your group, write a thank-you note. If his or her helpfulness rises above the call of duty, take the time to write a letter to that individual's supervisor. Go out of your way to find reasons to be helpful to others. The old saying that "no act of kindness is ever wasted" is true. We go the extra mile for our patients. Shouldn't we also do so for our colleagues?

Conduct a Disaster Drill

Whatever your specialty within forensic nursing, if a disaster occurs in your jurisdiction, you *will* be involved in some form in the management of that incident. Conducting an exercise will help you to prepare for a disaster. But the exercise cannot be developed until your area's emergency plan is studied. The emergency plan is a description of what personnel, in and out of government, should do in the event of an emergency. Furthermore, the plan indicates what resources, personnel, and procedures will be used during the incident. Your agency or organization should be included in the resources described in the plan. Exercises test performance, but it is the emergency plan that delineates the acceptable level of performance needed. If you are not familiar with your area's emergency plan, you should contact your jurisdictional emergency manager. In many jurisdictions this person will be a "direct report" to the senior elected official; in other areas he or she will be based in a fire department or a law enforcement agency.

To design an exercise that simulates a real emergency, you must know what responses are planned and assess what capabilities are needed to meet those responses. Ultimately, your exercise must factor in the types of disasters that have occurred in your area, what operations will have to be undertaken in similar future incidents, what the capability levels of the responders are, what equipment resources exist, and how all of these can be incorporated into the emergency plan. The exercise that you develop can be table-top, functional, or full-scale. Whichever type is selected will require a great deal of work to bring to fruition. However, the payoff for you and others in the forensic field is a better-integrated response and a quicker recovery for your community.

Look Outside Your Borders

This tip addresses two issues about "borders." First, it refers to the intellectual borders that may be present, which blind you to opportunities for your collaborative efforts. These borders are often verbalized as "we never did it that way before" or "it can't be done." Yet, many of the world's great pioneering efforts and innovations started out when just one person had the gumption to try to accomplish something in a different way. The second issue that this tip addresses is the fact that, as surely as you are wrestling with developing a collaborative effort to initiate your forensic task force, there is another nearby group (perhaps as close as your next jurisdiction) doing exactly the same thing. Are there "economies of motion" in working with them as well? Definitely. This is a chance to network with these other groups. Getting started may be as simple as offering to host an informal meeting in your offices. The advantages of such a meeting: You may discover the answer to a problem you are currently dealing with, you may expand your network of professional resources, and you may provide insights for others, as well.

Hold a Conference

Trainers aren't the only ones that can hold a conference. You and your colleagues can, too. Determine the content you will cover, the target audience, the training location, and the speakers, and you are ready to begin. In fact, your target audience may be those nearby forensic professionals that you unearthed as a result of looking outside your borders. If you require help with the details of conference planning, it may be provided by a nurse educator, a trainer on your local forensic task force, or a staff member at your local community college's continuing education department.

Job Rotation

Initially, you may not have the time to rotate jobs with someone else in the field of forensic nursing. However, you can probably arrange to set aside an hour or two to go to his or her job location and observe a typical morning's or afternoon's activities. A more extensive version of this allows you to actually trade jobs for a significant period of time (usually not exceeding a year). The British military and public safety services use this method, which they call "secondment," extensively to broaden the perspectives of employees on the fast track. In your case, such experiences can contribute to a comprehensive understanding of the forensic field.

For example, if you now work in an institutional or correctional setting, you could rotate jobs for a week with another nurse who now works in a criminal justice agency. Each of you would gain insights, make valuable contacts, and better understand how the entire forensic system works. Similar opportunities may exist for job rotation with other members of your forensic task force.

Benchmark the Best

The concept of "benchmarking" is well known in management circles, and it has value for forensic nurses as well. Find those community groups, businesses, and government organizations that are effectively collaborating, and analyze what makes them successful. Then judiciously select those activities that are a close match for what your group is trying to do. Finally, try a pilot test—a time-limited replication of that activity—to determine if it will work for your group. For example, if your area's Volunteer Organizations Active in Disasters (VOAD) group has been extremely successful in attracting community funding and you would like to obtain a similar type or level of funding, determine how VOAD accomplishes this (naturally, be sure to first assure your area's VOAD that you will not compete directly with it for funding). Benchmarking is a significant work-saver because it allows you to benefit from the hard-earned failures and successes of others.

FUTURE DIRECTIONS IN COLLABORATION

Fast-forward several years in your forensic nursing career: You have established yourself professionally, your major formal collaborative effort (the forensic task force) has performed flawlessly . . . what now? One option would be to further formalize the organization's structure at a higher level in the collaboration continuum. Given my earlier comments, that means that the group may be looking at consolidating or integrating. Because both of these require structural changes, they would also require input and authority from the highest levels of the involved agencies, companies, and jurisdictional powers.

Another option would be to consider developing or perpetuating a funding mechanism for the group. If the group decides to seek contributions, then nonprofit status may be worth considering. An excellent resource in determining how to attain nonprofit status would be an attorney willing to provide *pro bono* legal advice. If the group is trying to project its future work efforts—for example, how many patients will be treated in the next year—this can be accomplished in a number of ways. Certainly "data mining" on the Internet and with other forensic groups similar to your own will yield results. In addition, regression analysis, using a mathematical equation that can be done by hand or with a statistics package (such as SPSS), can determine the projected growth in the hypothetical patient load, based on the data about your patients from several prior years. Similarly, trend analysis can also help you to discover your future directions.

If there are several other active forensic task forces in your region or state then this may be an opportunity to initiate a region-wide or state-wide consortium. If travel distances are extensive, you may instead want to consider simply using an Internet list server function that can serve as your electronic bulletin board.

Finally, recognize that the transformational leadership process that was mentioned under "Leadership Teams" earlier in this chapter should have produced positive changes in you and your group. Use these newly developed skills as you seek new directions.

QUESTIONS FOR DISCUSSION

1. Define the concept of external collaboration. How does it differ from internal collaboration?
2. Given the collaboration continuum, how does cooperating differ from the four other types of collaboration?
3. What are the core elements in the "search for shared ground," and how can they be used in multidisciplinary collaboration?
4. How can the task force concept, taken from the incident command system, be used to develop collaboration?
5. Select two other practical tips for collaboration. How can each be used to foster multidisciplinary collaboration?

REFERENCES

Conger, J. A. (1998). *Winning 'em over: A new model for management in the age of persuasion.* New York: Simon and Schuster.

Federal Emergency Management Agency. (1999). *Incident command system, self study unit.* Washington, DC: U.S. Government Printing Office.

Fisher, R. & Ury, W. (1981). *Getting to yes: Negotiating agreement without giving in.* New York: Penguin.

Himmelman, A. T. (1994). Communities working collaboratively for a change. In Herrman, M. (Ed.), *Resolving conflict strategies for local government management.* Washington, DC: International City/County Management Assoc., p. 27–47.

Konrad, E. L. (1996). *The Elements of Collaboration.* In J. M. Marquart and E. L. Konrad (Eds.), *Evaluating initiatives to integrate human services. New directions for program evaluation, No. 69.* San Francisco: Jossey-Bass.

Lawrence, P. R. & Nohria, N. (2002). *Driven: How human nature shapes our choices.* San Francisco: Jossey-Bass.

McClintock, C. (1998). *Cross-agency collaboration: Research findings and practitioner experience.* Ithaca, NY: Cornell University.

Sociocultural Diversity

Nathan Light

Forensic nurses practice in cultural contexts that are far more complex, diverse, and challenging than those that most other nurses will encounter in their work. Forensic nursing clients bring widely varied backgrounds and expectations: Victims, offenders, and psychiatric patients have radically different needs and ways of engaging in the nurse–client relationship. Even if clients come from similar cultural and social backgrounds, those who suffer from crimes, those who may have committed them, and those with psychological difficulties will be involved in very different institutional processes, and their concerns and responses to treatment will vary widely. To properly treat people with such complex and varied backgrounds and issues, nurses must develop a sensitivity to the cultural and social factors that shape each nurse–client interaction.

Forensic nurses will rarely be able to carry out all their work solely within a single institution, such as a hospital, without some understanding and engagement with the cultures and institutional practices of other concerned organizations and their differing goals. Law enforcement, parole boards, correctional institutions, courts, and victim or substance abuser support groups are a few of the organizations that may become involved in a forensic nurse's work, in addition to the more familiar medical, family, and community contexts. Each context has its own cultural particularities, and offenders and victims will experience institutional interactions differently. They may deal with the same police, prosecutors, and medical personnel along the way, but their social roles and the significance of these contacts will differ greatly. Each client will move from crisis and separation from ordinary life through redress and reintegration into social life, but the actual processes will vary widely.

This chapter will introduce concepts needed to understand and deal effectively with culturally and socially diverse people and institutional contexts, and will offer models for understanding the particular cultural contexts that forensic nurses will find themselves in. This chapter will also describe the ways that cultural processes shape socialization so students will understand how childhood establishes the vital permanent connections between culture and the person that make transcultural nursing skills so important. To understand how and why client socialization affects behavior and thinking, this chapter provides a detailed discussion of the processes and effects of learning culture.

This chapter will also familiarize students with the ethical principles that guide transcultural nursing in order to better serve clients through communication and consideration of cultural preferences and concepts. The institutional contexts of nursing will be expanded to show how all clinical situations include transcultural elements, and how understanding this contributes to nursing practice.

CHAPTER FOCUS

Socialization and cultural learning
Cultural models
Subconscious and conscious culture
Culture and health
Cultural and social diversity
Transcultural communication
Transcultural nursing
Dominant and minority cultures
Ethnocentrism, prejudice, and discrimination
The institutional cultures of forensic nursing
Ritual process (separation, liminality, reintegration)
Cultural issues in forensic nursing
Ideas and practices related to institutions
Ideas and practices related to illness
Ideas and practices related to trauma
Ideas and practices related to mental illness

KEY TERMS

class
communicative norms
cultural awareness
cultural bias
cultural competence
culturally congruent

cultural integration
cultural model
cultural pain
cultural relativism
culture
culture-bound syndrome
culture care
ethnicity
ethnocentrism
ethnopsychology
gender
human rights
institutional culture
institutional discrimination
interpretation
macroculture
microculture
minority
multiculturalism
organizational subcultures
personal prejudice
pluralism
race
sexual orientation
situational identity
social control
stereotypes
symbols
tolerance
transcultural communication
transcultural nursing
Vega model

THE EXPERIENCE OF CULTURE

For practitioners of forensic nursing to work effectively in a multicultural society such as the United States, they must understand sociocultural diversity from a scientific perspective. Without an objective understanding of culture and social organization, professionals in positions of power tend to accept dominant European American middle-class values and norms and expect clients and colleagues to conform with them. Medical personnel may judge deviation from dominant culture expectations and values as social, emotional, intellectual, or medical failings.

In the medical and legal contexts within which forensic nurses work, many institutional values and practices are based on dominant culture expectations. If forensic nurses do not objectively understand the sociocultural processes in these institutions, they may provide inadequate service to clients because dominant culture assumptions about thinking, emotion, and behavior lead nurses to ignore, misunderstand, or reject a client's concerns.

This section will explain what culture is, how people experience it, and how these concepts can be applied to understanding the issues of sociocultural diversity in the context of forensic nursing.

What Is Culture?

Culture includes all of the concepts, beliefs, expectations, practices, abilities, and communicative skills acquired during life as a member of social groups. Despite this apparently simple definition, culture encompasses such a broad and complex spectrum of human learning and activity that it demands careful explanation and attention to overcome the many common misconceptions about it. Culture is learned, shared, adaptive, and symbolic (Schultz & Lavenda, 1998, p. 18), so to understand culture, we must understand each of these aspects of culture.

Anyone Can Learn Any Culture

Culture is learned by humans from birth. Any child with normal mental potential who enters a sociocultural context in childhood can acquire full symbolic and behavioral competence in that culture. Although the basic survival skills of an infant are products of instincts, the infant rapidly begins to expand upon abilities, and throughout childhood her brain acquires the vast range of skills and understandings that allow people to participate meaningfully in society. Through the course of human evolution, childhood has become longer specifically because humans survive better when they learn more cultural skills during this period of dependency. Because culture takes extended repeated experience to acquire, the human body and brain develop more slowly than those of other animals. Extended cultural experience allows mastery of complex skills that go far beyond what can be transmitted genetically as instincts (Bogin, 1995).

Culture Learning in the Brain

At the neurological level culture exists as neurons that are connected by synapses into patterns that link perceptions, experiences, memories, and behaviors. A child is born with highly interconnected neurons that respond to activity in the world through the five senses and to bodily processes through internal sensations such as pain, discomfort, or hunger. After an initial stage in which the infant's mind develops the ability to organize, process, and retain sense impressions, it begins to link different perceptions of objects or events that occur closely linked in time or space. At this stage the mind is open to and tends to record all impressions and make associations between anything and everything that occurs. For instance, until around 10 months of age the infant is able to hear and respond to the sound distinctions made in any language (Cole, 2001; Gopnik, Meltzoff, & Kuhl, 1999).

In infancy, the rich jumble of sensory experiences does not allow meaningful distinctions until the child learns to associate repeated perceptions and connect these into basic structures of cultural experience, while not retaining chance associations among experiences. Important childhood experiences are those that come in patterned associations that involve multiple senses in consistent ways; these patterned associations are the basic experiences of culture and establish the expectations and connections that make the world meaningful. For instance, repeated instances of parental speech become associated with certain actions; the child begins by recognizing such associated words and actions, and then gradually develops the ability to produce either words or actions to make or respond to requests.

After the extreme malleability of early childhood in which such cultural patterns become deeply rooted in the brain, at around age 6 or 7 the child's mind starts to reduce the number of synaptic connections among neurons in a process known as synaptic pruning. Only the synaptic connections that are reinforced by experience will remain active to provide associations and interpretations for the child. The more frequently experiences occur together, the more strongly the child will tend to associate them and expect one when experiencing the other (Bownds, 1999). Such linked experiences can be sequential patterns of action; linking words with objects; recognizing people by their voice, scent, appearance, or characteristic actions; linking the appearance of a food to its taste, and so on. New associations will also be formed and if reinforced can enter into the accumulated cultural understandings and behaviors. The pruning process does not impede new learning, although much that is learned in adolescence and beyond relies on physical and cognitive skills encoded in the earliest synaptic patterns. More diverse and complex early learned experiences provide more resources for the child to continue to acquire new understandings and skills in the world. Diverse sensory and physical experiences both lead directly to increased abilities to cope with cultural processes. Patterns of experiences also lead to the ability to retain conscious memories. Memories of events and objects are not retained perfectly over time, but are reconstructed during recall according to scripts or patterns of expected experience (Schacter, 2001).

Pruning is essential to effective learning: The brain has to reduce the complexity of connections until those that are reinforced by experience are the most easily accessible and useful associations. Without such pruning the brain becomes burdened with ambiguous and uncertain associations that interfere with effective cognition.

Neurobiology Facilitates Childhood Cultural Learning

Throughout adolescence, increasing biological constraints on cognitive flexibility make it more and more difficult for a child to become fully competent in all aspects of a new culture. One's childhood culture becomes the central structure of one's ways of thinking for neurological reasons: The mind permanently retains particular associations and knowledge. Emotions, ideas, and physical actions become neurologically set patterns that will remain important no matter what new cultural experiences one may learn from in later life. For example, in later life it becomes very difficult to learn a new language without retaining an accent that is based in the neurologically encoded pronunciations of one's native language, whereas learning a new language in early adolescence or before generally leads to native competence with essentially perfect pronunciation.

Culture Is Learned Through the Body

Culture consists of far more than verbal skills and practices that can be learned through words. Because most culture is learned through associations, it becomes hard-wired as part of cognitive skills, and difficult to explain or communicate outside of particular social environments. Early bodily experiences are obvious examples of this: Caregivers teach infants and young children not only how to eat and walk, but also how to regulate breathing and sleeping, how to clean themselves, sit, and so on. In fact, one of the most important learning experiences of early childhood is that all such activities are not solitary and individual, but ways that the person participates in and communicates with a community. Even later in life, personal care remains linked with social concerns, and bodily activities continue to have social meanings.

Many cultural skills are acquired more through bodily experience than by observation and explanation. Physical skills have to be acquired in activity, and in fact language itself cannot be learned through descriptive instruction, but has to be learned by example and use. Children with limited physical experiences of certain activities will learn them more slowly; for example, in U.S. society girls are often encouraged to be less physically competitive and therefore develop less of the confidence and motivation necessary to do well in some sports (Klomsten et al., 2004; Krombholz, 1997). Likewise, people who have not grown up riding in automobiles often take longer to learn the basic skills of driving because they have not internalized as children the physical experiences of smooth and effective clutching, accelerating, steering, and braking. The integration of such bodily experiences into one's sense of proper movement makes it easier to develop skills that produce the remembered patterns: A bodily sense of what one should feel when driving helps one regulate the vehicle's movement more readily.

Culture Shapes the Mind

In addition to somatic (bodily) culture, a child will also learn cognitive concepts and patterns of emotional responses and expressions that conform to cultural expectations. Concepts about time, food, dirt, clothing, physical affection, and so on, all become part of the nonverbal systems of feeling, order, and communication that have deep effects on how one responds in social situations. Most people are unable to learn to like foods that they have been taught from childhood are unpleasant or taboo; for example, although popular in many parts of the world, in most of U.S. society the idea of eating insects provokes strong distaste. This results from learned culture rather than anything intrinsic to insects (Douglas, 1966; Haidt et al., 1997).

Emotional responses and ideas vary widely from culture to culture. Systems of concepts about the relationship between self and society create and shape feelings of shame, anger, stress, love, desire, and so on. Emotions are extremely complex, and the study of cultural concepts of emotions and mental processes more generally has grown into a field known as *ethnopsychology* (Lutz, 1988). This field of cultural anthropology and cultural psychology has become highly relevant to health care because ethnopsychologists provide insights into *culture-bound syndromes* that arise when emotional and psychological states correlate with behavioral disorders that interfere with normal social life. Ethnopsychologists have extensively investigated the culture-bound syndrome of *nervios* found in Latin American cultures (Baer et al., 2003). Their research has helped refine understanding of such psychological conditions, and they are now included within the DSM IV diagnostic categories (Balick & Lee, 2003; Guarnaccia & Rogler, 1999). Because these conditions are understood in culturally specific ways, it is vital to understand the cultural framework in order to develop diagnoses and treatments (Pineros, Rosselli, & Calderon, 1998). The study of eating disorders has also revealed culture-bound aspects, and shows that ethnopsychological research can usefully supplement the conventional psychiatric categories and concepts applied in treating dominant culture conditions in the United States (Keel & Klump, 2003).

People Create Culture, Culture Creates People

Without interacting and communicating with other people in a mean-ingful social world, human children will not develop many basic capac-ities. A baby's mind will not become human without early social experiences. The biological potential for cognition has to be systemati-cally stimulated by other people before a baby can aquire basic commu-nicative competence, and yet as the examples of Helen Keller and children like her show, this stimulation need not be visual or auditory. The mind develops through interactive sensory experience with other people, especially caregivers, and if this stimulation does not occur in early childhood, the child has permanent limits to cultural competence because her mind is incapable of making social and cultural sense beyond a limited range (Skuse, 1988).

Cognitive abilities exist along a continuum, however; some require early social experience to develop at all, whereas others can be learned or relearned even after long atrophy. A recent study of visual processing in a man who lost his eyesight at age 3 and regained it surgically at age 43 showed that he could relearn to visually track objects and even catch them, but had irretrievably lost the ability to recognize faces. The most likely interpretation is that the object tracking skill was learned prior to age 3 and the ability remained potentiated in his brain, whereas recog-nition skills had not been as deeply learned by age 3, or depended on more extensive cultural reinforcement to prevent permanent atrophy (Fine et al., 2003; Johnson, 2001).

Cultures Are Highly Integrated

Cultural learning relies heavily on making systematic links among dif-ferent aspects of life and building logical models that connect these dif-ferent experiences. Because people who learn cultural patterns are themselves discovering and then reproducing them, culture becomes richly linked into networks of reinforcing conceptual patterns.

Without certain basic experiences within a social group—especially as a child—it may be difficult for someone to fully understand social inter-action. Because a person grows to understand relationships in the larger society from those he knows at home and within the fairly close com-munity of childhood, it is difficult to have the same integrated and spon-taneous sense of how social life works when some of the interpersonal patterns are unfamiliar.

For example, some widespread American caregiving behaviors are learned very early and have a strong emotional component. Children will extend these practices for use both in play and to provide comfort in a variety of situations that do not involve pain or injury. A child may consider kisses, ice, bandages, and comforting words to be important remedies for any accident, regardless of their symptoms, or they may use them with stuffed animals that cannot feel pain. Even further, these practices then establish expectations for kinds of treatment in later life: Both social attention to the feelings and physical attention to the injury will be expected as part of the caring process. The child's easy extension of such models from one situation to another leads to cultural integration because the patterns can be identified in many contexts, and children without the same practices will have different expectations about care for injuries.

Cultural Richness and Breadth Develop Through Creative Modeling and Metaphors

Throughout childhood, the child continues to learn new associations, making richer networks of connections among experiences. Humans are particularly skilled at making creative transfers from one domain of experience to another by using imitation, pretend play, and metaphorical comparisons to develop models. These models are tools to understand patterns in the world, and most develop subconsciously. There is usually no conscious "Aha!" moment when a child discovers the useful similarities between "adjusting" a radio volume control, a faucet, or a thermostat (Kempton, 1986).

Children in most societies learn through imitative play, but they are less concerned with exact imitation than with experimenting with models for manipulating the world. The malleability of the child's mind is reflected in the ease of their creative leaps from one domain to another. They are skilled at imagining an object or action as something very different. A more complex form of imaginative imitation comes when a child learns to understand a pattern of behavior or a personality in terms of a very different one; for instance, a child may learn that she can think of herself as one animal or another and take on the behaviors of that animal in play (Kahn, 1997; Tambiah, 1969).

This extension of experience from one area to another in the form of models is one way that cultures become integrated wholes. But cultural integration through imposing order and sense on the world also distorts experience. Cultural models and patterns make it difficult to observe reality without making it conform to expectations. In addition to helping understand new situations, imagination also organizes experience in ways that make more sense and are easier to recall and retain; new experiences are readily shaped to conform to known patterns or *cultural models*. The mind can reinterpret and distort experience to rationalize it and make it logical according to these cultural understandings (Schacter, 2001).

For example, in U.S. society the cultural model of property rights has been progressively extended from concepts about the autonomy of the person and his or her rights over concrete possessions and land in medieval times, to ideas about personal rights to controlling one's time, one's words, one's ideas, one's image, and so on. Such concepts are formalized in economic and legal contexts, and have become informal elements of negotiated exchange within interactions among family and friends in many U.S. communities. Many tribal societies, however, have very different ideas about personal autonomy and property rights within the family and community. The idea of exclusive ownership rights to objects and land is often incomprehensible, or at least causes great tension in such communities because sharing is expected or even obligatory, and private property rights are often only relevant in relations with strangers. In many societies the idea of denying people the use of land or withholding food or medicine from people because they lack money are highly contested innovations that arise from participating in market economies (Scott, 1985). Americans tend to extend these cultural models from everyday economic life to many personal relationships, and they are generally highly skilled in measuring the equivalent value of action, time, and object. Likewise, the idea of individual private property has become the foundation for ideas about collectively "owned" national territory, history, and culture in the system of modern nation-states; cultural integration results from such extensions of similar ideas to many different kinds of social contexts.

Culture Is Shared, But Not Fully

Although cultural integration results in widely shared expectations and understandings, culture is learned through many differing personal experiences, so not everyone in a social group shares the same culture. People have different experiences even in the same family, and in combination with variations in personal preferences, biochemistry, and differently created cognitive models, these generate widely varying individual tastes and abilities. This can be described as personal culture: the preferences, associations, ideas, and practices that individuals develop through the course of their lives. Much of personal culture arises in domains that are culturally defined and socially accepted as allowing room for expression of personal preferences. For instance, although it is considered usual in the United States for people to express a preference for coffee, tea, soft drinks, or—in the proper contexts—alcoholic drinks, members of the dominant culture do not often ask for hot water or roasted barley tea to drink. Preferences usually remain within areas of shared expectations or risk being ignored or misunderstood.

On the other hand, every group within a given culture develops its own shared experience and understandings, and if the group remains together over time, such as members of a workplace or school, they will develop shared cultural understandings that are not understood by the larger society. Such a group creates its own culture and institutional knowledge, and will use insider jargon in some of their communication. This can also happen with a group that shares identity features and experiences such as in a religious, gender, ethnic, or family group. Many aspects of sociocultural diversity are not necessarily inherited as different traditions, but develop among people who feel an in-group sense of belonging with each other, and thus develop shared cultural knowledge and patterns.

Culture and Its Symbols and Conventions Are Largely Unconscious

Because much cultural knowledge develops outside of conscious memory, people are never fully conscious of all the ways culture shapes their feelings and behavior. For example, when using language, people may understand that the association of a word and its meaning are arbitrary conventions within a society, but that does not help them use the language. In fact, it gets in the way if a person stops to make a conscious link between the word *dog* and the mental image of a dog, or more complexly, if she tries to figure out what "or" means in a concrete way. A word like *or,* which helps organize meanings but has no independent meaning, can only be understood as a way of thinking about the relationship between the two adjacent concepts.

Children learn symbolic culture such as language by acquiring the associations that they experience. Children may not use words in ways that parents expect, but they learn the associations they are exposed to. Words are tools, and the more expert one is with them, the less one thinks about how to use them and the more one gets done. Culture provides the tools for social life, and one learns to use most of these tools without conscious thought. In addition to tools of expression, cultural learning involves acquiring the physical skills, cultural knowledge, expectations, and assumptions that enable effective and meaningful social life. People speaking their native language do not have to consciously understand grammar to speak effectively, nor concentrate on balance when walking. These are learned in childhood and become part of the invisible background of life. The less concentration an activity demands the more likely that it will be a convenient and useful way to get something done. Only when cultural patterns do not have the expected consequences do people have to consciously focus on what is going on. For example, when people step onto slippery ice they have to concentrate on changing their gait, and when someone says "Hi Bob" to me and that is not my name, I have to rethink what is going on, and rapidly examine alternative interpretations. I quickly run through and test the alternatives: Either the person has forgotten my name, thinks I am someone else, is speaking to someone else behind me, or, these days, is talking on a hands-free cellphone that I have not noticed. My unconscious cultural models for interpersonal situations help me rapidly resolve and correct my misunderstanding of the situation.

Cultural Patterns Have Strong Emotional Meanings

Because culture begins to be learned within the most important relationships of a person's life, basic cultural patterns are strongly linked to emotions. If one's parents are associated with comfort and security, then the kinds of caregiving, food, and ways of talking they provide will be associated with feelings of comfort and security. Furthermore, familiarity and comprehensibility are extremely important to emotional well-being. When a person cannot make sense of the world around him, and does not know what to expect in a situation, he will experience confusion and anxiety.

This is the source of the psychological condition known as culture shock. When many of a person's experiences do not fit familiar patterns and expectations, there is a tendency to withdraw psychologically due to a feeling of loss of control. The sense-making skills that serve one so well in one's native culture are constantly challenged when living among people who do not share that cultural background, so communication does not work, one does not know what patterns of behavior are expected, and so on (Ward, Bochner, & Furnham, 2001).

Table 5–1 shows some relationships among the categories, skills, affective values, ideas and meanings, and models within some common cultural domains in U.S. dominant culture. Examining this list should make clear how complicated the interactions, in all social contexts, are among cultural categories, settings, skills, concepts, emotional responses, and symbolic meanings.

Explained Culture Is Harder to Learn Than Experienced Culture

Attempts to explain cultural rules, patterns, and expectations are often ineffective because children are attuned to learning through practice during their period of greatest cognitive flexibility. For example, the child acquires a complex set of caring practices through direct association that would be far harder to understand and apply if explained verbally. Similarly, riding a bike or playing baseball require physical practice. In fact, even overt correction of a child's language has very little effect on how he speaks: culture is learned by doing. Providing the correct grammatical form and insisting on its repetition will have little effect on a child's language acquisition because they do not think consciously about putting ideas or feelings into words.

The integration of culture allows children to learn to manage many different domains simultaneously, and in fact—just as with caring for injuries—they overextend or overgeneralize most of the techniques they learn when they first learn them. For instance, in learning language, children who master the making of plurals or past tense in English will impose the same rule even on irregular forms and talk about "mouses" or "deers" or say "he runned fast." Likewise, young children will apply narrow terms to broader categories, describing a man as "a daddy" and a woman as "a mommy" regardless of reproductive status. Children do not have to learn each example separately because of their great ability to generalize from a few examples or models to many similar situations. Their difficulty comes when they must learn from experience when not to generalize (Foster, 1990).

On the other hand, adults have similar difficulties learning from explanation, but rely on it more because they have lost much of the cognitive malleability that enables experiential learning to work so well in the child. Adult and adolescent learners are aided by their repertoires of existing skills, routines, and patterns that they can build upon, and they have a more conscious grasp of techniques of bodily and mental rehearsal. Nonetheless, because much adult learning relies on conscious remembering it is far more fallible and inefficient than the child's rapid subconscious acquisition of new information and ideas as integral parts of social activity.

Cultures Involve All-Encompassing Models That Give a Sense of Control

Culture shapes a person's emotions, cognition, beliefs, communication, skills, and understanding of self, society, and the relationship between them. Because culture is a part of all learning and communication, all understandings of the world are shaped by culture. This shaping includes ideas about logic, reasonableness, and validity that make it difficult to be objective and scientific. The world is culturally constructed. When coming up with new interpretations, those that bring on cognitive dissonance are avoided. Values and beliefs override experience because experience always has to be interpreted creatively, so people tend to interpret it to fit with what they already know.

Integrated cultural skills facilitate transfer from one domain to another, but they also make it easy to distort reality. Sociocultural conventions impose systematic order on lived bodily experience. For instance, most people have some health practices that are effective for subjective reasons. By regulating body and environment according to models, a person experiences a sense of enhanced health by controlling some of the uncertainties that

Table 5–1   Relationships Among Various Factors Within American Culture

Cultural Domains	Categories and Objects	Practices and Skills	Learning and Interaction Contexts	Affective Value	Meanings and Values	Concepts, Models, and Metaphors
Food	Fruits Vegetables Meats Grains Nuts	Gathering Shopping Preparation Cleaning Cooking	Learned informally in family and other social groups As part of self-care	High	Flavor Hunger Satiation Preferences Taboos	Food as shared social resource, ritual practice, and bodily fuel
Drink	Water Milk Juices Caffeinated Carbonated Alcoholic	Selection Preparation Rehydration Nourishment	Learned informally in family and other social groups As part of self-care	Moderate	Thirst Health Revival Intoxication	Drink to replenish body fluids, provide nutrients, or modify mental state
Clothing	Shirt Pants Dress Underwear Footwear	Dressing Shopping Washing Sewing	Learned informally Privately chosen Public presentation	High to moderate	Comfort Concealment Attractiveness Shame	"Clothes make person" Create and display identity and self-image
Motion and Transport	Walking Bicycling Driving	Balance Attention Signaling	Learned informally Mobility to reach social events	Moderate	Space Access Independence	"Watch your step" "Look before you leap" "Watch the road"
Games and Sports	Cards Dice Ball Skates Skis Swimming pool	Bidding Strategizing Calling plays Dribbling Shooting Swim strokes	Learned informally and formally Nonserious competition Public events and entertainment	Moderate	Fairness Shared enjoyment	"Team player" "Good sport" "eyes on the prize" Game tokens as proxies for people
Art	Tune Song Dance Poem Portrait	Singing Composition Performance Drawing Painting	Informal Formal Public audiences and events Recordings	Moderate	Emotional mastery Beauty Pleasure Expression Creativity Invention	"Follow your muse" "Art for art's sake" "1% inspiration and 99% perspiration"
Shelter and Built Environment	House Factory Office Roadway Waterway Utility	Creating home Cleaning Architecture Engineering Carpentry Excavation	Informal Formal On-the-job Living space Workplace Infrastructure	Moderate	Solidity Strength Protection from elements Usefulness Prestige Beauty	"Make a house a home" Decorating and landscaping Design for use

Table 5–1 Relationships Among Various Factors Within American Culture (*continued*)

Cultural Domains	Categories and Objects	Practices and Skills	Learning and Interaction Contexts	Affective Value	Meanings and Values	Concepts, Models, and Metaphors
Kinship	Parents Siblings Children Cousins In-laws	Caregiving Obedience Communication Sharing Cooperation Interdependence	Informal Family	Very high	Love Descent Inheritance Identity	"The apple doesn't fall far from the tree" "Be a credit to the family"
Health	Body Mind Injury Disease	Visiting Cleaning Exercising Caregiving Bandaging Medicating	Informal Formal Family Clinical settings	High	Treatment Pain relief Etiologies Healing Curing	"Sound body, sound mind" Wholeness Possessing one's faculties
Religion and Belief	Amulet Holy water Sign of the cross Scripture Zodiac signs	Magic Prophecy Divination Prayer Baptism Horoscope	Informal Formal Family Church Group rituals	High to moderate	Faith Respect Submission Retribution	The unseen controls the seen Everything happens for a reason
Economy	Profession Job Store Bank Money Property	Bargaining Shopping Saving Working Efficiency Paying taxes	Informal Formal Public markets Workplaces	Moderate	Honesty Diligence	"Time is money" "Watch your money" "Don't sell yourself short"
Nation	Flag Anthem Citizen Passport Immigrant Noncitizen Territory	Patriotism Defense Social Security	Formal	Moderate	History Solidarity Shared Reciprocal Interdependent	"American as apple pie" Bald Eagle
Politics	Vote Legislate Speech	Arguing Judgment Persuasion Policy making	Informal Media Public events	Moderate to weak	Honest Effective Trust Represent	Education Freedom Independence Democracy Human Rights

surround health. Awareness of objective experience is hard to achieve because culture gives people shared ways to conceive the world, and experiences that do not fit are readily ignored or explained away.

Because all people are quite capable of ignoring things that contradict their understandings, and inventing interpretations that reinforce the comfort and sense of control they derive from their cultural models, the extreme skepticism of science has become an important tool for overcoming the tendency to distort or misinterpret reality.

Tradition and Innovation in Culture Support Transcultural Communication

Culture is acquired through learning meaningful patterns among associated experiences and behaviors. Because each person creates his or her own associations and understandings, culture does not exist separately from the work of individuals to learn it. Culture is not a fixed set of unchanging practices or beliefs passed as a whole from parent to child, but part of the the ongoing process of making sense of the world. Cultural innovation makes transcultural communication possible.

In culture contact situations, new cultural forms emerge that help people deal with cultural difference. Understanding cultural differences depends on cultural values and cultural practices that facilitate such understanding. Transcultural understanding—like all interpersonal understanding—requires creative work and has to be nurtured. In most of the world, cultural values that stress hospitality, aid, and respect for others provide the foundation for creating tolerance and mutual understanding. When people do not show respect and hospitality towards others, they communicate less and create fewer of the shared understandings that facilitate tolerance.

Despite the widely varying lifeways and worldviews learned in sociocultural groups, because humans are creative they can invent new ideas and ways of communicating. People can creatively accomplish understanding, but only if they create the conditions for such understanding. The essential element is the will to understand, because when someone wants to understand and tries to understand, she calls upon her ability to creatively respond to others, and creative response creates meaningful associations. Each person can learn how others experience the world. Cultural creativity is regulated by cultural concepts and practices, just as values about respect and hospitality regulate contact.

APPLYING TRANSCULTURAL UNDERSTANDING IN FORENSIC NURSING

Although nursing science has developed a fairly comprehensive understanding of how to deliver nursing care when working with socioculturally diverse populations (Leininger & McFarland, 2002), the special concerns of forensic nurses have been far less carefully researched with respect to sociocultural diversity. We need a much more detailed understanding of cultural ideas about violence and culturally shaped responses to physically and mentally traumatic experience. This section will develop a discussion of the major issues within forensic nursing, as they relate both to health practices and cultural care and to dealing with trauma and violence.

Health Practices Within Cultural Life

Cultural health practices are complex and ubiquitous, and because they are only partially explained discursively, they are subconscious to a significant degree. Most discussions of health practices in a particular culture focus on those that are consciously recognized by participants in that culture, while the importance of other practices remains unrecognized until *cultural pain* and careful exploration of the issue bring out the underlying expectations that lead to the discomfort (Leininger, 1997).

From conception and pregnancy through birth, postnatal care, and throughout life, human existence in all cultures is guided by health concepts and practices. These include techniques for maintaining physical and mental health, preventing injury and disease, and restoring bodily and mental functioning when they are disrupted. Diet, movement, rest, body manipulation, cleanliness, security, warmth, and contamination avoidance are all part of daily health practices that are learned during childhood. Around the world people have widely varying beliefs about even simple substances such as air and water: Some people see night air as dangerous, others make sure they have adequate ventilation when they sleep; some people believe in daily washing, whereas others, such as Tibetan nomads, associate water washing with potential illness. Most Han Chinese avoid cold water and other cold drinks as potential sources of illness. Some Muslims in Central Asia believe that running water is pure and will not drink from bodies of standing water. Historically, people in Europe believed moonlight could cause mental illness, while in China the moon was valued as a reminder of distant loved ones, and in Persia it became a metaphor for great beauty.

Some of these beliefs have a certain validity—boiled water will not transmit intestinal illnesses and washing in cold water at the high altitudes where Tibetans live can be a threat to health—but the strongest motivation for these and many other beliefs is that maintaining consistent cultural practices helps maintain a sense of control and familiarity within life, and when such practices are changed uneasiness and cultural discomfort often result.

Since these practices start at the beginning of life, they are deeply embedded within understandings of a proper and balanced life, and it is difficult to separate health maintenance from food ways, bodily practices, and ideas about purity and contamination, which often include supernatural components. Most culturally shaped activities involve elements that can be felt to injure health if not conducted properly. Sociocultural health practices also include the processes of learning and maturation that are felt to create the properly adjusted and developed adult.

Health Practices and Nursing Communication

As mentioned earlier, the most important way to explore differing health practices and their effects on personal comfort and needs for care is through communication. The first goal of a nurse should be to facilitate communication concerning the client's emotional state and concerns, because this will usually reveal the earliest evidence of discomfort. Communication is very important in nursing, and every effort should be made to determine how to improve it. This includes assessing linguistic skills in English and in other languages, finding family or friends who can help a client communicate and help support the client in raising issues that he or she is reluctant or embarrassed to discuss, and finally, exploring what aspects of the clinical setting, activities, and personnel cause concern to the client.

Once effective means of communication have been established, the nurse should explore with the client any cultural discomforts he or she is experiencing, and attempt to identify their sources. As mentioned earlier, many aspects of cultural care are not consciously recognized but will affect how someone feels about the care they are receiving in the clinical context. In order to adequately support the client's needs, open-ended exploration of sources of vague discomfort or unease will help them to describe and understand how their cultural expectations are being thwarted (American Medical Association, 1999; Galanti, 1997; Luckmann, 1999).

A number of issues should be kept in mind in transcultural communication. First, recognize that ways of speaking to clients readily convey attitudes and prejudices. Because healthcare workers have the authority of institutionalized medical practices, they often establish power relationships through hierarchical modes of communication. Styles of speech that condescend to a client, especially minorities, women, and children, can effectively close off communication (Waitzkin et al., 1996).

Just as derogatory stereotypes and condescending attitudes have to be avoided to promote open communication, so too do ethnocentric and nationalist assumptions about history and tradition. The common identification of Mexicans as immigrants to the United States reveals a gap in many Americans' historical understanding: At the end of the U.S. Mexican War in 1848, Mexico ceded California, Arizona, New Mexico, Texas, and parts of Colorado, Nevada, and Utah, to the United States. Mexicans living in these areas became American citizens but were then confronted with violence, discriminatory voting laws, and fraudulent treatment that pushed them off their land. In the Southwest the border moved, not the Mexicans. Obviously, assuming that a Mexican has immigrated might only serve to remind her of the discrimination and ignorance perpetuated by some non-Mexicans in the United States.

Transcultural Nursing

The concepts and practices of transcultural nursing are widely used, but often in ways that imply that some nursing is not transcultural. In fact, all nursing should be seen as transcultural to the extent that the client is not a part of the healthcare community, and thus only partially shares the knowledge, expectations, and ways of thinking that are shared among medical personnel. When a patient from the dominant culture receives health care, the transcultural dimension remains largely unnoticed because healthcare workers accommodate dominant cultural expectations.

For instance, although nurses and doctors understand the biological differences between viral, bacterial, fungal, and parasitic infections, they do not expect the general public to make such clear distinctions, and they make allowances for this lack of understanding when they explain why an antibacterial drug is useless or even harmful in treating a viral or fungal infection. Likewise, although personal sanitation in the dominant culture of the United States involves certain shared concepts and practices—such as the germ theory of disease and the use of soap and disinfectants to control germs—the in-patient sanitation procedures in a hospital require additional explanation. These procedures are not part of the dominant culture's understanding, so they must be learned in order to participate properly as a patient in the hospital community. But the same courtesy is not automatically extended to people who do not bring dominant culture expectations with them when they arrive for health care. In such cases, nurses have to make sure that dominant culture assumptions about care are not getting in the way of proper treatment or causing cultural discomfort.

To perform the social role expected of a patient in a hospital, he or she acquires specialized knowledge from nurses and doctors, just as nurses and doctors acquire specialized knowledge to fulfill their roles. The patient goes through a necessarily transcultural socialization process when entering a hospital, although if caregivers assume that a patient shares their dominant cultural background, they will only explain how the hospital context differs from other dominant culture contexts, and resist seeing that this is a transcultural interaction. Because all patients are potentially new to the culture of the clinical context they have just entered, transcultural nursing is an integral part of explaining and carrying out healthcare procedures in cooperation with the patient. Communicating and explaining carefully are very important, and the patient's level of understanding must be closely monitored.

Assumptions should always be made overt and tested so they do not cause misunderstandings.

Cultural Pain Interferes with Communication

Culture helps people maintain meaningful and orderly social relations through shared understandings and expectations. When one person's social expectations and communicative practices do not conform to those of another, mutual avoidance may result because each feels that the other is a source of disorder. The only way to overcome the sense of alienation or unease someone feels when confronting the unexpected is to become aware of cultural sources of discomfort and to communicate about them. Nurses have to help people recognize when they are experiencing cultural discomfort, or what Margaret Leininger calls cultural pain (1997; 2002, p. 52), and understand ways to both cope with and reduce it. Coping with the unease resulting from differing cultural expectations can be particularly difficult in institutional contexts where one person has a lower status and is less respected, and thus has difficulty being heard when attempting to communicate about cultural discomfort. When an authority figure such as a nurse, doctor, or police officer assumes that their practices are not merely culturally distinct, but somehow more rational or moral, coping with cultural miscommunication becomes even more difficult.

Reducing Cultural Pain and Communication Barriers by Understanding Diversity

Properly understanding what sociocultural diversity means for healthcare practitioners is complex, and cannot be reduced to contrasts between the dominant culture and minority cultures. In fact, every person is a member of multiple cultures because ethnic and racial groups do not define the totality of cultural and social experiences. All people participate in a number of groups, from family and friends to local communities, to schools and places of work. Those people develop shared identities based on work, play, skill, age, handicap, sexual preference, participation in social organizations, and so forth.

A useful way to understand sociocultural diversity is to think of each individual as a member of multiple partially overlapping groups, as in Figure 5–1. Because most social groups that shape someone's identity consist of people who spend time together and have experiences in common, they develop shared cultural understandings and expectations. Communicative interaction and shared experience are the basis for any cultural sharing. Different sociocultural contexts have different emotional values for participants, and people usually become more attached to and deeply rooted and comfortable in culture learned within their family and community, and often less attached to the culture of their schools or workplaces, which are less encompassing experiences.

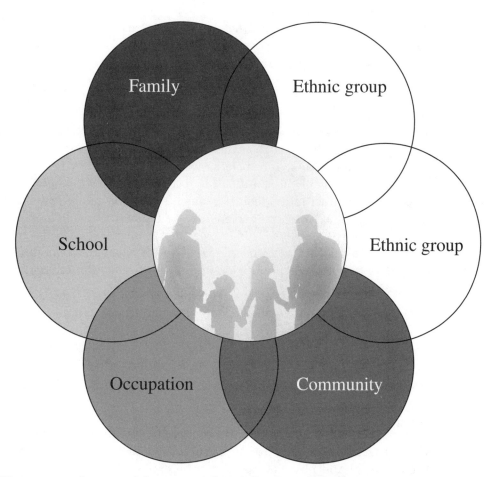

Figure 5–1 Some social contexts of socialization; through interactive participation the individual develops personal identity and culture.

Although a person's identity is often reduced to social categories known to sociologists as master statuses, such as ethnicity, race, age, or gender, human identities are complex products of experience in and affiliation with multiple communities and social contexts. Social scientists now recognize that identities are situational and strategic, and people can define themselves differently in different contexts by using relevant aspects of their background: In one situation someone may identify himself as African American, while in another he may say he is a New Yorker, and in yet another he may identify himself as a Red Sox fan. The identity someone chooses as salient in a social context depends on how he wants to be perceived, what he is there for, and what he wants to accomplish at any given moment. Very few people live within a single ethnic, class, or occupational identity without creating more differentiated and individualized identities within their families and among groups of friends or coworkers.

Nonetheless, most of us know that people assign us to groups by behavior, clothes, skin color, or language before they even know us, and make guesses about our background, lifestyle, economic status, and so on from this flimsy evidence. Such labels become part of our experience and we come to share more with people in the same ascriptive category, regardless of what we share in terms of other experience, simply because we are treated similarly in society. Obviously, such treatment can be negative and discriminatory, such as that often experienced by racial, ethnic, or sexual minorities, or lower-status workers. The underlying motivation is understandable: It is difficult to recognize and get to know every person as a distinct individual. It is much simpler to reduce the many dimensions of experience, personality, and identity to obvious and socially salient categories. This is particularly the case when the relationship one has with other people is the result of occupational duties. People try to limit and simplify job responsibilities by creating routines and categories.

When nurses or other healthcare workers feel they can assign people to particular categories, they may feel this increases their control and efficiency in clinical relationships. The risk is that such categories become self-fulfilling prophecies, as stereotypes fill in for real knowledge about a client gained through communicative interaction. Understanding people requires that they be seen as complexly connected to multiple groups and multiple intersecting sets of cultural experiences and beliefs. External markers should not be allowed to serve as indicators of identity or cultural patterns. Each patient has to be approached as an individual whose social and physical reality can be explored only through open communication.

Racial Categories Are Socially Constructed

As most students should already recognize, race is not a valid category within biological science, because it has no consistent genetic meaning. Race imagined as a biological category has no place in medical physiology and epidemiology (Cooper & David, 1986). The much vaunted associations between race and conditions such as sickle-cell anemia only work when race is used as a shorthand for assessing population genetics. Statistically in the United States many African Americans have West African ancestors and are thus somewhat more likely to have the sickle-cell trait. But West African ancestry is the genetic reason, and has no consistent expression in body type or skin color. Many people with West African ancestry are identified socially in the United States as white, and many people without West African ancestry are identified as black (including East Africans, South Africans, South Asians, and Pacific Islanders). In addition, the sickle-cell trait is found in other population groups from other parts of the world without recent genetic connections to West Africa (Cavalli-Sforza, Menozzi, & Piazza, 1994).

All human groups have widely ranging traits and have to be diagnosed according to standard procedures, not guesses about genetic background. Race is a social category defined according to cultural principles. Often in the United States, the principle of hypodescent—a social "rule," whereby children of a union between members of different socioeconomic groups are automatically placed into a less-privileged category—causes people to be identified as members of a non-white race when they are known to have any ancestor from that group (Harris, 1974). This illustrates that the genetic significance of socially-defined race is very limited.

Even the argument that race can be used as a proxy measure that stands in for cultural and social factors that affect health leads to careless assumptions because of the enormous range of cultural and social experience: Asian American, African American, or Native American experiences and lifestyles vary widely from place to place and depend upon income, urban or rural living, and geographic origins. Except for the very broadest statistical generalizations, racial categories are not useful in medicine. Instead, more precise characterizations of sociocultural and genetic groups should be used when attempting to construct groups for statistical study (Ikemoto, 1997; Krieger & Fee, 1994). When this is done, it is possible to make useful correlations among sociocultural background, culturally shaped health practices and ideas, and environmentally influenced health patterns. Otherwise, the genetic, environmental, cultural, and individual patterns cannot be usefully disentangled, and attempted generalizations based on race or sociocultural experience risk leading to prejudice and discrimination.

Prejudice and Discrimination

Racial attributions and ideas do affect treatment of people within hospital, court, school, and other public contexts. Although biological functioning and cultural behavior have no firm correlation with socially defined categories such as race, racism and discrimination do influence health. When someone's perceived racial identity affects how others treat them in social life or in clinical contexts, this may affect their health and the outcomes of medical care (Barbee, 1993). Similar effects result from the differing treatment people encounter because of their ethnicity, gender, sexual identity, age, or handicaps.

The Vega Model offers great insight into the workings of racism and discrimination in American society (Martin, 1992; Vega, 1978). The Vega Model describes the intersection of three dimensions of social relations: 1) cultural bias, 2) personal prejudice, and 3) institutional discrimination. In order to accurately understand how institutions discriminate one must understand how cultural biases shape images of people who belong to recognized social groups. Cultural bias can arise from any representations or ascriptions of particular behaviors and abilities to people because of their social identity. When such images become widespread, a cultural bias emerges that leads to personal prejudice.

For instance, if I hear from people I know or from media reports that Gypsies are involved in various petty crimes and I never know any Gypsies (properly known as Rom) from personal social experience—outside of institutional contexts that perpetuate biased interactions—I may form broad prejudices linking them to criminal activities. Rather than recognizing that rumor, media stereotypes, and outsider perspectives have biased my ideas about Gypsies, such ideas will replace the ignorance that I would otherwise have to acknowledge. Most people do not question their received cultural biases and hearsay "knowledge," but often rely upon it and end up discriminating against people that they know nothing about.

To avoid contributing to institutional discrimination, each individual must vigorously question the cultural biases that they are exposed to. Cultural biases are widespread and individuals cannot avoid being exposed to them, but people can prevent themselves from acting upon them or perpetuating their circulation. Individuals within an institution who carry out its policies and procedures should recognize that institutional discrimination remains potent in many contexts because people have failed to take responsibility for changing the ways that cultural bias, prejudice, and discrimination reinforce each other.

Examples of cultural biases that lead to prejudice and institutional discrimination are easily found: The witch trials in colonial New England and the Inquisition in Europe both resulted from Christian cultural biases about non-Christian religious practices that were interpreted as being evidence for dealings with Satan. The dominant cultural model provided biased interpretations of all non-Christian and heterodox religious activities as satanic practices, and the practitioners were punished and even executed, although they themselves explained that their beliefs and practices had nothing to do with Satan and were for the good of their community. Because of cultural bias, only the dominant official culture model of caring for a community's spiritual health were accepted, and practitioners of minority beliefs were harshly discriminated against and suppressed (Ginzburg, 1983).

Such witchcraft trials are not as far off as one might imagine: In the 1980s and early 1990s in the United States, Britain, and Australia a panic about satanic ritual abuse led to widespread mobilization of legal and psychological professionals against the perceived threat of a worldwide network of satanic cult members systematically attacking children. Despite the fact that there was never evidence for such a network, and many of the events were testified about by witnesses who had been coached by "experts" or were the work of teenagers using imagery borrowed from rock lyrics, hundreds of people were accused and many brought to trial. The mobilization against this supposed plague included many counselors, consultants, and police advisors who created a systematic cultural model of satanic rituals. Because they persuaded people these practices were ubiquitous, evidence was easy to bring together into the narrative they created: rock lyrics, kids' pranks on Halloween, communal lifestyles, and the practices of followers of beliefs such as Wicca and Santería were no longer seen as separate events, but as integral parts of a systematic satanic religion. The following quotes from two news stories show how easily law enforcement jumped from identifying a minority group to accusing them of satanic ritual abuse of children:

> Six unidentified children taken from two men believed to be members of a satanic cult were moved from a shelter when officials there received threatening phone calls, police said Saturday. The cult, known as the Finders, may have been accustomed to selling or smuggling its members' children out of the country, a police spokesman said. (Birk, 1987a)

Six days later, the police retreated from their accusations based in the cultural model of satanic ritual abuse:

> In a week's time, official descriptions of a secretive group called the Finders have softened from an animal-sacrificing satanic cult that might have trafficked in children to a 1960s-style commune. . . . [P]hotographs had been found on Finders property showing naked children and slaughtered goats. Suggestions were made that the goats were sacrificed. The animal slaughters turned out to be a routine part of life on a rural Virginia farm. (Birk, 1987b)

Such ideas were very widespread in the 1980s. The following year, on April 1—a date that suggests the story originated as a prank—the Associated Press reported the following from Pike County, Mississippi:

> Rumors that a satanic cult planned to sacrifice a virgin reached a peak this week, leading people to keep hundreds of children home from school and inundate police with calls.

> "We have a 30 percent absenteeism in the district." Sheriff Robert Lawson has said there are 22 members of a satanic cult in Pike County. "The story is that Good Friday is their Black Sabbath, and they need a sacrifice." (Associated Press, 1988)

Working from a biased cultural model, hypothetical narratives, and a few shreds of evidence, people can readily put things together into a believable explanation. The human mind strives to make narrative sense of the world, and people are often not willing to stop and question received models because the comprehensive explanation seems more reliable and enables decisive action. For this reason justice and science have to rely heavily on skepticism and the benefit of the doubt. Culturally biased models and stereotypes become traps, especially if based on hearsay and stories, because people frequently pass on stories without believing them simply for their entertainment value, and often encourage others to give them credence (Dégh, 2001). One person's funny story becomes another's truth. An excellent example of this is the wide credence people give to the—obviously culturally biased—stories about pets disappearing into the kitchens of Chinese restaurants.

The "crack baby" panic of the 1980s was similarly framed as a problem of poor minorities. Cultural biases against minorities led to discrimination that resulted in jail penalties for crack cocaine use that were more than 10 times as long as for non-crack cocaine, despite the lack of scientific evidence that crack was more destructive than other forms of cocaine (Hartman & Golub, 1999; Litt & McNeil, 1997). One has to assume that such "moral panics" will happen again and thus use critical thinking to resist urban legends and supposed "news" stories that promote cultural bias, because these will lead to personal prejudice and to participation in institutional discrimination (Goode & Ben-Yahuda, 1994).

In addition to cultural biases against people who are not members of the dominant culture, cultural biases can also provide images of positive behavior by members of the dominant culture. Pediatric doctors are more likely to assess nonwhite children for abuse injuries (Lane et al., 2002), although white offenders are more likely than nonwhite offenders to commit violence against children (Finkelhor & Ormrod, 2001, p. 4). The positive dominant culture image of middle-class, Anglo American families reduces education and healthcare professionals' willingness to recognize abuse when it occurs within such families. Child sexual abuse is common in all ethnic groups and social classes (Finkelhor, 1993), but biased intervention and prosecution tend to facilitate denial or concealment of abuse and the protection of dominant culture offenders, which in turn perpetuates the belief that such cases are less common. Assumptions about the infrequent occurrence of and the milder consequences for child sexual abuse by female perpetrators likewise motivates social workers and the police to provide less protection to victims of such cases (Hetherton & Beardsall, 1998).

Clearly institutional cultures are important places to prevent discrimination through systematic questioning of the biases and stereotypes that shape personal prejudice. The following section will consider some of the ways that institutional cultures form, and how these affect client experiences.

Institutions Create Their Own Cultures

Much of what people feel to be the shared and unspoken cultural understandings of a group are often quite weakly shared. People usually assume they can make themselves understood to people who share their language, but within organizations interaction can be complex for outsiders who do not understand the organizational culture very well. Any complex institution, such as a university, bank, or hospital, develops complex systems and specialized language, whether about research procedures, insurance, mortgages, or medical procedures. Even straightforward procedures are highly technical in unsuspected ways. When someone wants to know why the bank has not processed a check yet, she discovers the complexities of financial processes. Every institution has complex procedures that are obscure to outsiders pursuing their particular goals, and insiders may take the procedures so completely for granted that they cannot explain them to outsiders.

Expert knowledge consists of both the formal and explicit systematic knowledge of how to practice a particular skill, such as nursing, as well as extensive informal knowledge acquired piecemeal through experiences that would be difficult to systematize and explain. This kind of sociocultural knowledge develops through long participation in a work context.

Upon arriving for the first day of a new job in a healthcare institution, such as a hospital, one begins a very steep learning curve of discovering its formal and informal culture. Over the course of weeks and months one builds a fairly accurate knowledge of job responsibilities and social expectations in most circumstances. But only over the course of years does one become aware of the political, historical, and institutional forces shaping the policies, attitudes, and practices of the hospital. Like any large institution, hospitals are complex social systems with diverse cultures that outsiders know little about. Wards, departments, and offices within a hospital develop idiosyncratic patterns. The people within the hospital bring characteristic modes of behavior from their prior experiences into their present interactions with others, creating patterns sometimes described as organizational subcultures (Brooks & MacDonald, 2000; Costello, 2001; Jermier et al., 1991; Louis, 1980; Mason, 2002; Secker et al., 2004; Walker, 1967).

A client's arrival in a new medical context is likewise a complex learning experience. New clients do not know what to do, what to expect, who to ask for information, or how they will be treated. They will likely expect some highly structured bureaucratic and medical procedures that bestow patient status on outsiders, and they will understand that attaining this new status is a prerequisite for getting the diagnosis and treatment that they came for, but the power and knowledge differential makes a productive clinical experience problematic. The rituals of entering a new organization and negotiating to resolve concerns are important components of care-seeking processes (Lock & Scheper-Hughes, 1996; Rimal, 2001).

Madeleine Leininger points to many ways that different cultures arise in clinical and hospital contexts, and that differences between the cultures of nursing and medicine can lead to conflicts within nurse–physician interactions and hierarchies. The recognized authority and expertise of physicians facilitates their professional autonomy and exercise of decision-making power. "Physicians tend to communicate that they 'always know what is best' for the client" despite seeing the client only briefly in care settings and hospitals. Leininger argues that most hospitals and physicians rely on a technoscientific model of disease treatment and symptom management, and finds that problems arise when the nurses do not retain their own autonomy in care and instead allow the physicians' model to be imposed on them. Further, public media support the dominance of the physicians' model, so "nursing's unique and valuable discoveries" to healing and well-being remain little noted, and the hegemonic practices of medicine perpetuate clients' "cultural pain and distrust" (Leininger & McFarland, 2002, p. 202). The physician model of technoscientific medicine significantly impedes client treatment when it overwhelms or leads to rejection of client concerns. The symbolic rituals of technoscience tend to subordinate client needs to those of the institution and its procedures. Studying these rituals has become an important part of overcoming obstacles that prevent culturally sensitive client care.

The Ritual Process of Medicine

The conflicts between technoscience and care models may be largely invisible to clients, who tend to perceive the institution's staff and their policies and activities as integrated parts of a homogeneous and impenetrable system. In fact, the client experience of medical institutions usually revolves around the ritualized aspects of admission, treatment, and discharge, which have been interpreted from the perspective of Arnold van Gennep's theory of rites of passage (Davis-Floyd, 1992). Using this approach, filling out forms, changing into a hospital gown, transportation by wheelchair, submission to an admission physical, and being assigned to a room and a bed serve as the ritual stage of separation during which the client leaves the everyday world of individuated identities to become one of many patients under the care of authoritative ritual experts whose tutelage they must follow for successful treatment and transition back to the everyday world.

Many aspects of hospital treatment have more to do with controlling patient individuality, freedom, and options, and enforcing their obedience to ritual specialists than with medically necessary activities. Sitting in a wheelchair for transport, bodily exposure and accessibility enforced by the hospital gown, and catheterization with a saline drip "just in case" intravenous access is needed are all examples of rendering the body the object of technoscientific ritual and taking away comfort and freedom. Such practices remind the "patient" that she is there to wait, to suffer, and to be passive (all root meanings of the word *patient*).

The ritual and symbolic aspects of hospital technoscience have been extensively documented by Robbie Davis-Floyd in her study of the "technocratic model of birth": She finds that hospital birth ritual treats the mother as if she is suffering from a dangerous condition and is dependent on medical technology to avoid the impending disaster threatened by a natural body. "The intravenous drips are umbilical cords to the hospital" and make her "dependent on the institution for her life." The patient is expected to subordinate her needs to those of the hospital staff, who often seem to want childbirth to be a calm and well-managed affair, like other institutional procedures. The mother's body is subjected to an unnatural birth position for the convenience of the doctor and for many years the mother was expected to undergo anesthesia in order that her experience of pain would not disturb the doctor's concentration (Davis-Floyd, 1992, p. 52).

Davis-Floyd's description can be expanded to include other interventionist medical procedures: hazardous screening tools such as X-rays, CT scans, and procedures requiring anesthesia are routinely ordered merely to eliminate unlikely conditions. Inadequate risk-reward analysis plagues medical diagnostic procedures. The dominant interpretation of technology as solving problems overwhelms the recognition of the risks and possibility of medical error that come with its use. Risk assessment is rarely carried out despite the incidence of complications with even the most routine medical procedures and prescriptions. When a patient rejects a treatment as too invasive or dangerous, strong pressure is often applied to encourage compliance.

The patient experiences treatment rituals imposed from outside with few choices about the process. It is taken for granted that the doctor's expertise outweighs patient concerns or preferences, so the patient's role is often reduced to consenting to the treatment plan presented. After the *liminal* period in which the treatment and its outcome, and hence the patient's health status itself, remain indefinite and monitored, the healing process begins and the patient gradually transitions back to normal social roles through rituals of *reintegration*, such as removal from intravenous or breathing support, or starting physical therapy. The passage through ritual separation, liminal uncertainty in which the patient's body is subjected to symbolic domination by technological and bureaucratic means, and finally the declaration that one is healing and can be reintegrated back into ordinary life, are all part of the technoscientific control of medical crisis, and as Davis-Floyd points out, such rituals function to reinforce social values (1992).

It is important to understand how client experience involves ritual processes because technoscientific medical training and clinical practices often deny the sociocultural effects of medical ritual, and rely primarily on medical and institutional necessities to legitimize procedures. But ritual techniques are used in all cultures for giving a sense of control over uncertain or dangerous processes (Glicksman, 2003; Gmelch, 2003; Malinowski, 1948). Although the uncertainties of medical diagnosis and treatment involve many complex and demanding ritual practices, the psychosocial effects are subordinated to more objective demands such as sterility, standardization, rational procedures, and the catch-all "placebo effect." The concept of the placebo effect has the added benefit of implying that only patients may be influenced by rituals while practitioners preserve their scientific rationality. Even the broadest studies of so-called "context effects" in healing situations avoid examining how treatment rituals may influence the caregivers themselves to reduce anxiety and improve outcomes (e.g., Christakis, 2003; Di Blasi et al., 2001; Kaptchuk, 2002).

It seems obvious that medical rituals reassure both patients and practitioners that the best possible treatments are being identified and carried out in the best possible way. Rituals create a sense of control that alleviates anxieties about injury, trauma, pain, illness, and outcomes that can promote recovery in patients and preserve a sense of effectiveness in practitioners. Research on pain shows that pain is subjectively experienced as much worse when the patient does not know how long and how painful a condition will become. If a patient has some certainty about the duration and severity of the pain that he or she will feel, he or she actually feels less pain (Goldberg & Remy-St. Louis, 1998). Similarly, physicians who focus their attention and work in controlled and ritualized contexts "with well-defined sequences of actions," "precise expectations," and limits on sources of variation are able to feel confident and effective (Delle Fave & Massimini, 2003; p. 335; see also Csikszentmihalyi, 2000).

Forensic nursing clients experience multiple crises and encounter numerous institutional procedures that are meant to help them regain control. Understanding how these processes involve elements of ritual (especially separation, liminality, and reintegration) will aid communication with and treatment of clients. Medical procedures not only serve to restore physical and mental health, but also can support or impede the psychosocial recovery process by helping clients make sense out of traumatic and disabling events and regain control over their lives.

Client Experiences in the Institutional Contexts of Forensic Nursing

The forensic nursing client faces complex institutional involvements that are not limited to nursing and medicine, but can include police, courts, and therapists, among others. This added complexity is less common in other fields of nursing: The different organizational cultures of these institutions place demands on both the client and the nurse. The nurse will often have to mediate and explain these demands for clients, because the client will not understand the various institutional expectations.

In order to understand client experiences of the overlapping cultural processes pertaining to a victim of domestic violence or sexual assault, one needs to think of the ways that each social context has its own culture. The shared dominant culture within which these groups exist can be described as a *macroculture*, with each professional group having its own *microculture* within that macroculture. The client will have to interact with and learn the concerns, rules, and expectations of the unfamiliar cultures of police, doctors, courts, and nurses, among others. In addition, they have to maintain relations with their family and community while in a period of crisis that will profoundly affect expectations and interactions. The assault itself and any court proceedings will bring victims into contact with the offender, and the healing process will potentially bring the victims into contact with other victims. One way of understanding how these intersecting microcultures are experienced is represented graphically in Figure 5–2.

To understand the relationship of macroculture and these microcultures, it is best to see the macroculture as the shared national culture, including all the general expectations and understandings of the roles of the police, doctors, nurses, and courts; the sense of a shared project of maintaining social order; and even the exploitative ideologies that contribute to violence or sexual assault as anti-social attempts to attain culturally idealized power. The macroculture cannot be said to be as deeply learned or completely shared by its members, but brings general understandings and language, while each microculture develops more specific cultural expectations as well as ways of using language.

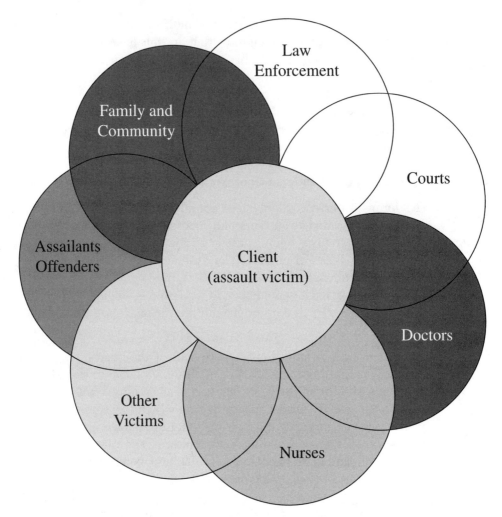

Figure 5–2 The interacting sociocultural contexts for a victim client with the larger macroculture in the background.

Similar diagrams for understanding the interacting sociocultural contexts for incarcerated or psychiatric clients can be seen in Figures 5–3 and 5–4. These diagrams only suggest the complexity of intersections among these contexts because in many there will be more than the three subcultures or identities overlapping.

A CULTURAL PROCESS MODEL OF RECOVERY

Understanding the client experience in terms of overlapping institutional contexts, each with their own cultural models of events, methods, and goals, can guide practitioners who wish to promote integration and

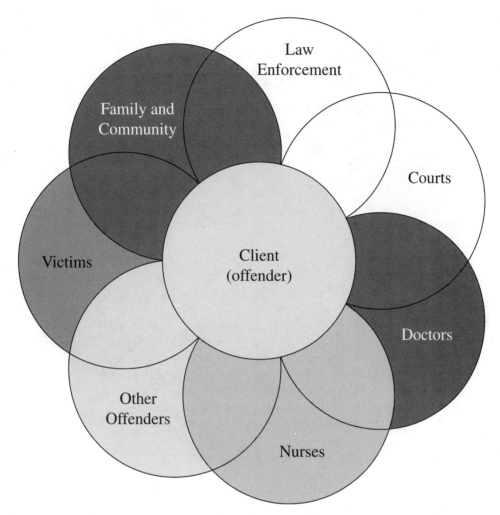

Figure 5–3 The interacting sociocultural contexts for an incarcerated client.

communication among these processes. Despite the great differences among these institutions and their goals, the overall processes are comparable. Understanding these processes will help the forensic nurse understand the situation of the clients he or she works with, and will facilitate supporting clients in dealing with these overlapping institutional cultures.

The Model

In forensic nursing, the client is generally in a crisis or has undergone traumatic experiences that make trust and communication difficult. In any sociocultural context, crisis creates an unexpected and dangerous sit-

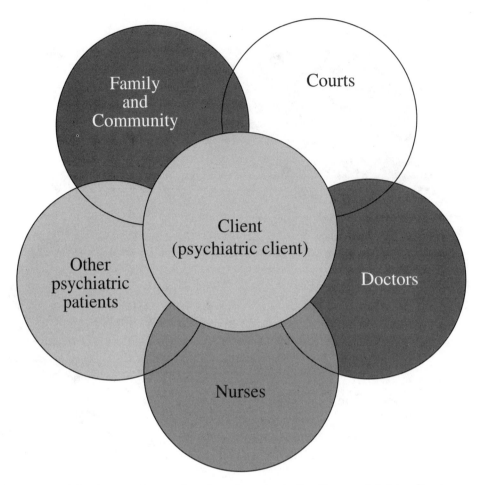

Figure 5–4   The interacting sociocultural contexts for the psychiatric client.

uation that cannot be dealt with by ordinary means—by its very nature there are few cultural responses and expectations to draw upon because culture consists of familiar and usual social activities. To gain sociocultural control over unusual natural or social crises or disasters depends upon specialists. In U.S. society, these specialists can include police, fire-fighters, EMTs, Red Cross personnel, the National Guard, news reporters, politicians, and nurses and doctors (Vaughan, 1999, in press).

These specialists are responsible for identifying the components of the crisis, seeking out its causes, healing its symptoms, and resolving long-term consequences. As can be seen from Table 5–2, in a medical emergency involving a crime victim, each specialist not only focuses on particular

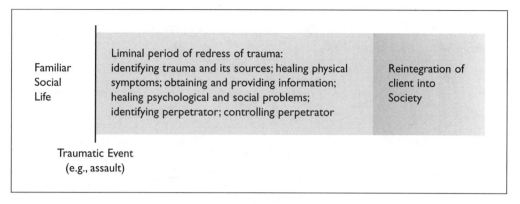

Figure 5–5   The overall sociocultural model of the trauma process.

aspects of crises, but also provides certain kinds of remedies and redress. Although the client is the central subject of the remedies and redress of a crisis, he or she generally knows little about the roles and work of these specialists, and must discover the procedures and expectations as the specialists do their work. Although overlapping in many ways, the client's concerns can be quite different from those of the specialists.

The sociocultural process that a client undergoes as part of a traumatic experience can be narrated as a sequence consisting of a prehistory of relative normalcy and meaningful participation in a familiar social order, followed by a personally disruptive event or events that occur with little or no warning and disconnect the client from meaningful and orderly existence. The client is thrown into a liminal or crisis period in which expectations about social relations and physical experience break down. The changed behavior or concerns of significant others and the unfamiliar language of crisis specialists can add to the sense of separation and result in loss of stability, safety, and trust.

Coping with a crisis has to include institutional processes of redress, psychosocial processes of reestablishing familiarity and trust, and sociocultural processes of reclaiming one's former roles, relationships, and identity. The social complexity of these overlapping processes indicates the degree of importance society places on controlling such events and finding multiple kinds of redress for these disruptions. Social order and cultural consistency are highly valued by most members of society. Violence, trauma, crisis, and disaster that threaten sociocultural order must be dealt with as effectively as possible. The work of specialists involves discovering the causes and resulting symptoms of the crisis to remedy them, and applying specialist cultural models to restore order and stability. Victims generally have fewer models, and must rely on others to provide explanatory narratives that help make sense of the crisis. Figure 5–5 offers one way to understand this process in overview for victims of violent trauma, and Table 5–2 shows the many different

Table 5–2   The Culturally Shaped Concerns of Client and Specialists Through the Course of the Trauma and Recovery Process; the Client Is a Sexual Assault Victim in This Example (see also Helman, 2000)

Identity and Institutions	Pre-event Social Life	Trauma or Crisis Event	Identify Events, Causes, Agents, Models	Apply Models in Planning Redress	Perform Redress	Resolve Remaining Issues	Reintegrate into Social Life
Client (victim of assault)	Meaningful multidimensional participation in a variety of social groups and contexts	Injury and confusion about what, how, and why Seek safety Emotions: fear, stress, anxiety, frustration, feel trapped by event and aftermath of violated privacy Potential culturally-shaped feelings: guilt, shame, anger, hatred, or distrust of others	Seek reasons, causes, responsibility, models, and understanding Flashbacks to events Identify sources of social and emotional support; seek narrative knowledge from others with similar experiences Begin to identify as "victim of this event"	Engage with significant others; explore physical, emotional, and legal solutions; use others' narrative knowledge to develop a probable course to recovery; develop a narrative of this new identity; develop symbolic representations of this "trial," this "burden," this "chaos"	Find support; rebuild trust in others Pursue medical, emotional, legal redress Attempt to follow models of recovery Find more positive, active symbolic identity to separate from event	Separate more fully from the event Return to other identities and roles Rebuild integrity and stability of social relations Return to social participation and to self-concept from before the event	Come to see self as once again having multidimensional social identity within one's community
Police (from client perspective)	Facilitate and organize daily community life; enforce laws and court orders	Emergency response	Identify and investigate crime; identify suspects	Build case against suspects; attempt to arrest suspect	Incarcerate offender; monitor offenders in the community	Inform and educate community to help avoid similar events; provide continuing protection	Promote safety and order; facilitate community activities
Courts and prosecutors (from client perspective)	Carry out justice procedures	Limited role	Determine legal issues; identify suspects	Develop case; prosecute suspect; hold trial	Reach judgment; sentence and punish culprit	Restrict offender's recidivism potential; consider victim's concerns	Carry out justice procedures
Medical personnel (from client perspective)	Promote health; identify and resolve medical issues	EMTs; emergency room treatment: return client to physical and mental integrity	Diagnose medical condition; identify concerns	Determine treatments; alleviate symptoms	Apply medical remedies; support bodily healing; evaluate prognosis; plan management	Psychological support and counseling for emotional recovery and reintegration; aid in restoring social integrity	Promote health; identify and resolve medical issues
Nurses (from client perspective)	Promote health; facilitate prevention; mediate contact with physicians	Relieve trauma; carry out SANE protocol; convey and gather vital information; understand client needs	Determine client care needs Identify cultural, social, personal issues Begin to provide culturally congruent care	Expand communication with client and explain procedures and resources; help find narrative understanding Monitor and help resolve patient concerns about physical, mental, and social situation	Perform procedures; support bodily, social, and emotional healing; facilitate interaction with physicians and with significant others	Monitor client's healing; educate about issues and options; facilitate contact with psychological support staff	Promote health; facilitate prevention; mediate contact with physicians

specialist roles and activities that can be identified within each stage of the process.

Table 5–2 helps us to understand that the complexity of experiencing violent trauma is only one generalized model of the experience, but it suggests the value of seeing it as a multilayered process. Its complexity is even more pronounced when the client is not a member of the dominant culture or is unfamiliar with the cultural patterns of personnel in these institutions. If the client has to have everything translated into his or her native language and learn unfamiliar interaction patterns and expectations, cultural pain can be added to already existing trauma.

When we add these stages to the earlier discussion of the ways in which the ritual process is experienced in the hospital as a loss of control to technoscientific procedures, we can begin to understand why the cultural and symbolic meanings of the experience can be as important as the physical reality of the trauma itself. The ritual helps bring a sense of control over a crisis, but at the cost of relinquishing personal control to ritual specialists to whom we turn when we cannot deal with a crisis as individuals. One result of Table 5–2 is that we see that the opportunity to take time planning redress is more pertinent to the doctor, therapist, and prosecutor roles, while the police, EMT, emergency room doctor, and nurse roles require that more immediate care be given to a client. Despite these differing orientations, a planned, integrated, and systematic organization of treatment within an environment of open communication with the client will be extremely helpful in healing and regaining a sense of control over her life.

This model is not comprehensive because every situation is different, but the processes of healing body, mind, and social relations are central to recovery. In fact, these are overlapping phases rather than the tidy stages represented in the table. But healing requires not simply a return to prior bodily, mental, and social wholeness; it also requires finding labels, explanations, and resolutions to use to give meaning to traumatic experience. The resolution of disorder involves identifying and naming the pieces of that disorder, explaining the causes and effects, and beginning to resolve ongoing problems with normal social functioning.

Trauma Process and Ethnomedical Techniques in Folk Healing

The trauma process model can help understanding of healing rituals in other cultures. One of the most important steps in healing is the diagnosis. In technoscientific medicine this is presented as a way to systematically classify and describe the etiology and symptoms of a condition, but more generally this serves to label and explain the problem. The ritual process moves beyond disorder and ambiguity by labeling and explaining the condition and then seeking remedies. In the case of many healing traditions, diagnosis includes identifying supernatural explanations for a condition. However, the diagnosis of the cause is usually less important than characterizing the severity of the injuries and the probable prognosis for treatment and healing. Such diagnosis moves patient and medical staff from a condition of lacking information to one of having a somewhat elaborate description of the condition that helps return the patient to the meaningful world of cultural understandings.

The feeling that a bodily or mental crisis has brought loss of control can begin to be overcome as soon as the mysterious is put into familiar and *culturally congruent* terms. When Madeleine Leininger advocates culturally congruent care, she means not only care that fits within patient expectations and experiences, but also care that begins by making culturally reasonable sense of the condition from which the patient suffers (Leininger & McFarland, 2002). Within forensic nursing, the conditions of uncertainty and crisis that a nurse will likely provide care for clearly extend beyond medical or psychological to the social liminality that crime victims, offenders, and psychiatric patients all experience in one way or another. An important aspect of care is labeling and explaining the condition in order to promote healing. This involves finding answers to the questions: What happened? Why has the event disconnected the client from society? What processes of recovery and reintegration will be most effective? These questions arise in all medical treatment because all clients need to be reassured about when they will get out of the hospital, but the multi-institutional nature of victim and offender experiences makes the uncertainties greater in their cases, as they deal with intersecting processes.

Cultural care techniques from many different societies have been described for illnesses and psychiatric conditions, but there are far fewer studies of traditional healing methods used for injuries. Thus it is rather difficult to describe in much detail examples of techniques clients may be familiar with. Beyond ethnomedical rituals that assist in injury diagnosis, treatments for injuries can include plant or other substances, ritual recitations, offerings, and so on. The trauma itself will be less important than engaging and appeasing the supernatural forces who allowed it to happen so that they do not allow further injury, as well as seeking supernatural aid to promote healing. Ideas about dealing with the evil eye, making offerings to helpful spirits, or warding off witchcraft are often part of traditional medical practices and should not be interfered with because they often provide clients with a sense of added security in the face of uncertainty.

Although folk healing techniques for dealing with injuries are not very highly elaborated and have not been studied adequately in most cases, the techniques for dealing with psychological conditions are often quite complex, and may well be encountered by forensic nurses. Beliefs about supernatural influences or strong emotions leading to culture-bound conditions such as *locura* (psychosis), *susto* (fright illness), and *nervios* among Hispanics; *ceeb* (fright illness) and soul wandering among the Hmong; *shenkui* (panic with somatic conditions) among Chinese; and *zar* (spirit possession) among people from North Africa and the Middle East (Simons & Hughes, 1985). It has been pointed out that hypoglycemia has similarly entered popular thinking as an ambiguous and flexible illness construct because those who claim to suffer from it far outnumber those who have been clinically diagnosed with it (Hunt, Browner, & Jordan, 1990).

All of these conditions can be diagnosed and treated by folk healers using a variety of ways to gain information about supernatural and emotional events that influence a person. Extensive studies have explored how shamans in Native American, Siberian, Hmong, Korean, and Balinese societies, among many others, provide important diagnostic and healing practices to help cure a wide range of mental and physical conditions, ranging from infertility to epilepsy (Connor, Asch, & Asch, 1986; Grim, 1983; Thao, 1989). Most shamans rely on knowledge gained through interaction with spirits, who diagnose the problem in terms of bodily, supernatural, or social causes, and then prescribe treatment. Such consultation of the spirits often involves the shaman going into a trance and inviting spirits to speak through him or her as a medium or channel. When the shaman comes out of the trance, he or she often has to ask those present what the spirit has said. Thus the shaman does not claim medical expertise, but has authority that comes from intimate connections with spirits who can explain unseen causes and effects (Kendall, 1985).

It is very important to recognize that although shamans and other healers are generally expert in interaction with the supernatural, they do not necessarily have a narrow medical specialization or a consistent style of performing their rituals. Each shaman and supernatural healer develops his or her own relationship with particular spirits, and they tend to expand their repertoire of supernatural services to deal with almost all problems or concerns clients might bring, from explaining the causes of bad luck and preventing further bad luck to predicting the future to providing healing services. Although any given culture will have certain patterns of interaction and typical kinds of conditions that healers can treat, there is extensive personal variety, especially in larger societies and more urban settings where many different traditions come together and healers tend to pick and choose among practices that they feel work best. For instance, the Balinese medium and healer Jero Tapakan both goes into trances, so that clients could "ask for speech" from the spirits to determine the source of medical problems and misfortunes, and provides therapeutic massage and medicines to heal people after they have been diagnosed by the spirits. In contrast to the traditions of *curanderismo* in Latin America, where the *curandero* usually does diagnose and prescribe based on personal expertise (Press, 1971), Jero Tapakan could not herself diagnose a problem or prescribe medicine. When asked the diagnosis for one patient she says "In my opinion—well, I don't know anything, but according to my guardian deity, the Balinese diagnosis is called *babai*. But I don't know, it's not visible." On the other hand, Tapakan does display extensive traditional knowledge about bodily "forces" and "channels" when she discusses her clients' conditions and treats them by massage (Connor, Asch, & Asch, 1986, p. 202).

These are only a few examples of the endless array of healing alternatives available in any urban setting around the world. As Irwin Press describes for residents of Bogota, there are healers who diagnose through bodily examination, divination, pseudoscientific instruments, and religious practices. Treatments can include homeopathy, patent medicines, charms, amulets, prayer and saints' images, holy water, injections, and prescriptions to restore humoral imbalance (Press, 1971). One mile from the university where I am writing this in the midwestern United States, I can walk into a "health food" store and ask one of the several prescribing salespeople about any condition I might believe I have, and they will offer me a vitamin, mineral, herb, or extract that they believe will cure or alleviate it. I could just as easily consult with nearby chiropractors, and would not have to go much further to find fortunetellers or faith healers who would suggest other treatments. Many people in North America rely on practitioners of Wicca and religious healing systems derived from West African traditions, including Santería, Vodun, and Candomblé. Or I could go to one of the two local hospitals both less than two miles from here, that rely on biomedical principles. The human capacity to feel ill or otherwise out of balance far exceeds the ability of medical science to manage, and people rely on many treatments that seem to offer control over the complex uncertainties of bodily and mental life, as long as the practices are culturally congruent with their understanding of the connections among themselves, their society, and the world around them.

In addition to many curing processes that include supernatural components or placebo effects, research has revealed that many folk remedies prove to be effective therapies in double-blind studies and thus offer alternatives to more expensive patented medicines. Such substances rarely find a place in technoscientific medicine because the drug approval process is very costly and hence only worthwhile for companies when they know they can make a profit from patent-protected drug innovations. Since it is not possible to patent natural products, these are rarely shepherded through the FDA approval process, and thus remain folk or herbal remedies that people rely on as alternatives to high priced drugs.

Sociocultural Concerns in Treating Injuries

Perhaps because they have less mysterious origins and heal with somewhat less mystery than bodily and mental illness, injuries are more often the subject of self-care, which is not as well studied as the practices of professional healers. There are few descriptions in the literature of techniques used to diagnose injuries, trauma, blood loss, and the like, but many medical techniques used to treat them.

Traditional treatments for injury and trauma include applying mineral, plant, and animal products; rituals and incantations; mechanical treatments; and bodily manipulation. A comprehensive review of the literature on the botanical pharmacopeia used in Ayurvedic medicine (from India) showed that only 8% of the 166 plants described had uses for controlling pain and inflammation, and none were described as being used to aid treating other trauma (Khan & Balick, 2001). In eastern Indonesia, palm oil, betel nut, turmeric, and papaya are all used to treat wounds. Papaya is similarly used by Native Americans (Dweck, 1997). Aloe vera has also been used to treat wounds in some areas, but research shows it has little effectiveness. Acupuncture is an alternative therapy with considerable effectiveness for treating pain.

Although many injury treatments that will be part of the cultural repertoire of many patients are little known, there has been considerable study of how people from different cultural backgrounds respond to and express pain (Edwards, Fillingim, & Keefe, 2001). This is an important dimension of nursing because pain sensations have important effects on well-being and healing, and serves to alert caregivers to problems that may need further assessment. The clinical assessment of pain and its cultural variability have been extensively studied. Many examples of how people in different societies cope with pain have been combined into a model that attempts to predict the experience and expression of pain in terms of cultural values and social conditioning that influence choices among the options of stoicism versus expression, extroversion versus introversion, anticipatory anxiety about pain, emotional state, accurate understanding of the probable degree of pain, and narrative understanding and explanation of pain (Goldberg & Remy-St. Louis, 1998).

There is also complex literature on the many biological pathways that generate pain. It shows that although there are no fundamental biological differences in pain experience around the world, culture does profoundly shape pain sensations. It has also been found that in many treatment contexts in the United States, minorities are not given adequate pain management, especially if they receive care from people who do not share their native language (Lasch, 2002). Pain assessment clearly depends heavily upon culturally sensitive communication and empathy, including the willingness to find the means to communicate in the client's native language so that full and open assessment of pain can be attained (Davidhizar & Giger, 2004). The McGill Pain Questionnaire is an important tool for assessing pain by dividing assessment terms into the semantic fields of sensation, affective or emotional impact, evaluation, and temporal pattern. In nursing, culturally appropriate pain assessment tools such as translated versions of the McGill Pain Questionnaire should be available to make accurate evaluation and treatment of client pain (van Duijn, 1995). In addition, nurses should be sensitive to client behaviors and expressions such as limping or grimaces that indicate pain.

Cultural Practices and Forensic Nursing

A few issues remain about the connections between forensic nursing and cultural practices. Although there has been very little systematic study of the legal and medical dimensions of the wide variety of religious, educational, ritual, and folk healing practices, a number of relevant examples have been studied by anthropologists and medical researchers.

Folk medical practices can be fairly invasive and often result in injuries or leave lasting marks on the body. Since medical practices are often done to children by adults, some instances result in injury that may lead to questions about child abuse. In one case an infant who died of unknown causes later ascribed to SIDS was examined and found to have healing clavicular fractures. The parents were initially suspected of child abuse, but further investigation revealed that the child had been treated by an unlicensed chiropractor three or four weeks before the death (Sperry & Pfalzgraf, 1990). In rare cases injuries have resulted from acupuncture techniques, and these might be more likely in small children because the needle depth would have to be adjusted to account for smaller body size. Another Asian medical tradition, moxibustion, has also been misinterpreted as child abuse because it can leave burn marks (Feldman, 1984).

Faith healing and Christian Science practices raise deep questions about parental rights to refuse medical treatment to a child, and generate numerous legal cases each year, when states try to impose treatment by having a parent declared negligent and then taking custody of the child, or when a state presses criminal charges against a parent for not seeking medical treatment for a child who suffers permanent harm or death.

Although there were legal statutes that protected the rights of Christian Scientists to provide alternative medical care without being considered negligent, most have been eliminated in the past few decades, so it is now easier for states to prosecute parents for neglect when they do not seek medical care for children (Merrick, 1994, 2003; Swan, 1983).

Another dimension of religious healing involves practices that are designed to eliminate supernatural causes of possession. This can take many forms, including the shamanism described earlier. In the case of certain forms of faith healing based on the Christian Bible, people can be subjected to physical practices that can cause harm and even death. A recent example from Milwaukee concerns a faith healing service to rid an autistic boy of spirits. The healing practices allegedly involved physical restraint that resulted in the boy's death (McCord, 2003). Religious worship can also involve other hazardous practices such as snake handling, fire walking, or piercing the body to show imperviousness to pain due to supernatural protective powers. In general, such practices are not protected religious expression if they result in harm to a child, so investigation and prosecution are standard responses in the United States. Another example of practices that can result in injury include some of those that are used to rid a child of the influences of the evil eye (Bottoms, Shaver, Goodman, & Qin, 1995).

In general, however, religious and faith healing practices involve little threat to the body or mind and do not result in injury. There are a number of initiation rituals that can easily involve injury to a child, especially those that involve physical modification of the body such as circumcision. Already widely recognized are the dangers of female genital cutting in many parts of the world. Less well publicized are the dangers of male circumcision and subincision. Other ritual practices involve body modification, scarification, and tattoo. As with religious healing practices, there are cultural and religious motivations for these practices that make it difficult to interfere without being accused of discriminatory treatment. In general, there has to be a risk of serious harm before legal sanctions can be used to challenge a traditional custom. Worldwide, the campaign against more extreme forms of female genital mutilation has only been successful when people from the local culture are enlisted to support changes to the practice. One positive aspect of changing such rituals is that often the initiation aspect of the rite of passage can be accomplished symbolically without significant body modification. Few people consider the standard circumcision of male babies after birth in the United States to be a major body modification—although it is not medically necessary—so there is little effort to change it. Female-genital-cutting rituals are being replaced in Africa and elsewhere by less extreme symbolic acts, with role models provided by activists who publicly reject the practices and promote the alternatives.

SUMMARY

Dealing with client experiences and ideas about cultural and social dimensions of life are complex responsibilities that depend upon caregivers' sensitivity, skillful and attentive communication, and open-minded willingness to understand clients' concerns. Healthcare practitioners have to be careful to avoid bringing their own cultural biases or personal prejudices into their institutional practices.

Physical and mental experience do not exist outside of the cultural interpretations, concepts, and needs that people begin learning in early childhood, and continue to develop throughout their lives. Effective, nondiscriminatory communication about emotional, physical, or cognitive experience, and cultural meanings requires creative work to bridge the gap between those different experiences. This is particularly true with transitions into new organizational subcultures, such as those found in hospitals.

In addition to trauma experienced before arriving at an institution, the clinical experience itself, along with encounters with law enforcement and the courts, can contribute to separation of the patient from ordinary social functioning. Treatment has to take into account psychosocial needs in order for the patient to deal with this new state of liminality. Through complex ritual processes many specialists will participate in aiding a patient in accomplishing redress and reintegration with society at large.

Biomedical procedures—like those of most healing traditions—depend upon ritual practices to help control anxiety and uncertainty. Although there has been extensive work on how healthcare provider rituals can influence patient experiences and outcomes, there remains a reluctance to consider the ways ritual in the healing situation also significantly effects practitioners. Acknowledging the significant contribution that ritual processes make to controlling uncertainty and restoring social order in the face of crisis would go a long way towards linking patient experiences more closely to physician and nurse experiences, and in adding to our understanding of the complexity of these social processes.

Perhaps the most important influences on caregiving interactions are the aspects of technocratic and bureaucratic ritual and symbolism that prevent effective therapeutic communication. The hierarchical effects of depending on medical technology and procedures to control uncertainty in the clinical context can suppress the mutual respect that will help a client regain control over his or her situation.

In addition, patients' own care traditions should be understood and respected as techniques that help them introduce familiar cultural order in unfamiliar situations. Practitioners should work to be aware of the variety of different cultural practices and communicate openly with patients about the effects and concerns of alternative treatments.

Cultural concepts and expectations about communication, health, food, and bodily comfort are diverse and have a deep impact on the feelings of people made vulnerable by the conditions or experiences that bring them into forensic healthcare settings. Forensic healthcare patients should be understood as individual members of a number of different subcultures that shape complex sociocultural concerns in ways that must be explored through attentive interaction and caregiving.

QUESTIONS FOR DISCUSSION

1. What is culture and how does it impact social life?
2. What are class, race, and ethnicity and what role do they play in social life?
3. How do people learn culture?
4. How and when do people use culture in daily life to communicate, judge, make choices, and act?
5. What aspects of culture are the hardest to recognize?
6. How do people become attached to culture and impose it on social interaction?
7. How do people respond to violations of cultural norms and values?
8. How do institutions create, propagate, and use culture?
9. What cultural patterns and practices will be encountered in forensic nursing?
10. When, why, and how will cultural assumptions have to be made overt in forensic nursing?
11. What tools can you use to visualize cultural and social domains?
12. How can one evaluate cultural knowledge, expectations, and communication strategies?
13. How can one recognize when cultural differences are distorting communication?
14. How do rituals and cultural models shape the practice of medicine?

ACKNOWLEDGMENTS

I wish to thank Barbara Chesney, Lynne Hamer, and Seamus Metress for discussing this chapter with me and suggesting issues and resources I should include.

REFERENCES

American Medical Association. (1999). *Cultural competence compendium.* Chicago, IL: American Medical Association.

Associated Press. (April 1, 1988). *Devil getting unwarranted publicity in McComb.* Associated Press Wire Story. Retrieved from Lexis/Nexis database January 12, 2004.

Baer, R. D., Weller, S. C., Garcia, J. G. D., Glazer, M., Trotter, R., Pachter, L., & Klein, R. E. (2003). A cross-cultural approach to the study of the folk illness nervios. *Culture Medicine and Psychiatry 27*(3), 315–337.

Balick, M. J. & Lee, R. (2003). Stealing the soul, Soumwahu en Naniak, and Susto: Understanding culturally-specific illnesses, their origins and treatment. *Alternative Therapies in Health and Medicine 9*(3), 106–109.

Barbee, E. L. (1993). Racism in U.S. nursing. *Medical Anthropology Quarterly, New Series 7*(4), 346–362.

Birk, E. (February 14, 1987a). Authorities Tone Down Description of Finders. Associated Press Wire Story. Retrieved from Lexis/Nexis database January 12, 2004.

Birk, E. (February 8, 1987b). *Threats phoned to tattered kids; Police on alert.* Associated Press Wire Story. Retrieved from Lexis/Nexis database January 12, 2004.

Bogin, B. (1995). Growth and development: Recent evolutionary and biocultural research. In N. T. Boaz & L. D. Wolfe (Eds.), *Biological anthropology: The state of the science* (pp. 49–70). Bend, OR: International Institute for Human Evolutionary Research.

Bottoms, B. L. & Davis, S. L. (1997). The creation of satanic ritual abuse. *Journal of Social and Clinical Psychology 16,* 112–132.

Bottoms, B. L., Shaver, P. R., & Goodman, G. S. (1996). An analysis of ritualistic and religion-related child abuse allegations. *Law and Human Behavior 20,* 1–34.

Bottoms, B. L., Shaver, P. R., Goodman, G. S., & Qin, J. J. (1995). In the name of God: A profile of religion-related child abuse. *Journal of Social Issues 51,* 85–111.

Bownds, D. (1999). *The biology of mind: Origins and structures of mind, brain, and consciousness.* Bethesda, MD: Fitzgerald Science Press.

Brooks, I. & MacDonald, S. (2000). "Doing life": Gender relations in a night nursing sub-culture. *Gender, Work and Organization 7*(4), 221–229.

Cavalli-Sforza, L. L., Menozzi, P., & Piazza, A. (1994) *The history and geography of human genes.* Princeton, NJ: Princeton University Press.

Christakis, N. A. (2003). On the sociological anxiety of physicians. In C. Messikomer, J. Swazey, & A. Glicksman (Eds.), *Society and medicine: Essays in honor of Renée C Fox* (pp. 135–144). New Brunswick, NJ: Transaction.

Cole, M. (2001). Culture in development. In N. J. Smelser & P. B. Baltes (Eds.), *International Encyclopedia of the Social & Behavioral Sciences* (pp. 3159–3164). New York: Elsevier.

Connor, L. H., Asch, P., & Asch, T. (1986). *Jero Tapakan: Balinese Healer, An Ethnographic Monograph.* Cambridge, UK: Cambridge University Press.

Cooper, R. & David, R. (1986). The biological concept of race and its application to public health and epidemiology. *Journal of Health Politics, Policy and Law* 11(1), 97–116.

Costello, John. (2001). Nursing older dying patients: Findings from an ethnographic study of death and dying in elderly care wards. *Journal of Advanced Nursing 35*(1), 59–68.

Csikszentmihalyi, M. (2000). *Beyond boredom and anxiety: Experiencing flow in work and play.* San Francisco: Jossey-Bass.

Davidhizar, R. & Giger, J. N. (2004). A review of the literature on care of clients in pain who are culturally diverse. *International Nursing Review 51*(1), 47–55.

Davis-Floyd, R. (1992). *Birth as an American rite of passage.* Berkeley, CA: University of California Press.

Dégh, L. (2001). *Legend and belief: Dialectics of a folklore genre.* Bloomington, IN: Indiana University Press.

Delle Fave, A. & Massimini, F. (2003). Optimal experience in work and leisure among teachers and physicians: Individual and bio-cultural implications. *Leisure Studies 22,* 323–342.

Di Blasi, Z., Harkness, E., Ernst, E., Georgiou, A., & Kleijnen, J. (2001). Influence of context effects on health outcomes: A systematic review. *Lancet 357*(9258), 757–762.

Douglas, M. (1966). *Purity and danger: An analysis of concepts of pollution and taboo.* London: Routledge & Kegan Paul.

Dweck, A. C. (1997). Ethnobotanical use of plants. Part 4. The American Continent. *Cosmetics and Toiletries 112*(11) 1–12. Online at http://www.dweckdata.com/Published_papers/American_Indians.pdf.

Edwards, C. L., Fillingim, R. B., & Keefe, F. (2001). Race, ethnicity and pain. *Pain 94*(2) 133–137.

Feldman, K. W. (1984). Pseudoabusive burns in Asian refugees. *American Journal of the Diseases of Children 138,* 768–769.

Fine, I., Wade, A. R., Brewer, A. A., May, M. G., Goodman, D. F., Boynton, G. M., Wandell, B. A., & MacLeod, D. I. A. (2003). Long-term deprivation affects visual perception and cortex. *Nature Neuroscience 6*(9), 915–916.

Finkelhor D. (1993). Epidemiological factors in the clinical identification of child sexual abuse. *Child Abuse and Neglect 17*(1), 67–70.

Finkelhor, D. & Ormrod, R. (2001). *Offenders incarcerated for crimes against juveniles.* Washington, DC: U.S. Department of Justice. Office of Juvenile Justice and Delinquency Prevention. Online at http://www.unh.edu/ccrc/pdf/offendersincarcerated.pdf.

Foster, S. H. (1990). *The communicative competence of young children.* London and New York: Longman.

Galanti, G. (1997). *Caring for patients from different cultures: Case studies from American hospitals.* Philadelphia: University of Pennsylvania Press.

Ginzburg, C. (1983). *Night battles: Witchcraft and agrarian cults in the sixteenth and seventeenth centuries.* Baltimore: Johns Hopkins University Press.

Glicksman, G. G. (2003). It Couldn't Hurt: An Ethnographic Study of a Ritual for Healing. *Society and Medicine: Essays in Honor of Renée C Fox.* New Brunswick, NJ: Transaction Publishers, 59–68.

Gmelch, G. (2003). Baseball magic. In J. Spradley & D. M. McCurdy (Eds.), *Conformity and conflict: Readings in cultural anthropology.* Boston: Allyn and Bacon, 348–357.

Goldberg, M. A. & Remy-St. Louis, G. (1998). Understanding and treating pain in ethnically diverse patients. *Journal of Clinical Psychology in Medical Settings 5*(3), 343–356.

Goode, E. & Ben-Yahuda, N. (1994). *Moral panics: The social construction of deviance.* Cambridge, UK: Blackwell.

Gopnik, A., Meltzoff, A. N., & Kuhl, P. K. (1999). *The scientist in the crib: Minds, brains, and how children learn.* New York: William Morrow.

Grim, J. (1983). *The shaman: Patterns of Siberian and Ojibway healing.* Civilization of the American Indian Series, vol. 165. Norman, OK: University of Oklahoma Press.

Guarnaccia, P. J. & Rogler, L. H. (1999). Research on culture-bound syndromes: New directions. *American Journal of Psychiatry 156*(9), 1322–1327.

Haidt, J., Rozin, P., McCauley, C., & Imada, S. (1997). Body, psyche, and culture: The relationship between disgust and morality. *Psychology and Developing Societies 9*, 107–131.

Harris, M. (1974). *Patterns of race in the Americas.* New York: Norton.

Hartman D. M. & Golub, A. (1999). The social construction of the crack epidemic in the print media. *Journal of Psychoactive Drugs 31*(4): 423–433.

Helman, C. G. (2000). Ritual and the management of misfortune. *Culture, Health and Illness.* (4th ed.). Boston: Butterworth-Heinemann, 156–169.

Hetherton, J. & Beardsall, L. (1998). Decisions and attitudes concerning child sexual abuse: Does the gender of the perpetrator make a difference to child protection professionals? *Child Abuse & Neglect 22*(12), 1265–1283.

Hunt, L. M., Browner, C. H., & Jordan, B. (1990). Hypoglycemia: Portrait of an illness construct in everyday use. *Medical Anthropology Quarterly 4*(2) 191–210.

Ikemoto, L. C. (1997). The fuzzy logic of race and gender in the mismeasure of Asian American women's health needs. *University of Cincinnati Law Review 65*(Spring), 799–824.

Jermier, J. M., Slocum, J. W., Fry, L. W., & Gaines, J. (1991). Organizational subcultures in a soft bureaucracy: Resistance behind the myth and facade of an official culture. *Organization Science 2*(2), 170–194.

Johnson, M. H. (2001). Functional brain development in humans. *Nature Reviews Neuroscience 2*(7), 475–483.

Kahn, P. H. (1997). Developmental psychology and the biophilia hypothesis: Children's affiliation with nature. *Developmental Review 17*, 1–61.

Kaptchuk, T. J. (2002). The placebo effect in alternative medicine: Can the performance of a healing ritual have clinical significance? *Annals of Internal Medicine 136*(11), 817–825.

Kempton, W. (1986). Two theories of home heat control. *Cognitive Science 10*(1), 75–90.

Kendall, L. (1985). *Shamans, housewives, and other restless spirits: Women in Korean ritual life.* Honolulu: University of Hawaii Press.

Khan, S. & Balick, M. J. (2001). Therapeutic plants of Ayurveda: A review of selected clinical and other studies for 166 species. *The Journal of Alternative and Complementary Medicine 7*(5), 405–515.

Klomsten, A. T., Skaalvik, E. M., & Espnes, G. A. (2004). Physical self-concept and sports: Do gender differences still exist? *Sex Roles 50*(1–2), 119–127.

Krieger, N. & Fee, E. (1994). Man-made medicine and women's health: The biopolitics of sex/gender and race/ethnicity. *International Journal of Health Services 24*(2), 265–283.

Krombholz, H. (1997). Physical performance in relation to age, sex, social class and sports activities in kindergarten and elementary school. *Perceptual and Motor Skills 84*(3), 1168–1170.

Lane, W. G., Rubin, D. M., Monteith, R., & Christian, C. W. (2002). Racial differences in the evaluation of pediatric fractures for physical abuse. *Journal of the American Medical Association 288*(13), 1603–1609.

Lasch, K. (2002). Culture and pain. *Pain: Clinical Updates 10*(5). Retrieved February 02, 2005 from http://www.iasp-pain.org/PCU02-5.html.

Leininger M. (1997). Understanding cultural pain for improved health care. *Journal of Transcultural Nursing 9*(1), 32–35.

Leininger, M. & McFarland, M. R. (2002). *Transcultural nursing: Concepts, theories, research and practice.* New York: McGraw-Hill.

Litt, J. & McNeil, M. (1997). Biological markers and social differentiation: Crack babies and the construction of the dangerous mother. *Health Care for Women International 18*(1), 31–41.

Lock, M. & Scheper-Hughes, N. (1996). Critical-interpretive approach in medical anthropology: Rituals and routines of discipline and dissent. In Carolyn F. Sargent & Thomas M. Johnson (Eds.), *Medical anthropology: Contemporary theory and method* (pp. 41–70). Westport, CT: Praeger.

Louis, M. (1980). Surprise and sense making: What newcomers experience in entering unfamiliar organizational settings. *Administrative Science Quarterly 25,* 226–251.

Luckmann, J. (1999). *Transcultural communication in nursing.* Albany, NY: Delmar.

Lutz, C. A. (1988). *Unnatural emotions: Everyday sentiments on a Micronesian atoll & their challenge to Western theory.* Chicago: University of Chicago Press.

Malinowski, Bronislaw (1948). *Magic, Science, and Religion.* Garden City, NY: Doubleday.

Martin, R. J. (1992). A model for studying the effects of social policy on education: Gauging the impact of race, sex, and class diversity. *Equity & Excellence 25,* 53–56.

Mason, T. (2002). Forensic psychiatric nursing: A literature review and thematic analysis of role tensions. *Journal of Psychiatric and Mental Health Nursing 9,* 511–520.

McCord, M. (August 25, 2003). *Autistic boy dies during prayer service; man arrested in connection with death.* Associated Press wire report.

Merrick J. C. (1994). Christian-Science healing of minor children–spiritual exemption statutes, first-amendment rights, and fair notice. *Issues in Law & Medicine 10*(3), 321–342.

Merrick J. C. (2003). Spiritual healing, sick kids and the law: Inequities in the American healthcare system. *American Journal of Law & Medicine 29*(2–3), 269–299.

Pineros M., Rosselli D., & Calderon C. (1998). An epidemic of collective conversion and dissociation disorder in an indigenous group of Colombia: Its relation to cultural change. *Social Science & Medicine 46*(11), 1425–1428.

Press, I. (1971). The urban curandero. *American Anthropologist, New Series 73*(3), 741–756.

Rimal, R. (2001). Analyzing the physician–patient interaction: An overview of six methods and future research directions. *Health Communication 13*(1), 89–99.

Schacter, D. (2001). *The seven sins of memory: How the mind forgets and remembers.* Boston: Houghton Mifflin.

Schultz, E. A. & Lavenda, R. H. (1998). *Anthropology: A perspective on the human condition* (4th ed.). Toronto: Mayfield.

Scott, J. C. (1985). *Weapons of the weak: Everyday forms of peasant resistance.* New Haven, CT: Yale University Press.

Secker, J., Benson, A., Balfe, E., Lipsedge, M., Robinson, S., & Walker, J. (2004). Understanding the social context of violent and aggressive incidents on an inpatient unit. *Journal of Psychiatric & Mental Health Nursing 11*(2), 172–178.

Simons, R. C. & Hughes, C. C., Eds. (1985). *The culture-bound syndromes: Folk illnesses of psychiatric and anthropological interest.* Dordrecht, the Netherlands: D. Reidel.

Skuse, D. H. (1988). Extreme deprivation in early childhood. In D. Bishop & K. Mogford (Eds.), *Language Development in Exceptional Circumstances* (pp. 29–46). New York: Churchill Livingstone.

Sperry K. & Pfalzgraf, R. (1990). Inadvertent clavicular fractures caused by "chiropractic" manipulations in an infant: An unusual form of pseudoabuse. *Journal of Forensic Science 35*(5), 1211–1216.

Swan, N. R. (1983). Faith healing, Christian Science, and the medical-care of children. *New England Journal of Medicine 309*(26), 1639–1641.

Tambiah, S. J. (1969). Animals are good to think and good to prohibit. *Ethnology 8*(4), 423–459.

Thao, P. (1989). *I am a shaman: A Hmong life story with ethnographic commentary.* (D. Conquergood & X. Thao, Trans.) Minneapolis: Southeast Asian Refugee Studies Project, Center for Urban and Regional Affairs, University of Minnesota.

van Duijn, N.P., (1995). Translations and use of the McGill Pain Questionnaire. *Quality of Life Newsletter 12,* pp. 7–9. Online at http://www.mapi-research-inst.com/mapi/pdf/art/qol12_7.pdf.

Vaughan, D. (in press). Organizational rituals of risk and error. In Bridget Hutter & Michael Power (eds.) *Organizational encounters with risk.* Cambridge, UK: Cambridge University Press.

Vaughan, D. (1999). The dark side of organizations: Mistake, misconduct, and disaster. *Annual Review of Sociology 25,* 271–305.

Vega, F. (1978). *The effect of human and intergroup relations education on the race/sex attitudes of education majors.* Dissertation, University of Minnesota.

Waitzkin, H., Cabrera, A., deCabrera, E. A., Radlow, M., & Rodriguez, F. (1996). Patient-doctor communication in cross-national perspective—A study in Mexico. *Medical Care 34*(7), 641–671.

Ward, C., Bochner, S., & Furnham, A. (2001). *The psychology of culture shock.* 2nd ed. Philadelphia: Routledge.

Walker, V. H. (1967). *Nursing and ritualistic practices.* New York: Macmillan.

Wolf, Z. R. (1988). *Nurses' work: The sacred and the profane.* Philadelphia: University of Pennsylvania Press.

Ethical Considerations in Forensic Nursing

Douglas Olsen

Many definitions and descriptions have been offered for forensic nursing, varying in emphasis on treatment of victims, treatment of offenders, and the nurse's role in developing forensic information (Mason, 2002). This consideration of ethics in forensic nursing will bypass that debate and use Mason's characterization of the discipline, "... forensic nursing ... where crime interfaces with human suffering" (Mason, p. 512). As the field involves crime which, by definition, involves behavior that society has determined is unacceptable and contrary to the social good, defining ethical comportment in forensic nursing will require careful consideration of the nurse's relationship to both the patient/subject and the community.

CHAPTER FOCUS

Principles
Recurring Concepts in Ethical Discourse of Forensic Nursing Practice
Points of Ethical Tension in Forensic Practice

KEY TERMS

autonomy
beneficence
contextual caring
distributive justice
ethical comportment
ethical tension
ethics
fiduciary
retributive justice
values-based decisions

INTRODUCTION

The study and practice of clinical ethics can be thought of as having two components. First, ethics provides tools for solving dilemmas involving personal or social values, in contrast to clinical decisions based on empirical evidence. For example, whether a nurse should report criminal intent revealed in the context of a clinical relationship is an ethical dilemma because it involves a conflict between the nurse's value of patient confidentiality and his or her value of society's right to safety. In contrast, the decision to withhold or give an antihypertensive is made on the basis of clinical data—measurements of the patient's blood pressure, the patient's health history, and knowledge of the efficacy of various interventions. Despite this apparent distinction, the line between values-based decisions and clinically based or data-based decisions is anything but clear. Indeed, in a real sense all decisions are values-based, in that clinical nursing practice is based on the value of reducing human suffering; so, in the example of giving or withholding the antihypertensive, ultimately the decision is made from the value that a nurse should do good for the patient.

The second aspect of clinical ethics is to guide clinicians in ethical comportment. This aspect of ethics is concerned with ongoing moral relationships and behavior. For example, in forensic practice the development of a therapeutic relationship with a potentially dangerous patient is a question of ethical comportment. Ethical considerations of both types should be used to anticipate problems, and to frame problems that do occur in order to design policy.

The discipline of healthcare ethics is related to the law but is not the same as the law. Ethics is the study of how one ought to act; it provides rationales as to why one course of action is better than another and finds a basis on which to agree about right and wrong action. Ethics examines values and ways to enact them, as well as ways in which values are not enacted. The language of values includes words that are often avoided in social situations, such as *ought, should, right, wrong,* and *better* (in the sense of more worthy, not more efficacious). The law is presumed to be an attempt to enact the value of fairness, and thus often coincides with what we think of as ethical. Further, the law circumscribes what can be done and therefore is vital to ethics as applied to health care. Also, when a recurring situation is identified as unethical the remedy is often a change in the law. However, the study of how to understand values in health care is different from knowing the law; this chapter will concentrate on ethical and not legal understanding. This distinction needs to be clear in the field of forensic nursing because a detailed understanding of the law is vital to practice; this chapter will help the forensic nurse distinguish how ethics coincides with, differs from, and comments on the law.

Table 6–1   Principles Guiding Forensic Nursing Practice

Respect for persons
Beneficence
Distributive justice
Respect for community
Contextual caring

Source: Working Group for the Study of Ethics in International Nursing Research, 2003.

An ethical approach to forensic nursing will be proposed by offering five principles (Table 6–1) to guide forensic practice; explicating three conceptual areas that occur regularly in ethical discussion of forensic issues; conceiving and labeling pathology and deviance, the nurse–patient relationship, and the assignation of responsibility; and then examining specific points of ethical tension in forensic nursing practice.

PRINCIPLES

The principles offered here are intended to assist clinicians both in dilemma situations and in guiding ethical comportment. However, different principles will be more directed toward considering one of the two aspects in particular situations. For example, respect for person is a central consideration in dilemma situations involving the possible need to breach an individual's right of liberty, whereas contextual caring may be more helpful in considering how to respond to a violent patient's depression. However, all five principles have some relevance to all situations.

The articulation of principles has come under criticism in recent years because of fears that certain principles will be applied dogmatically in the manner of rules or laws, without regard to ethically relevant context (Strong, 2000). Many of these problems are avoided by understanding that principles are not prescriptive rules, but broad guides in how to consider ethically difficult situations. Such guides can be useful to the nurse attempting to be rigorous in difficult complex situations, so long as principles are not confused with prescriptions and applied rigidly as rules.

These five principles are adapted from the consideration of ethics in international nursing research because these two situations share several points of similarity, including relationships with legitimate considerations beyond the individual patient/subject, the need for particular attention to the community aside from considerations of resource allocation, and the difficulties of actualizing caring concern in situations of divided obligation.

Respect for Person

The first three principles, respect for persons, beneficence, and distributive justice, are derived from the standard Western canon of ethics as interpreted by Beauchamp and Childress (2001). Respect for person holds that personhood is a privileged category; that is, persons deserve special consideration. The principle of respect for person is based on the irreducible value of personhood, the concept of which reaches an apex of articulation in Kant's second formulation of his categorical imperative, "Act so that you treat humanity, whether in your own person or in that of another, always as an end and never as a means only" (1959, p. 47). Although there is considerable latitude for debate—Is a fetus a person? What is it about being a person that is special? Do any animals have this special quality to some degree?—there is broad social consensus that human life has intrinsic value. Therefore, furthering the respect shown for an individual is a valid ethical justification.

Respect for person incorporates both respect for autonomy and protection of vulnerable persons (National Commission for the Protection of Human Subjects of Biomedical and Behavioral Research, 1979). Granting and respecting personal autonomy is the chief way of expressing respect for person in Western societies. This is because autonomy—that is, the ability to rationally self-direct or self-govern—is widely treated as the morally significant and unique feature of being human. If each individual has intrinsic ultimate value and is self-governing, then each person has equal moral worth. It further follows that the right of liberty, as the freedom to pursue those goals without interference, is essential. In everyday social interaction autonomy is recognized and liberty granted passively by not actively interfering with others. But in health care, clinicians have an ethical obligation to go beyond merely recognizing autonomy and granting liberty to respecting and enhancing the patient's autonomy (Beauchamp & Childress, 2001; Cassel, 1976). This requires clinicians to take an active role using expert knowledge to make patients more aware of the possibilities and shortcomings of medical science in defining their goals, and at times, working with patients to define their goals and increase their voice in articulating those goals.

It also follows that if being human has intrinsic value, then those persons who by virtue of some vulnerability, internal (e.g., mental illness) or external (e.g., oppression), cannot govern themselves in their own best interests should be protected. Clinicians need to be highly aware of what conditions—medical, social, and otherwise—interfere with a person's autonomy.

Autonomy and liberty are central concepts in ethical consideration of forensics because limiting liberty is the primary technique for dealing with criminal behavior. Many of the current ethical dilemmas in forensic mental health involve issues of autonomy, for example, implementation of the death penalty with the mentally retarded and children and involuntary restoration of competency. Decisions central to a forensic practice are conceptually based on the work of the enlightenment era philosophers (especially Kant and Mill), who held individual autonomy and liberty to be the starting point of ethics. Decisions such as competency, dangerousness, and responsibility are all tied to the belief that autonomous action is central to personhood.

Acts of coercion must be justified as exceptions to the clinician's obligation to respect patient autonomy. The form of currently accepted standards for forcing treatment in psychiatry can be found in John Stuart Mill's *On Liberty*, first published in 1985. The two justifications for denying a patient's choice of treatment are that the patient lacks capacity to make the decision or that the patient's choice could result in harm, either to the patient or others. Mill (1985) gives an example that invokes both criteria. A man is about to walk over a bridge that will collapse under his weight, sending him to his death. A bystander does not have time to warn him and so pushes him out of the way. At first the walker is angry, but when fully informed of the situation, he concurs that pushing him was the proper action.

The legal justification for psychiatric commitment and many other forms of forced treatment in all fifty U.S. states requires the presence of mental illness, which no longer implies legal loss of competence but represents a transformation of Mill's requirement of impaired capacity, coupled with potential danger, either to one's self or others (Tasman, Kay, & Lieberman 1997). The commitment criterion of "gravely disabled" is conceptually grounded as an extension of potential danger to self, providing ethical justification of the forced treatment.

In Mill's case, the bystander's assumption that the walker lacked competence is confirmed by the walker's approval of being pushed when he is fully informed of the bridge's condition. This information restores his competence. Thus the walker's liberty was not violated. The analogy in psychiatric treatment is that the noncompetent (i.e., mentally ill) patient who is restrained, committed, or force-medicated will concur after a course of treatment has restored the patient to a competent mental state. Allen Stone has labeled this the "thank you" theory of civil commitment (Alexander et al., 1991).

However, the actual situation of seeking concordance or a "thank you" regarding both forced treatment and treatment in coercive situations, like prison, presents two problems likely to result in the clinician having an inflated sense of the patient's agreement with the necessity of forcing treatment. First, clinicians believe that they act in a patient's best interest, so they will be biased toward interpreting the patient's discussion of an incident as agreement. The second barrier to assessing the patient's retrospective endorsement of coerced treatment is that asking from the position of the treating clinician, particularly when backed by repressive authority, is inherently coercive. Patients expecting to continue in treatment or gain institutional privileges are likely to feel that their endorsement of the treatment demonstrates cooperativeness and improved "health." A study by Soliday (1985) found that patients who endorsed the need for seclusion provoked this response: "Many patients after an episode of solitary confinement will learn that the best way to avoid another is to acknowledge therapeutic benefit, even if this is not how they really feel" (Chamberlain, 1985, p. 290).

The second justification for overruling a patient's stated wishes is to prevent harm. An example is when a homicidal patient refuses inpatient admission and is civilly committed rather than left at liberty in the community.

Autonomy is an essential concept in forensics in a way not found in other areas of health care. The determination of responsibility hinges, in part, on a subject being autonomous, that is, self-directing. People are not considered morally responsible unless they are acting autonomously, and their responsibility may be mitigated if autonomy is felt to be compromised. Forensic nurses may be called upon to assist the court in determining if a person's mental status was compromised to determine the degree of culpability, which may involve appropriate sentencing. In nonforensic practice, nurses are specifically warned that a patient's responsibility for the clinical problem should not influence clinical care. When providing health care, nurses should not determine the degree or type of care a patient deserves based on an assessment of the patient's responsibility (Olsen, 1997a). In some forensic situations, however, the nurse may be assessing a person's mental state in order to help the justice system determine what conditions and handling are just and deserved by the person. Nurses need to be clear with patient–prisoners when they are in a situation where the nurse's assessments may be used to determine responsibility—such as an evaluation prior to sentencing—and when those assessments are for clinical purposes. For example, in prison nursing, as in nonforensic health care, the patient's responsibility for either the crime or the clinical problem should not influence a patient–prisoner's nursing care. Because relationships are part of good nursing care, these also should not be negatively affected by responsibility. For example, smokers with emphysema should not receive inferior care, either in terms of physical care or in terms of the quality of the nurse–patient relationship. Although this is relatively clear and easy for most clinicians to implement in the case of smokers, forensics can present special difficulties, such as a child molester with depression or a surly gang member with a knife wound. In summary, patient responsibility for problems should never be a consideration in giving health care, except as an adjunct for self-healing. However, assessments regarding responsibility may be a consideration in certain forensic situations to help the justice system determine appropriate responses to criminal behavior.

Beneficence

This is the principle that one should act for the benefit of others, maximizing positive good and minimizing or preventing harm (Beauchamp & Childress, 2001). In nonforensic health care many ethicists posit a fiduciary relationship with patients. A fiduciary is one in whom a person has placed special trust and confidence and who is required to watch out for the person's best interests. Such a relationship acknowledges a differential in power and knowledge requiring special loyalty on the part of the clinician. Many of the ethical dilemmas in health care are framed as a conflict between respect for a patient's autonomy and the duty to act beneficently toward the patient, that is, in the patient's best interests. This conflict is particularly pertinent to mental health as a specialty because many of the disorders encountered include denial of disorder or dysfunction as an integral aspect of the disorder. Much of the mental health clinician's effort is often directed toward having the patient acknowledge the problem and commit to working toward change. This takes on an added dimension in forensic practice where people are often compelled into treatment situations.

Justice

Distributive justice is the principle dealing with the fair distribution of goods and resources. The goal of this principle is to determine just ways to distribute goods and resources and to develop polices for determining distribution. Frankena says, "The paradigm case of injustice is that in which there are two similar individuals in similar circumstances and one of them is treated better or worse than the other" (1973, p. 49). As with other ethical principles, the difficulty is often in how key terms are interpreted. In Frankena's definition, many decisions hinge on what are considered the ethically relevant features of "treatment" and "circumstances" to determine "similarity." For example, gender is no longer considered ethically relevant in determining the appropriate level of education a child should receive, but historically gender was considered a relevant circumstance in determining education.

Another form of justice is retributive justice—the ethics of determining just punishment. Punishment is not a part of healthcare ethics, but is an integral concept of the criminal justice system. The use of certain healthcare techniques, such as administering a lethal injection to carry out the death penalty, and the denial of health care are not appropriate forms of punishment, and nurses should never be involved in these actions (American Nurses Association, 1995).

Respect for Community

The fourth ethical principle suggested for forensic nursing practice, respect for community, departs somewhat from standard Western canon. This principle suggests that a wider context of concern than the individual should come under consideration.

Although ethics in nursing always requires attention to the clinical relationship, the consideration of the community as a context in the forensic situation has unique features, including: 1) Persons who have committed crimes are not always easy people with whom to form relationships that nurses consider ethically ideal or therapeutic (Peternelj-Taylor & Johnson, 1995); 2) the community has substantial legitimate interests that may conflict with the patient's wishes and perceived interests; 3) the nurse may have substantial personal safety concerns; 4) therapeutic interaction or community interests may require nurses to go beyond simple advocacy in working with victims; 5) diagnostic entities common in the forensic situation are often blurred by social conceptions of the meanings and implications of deviance and volition; 6) forensic nurses often work with society's outcasts in marginalized institutions; and 7) some roles confer legitimate obligations to the community that conflict with an offender's perceived best interests.

Ethical actions in forensic practice should consider a community's self-conception, how perceptions outside the community might be altered, and policy questions arising from particularly difficult situations. These considerations go beyond justice because they are not simply questions of the distribution of goods and services. The consideration of any effect on the community has become increasingly important in today's climate of media coverage where particular crimes capture the imagination of the entire nation. These situations often go beyond news coverage and influence policy, as in the case of such named laws as Megan's law or the Amber alert legislation.

Contextual Caring

The final guiding principle, contextual caring, entreats the forensic nurse to interact with each patient, whether criminal or victim, as a person within an ethical relationship of caring concern grounded in the nurse's personal values. This differs from beneficence, where the actions are abstractly guided by the principle of acting in the patient's best interest. In contextual caring the nurse acts in accord with personal caring concern for the concrete specific other within the context of a particular relation-

Table 6–2 Comparison of Ethical Principles in Clinical Relationships and in Relationships in Forensic Evaluation

Principle	Clinical	Forensic Evaluation
Respect for autonomy	Patient sets treatment goal.	Person is made aware of the purpose of the evaluation.
Justification for overriding autonomy	Patient's best interests when competence is impaired.	Compelling offenders to undergo evaluation is justified by their potential for harm to society.
Beneficence	Do the best thing for the patient.	Person should not be deliberately harmed or any potential for benefit from the evaluation minimized.
Justice	1. Fair access to health care.	1. Due process in ordering the evaluation and the use of the information.
	2. Fair distribution of healthcare resources.	2. Qualified evaluators.
Goal	Best treatment for individual patient.	Benefit society by: 1. Minimizing harm that person might cause. 2. Helping to determine justly deserved treatment.
Nature of relationship	Assistive.	Coercive.
Offender's motivation	Meet healthcare goals.	1. Evaluation may help person. 2. Person may be actively opposed to evaluation.
Nurse's motivation	Help individual patients.	Benefit society through the court.

ship. Caring is more difficult to prescribe than beneficence because it is more closely bound to the nurse's emotional reactions; however, there is increasing recognition that emotion is inextricably bound to moral good (Nortvedt, 1996; Vetlesen, 1994). The principle of caring concern encourages the consideration of what good can and may be done for the patient to whom one is responsible beyond the obligatory dictates of patients' rights (Benner & Wrubel, 1989; Gastmans, 1999; Gastmans, Dierckx de Casterlé, & Schotsmans, 1998). Although all health care should be guided by a caring concern for the specific patient, care as a guide to practice has special import in forensic practice because of the patient and the type of problems encountered. First, there is the difficult question of how one cares for a patient who either denies the problem, seems to takes a volitional role in the problem, or is threatening or belligerent. Second is the other side of this issue: Should victims receive special caring and concern in their health care? (For a comparison between clinical and forensic application of these principles, see Table 6–2.)

RECURRING CONCEPTS IN ETHICAL DISCOURSE OF FORENSIC NURSING PRACTICE

In examining ethical practice and dilemmas in forensic practice or in creating policy to anticipate dilemmas and foster ethical practice, three conceptually dense quandaries repeatedly recur. First is the problem of diagnostic labels and their meanings, which define what is considered pathology, what is deviance, and what these distinctions should mean in terms of responsibility, culpability, clinical treatment, and treatment by the justice system. The second issue is that of relationship. This is an especially complex issue in forensics because of the difficult population served and because some forensic roles have legitimate concerns other than the patient's welfare. The last is the issue of responsibility, which has two aspects, the determining of individual responsibility for acts and the effect on the nurse of the offender's responsibility. These issues are too large and complex to be completely separate; discussion of each includes aspects of the other two.

Labeling Issues

Labeling issues are of particular concern to forensics because many legal decisions, particularly those relating to culpability and punishment, are influenced by social assumptions regarding the nature of disease. Mental health experts may be called upon to report the existence of various disorders and their relationship to a person's mental status in determining an individual's culpability. Figure 6–1 diagrams in simplified form the implications of distinctions between problem behavior arising from "illness" and that arising from "badness."

Society is increasingly alert to the relationship between psychiatric issues and the work of the justice system, both sides showing concern about inappropriate use of mental disorder to avoid responsibility and the alarming rate at which the mentally ill are being incarcerated for minor crimes (though the latter gets bigger headlines).

Despite advances in understanding the biology of the brain, diagnosis in psychiatry remains phenomenological. Patients are given diagnostic labels based on what the clinician sees, what the patient reports, and what is reported about the patient. As of yet there are no objective (observable physical criteria that are relatively uninfluenced by the desires and volition of the patient) or laboratory tests for mental disorders, although there are known statistical differences between "normal" people and those with certain disorders. For example, it is well known that, on average, people with schizophrenia exhibit ventricular volume abnormalities (Andreasen et al., 1990).

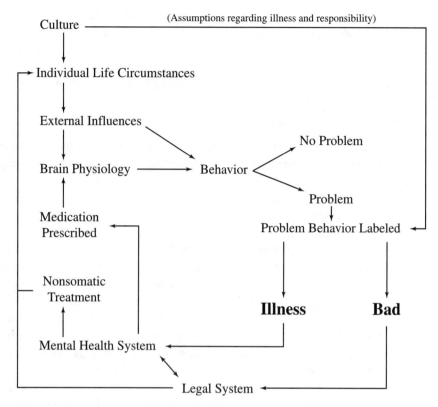

Figure 6–1   Schematic of Behavior, Culture, and Treatment

Mental health care provides three rationales for labeling a person as having psychopathology—distress, dysfunction, and deviance. None of these alone serves as a complete guide to identifying psychopathology in an individual. Distress can be thought of as personal discomfort or pain. The patient complains and wants the condition changed. However, all forms of mental distress are not mental disorders: grief, for example, is not a disorder and should not be treated as such. The example of prisoners reporting feelings of depression highlights the difficulty of diagnostic issues in forensics, because one expects prisoners to experience distress, indeed for many in our society this is the purpose of incarceration. Thus, more than distress must go into the determination of pathology in a context where distress is anticipated as normal.

Dysfunction can be thought of as an impaired ability to perform one's social or family role. The person may complain of the condition causing dysfunction, as with distress, or the person may deny the condition but others who interact with the person, like an employer or family member, may report dysfunction related to the condition. Many mental disorders are characterized by the person's denial of the disorder or any associated dysfunction, for example, alcohol dependence and mania. In some cases the person denies both the disorder and the dysfunction, whereas in other cases the person attributes the dysfunction to other causes. Although denial is inherent to the nature of some disorders, the tendency to deny and minimize is severely exacerbated by the stigma society puts on mental illness, causing many people with more "distress-based" disorders, like depression, to deny and actively resist the possibility that their problems are a mental disorder.

Deviance can be thought of as behavior outside accepted social norms. The family, employer, police, or members of the general public may complain about the deviant person's behavior. In those cases where the deviant behavior causes distress, the person may complain. However, in many cases the deviant behavior is pleasurable or is perceived by the person as creating an advantage. Deviance as a determinant of psychopathology brings the field of mental health close to forensics because criminal behavior is deviant behavior. Some psychiatric diagnoses, including antisocial personality disorder, substance abuse disorders, and conduct disorder, are closely related to criminal behavior. Although deviance is an essential aspect of identifying psychopathology, it must be viewed cautiously because not all deviant behavior is criminal or pathological. Simple deviation from accepted norms is not sufficient to define criminality or mental disorder. As Altman (1982) points out, "There is no such thing as a value-free concept of deviance; to say homosexuals are deviant because they are a statistical minority is, in practice, to stigmatize them. Nuns are rarely classed as deviants for the same reason, although if they obey their vows they clearly differ very significantly from the great majority of people" (p. 5). A society that values personal freedom and harbors a strong concept of individual rights could never equate deviance with mental illness and conformity with mental health. Deviance as a determinant of pathology underscores the inevitable element of social construction in defining pathology. Society cannot give up its function in defining acceptable and unacceptable behavior, because this is one function of the community. Therefore there is a social responsibility to make moral decisions regarding what are acceptable and unacceptable variations in behavior, and whether the unacceptable behavior is an "illness" or criminal. Current Western society is based on the concept that free and open discussion of the issues combined with power sharing throughout the population will result in fair and reasonable norms and humane categorization of deviance.

Relationship

There are two different reasons for focusing on nurse–client relationships in forensic practice—the often difficult nature of the population and the fact that clinicians have legitimate goals other than the welfare of the person under consideration. The patient population in forensic practice has, by definition, some involvement with crime either as per-petrators or victims, and each group presents relationship problems.

Working with Offenders

For many nurses a forensic practice means working directly with con-victed criminals, persons accused of a crime, persons who committed crimes but are found not guilty by reason of insanity, or persons who are believed to have committed crimes but are incompetent to bring to trial. The criteria for some DSM-IV diagnoses specify criminal or violent behavior, whereas in others it is easily inferred. Antisocial personality disorder is the most well-known diagnosis, but the implication of crim-inal or violent behavior is also found in the criteria for conduct disorder, some impulse control disorders, intermittent explosive disorder, and some paraphilias. In addition to antisocial personality disorder, other Cluster B personality disorders (narcissistic, borderline, and histrionic) can be expected among people who use violent or criminal behavior, because these disorders consist mainly of difficulties with interpersonal relations. Further, many individuals without clear personality disorders rely on some immature and dysfunctional personality traits like intimi-dation and splitting. Peternelj-Taylor and Johnson (1995) are quite dis-couraging regarding the possibility of the usual nurse–patient relationship in an institutional setting, stating, "the relationships that are formed are dubious at best; offenders regard the professional as a friend or confidant when requests are approved, and as a member of the establishment or the system when requests are denied" (p. 16).

One could even argue that the nature of forensic settings like prisons encourage antisocial traits as a survival mechanism. In addition, the connection between the lifestyle involved in substance abuse and crim-inal activity is well established, although criminal behavior is not inher-ent in the DSM diagnostic of substance abuse disorder. The U.S. Department of Justice reports that 36% of all crimes are committed by someone under the influence of alcohol (Greenfield, 1998), and one study showed that 64% of adult males arrested had one of five drugs in their blood: cocaine, marijuana, opiates, methamphetamine, or PCP (Arrestee Drug Abuse Monitoring Program, 2000).

One concern when working with a criminal population is the potential for violence. Nurses certainly have the right to safety in their working environment. At the same time, even potentially violent individuals have a right to health care.

Many measures intended to ensure the safety of the community and healthcare staff in an institution are repressive to the inmates. As with other forms of security, such measures will be unnecessary much of the time for most individuals. In many cases, when security serves a preventive function one cannot know of specific incidences of violence that were averted. Retrospective analysis showing an overall reduction of incidents is the only way to evaluate specific techniques for reducing violent incidents and other breaches of security. Airport security provides a good illustration of this problem. Very few of the people searched will be terrorists, and no one knows how many prospective terrorists are deterred by airport searches, but most agree that searches are needed. (The analogy is not perfect because incidents of violence in a prison can be expected to be far more frequent than incidents of terrorism on airplanes.) This essential overdone quality of security makes it feel repressive to the recipient, conveying a lack of trust and certainly reinforcing the power differential between staff and inmate. Again, it is similar to the case when typical business travelers are pulled out of line while boarding a plane for a more extensive search. Such travelers know that they are not terrorists and that the search is a waste of time, at least as far as the threat from them. It requires some degree of maturity on the part of such travelers to acknowledge that although they are not threats, tight security benefits everyone through prevention, including them. This maturity is much more difficult for an inmate inside a prison, where the message of distrust and lack of power is not a one-time event but a continuous feature in all aspects of life. Also, inmates with personality disorders and other forms of mental disorder may lack the maturity and foresight to see repressive security as a benefit to them by deterring others. Beyond the effect of any diagnoses on particular prisoners, many inmates come from oppressed segments of society where messages of power and distrust, such as racial profiling by police and the extreme security in many inner city stores, are rampant. Indeed, the issue of diagnosis and effect of social repression are not separate and additive, but interactive. People raised in oppressive or traumatic circumstances will develop ways of surviving that may be labeled as pathological or deviant by the dominant society; further, such individuals may interact with the larger society in ways that become labeled symptomatic. People who perceive themselves as outsiders to a dominant, more powerful group will often act in ways that are labeled paranoid.

The need to ensure safety must be balanced with the inmate's right to health care and a desire to show respect to the individual. Stringent security measures during the provision of health care should be driven only by the degree of actual threat and not by an impulse to punish the offender. The appropriateness of punishment as a motivation for harsh measures elsewhere in prison life is a separate and controversial issue.

Another difficult ethical question occurs at the level of the individual. Clinicians and authorities must decide the proper response to the individual who has used violence or intimidation in dealing with clinicians. The consideration of an ethical response to violence by the patient will vary depending on how certain controversial ethical issues are viewed. For example, consider the question of whether health care for inmates is considered a privilege or a basic right. Some aspects of health care, such as prevention, may be seen more as privilege, whereas other aspects, such as wound care, are more concerned with basic rights. In some cases intimidation may be an issue of respect for autonomy. If intimidation is used to refuse a treatment, then clearly the treatment is unwanted and perhaps autonomy should be respected by allowing the person to refuse. This is more complex in cases where the person's competence and understanding of the treatment is questionable or where the treatment is psychiatric medications that help maintain the competency needed for an autonomous refusal. Clearly respect for autonomy is not an issue where intimidation is being used to obtain medications the clinician has determined are not needed.

Security and care need to be balanced in terms of the environment, but a nurse providing health care in that environment is left with an even more difficult balance to resolve. Nurses working with intimidating and potentially violent persons still need to develop a clinical relationship in as ethical and therapeutic a manner as possible despite the considerable constraints to good relations. Constraints can be external, like a security environment conducive to distrust; internal, such as patients with personality structures/disorders that make connection difficult; and social, as in the culture of oppression and bias from which many inmates originate.

In nursing, therapeutic and ethical relationships are generally held to involve an empathetic regard for the patient. In seeking to form such relationships with perpetrators, nurses in forensic practice face the obstacle of an intrinsic social bias against feeling sympathetic toward persons believed to have caused the problem. One need only reflect on certain everyday formulations of expression to see how deeply embedded is the assumption that it is correct to feel less sympathy when a person is responsible for their troubles. Consider, for example, the mother who scolds a child running at poolside, "Don't come crying to me when you fall, I told you not to run," or when a person asked his or her feelings regarding the plight of another responds by saying, "They brought this on themselves." This formulation of responsibility is so commonly understood to convey a negative feeling that reflection is required to realize that it is not an expression of feeling at all.

Nurses are not immune to this way of thinking. In one study, 50% of nurses specifically stated that their empathetic regard for patients was tied to their sense of the patient's responsibility for the clinical problem (Olsen, 1997b). In nonforensic practice it is clear that the clinician's role never involves deciding whether and how much care a patient deserves based on the patient's responsibility. Nurses are quite clear that smokers with lung cancer don't deserve any less care, including empathetic regard, than nonsmokers with lung cancer. However, a forensic practice with offenders can push this boundary because of the extremity of the acts committed. Some mental disorders found in criminal offenders actually involve harm to others; for example, pedophilia, by definition, involves either having harmed children or wanting to harm children, and other disorders like antisocial personality imply the possibility of harm to others as part of the disorder. Personal feelings about acts like murder, rape, and child molesting are much harder for the nurse to put aside in the name of an abstract duty to care for all, regardless of how they came to need care, than feelings about smokers and those with a poor diet.

Nurses working with offenders have an ethical duty to reflect honestly on their feelings and strive for personal growth in their regard for others. Nurses working in this environment are cautioned against a facile use of the concept of the "nonjudgmental attitude." The first problem is that the formulation, nonjudgmental attitude, can easily become a rationalization for perfunctory physical care given to personally distasteful patients without reflection on the patient's suffering and ways to help. The second problem with a nonjudgmental attitude is that when behavior related to a mental disorder is morally wrong, healing for the patient means facing and accepting responsibility for the behavior and for changing it. The Alcoholics Anonymous philosophy provides an excellent example of how personal responsibility can be construed in the context of a disease model. Nurses should not be judgmental or condemn patients, but should be able to tolerate the moral evaluation of behavior by the patient. It may seem odd to suggest simultaneously that nurses should not be judgmental and that nurses should not rely on the concept of the nonjudgmental attitude, but as these terms are commonly used they are not diametric. Judgmental implies a critical and dismissing attitude that is certainly not a good attitude for clinicians, whereas nonjudgmental implies the acceptance of all patient behaviors as morally equal. That the latter is not humanly possible provides another argument against the over-reliance on the concept.

An over-interpretation of the nonjudgmental attitude can be problematic when combined with the social bias of connecting sympathetic regard to responsibility. The nurse may mitigate a patient's responsibility in an attempt to develop a more positive connection with the patient than is possible if the patient is seen as responsible. The result is an inability to hear and accept the patient's own moral assessment of the behavior, which if accurate is a needed step to change. The attitude recommended here is to break through social bias and separate a moral assessment of the patient's behavior from concern for the person's suffering. One must try to simultaneously understand the moral weight of the offender's behavior, which is clinically essential, and empathize with the person's real suffering, which is essential for therapeutic and ethical relations.

Working with Victims

A patient's status as victim presents related problems in developing helpful relationships. One's natural sympathy for people harmed through no fault of their own or even actively wronged by another should not be allowed to interfere with what is best for the person. One must tread a fine line and not "blame the victim" while simultaneously not being blind to any role the victim's behavior may have played. Further, the nurse must understand the particular role he or she plays in the victim's treatment. Even when a victim's behavior has played a significant role in current troubles, that aspect is generally not the initial focus with a victimized individual, and harm can be done if this concept is introduced clumsily or at the wrong time.

In working with victims, social advocacy can be seen as the enactment of one's respect for the community. When working with a victim population, the nurse will gain inside knowledge of the social condition of victims and of problems leading to certain types of crimes. This knowledge leads to a responsibility to act on one's knowledge and expertise in advocating changes for the community's benefit. For example, nurses counseling rape victims may be thought of as having an obligation to use their expertise for the benefit of the larger community.

Community advocacy may be needed when working with either victims or perpetrators. Social conditions such as poverty, inequitable treatment, and oppression create an environment that enhances the possibility of specific types of individuals becoming perpetrators. When this happens it is often members of that same community who are victimized. This is amply demonstrated by the overrepresentation of African Americans in both the prison population and the victim population (U.S. Department of Justice, 2000a, 2000b). Many forms of social advocacy don't require a distinction between victim and perpetrator to argue for community change that will help decrease the incidence of both. Understanding that social conditions are linked to the incidence of crime does not necessarily mitigate any specific individual's responsibility; this is a controversial argument that has well-meaning adherents on both sides. However, nurses can advocate for social change without the implication that individual responsibility is lessened.

Special Forensic Relationships

In some roles, nurses working in a forensic practice will bring clinical techniques, particularly assessment skills, to bear on individuals where the goal of the encounter or intervention is not the person's welfare. This is drastically different from normal clinical nursing practice where there is broad consensus that ethical conduct demands that the patient's welfare be the nurse's primary and overriding goal. Even in those cases where patient autonomy is denied, the justification rests on the patient's being unable to choose in his or her best interest.

There are at least two specific instances where forensic practice has legitimate goals that are not necessarily the same as the person's and may actually work to harm the patient, at least from the person's perspective: court-ordered evaluation and restoration to competency.

There are many reasons why a court may order an evaluation of a person's mental status, including to determine the person's competence to stand trial, to help evaluate not guilty by reason of insanity claims, and to help determine appropriate sentencing and disposition. The nurse's primary obligation in performing an evaluation for the court is to serve the needs of society as determined by the court. The nurse is not performing the evaluation for the person's benefit, and may make assessments that the person and the person's legal counsel feel are against the person's interests.

The nurse makes an assessment based strictly on observations and reports it to the court. These assessments may favor the person's position or not. However, in these situations nurses are specifically charged to use their clinical skills to benefit society and not to be acting solely in the person's interests. Therefore, the usual strictures of privacy are not in effect with regard to the court. The nurse is acting as an extension of the legal system, which is balancing society's safety, society's interest in just treatment of the offender, and the person's rights and interests. Although the goal of the evaluation is not the person's benefit, people under evaluation must still be shown respect as people and so should be aware of the circumstances and purpose of the evaluation (American Academy of Psychiatry and the Law, 1995).

Another situation requiring coercive treatment that is done at the behest of the legal system is competency restoration, particularly in cases where the person is refusing the treatment. In these cases people may not wish to be declared competent because that will allow them to stand for trial, or they may not want treatment because they lack the insight needed to see that treatment is required or that they are acting on delusional beliefs. (See Table 6–2 for a comparison of the application of ethical principles between clinical and forensic care.)

Responsibility

The nurse in forensic practice needs a grasp of the conceptual basis of responsibility for three reasons. The first reason is because court evaluations and expert testimony are often part of the court's attempt to determine responsibility or assign the appropriate degree of responsibility for an offender's action. Although the nurse may not be asked directly to assign the degree of responsibility, the court's determination will likely be influenced by the evaluation. Many aspects of mental status sought by courts bear directly on the formulation of the offender's responsibility, for example, "irresistible impulse" and "reduced mental capacity." The formulation "not guilty by reason of insanity" directly connects mental state and moral responsibility for a criminal act. Beecher-Monas and Garcia-Rill stress the connection between psychiatry and responsibility determinations, saying, "Mental state is such an important facet of our understanding of criminal responsibility that judges need to be open to the new ideas emerging in the field of brain science" (1999, p. 260).

The second reason is the effect the patient's responsibility can have on the clinical relationship. Although nurses should work to keep notions of responsibility separate from caring concern in the clinical relationship, this will best be accomplished if the nurse understands the nature of responsibility. Further, only through understanding can the forensic nurse take the lead with other clinicians to examine the effect of the patient's responsibility and formulate an ethical approach.

The third reason is clinical: Patients who are offenders will need to examine and accept responsibility for their actions as part of healing. Forensic nurses can only act as a guide and help in this process through understanding the nature of responsibility.

The concept of personal responsibility forms a fundamental background assumption to personal relations in the same way gravity is a background concept in our understanding of how to handle physical objects. However, a slight scratch of the surface shows responsibility to be a difficult, controversial topic, the nature of which has been debated throughout history. Plato felt bad action resulted from ignorance, stating, "But if justice be power as well as knowledge—then will not the soul which has both knowledge and power be the more just, and that which is the more ignorant be the more unjust?" (1926, p. 425). Aristotle, however, felt that bad actions could be willful: ". . . the virtues are voluntary (for we are ourselves somehow partly responsible for our states of character . . .), the vices also will be voluntary; for the same is true of them" (1935, p. 215).

The first distinction to address in understanding responsibility is that between being responsible *for* (that is, liable or culpable) and responsible *to* (that is, owing an obligation). Although there is a distinction, the two in a sense are related in that when one is responsible for a negative or harmful act, one is often thought of as also being responsible to the person harmed and sometimes to society at large. In the case of a crime, an offender is held to be responsible *for* committing the act that is the offense, and in committing the act the offender has breached a responsibility *to* society and the victim—that is, the responsibility to honor the rights of others. In some cases, victims will even stake a legal claim on the offender's social obligation through civil action. We intuitively sense responsibility as occurring on a continuum, with the severity of our moral condemnation corresponding to the assessment of degree. Responsibility can be seen to be shared with another person or persons, acts of nature, or society and culture. Indeed, most sophisticated assessments of responsibility are multifactorial. However, in Morse's estimation the law has difficulty accounting for partial responsibility, saying, "Although insanity defense rules do draw such an (admittedly blurry) 'bright' line, in principle and in fact rationality is distributed along a continuum in the population at large" (1999, p. 160).

Another inherent aspect of the concept of responsibility is the connection to consequences. One test of responsibility is to see what and where consequences actually lie and where one feels they should lie. Our intuitive sense of responsibility is tied to the sense that responsible parties ought to bear the consequences. Our sense that consequences are closely tied to responsibility is so strong that people often must be reminded that you cannot work backward from all consequences to reveal responsibility. People must be reminded that "bad things happen to good people" without apparent reason (Kushner, 1997). Much early religion is based on the notion that one's fortune in life, including health, is tied to the morality of one's character.

Consequences have two sources, natural and imposed. Emphysema is a natural consequence of smoking; time in prison is an imposed consequence for burglary. When consequences are imposed, the legitimacy of the imposing agency is vital. In the legal system the imposition of consequences is an issue of retributive justice or deservedness, but there are other forms of consequence imposition. For example, "sin taxes" are a consequence imposed on smokers and drinkers, and other financial incentives are manipulated by the government to alter behavior.

This shows one aspect of the ethical reasoning behind not penalizing smokers in their health care. Smokers bear the burden of the consequences of their actions by getting ill; to impose consequences beyond those that occur naturally would require greater justification in the realm of retributive justice, showing that smokers deserved more consequences than those inherent in the act.

Hans Jonas (1984) provides a straightforward set of criteria for determining the responsibility for particular actions:

1. *Causality:* The act must cause the consequence.
2. *Control:* The agent must control the act.
3. *Foresight:* The agent must foresee the consequence.

All three conditions must be met to consider a person responsible for a specific act. Many legal tests of criminal responsibility can be related to these criteria. For example, the irresistible impulse standard used in about five states (Levine, 1998) for determining insanity clearly echoes Jonas's control criteria. Also, the M'Naghten test for insanity, which requires that the defendant lack the capacity to appreciate the difference between right and wrong, coincides with the Jonas requirement of foresight for responsibility (Slovenko, 1998). In this case, foresight is understood as the ability to see a moral wrong occurring as a consequence of the act. The model penal code for determining insanity in the United States combines both these criteria (Slovenko). An interesting additional test of insanity used only in New Hampshire, called the Durham test (Levine), finds that "a person is relieved of liability if his unlawful act is the product of a mental disease or defect" (Bienstock, 2003, p. 482), which essentially repeats Jonas's causality criteria by separating the person from his or her disorder. Using this standard, the mental disease is responsible, not the person.

The concepts of autonomy and responsibility are closely related. Beauchamp and Childress (2001) state that for a decision to be considered autonomous it must be intentional, occur with understanding, and be made without controlling influences. In these criteria, intention, which requires rationality and thus competence, is internal to the person whereas understanding and lack of influence are essential in the decision environment. Understanding is internal, but the information must be provided from the outside; the ability to understand and form intentions, that is to be competent, is internal. Responsibility requires competence to achieve foresight and lack of coercion to achieve control. Essentially, one must be acting autonomously to be responsible for an act. (See Table 6–3 for a comparison of the Jonas criteria with the criteria for autonomy and various criteria used to determine criminal responsibility. The elements of informed consent are also included in Table 6–3 because informed consent is the principle means for respecting autonomy.)

Table 6–3 Autonomy and Responsibility

	Criteria for:			
Autonomy	Informed Consent	Responsibility	Criminal Responsibility	Comments
		Causality	Did the person perform the act?	Criteria of autonomy and criminal responsibility bear on teleologic cause (i.e., intention)—why an act was done.
			Actus Reus (bad action)	
Intentional (competence)	Competent and gives authorization	Foresight	*Mens rea* (bad intent)	More knowledge confers greater responsibility. However, as the severity of consequences in-
With understanding	Clinician gives proper disclosure		Appreciation of wrongfulness	creases we tend to imbue more responsibility at lower levels of understanding.
Without coercion	Without coercion	Control	Irresistible impulse	The less influence, the more autonomous the decision. (That one's
			Act a product of mental disorder	decisions cannot be entirely without influence is a critique auton-
			Under duress?	omy; to decide is to sort among influences.)

POINTS OF ETHICAL TENSION IN FORENSIC PRACTICE

The principles and concepts presented in this chapter can be used to identify and categorize points needing discussion and clarification when facing specific situations or dilemmas or when formulating policy. In ethics, one proceeds by clarifying who the interested parties are; their interests, which can be based in the five principles; and precedent practice, and then discerning distinctions that need to be made using the key concepts. For example, for ethical justification of decisions regarding how much and what types of control are needed to maintain safety in specific situations with prisoners, a nurse may need to be able to distinguish between those who are dangerous and nondangerous, responsible and nonresponsible, and competent and noncompetent, as well as behavior indicating disorder from other kinds of bad behavior. This section will review some situations where an ethical decision must be made between alternative courses of action in forensic practice, including treatment vs. containment, privacy vs. safety, and treating vs. placating.

Treatment vs. Containment

Power is not equally distributed in the clinical relationship; the nurse has the power of greater knowledge and experience, whereas patients control specific knowledge of their condition and the emotional character of encounters. In addition to the usual power held by clinicians, mental health and forensic nurses can also bring socially sanctioned forms of physical force to bear. Although the nurse has most of what is considered the traditional power in the clinical relationship, the patient retains certain types of power that are always available to oppressed people. The patient can cooperate and create a situation where the encounter runs smoothly or the patient can be difficult and passive-aggressive, making the encounter difficult from the nurse's perspective. Although it seems counterproductive for patients to make life difficult for the clinician helping them, patients are often not willing participants, especially in mental health and forensic situations. Further, mere recognition of being in the lower position of an encounter is often enough to evoke an exertion of whatever power one does have available. Compliance issues can be viewed in this way.

In all clinical situations nurses are continuously making assessments regarding how much and what types of influence are appropriate to exert. Titrating the proper amount of influence is a central concern in mental health practice, where patients are habitually considered to have an impaired ability to make rational decisions in their own best interests, and so coercive treatment is routine. The concern over coercion is compounded in forensic practice with criminals because the severe coercion of incarceration is considered essential to community safety. Forensic nurses in prisons and similar settings must not only balance respecting patient–inmates' autonomy with a duty to act in their best interests and with a sense of caring concern, but also consider the safety interests of the community, including the prison community, which may be most at risk from an inmate's poorly controlled behavior. A further complication is that patient–inmates are in an exceptionally oppressive environment prior to and surrounding the clinical encounter. This environment colors and pervades all encounters in the prisoner's life, health-related and otherwise. So although the nurses have some control over the amount of influence that can be brought to bear depending on their clinical assessment and judgment, the patient–inmate remains in a highly coercive environment.

A relational approach can help the nurse examine a wide variety of factors that bear on the decision of how much influence is appropriate in specific situations. Briefly, the relational approach is a shift in emphasis onto the maintenance of an ethical relationship entailing positive obligation to the patient extending beyond simple honoring of patient rights. The relational approach makes these assumptions:

- *Influence is inherent in the clinical relationship:* The patient cannot be without influence from the clinician. If the focus is set too narrowly on respect for autonomy and liberty rights, then all forms of influence seem negative. However, a wider focus on clinical relations recognizes that patients want the nurse to use influence for their benefit. Influence is inherent in the concept of treatment. This confers a responsibility on the nurse to wield such influence ethically.
- *The factors relevant to treatment decisions and the use of influence are continuous, not dichotomous:* A too-narrow focus on preserving patient rights forces clinicians to consider relevant factors dichotomously. For example, competent patients have a right to refuse treatment, so to honor this right one must know whether the patient is competent or incompetent; no answer in between will do. Of course, this is not the way mental status and competence occur. To maintain an ethical relationship the nurse must recognize and balance competence and all other ethical factors as they occur on a continuum without imposing false dichotomy.
- *All decisions are subjective, and so the clinician, as a person, is a fundamental component of the situation:* Decisions made with a narrow focus on rights have the character of objectivity. In the relational approach, the application of influence in clinical relations arises from a particular relationship between that provider and that patient. Thus, determining ethical action is connected to the personhood of the clinician in the context of each unique relationship, highlighting the need to include the principle of caring concern (Olsen, 2003).

In many situations a nurse must consider increasing or decreasing the degree of influence exerted; in the prison setting influence may be contemplated for clinical care or for security. For example, finding that an patient–inmate who was previously undiagnosed with a mental disorder is now psychotic but declining treatment would prompt the nurse to bring increased influence to bear with the goal of better clinical treatment. In contrast, assessing that a patient–inmate with antisocial personality felt violent toward another inmate would prompt increased influence for security purposes. Assessing that a patient–inmate with schizophrenia had decompensated, possibly to a point where fellow inmates were at risk from delusional violence, would require the nurse to bring some influence to bear for both clinical and security reasons. A

Table 6–4 Ethical Justification of Clinical Decisions

Strength and nature of clinical relationship
The patient's mental state
The patient's willingness to participate
Potential for harm if treatment is not instituted
Degree of benefit from an intervention
Intensity of restriction or intrusion from the intervention
Intensity of the method used to exert influence
Degree of confidence in the intervention's efficacy

list of factors that can be brought to bear in considering the ethical justification of clinical decisions is found in Table 6–4.

- *Strength and nature of clinical relationship:* This provides the context within which all other factors are evaluated. Decisions made by a clinician who has just met a patient and spent an hour assessing him or her are different contextually from those made by a primary care provider who knows the patient well. In the relational approach all considerations are embedded in the actual relationship. Too strong a focus on patient rights deemphasizes differences in relationships, seeking a right answer that would apply regardless of the specific relationship.
- *The patient's mental state:* Greater impairment in a patient's mental status provides more justification for overriding a patient's decision. This is an area where the quality of the clinical relationship makes a critical difference. The nurse must take care to distinguish poor judgment due to impaired mental function from decisions with which the nurse disagrees. The greatest ethical error regarding this factor is to equate sound judgment with the agreement with the treatment plan.
- *The patient's willingness to participate:* More intensive interventions are justified when patients are willing recipients. Even restraint, the most restrictive intervention, can be applied without ethical conflict if the patient desires the intervention. This excludes cases where the intervention is clinically inappropriate or the patient's motives are not congruent with the therapeutic use of the intervention. However, assessing willingness must be an ongoing, open process because of the coercion inherent in clinical relationships and clinicians' bias to perceive patients as willing.
- *Potential for harm if a treatment is not instituted:* The greater the potential for harm, the more intensive the influence that is justified. This includes harm to the patient, others, and the community.
- *Degree of benefit from an intervention:* The greater the benefit, the more intense the influence that is justified.

- *Intensity of restriction or intrusion from the intervention:* More intrusive treatment requires stronger justification. A rough hierarchy of intensity of influence follows:
  1. Body movement (e.g., four-point restraint)
  2. Movement in space (e.g., seclusion rooms)
  3. Decisions of daily life (e.g., food, television, when to smoke, with whom to socialize, what to keep private)
  4. Meaningful activities (e.g., housing, work)
  5. Treatment choice (e.g., court-mandated treatment)
  6. Control of resources (e.g., use of money)
  7. Emotional or verbal expression (e.g., censorship, social expectation) (Olsen, 1998)

Restraint is the most intensely restrictive and intrusive intervention available to the clinician, so it requires the highest level of justification.

- *Intensity of the method used to exert influence:* More intensive forms of exerting influence require a higher level justification. A rough hierarchy of intensity in methods used to influence a patient might be:
  1. Physical force
  2. Manipulation of resources (e.g., access to privileges)
  3. Manipulation of social forces (e.g., access to other inmates, telling inmates that compliance with treatment reflects well on them)
  4. Social pressure (e.g., arranging peer pressure, men wear neckties and not skirts); some mental disorders might be seen as an insensitivity to this influence
  5. Advice (e.g., psychotherapy) (Olsen, 1998)

Again, as the most restrictive measure, physical force requires the strongest justification, usually eminent substantial harm to specific persons.

- *Degree of confidence in the intervention's efficacy:* The lower the probability of an intervention's beneficial effect, the less justification for coercion.

In making a decision regarding the increase or decrease in the use of influence, including extreme forms of coercion, seclusion from others, restraint, or forced medication, all relevant factors should be considered. In this list of relevant factors the patient's position on the continuum represented by each factor bears on the justification of an intervention exerting influence, but no single factor is definitive. Nor is a simple formula sufficient when factors are seen as continuous rather than dichotomous. The balance of all relevant factors should be weighed. The list presented here is not necessarily exhaustive. Each use of influence changes the moral tone of the relationship. So although putting a patient–inmate in restraints may be justified, the nurse must maintain an ethical relationship with that person. The nurse bears the moral weight of the responsibility inherent in holding great power over others and the charge to use that power for their good.

Privacy vs. Safety

The two broad areas where privacy is considered are privacy of information and privacy of person. Privacy of information, also referred to as confidentiality, is most closely tied to respect for autonomy because it is maintained by giving patients control over the flow of information about them. Privacy of person is closely tied to contextual caring in that the bodily exposure and exposure of the most intimate and personal aspects of daily life, such as excretion and bathing, that occur in nursing care require the nurse to extend deep personal trust, at times compelling a type of closeness the patient will have with few others.

Control over personal presentation is a central mechanism of identity, serving as a basis for social relations (Bok, 1983; Goffman, 1973). Thus some privacy of person is needed to develop and maintain a sense of personhood (Reiman, 1984). Privacy provides a boundary between self and others and allows limitations and controls to be placed on what is presented publicly and what is shown to intimates. Private time and space allows expression of characteristics and desires that one does not wish to reveal publicly. When others view what the society considers private, embarrassment and shame are experienced (Levy, 1983; Lynd, 1958). An inability to maintain some secrecy about aspects of the self can result in a profound loss of identity (Bok). The experience of shame and embarrassment from public exposure of the private is a cross-cultural phenomenon (Levy), and virtually all cultures have some accommodation for individual privacy (Moore, 1984).

Although prisoners may have issues with privacy of information, it is privacy of person that is especially compelling during incarceration. Prison is extraordinary in the degree to which privacy of person is denied. Indeed, extreme denials of privacy have been used as a method of breaking down political prisoners (Caplan, 1982).

As with other constraints on forensic practice, nurses working in prisons will make ethical decisions regarding patient privacy embedded within a context of unusually little privacy of both information and person. This will influence not only the nurse's decisions, but also the way the nurse's behavior is viewed by the patient–inmates. The forensic nurse will want to maintain privacy of person to the greatest degree feasible as a sign of respect for the patient. However, this will be significantly curtailed from what is expected in nonforensic clinical encounters. Patient–inmates may be required to undergo searches or observation by nonclinicians that would be unthinkable in nonforensic practice.

Incursions on privacy can be considered a form of influence because the exposure of person or revelation of information that a patient–inmate prefers to keep private denies autonomy and restricts choices. This means the guide to considering other forms of influence can be used. Anticipation is the best way to keep losses of privacy respectful and for the loss of privacy to be distributed fairly among the entire prison population. All parties should be aware in advance what information and in what situations the patient–inmate can expect privacy to be maintained, the extent and types of exposure that will occur during clinical encounters, and what information the nurse will feel compelled to report.

Treating vs. Placating

Incarcerated people have higher rates of diagnosable mental illnesses, including depression and anxiety disorders, than the general population (Baillargeon et al., 2000; Teplin, 1990). In the United Kingdom, 16% of inmates were found to suffer from depression (Mitchison et al., 1994). Further, the rate of treatment for those with depressive disorders in prison was found to be higher than the treatment rate in the general population (Baillargeon et al., 2001).

However, the circumstances resulting in incarceration and the situation of the imprisonment itself can be expected to produce reactions much like many of those described in DSM-IV for the identification of a depressed patient—difficulty sleeping, irritability, depressed mood, alterations in weight, feelings of worthlessness, and difficulty concentrating (American Psychiatric Association, 2000). The current recommendation regarding the diagnosing of depression is to treat the disorder where the symptoms exist, even in the context of extreme life circumstances such as terminal illness (Massie, Gagnon, & Holland, 1994).

Patient–inmates may want to take medications for a variety of reasons— to cure or ameliorate symptoms, which is the usual socially accepted motivation; out of boredom; or to continue a pattern of using substances as a panacea begun and reinforced by participation in a drug-abusing subculture. Simply raising the issue creates awareness that there is no firm line between symptoms and reactions to life circumstances. Further, particularly in regard to mental disorders, reactions to life circumstances may be the disorder. Indeed, this is the definition of post-traumatic stress disorder (APA, 2000).

The epistemological maneuver that real illnesses are biological is unsatisfactory because all behaviors, even malingering, reflect biologically distinct brain states (Olsen, 2000). This controversy has been avoided by some managed care companies in reference to decisions about what treatment for aberrant behaviors should be reimbursed as "mental disorders" by saying that "real" disorders are those found in the DSM (Sabin & Daniels, 1994).

The forensic nurse confronted with a request for psychotropic medications may sense that the patient desires the drugs for inappropriate reasons, particularly when certain categories of medications, such as benzodiazepines, are requested. The nurse faces several difficult issues in distinguishing appropriate from inappropriate motivations—respecting the patient's autonomy; demonstrating care for the patient despite denying a request; beneficence, in the sense that the nurse wants to address any underlying problem; and care of the community, because overly easy or restrictive access to medications will adversely affect the entire inmate population.

As discussed earlier, the nurse should be willing to examine his or her own feelings about whether perception of patient volition in creating or bringing about the clinical circumstances affects judgments regarding the "reality" of the condition. Fabrication of symptoms should not result in medicating the fabricated symptoms, but the nurse should remain aware that the motivation to fabricate symptoms is itself a cause for concern and possibly a "legitimate" disorder—just not the one the patient is reporting. Unfortunately, many cases will be clouded—not complete fabrication, but not fully forthright disclosure. Further, the nurse should be aware that some reports may result from differing assumptions between the nurse and the patient–inmate regarding the level and type of distress for which medication is appropriate, particularly symptoms like anxiety or insomnia that are ubiquitous problems and are often identified as disorders by degree of severity.

THE UNHAPPY PRISONER

The following case brings together many of the issues discussed in this chapter: the balance of respect for autonomy and beneficence, deciding the correct degree of coercion in treatment, contextual caring in the face of difficult or even repulsive behavior, the effect on the clinician of feeling the patient–inmate is deliberately causing a problem, what is illness and what is bad behavior, and honoring or denying a patient–inmate's request for medications. This case is not far-fetched, unusual, or exotic, and is drawn from actual practice. There are no easy answers, but reflection on the events in light of the issues raised in this chapter will help the reader to clarify his or her feelings about the issues.

Johnny was a 25-year-old Black Haitian man who was in the custody of the State Department of Corrections for 3 years following a conviction on a robbery charge. His incarceration ended with suicide 2 months after being transferred to the state's oldest and most secure facility. Prior to transfer he was prescribed psychotropic medication; following transfer medication was discontinued.

Johnny had two prior arrests on unknown charges. He was also in and out of treatment at his local community mental health center and had three documented inpatient psychiatric admissions for unknown diagnoses. Shortly after his arrest he was sent to the State Hospital for the Criminally Insane. He spent 2 months at this facility. His discharge diagnoses were: Depression, Alcohol Abuse, Cocaine Abuse, Opiod Abuse, Malingering, and Borderline Personality with Histrionic and Narcissistic Traits.

Johnny's time in prison was marked by severe behavioral and social problems. He frequently demonstrated intimidation, violence, self-mutilation, threats of self-mutilation, and feigned symptoms. His prison record reveals numerous offenses for which he was disciplined. Over a period of 2.5 years there were 35 infractions including:

Five assaults
Seven fighting
Six destruction of property
Six self-mutilation
Two arson
Disobedience
Malingering
Theft
Contraband

The 6 months prior to his death were a particularly difficult period. He spent most of this time in isolation. His record while in isolation reflects numerous requests for medication, and behavioral acting out. He was frequently noted in the medical record to be feigning symptoms, including EPS and psychosis. He often refused medications in whole or in part.

When his wishes were not gratified he would lash out at staff with spiteful anger, for example, ripping up his isolation mattress or defecating on the floor. Staffs' attitude is illustrated in the following nurse's note, "He likes to whine a lot and tries to get other people to feel sorry for him."

During the period prior to his transfer to maximum security, an effort was made to keep him compliant by tying medications to privileges. Despite this, his compliance was sporadic and the medications became the focus of intense struggle. Johnny sometimes reported that the medications helped him "calm down."

During this period the nurse practitioner supervising his care, Ms. Green, repeatedly documented that the vigor of his acting out was significantly less when on medication. In the medical record she stated:

- *"Pt. has been compliant to meds for at least 48 hours. He now reports being aware of his aggression and impulsivity and articulates that his meds help this."*
- *"He becomes more impulsive and more assaultive the longer he is non-compliant to prescribed medication regime including Klonapin, Tegretol or a neuroleptic. . . ."*

After transfer to the maximum security facility his new clinician, Ms. Blue, PNP, made the following notations in the medical record:

- *At transfer: "I think that routine, somewhat impersonal, handling might help this individual grow up."*
- *A month later and a week prior to his suicide on a form titled "Prisoner Request for Mental Health Services": "Meds discontinued due to non-compliance. Will monitor off meds and make appropriate diagnosis."*

SUMMARY

Forensic practice is by necessity very close to legal matters, but the forensic nurse should remain mindful that ethics and law, although closely related, are different. Lawful practice requires knowing the laws and following them. Ethical practice is a process best conducted by knowing and using the available tools, principles, and concepts to guide daily behavior and clinical relationships, and to reason through and justify actions and solutions. Memorizing what is right and what is wrong and then acting in accordance will not do; one must engage in the process. The best approach to creating an ethical practice environment is to anticipate problems and react to the inevitable occurrence of problems. This can be done by widely discussing the social and personal values and ethical issues either in advance or as they arise within an agreed-on, fair procedure for achieving consensus regarding how specific situations will be approached within that practice environment, creating policies where needed.

QUESTIONS FOR DISCUSSION

1. If caring concern for patients is one of the benefits of good nursing care, are there potential barriers to achieving this when caring for forensic patients? And how might a nurse overcome the barriers?
2. What are some problems that might occur when applying Western bioethical principles to persons from non-Western cultures?
3. How does recognition that psychiatric diagnosis is, at least in part, socially constructed inform the practice of forensic nursing?
4. How would you balance the community's need for security and the individual's right to treatment in the case of "the unhappy prisoner" found at the end of this chapter?
5. Use the factors for considering the ethical justification of clinical decisions to discuss the decisions made about "the unhappy prisoner."
6. How would you use ethical principles and justifications in deciding on a course of action in the case of a patient making a questionable request for medication?

REFERENCES

Alexander, V., Bursztajn, H., Brodsky, A., Hamm, R., Gutheil, T., & Levi, L. (1991). Involuntary commitment. In: T. Gutheil, H. Bursztajn, A. Brodsky & V. Alexander (Eds). *Decision making in psychiatry and the law.* Baltimore: Williams & Wilkins, pp. 89–107.

Altman, D. (1982). *The homosexualization of America.* New York: St. Martin's Press.

American Academy of Psychiatry and the Law. (1995). *Ethical guidelines for the practice of forensic psychiatry.* Bloomfield, CT: AAPL.

American Nurses Association. (1995*). Position statement: Nurses' participation in capital punishment.* Washington, DC: American Nurses Publishing.

American Psychiatric Association. (2000). *Diagnostic and statistical manual of mental disorders* (4th ed., text rev). Washington, DC: American Psychiatric Association.

Andreasen, N., Swayze, V., Flaum, M., Yates, W., Arndt, S., & McChesney, C. (1990). Ventricular enlargement in schizophrenia evaluated with computed tomographic scanning. Effects of gender, age, and stage of illness. *Archives of General Psychiatry, 47,* 1008–1015.

Aristotle. (1935). *Aristotle.* (Wheelwright, P., Trans.) New York: Odyssey Press.

Arrestee Drug Abuse Monitoring Program. (2000). Annual report 2000. U.S. Justice Department, Washington, DC. Retrieved August 27, 2003, from http://www.ncjrs.org/pdffiles1/nij/193013.pdf.

Baillargeon, J., Black, S., Contreras, S., Grady, J., & Pulvino, J. (2001). Antidepressant prescribing patterns for prison inmates with depressive disorders. *Journal of Affective Disorders, 63*(1–3), 225–231.

Baillargeon, J., Black, S., Pulvino, J., & Dunn, K. (2000). The disease profile of Texas prison inmates. *Annals of Epidemiology, 10,* 74–80.

Beauchamp T. & Childress J. (2001). *Principles of biomedical ethics* (5th ed). New York: Oxford University Press.

Beecher-Monas, E. & Garcia-Rill, E. (1999). The law and the brain: Judging scientific evidence of intent. *The Journal of Appellate Practice and Process, 1,* 243–277.

Benner P. & Wrubel J. (1989). *The primacy of caring.* Menlo Park, CA: Addison-Wesley.

Bienstock, S. (2003). Mothers who kill their children and postpartum psychosis. *Southwestern University Law Review, 32,* 451–499.

Bok, S. (1983). *Secrets: On the ethics of concealment and revelation.* New York: Vintage.

Caplan, A. (1982). On privacy and confidentiality in social science research. In T. Beauchamp, R. Faden, R. Wallace, & L. Walters (Eds.), *Ethical Issues in Social Science Research.* Baltimore, MD: Johns Hopkins Press, pp. 315–325.

Cassel, E. (1976). What is the function of medicine? In S. Gorovitz, R. Macklin, A. Jameton, J. Oconnor, & S. Sherwin (Eds.), *Moral Problems in Medicine* (2nd ed.). Englewood Cliffs, NJ: Prentice-Hall, pp. 73–78.

Chamberlain, J. (1985). An ex-patient's response to Soliday. *The Journal of Nervous and Mental Disease, 173,* 289–290.

Frankena, W. (1973). *Ethics* (2nd ed.). Englewood Cliffs, NJ: Prentice-Hall.

Gastmans, C. (1999). Care as a moral attitude in nursing. *Nursing Ethics, 6,* 214–223.

Gastmans, C., Dierckx de Casterlé, B., & Schotsmans, P. (1998). Nursing considered as moral practice: A philosophical-ethical interpretation of nursing. *Kennedy Institute Ethics Journal, 8,* 43–69.

Goffman, E. (1973). *The presentation of self in everyday life.* Woodstock, NY: Overlook Press.

Greenfield, L. (1998). An analysis of national data on the prevalence of alcohol involvement in crime. National Symposium on Alcohol Abuse and Crime, U.S. Department of Justice. Retrieved April 27, 2003, from http://www.ojp.usdoj.gov/bjs/pub/pdf/ac.pdf.

Jonas, H. (1984). *The imperative of responsibility: In search of an ethics for a technological age.* Chicago: University of Chicago Press.

Kant, I. (1959). Foundations of the metaphysics of morals. (L. Beck, Trans.). New York: Macmillan. (Original work published 1785.)

Kushner, H. (1997). *When bad things happen to good people.* New York: Schocken Books.

Levine, A. (1998). Denying the settled insanity defense: Another necessary step in dealing with drug and alcohol abuse. *Boston University Law Review, 75,* 78–103.

Levy, R. (1983). Self and emotion. *Ethos—Journal of the Society for Psychological Anthropology, 11*(3), 128–134.

Lynd, H. (1958). *On shame and the search for identity.* New York: Harcourt Brace.

Mason, T. (2002). Forensic psychiatric nursing: A literature review and thematic analysis of role tensions. *Journal of Psychiatric and Mental Health Nursing, 9,* 511–520.

Massie, M., Gagnon, P., & Holland, J. (1994). Depression and suicide in patients with cancer. *Journal of Pain & Symptom Management, 9*(5), 325–340.

Mill J. (1985). *On liberty.* New York: Penguin.

Moore, B. (1984). *Privacy: Studies in social and cultural history.* Armonk, NY: M.E. Sharpe.

Morse, S. (1999). Craziness and criminal responsibility. *Behavioral Sciences & the Law, 17*(2), 147–164.

National Commission for the Protection of Human Subjects of Biomedical and Behavioral Research. (1979). *The Belmont report: Ethical principles and guidelines for the protection of human participants of research.* Washington, DC: OPPR Reports. A6-14. Retrieved August 27, 2003, from http://ohrp.osophs.dhhs.gov/humanparticipants/guidance/belmont.htm.

Nortvedt, P. (1996). *Sensitive judgment: Nursing moral philosophy and the ethics of care.* Oslo: Tano Aschehoug.

Olsen, D. (1997a). The development of an instrument measuring the cognitive structure used to understand personhood in patients. *Nursing Research, 46,* 78–83.

Olsen, D. (1997b). When the patient causes the problem: The effect of patient responsibility on the nurse-patient relationship. *Journal of Advanced Nursing, 26,* 515–522.

Olsen, D. (1998). Toward an ethical standard for coerced mental health treatment: Least restrictive or most therapeutic? *Journal of Clinical Ethics, 9,* 235–246.

Olsen, D. (2000). Policy implications of the biological model of mental disorder. *Nursing Ethics, 7,* 412–424.

Olsen, D. (2003). Influence and coercion: Relational and rights based ethical approaches to forced psychiatric treatment. *Journal of Psychiatric and Mental Health Nursing, 10,* 705–711.

Peternelj-Taylor C. & Johnson R. (1995). Serving time: Psychiatric mental health nursing in corrections. *Journal of Psychosocial Nursing, 33*(3), 12–19.

Plato. (1926). *Plato: Cratylus, Parmenides, Greater Hippias, Lesser Hippias* (H. Fowler, Trans.). (Loeb Classical Library, No 167). St. Edmundsbury, Suffolk, UK: St. Edmundsbury Press.

Reiman, J. (1984). Privacy, intimacy, and personhood. In F. Schoeman (Ed.), *Philosophical dimensions of privacy.* London: Cambridge University Press, pp. 330–316.

Sabin, J. & Daniels, N. (1994). Determining "medical necessity" in mental health practice. *Hastings Center Report, 24*(6), 5–13.

Slovenko, R. (1998). The mental disability requirement in the insanity defense. *Behavioral Sciences & the Law, 17,* 165–180.

Soliday, S. (1985). A comparison of patient and staff attitudes toward seclusion. *The Journal of Nervous and Mental Disease 173,* 282–286.

Strong, C. (2000). Specified principlism: What is it, and does it really resolve cases better than casuistry? *The Journal of Medicine and Philosophy 25*(3), 323–341.

Tasman A., Kay J., & Lieberman J. (1997) *Psychiatry.* Philadelphia: Harcourt Brace.

Teplin, L. (1990). The prevalence of severe mental disorder among male urban jail detainees: Comparison with the epidemiologic catchment area program. *American Journal of Public Health, 80,* 663–669.

U.S. Department of Justice. (2000a). *Jail populations by race and ethnicity, 1990–2000.* Retrieved September 27, 2003, from http://www.ojp.usdoj.gov/bjs/glance/tables/jailracetab.htm.

U.S. Department of Justice. (2000b). *Violent crimes by race of victim.* Retrieved September 27, 2003, from http://www.ojp.usdoj.gov/bjs/glance/race.htm.

Vetlesen, A. (1994). *Perception, empathy, and judgment: An inquiry into the preconditions of moral performance.* University Park, PA: Pennsylvania State University Press.

Working Group for the Study of Ethics in International Nursing Research. (2003). Ethical considerations in international nursing research: A report from the International Centre for Nursing Ethics. *Nursing Ethics, 10,* 122–137.

Overview of the American Justice System

Bonnie R. Bentley Cewe

By its very nature, forensic nursing requires regular interaction with some aspect of the American justice system. A clear understanding of the various courts, their jurisdictions, and the stages of proceedings is vital. This chapter provides an overview of the trial process and the requirements for admissibility of evidence. The standards for expert witness testimony are also addressed.

CHAPTER FOCUS

History of the Anglo-American justice system
Sources of lawmaking power and laws
Overview of the federal and state court systems
Case procedure
Evidence standards
Overview of criminal procedure
Civil litigation

KEY TERMS

case in chief
civil litigation
closing argument
competence
Daubert
evidence
expert witness
Frye

habeas corpus
jurisdiction
jury nullification
lay witness
opening statement
relevance
reliability
venue
voire dire

INTRODUCTION

Students of forensic nursing likely will, at some point during their careers, be called upon to testify in a court of law and, thus, should possess at least a basic understanding of the American system of justice and court structure. Insight into the processing of cases and the application of the information presented in this chapter will undoubtedly aid the forensic nurse by providing the legal context within which forensic nursing is practiced. The forensic nurse's credibility within the legal system, with other practicing professionals, and with a judge or jury might seriously be diminished by an unfortunate display of lack of awareness of the details of the legal system.

Time and space constraints limit this discussion to a basic overview of the justice system, both federal and state, civil and criminal. Ideally a more specific understanding of the legal system and a rudimentary appreciation for the laws of a particular jurisdiction in which the forensic nurse will practice should be sought. The most effective way to become familiar with the workings of the legal system is to spend some time observing the proceedings in criminal and civil courtrooms during daily court activities and especially during trials. The roles of the forensic nurse as consultant and expert witness require a thorough understanding of the proceedings and procedures of the court, as well as the statutory requirements that must be met for a case to go forward in either criminal or civil court. The roles of the expert witness within the legal system are discussed in more detail in Chapter 22.

HISTORY

After some early colonial attempts at legal systems based on the philosophies, customs, and needs of the particular colonies, convenience and necessity led colonists ultimately to pattern early American jurisprudence on the legal system of England. That system, based on the rights of the individual granted in the Magna Carta, was further developed to encompass the fundamental freedoms outlined in the Bill of Rights of the U.S. Constitution. Those rights, including the right not to be deprived of life, liberty, or property without due process of law; the right to equal protection under the law; the right to an impartial jury; and the right to confront one's accusers, serve as linchpins of our American justice system.

The system of justice in the United States is an "adversarial" system; that is, there exist two sides in a case, each of which presents its own point of view. *Black's Law Dictionary* defines an adversarial system as "characterized by opposing parties who contend against each other for a result favorable to themselves" (*Black's*, 1999). Consequently, each side of a dispute must present evidence in support of his or her side of the case. Simultaneously, each side strives to challenge, limit, or object to the evidence presented by the other side. Courtroom and evidence rules and procedures help to keep the proceedings fair and to prevent questionable facts from being presented to the jury. The case is carried out in front of a neutral judge whose job is to ensure that such rules and procedures are followed. When all the facts have been presented it is up to the trier of fact, usually a jury, to weigh the facts and reach a conclusion about the case.

Some countries have what is called an "inquisitional" type of justice system. This means that in those countries the defendant is assumed to be guilty. Questions and proceedings may follow any number of tactics, but the accused essentially must prove his or her innocence. Conversely, the American justice system, as an "accusatorial system," assumes the defendant is innocent unless and until guilt is proven. In an accusatorial system the defendant is identified as having caused a harm, either civil or criminal, but the burden of proof rests on the accuser to prove guilt.

In a criminal trial the justice system has developed a series of steps that must be followed according to specific rules so the rights of the parties are upheld while society attempts to prove the case against the defendant. As everyone who watches television knows, the standard of proof for a criminal trial is "beyond a reasonable doubt." That proof must be in the form of evidence that is obtained in an appropriate manner without violating the rights of the accused. Also, the constitutional right against self-incrimination means that the defendant has an absolute right to remain silent concerning criminal charges. It cannot be stressed enough that a defendant's silence cannot be interpreted negatively. The state also has the burden of persuasion in most instances in a criminal trial because of the defendant's fundamental rights.

Civil trials proceed differently than criminal trials, as will be discussed briefly in this chapter. Because there is no criminal wrongdoing at question and the state is not bringing the charges, many of the individual protections of the Bill of Rights do not apply. In addition, the burden of proof in a civil case is "more likely than not." Thus, because the accusation must be proved only by a predominance of the evidence, a person could be found liable in civil court using evidence that would not meet the burden of proof in a criminal case. One of the most prominent examples of this potential disparity in trial outcome is the O.J. Simpson cases. O.J. Simpson was tried for the murders of his ex-wife, Nicole Brown, and an acquaintance. After months of highly publicized testimony, Simpson was acquitted of all criminal charges related to their deaths. Several months later a civil case was held, charging Simpson with the two untimely deaths. A jury found Simpson civilly liable for the two deaths and awarded the families $30 million (*Louis H. Brown, Estate of Nicole Brown Simpson v. Orenthal James Simpson,* 1995).

SOURCES OF LAWMAKING POWERS AND LAWS

The United States Constitution establishes the framework for our federal system of government by allocating power between the federal and state governments. Likewise, the constitution of each state creates the framework for that state's government. A fundamental principle in both the federal and state constitutions is the separation of powers between the legislative, judicial, and executive branches of government. Although lawmaking powers primarily are the province of the legislative branch, in practice, all three branches perform some manner of lawmaking function.

The federal and state legislatures create law by enacting statutes in accordance with the authority granted to them by the federal and state constitutions. The legislatures frequently delegate lawmaking power to the executive branch by statutorily authorizing executive agencies to issue rules and regulations designed to help implement statutory schemes. The judicial branch, in the context of legal disputes between or among parties, develops law by interpreting and applying the provisions of constitutions and statutes and by developing and applying common law.

The federal and state courts administer laws that actually originate from several sources. These various sources of law—constitutional, statutory, common, and case—often must be synthesized. Synthesis requires that the various sources are read together and in light of each other in order to obtain a full and clear understanding of how a particular "law" is to be interpreted and applied.

Sources of Constitutional Law

The U.S. Constitution enumerates rights to which the citizens of this nation are entitled, including certain rights applicable in any federal or state courts of law. The U.S. Constitution was drafted in response to actions by the government upon the citizenry. The federal system was designed to limit such governmental intrusion by dividing sovereign power between a central (federal) government, which would coordinate issues of interest to all the states, and state governments, recognized as representing local interests and opinions. Although the U.S. Constitution clearly identifies and guarantees certain rights of the people under the federal sovereign, when the Bill of Rights was written it applied only to the actions of the federal government; initially, states were not required to guarantee these enumerated rights. Subsequent amendment of the Constitution required that states act in accordance with maintaining those basic, individual rights. In addition to the U.S. Constitution, the constitutions of individual states set forth the rights of persons in each state. Although state constitutions may provide protections equal to or greater than those afforded by the federal Constitution, they cannot infringe upon or eliminate any right granted by the U.S. Constitution. In fact, many state constitutions currently provide greater rights and protections to individuals residing in those states than the U.S. Constitution. These constitutional protections form the standard against which all statutes, regulations, rules, and procedures must be measured.

Common Law

Common law, or "judge-made" law, as it also is known, was developed over centuries. Numerous cases, involving different factual situations, came before judges for decision. Eventually judgments became more uniform, reflecting legal principles that were derived from the usages and customs of the people, affirmed and enforced by the courts. Common law consists of legal principles created and developed by the courts independent of legislative enactments. The common law developed and applied by American courts has its roots in the English common law. In England such law came to be known as "common law" because it applied generally throughout medieval England and, thus, replaced a less uniform system of customary law dispensed in local or regional courts and in the private courts of feudal lords.

Although the courts in each state are free to develop the common law of that state in a manner that reflects local policies, to a surprising degree, federal courts and courts in different states share common views on general principles of law. Although some variation is inevitable, the legal methods employed by courts in deciding and developing common law do not vary substantially. This consistency is due in part to the fact that the decisions of the court are "inspired by natural reason and an innate sense of justice" (Mosk, 1988). In addition, the consistency with which cases are decided results in large part from the doctrine of *stare decisis*, which is grounded in the belief that "security and certainty require that accepted and established legal principles, under which rights may accrue, be recognized and followed" (*Otter Trail Power Co. v. Von Bank,* 1942). Accordingly, once a court has established a principle of law that is applicable to a certain set of facts, future courts should adhere to that principle and apply it in similar future cases unless the court subsequently finds that justice requires otherwise.

Legislation

The third source of law in the United States is the legislatures. Consistent with their role as the primary policy-making body, federal and state legislatures enact laws, known as statutes, to address problems that they have concluded were not adequately addressed by the common law. Some statutes were enacted to fill gaps in the body of common law; some statutes altered rights or obligations as defined by common law. Because the legislature is the paramount lawmaking authority, a legislative enactment supersedes common law if a discrepancy exists between the sources of law. Today, the causes of action in civil cases and criminal charges are primarily outlined in state statutes. Over time, legislatures have created comprehensive bodies of legislation known as codes. A code, as distinguished from a statute, contains a systematic compilation of related enactments. Today, federal and state legislation has so proliferated that most American jurisdictions are now code jurisdictions. Every forensic nurse is likely familiar with the codes that establish licensing and professional standards within each state.

The forensic nurse is often called upon to act as an advocate to the legislature during the development of its laws and regulations. For example, testimony by nurses at a hearing committee before a final vote has had significant impact on legislation in areas such as victim's rights, domestic violence and partner abuse, and standardization of sexual assault examinations. Recent testimony before U.S. Senate subcommittees regarding the need for mandated training and funding for sexual assault examiners is another way in which the forensic nurse has had an impact on important legislation.

Case Law

As federal and state courts are called upon to decide disputes brought before them, they must often interpret the necessarily general terms of constitutional and statutory law and apply those terms to the facts of a dispute. The opinions of such courts serve as vehicles for developing and articulating general legal rules or principles, known as case law. Constitutional provisions and statutes, federal or state, thus must be read in conjunction with the decisions of the courts that have issued opinions pertaining to those provisions or statutes. Decisions by higher courts establish precedent upon which case law is built. Once an issue has been decided by a higher court for a particular factual scenario, all lower courts within that jurisdiction are required to follow that decision in cases of similar facts. The decision of the higher court is said to be "binding authority" for the lower courts. The decisions of one state are not binding on the courts of other states; however, if a state court is confronted with a legal question novel to that jurisdiction, decisions in other states may provide guidance and serve as a basis for a new rule of law.

OVERVIEW OF THE FEDERAL AND STATE COURT SYSTEMS

Two separate but interrelated court systems coexist in the United States. Article III of the U.S. Constitution establishes the federal courts and the areas of law that can be tried in those courts. The federal system includes the United States Supreme Court, established by the U.S. Constitution, and the federal district courts, courts of appeal, and several specialized courts of limited jurisdiction, allowed for in the U.S. Constitution and established by Congress. State courts, created by the states, hold the residuum of jurisdiction. State court structure and jurisdiction is the sole responsibility of the states. State decisions cannot be overturned by the federal court unless the state has based its decision on an erroneous interpretation of the U.S. Constitution.

Most court systems in the United States function as a hierarchy; that is, there are "supreme" courts that make final decisions in appeals of disputes brought to lower courts. Most states and the federal system also have an intermediate court to which a party can appeal if there are questions about the verdict in a case. Cases are first heard at the "entry level." In the federal system, these are the district courts. In states, lawsuits or prosecutions are brought in courts of "limited jurisdiction" or "general jurisdiction." Limited jurisdiction includes minor courts that hear a wide range of cases, such as police courts, small claims courts, and magistrate's courts. General jurisdiction courts hear most of the criminal cases in the states. All trial courts, whether federal or state, are "courts of record." This means that a verbatim record is kept of each proceeding.

Federal Court Jurisdiction

The intricacies of federal jurisdiction are such that most schools of law offer a separate course on the subject. Thus, this section merely contains an overview of the federal court system and the jurisdiction of those courts. In general, the U.S. Constitution limits the jurisdiction of the federal courts to: cases arising under the U.S. Constitution and laws of the United States, and treaties made under their authority; cases affecting ambassadors, consuls, and public ministers; admiralty and maritime cases; and cases in which a citizen of one state is suing a citizen of another state.

The basic structure of the federal court system consists of three layers: the trial courts of general federal jurisdiction known as district courts, the 13 courts of appeals known as circuit courts, and the Supreme Court. There also are specialized trial courts, such as the Claims Court, the Tax Court, and the Court of International Trade, and appellate courts, such as the Court of Military Appeals and the Temporary Emergency Court of Appeals.

The United States District Courts

All 50 states have at least one federal district court within their borders. A greater volume of cases in some states, including New York and California, necessitated the creation of additional federal districts within the state. In addition, there are federal district courts in the District of Columbia and the United States territories of Puerto Rico, Guam, the Virgin Islands, and the Northern Mariana Islands. In all, there are 99 federal district courts in the United States and its territories.

In order for a civil case to be brought in a federal district court the case must "arise under" federal law, involve a "federal question," or involve maritime law or parties from different states. An action "arises under" federal law only if the complaint seeks a remedy expressly granted by a federal statute or if resolution of the issue requires construction of the statute, or if the statute embodies a distinct policy that requires federal legal principles to control its disposition (*Black's,* 1999). "Federal question jurisdiction includes cases arising under the United States Constitution, Acts of Congress, or treaties, and involving their interpretation and application" (*Black's*). Additionally, with the exception of crimes committed by members of the military, all criminal prosecutions for violations of federal law are brought in federal district courts. District court cases are heard by a single judge (with a jury where one has been rightfully demanded) except in rare types of cases where a three-judge panel may hear the case, or in cases of special significance, where all the judges of a particular district may choose to sit together on a case *en banc,* or "as one."

The United States Circuit Courts

The United States circuit courts derive their name from the early days of the federal court system when circuit judges literally "rode circuit," traveling throughout the area of the court and holding sessions in the major towns and cities therein. There are 13 courts of appeals assigned to the 11 "circuits" or areas into which the country is divided, plus a circuit for the District of Columbia and a special appellate court called the Federal Circuit. This Federal Circuit has limited jurisdiction to hear appeals involving patents or contract claims against the federal government, all appeals from the Claims Court and the Court of International Trade, plus several other special categories of cases.

The caseload of the circuit courts consists of the appeals brought by litigants who lost in the federal district courts. Such litigants may take an appeal as a matter of right to the court of appeals serving that particular district. The circuit, or appellate, courts do not hear such cases anew, or *de novo,* rather, they review the records of district court cases to determine whether errors were made during the trial. Thus, the appellate courts consider legal issues in the context of little more than a bare outline of the human drama that has preceded the appellate litigation. Normally, cases are heard by panels of three judges in the circuit courts, although, in certain cases of particular importance, all or a substantial number of judges may sit *en banc.*

The United States Supreme Court

As the only court in the federal court system to be specifically established by the U.S. Constitution, the U.S. Supreme Court sits atop the federal court hierarchy. Although certain cases may be filed directly in the Supreme Court, such as cases in which one state is suing another state, most cases brought to the Supreme Court seek review of the judgments of lower courts. Figure 7–1 depicts the flow of cases to the Supreme Court. Most of these cases are appeals from the judgments of either federal courts of appeals or of state courts of last resort that dealt with questions of federal law. In a few types of cases, which are becoming increasingly rare, the Supreme Court hears an appeal from a district court without any intermediate appeal to the circuit court. The Supreme Court has the discretion to refuse to hear the vast majority of cases in which review is sought. Most cases that are appealed to the Supreme Court are refused a hearing. Each case is heard in the Supreme Court by the nine Supreme Court justices. On rare occasions a case may be heard by fewer justices,

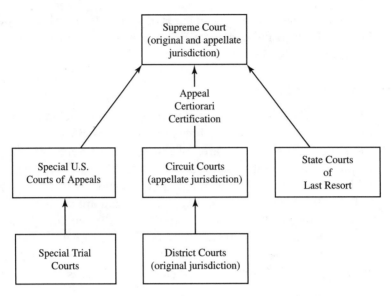

Figure 7–1   The flow of cases to the United States Supreme Court.

but the quorum is never fewer than six. The U.S. Supreme Court is the final arbiter of federal law and federal constitutional issues.

State Court Jurisdiction

State courts are courts of general jurisdiction and are governed by state law. They are subject only to specific limitations set forth in the U.S. Constitution or by acts of Congress. Most states have a tri-level court structure that is similar to the federal court system: trial-level courts that possess general jurisdiction; intermediate appellate-level courts that hear appeals taken from trial-level cases; and a high appellate court, often called the state supreme court, or court of last resort. Figure 7–2 shows the structure of the tri-level state court system established in Connecticut, which is typical of many state systems. Some states have only a high appellate court, with no intermediate appellate courts. Like the federal court system, state court systems also typically have several courts of limited jurisdiction called "inferior courts," which hear only specified matters.

State Trial (Superior) Courts

State trial-level courts generally have concurrent jurisdiction with the federal courts to enforce federal claims, although Congress has exercised its authority to vest exclusive jurisdiction involving certain areas of federal law in the federal courts. State trial courts, commonly called superior courts, are the courts in which most criminal and civil matters are heard. There may be some difference in the terminology used as related

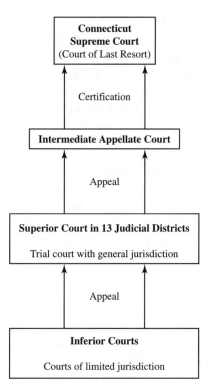

Figure 7–2   The Connecticut state court system.

to these levels in the state systems. For example, in New York the trial-level court is known as the New York Supreme Court. The Appellate Division of the New York Supreme Court operates as the intermediate appellate court, and the highest state court in New York is called the Court of Appeals. When a case is heard in a state trial court, the evidence and procedural rules of that state apply. One judge typically presides over a case whenever a case is tried before a jury. When a bench trial is chosen, the case may be tried before one judge or a panel of judges, depending on the type of case and the applicable rules of procedure in that state.

In the federal trial court system, the United States are divided into jurisdictions, called districts, that are based primarily on state boundaries. Similarly, there are jurisdictional divisions in the state court systems. The method of determining those state jurisdictions varies from state to state. In some states, jurisdictions are based on county, or even city boundaries. In others, arbitrary judicial districts have been created. An appeal in a case heard in a state superior court is brought to one of that state's appellate courts.

In addition to trial-level courts, most state court systems include courts of limited jurisdiction, known as inferior courts. These courts typically are less formal than superior courts and often are not courts of record; that is, detailed transcripts of court proceedings are not regularly kept. Examples of inferior courts are probate courts, traffic courts, administrative courts, and small claims courts. Jurisdictional divisions among inferior courts vary widely. In some instances, appeals can be taken from an inferior court to be heard in a superior court.

State Appellate Courts

Each state has its own system of appellate courts. As previously mentioned, some states have an intermediate appellate level and a high appellate court, whereas some have only a high appellate court. Some states, especially those with an intermediate-level appellate court, provide for an appeal as a matter of right from a trial court decision. Other states provide for appeals only in certain circumstances. State high appellate courts generally select from among the applications those cases that it considers appropriate for consideration. An appellate court may decide to hear a case because it presents an important issue, perhaps of constitutional magnitude, or perhaps poses an important question that requires a rule binding on all lesser courts within that state in order to ensure judicial consistency.

State High Appellate (Supreme) Courts

Every state has a high appellate court that serves as the ultimate authority of issues of state law within that state. Generally, in states with intermediate appellate courts, high appellate courts consider appeals only from those intermediate courts. Appeals from intermediate appellate courts to high appellate courts typically require some type of application process, sometimes called certification or *certiorari*. In states without intermediate courts, appeals to high appellate courts are taken directly from trial court decisions. High appellate courts also can exercise their authority to take appeals directly from trial courts whenever the high court considers the case to be one of special interest to the court.

THE CASE PROCEDURE

All legal disputes or cases arise out of some type of event. In a criminal case the event is the commission or omission of an act that constitutes a crime. In a civil case it might be the commission of a negligent or intentional act that causes harm to an aggrieved party, the breach of a contract between parties, or even the dissolution of a marriage. The type of event matters with regard to whether the result is a criminal action or a civil action. Ultimately, in either type of action the case must be proven by the presentation of evidence pertaining to the event.

The Role of Evidence

Evidence is defined as any physical, circumstantial, or direct information that is offered in a proceeding to prove or disprove an issue in dispute. Evidence may include all statements, perceptions, physical evidence, and knowledge presented that pertains to the elements of a case. As described earlier, the adversarial system allows each side to present evidence that is most favorable to its side, while allowing challenges to the evidence of the other side. Generally, unless the opposing side objects successfully to its admission, proferred evidence will be available for the trier of fact (judge or jury) to consider in its deliberations. In some circumstances, the judge may decide to admit for a limited purpose evidence that has been objected to. When that occurs, the judge will instruct the jury to consider such evidence only for a specified purpose. Otherwise, once evidence is admitted at trial, the jury has sole discretion and responsibility to decide what weight to accord each item of evidence and to determine what evidence is credible.

After centuries of looking to the common law rules of evidence, the federal government determined that a more uniform set of evidence rules was necessary. In 1975 Congress enacted the Federal Rules of Evidence (FRE), which were, for the most part, standardized versions of the existing common law rules. In order to create workable rules that allowed for the flexibility necessary to address the myriad evidentiary questions facing judges every day, the FRE were drafted using general language that allows judges a great deal of discretion. Hence, judges must still rely on the vast body of the common law for application of the FRE in specific circumstances. In addition, the FRE did not address certain evidentiary issues, such as spousal privileges. Like the rules of procedure, the FRE are dynamic. For example, the FRE were recently revised to reflect the current federal admissibility standards for scientific evidence outlined in *Daubert v. Merrell Dow Pharmaceuticals* (1993).

In general, evidence can be divided into four categories: 1) witness testimony; 2) real, or physical, evidence; 3) documents or writings; and 4) demonstrative evidence (i.e., visual or audio materials presented to assist the jury). Such broad categories inevitably allow for many types of evidence in many formats to be presented during a trial. Although the actual form and origin of the evidence may influence the judge's decision regarding whether it can be used in a particular proceeding, three basic requirements must be considered by the court: relevance, reliability, and competence. Evidence that is not relevant, reliable, and competent cannot be effectively tested by the opposing side and, therefore, is not an appropriate part of a fair trial process.

Relevant Evidence

According to common law and FRE 401, relevant evidence is "any evidence" that has "any tendency to make the existence of any fact . . . more probable or less probable than it would be without the evidence" (FRE, 2003). For evidence to be relevant it must pertain to the case at hand in such a way that the trier of fact could find this information useful during deliberations. Although this is necessarily a somewhat vague concept, relevancy is essentially a logical evaluation of the evidence. The court may consider many facts and arguments about the relevancy of the evidence and ultimately will decide whether this evidence has "any tendency" to affect the determination of the fact finder. Usually if there is a logical relationship between the evidence and the case the judge will allow its presentation. Admitting relevant and excluding irrelevant evidence is a practical rule, as well. The relevancy rule limits the scope of the topics that can be addressed during trial. Thus, the need for relevancy saves time during both case preparation and the actual court proceedings. Relevancy also helps to prevent the admission of evidence that may be misleading or confusing to the fact finder. Some experts have suggested that the relevancy rule also improves society's perception of a trial by requiring that the proceedings actually have something to do with the charge (Best, 2000).

Relevancy functions as the initial filter of evidence, based on the particular case scenario. For example, if J.J. is charged with forging checks, and during the investigation it is found that he has been carrying out a business in a residential zone, that evidence would likely be found inadmissible because it is irrelevant. Although some may consider J.J.'s acts as proof of his willingness to disregard the zoning law, this fact is not relevant because it is not of consequence to the determination of whether J.J. forged checks. On the other hand, if J.J. has a broken hand at the time of his arrest, the court may allow medical testimony from a nurse or physician to establish whether J.J. had a broken hand at the time the checks were forged. Another example of an evidence rule based on the concept of relevancy is the "rape shield" rule. (This rule has been codified by Congress and most state legislatures.) Generally, evidence of a sexual assault victim's prior sexual history is considered not relevant to the determination of whether she or he was sexually assaulted by the accused. However, in some instances, such as when the prosecution presents evidence that semen was found during a forensic examination of the victim, the court may allow the defendant to present scientific evidence that the recovered semen came from someone with whom the victim had consensual relations.

Reliable Evidence

Evidence must also be reliable to be admissible. Reliability of evidence may be established in several ways, depending on the nature of the evidence presented. Witnesses generally may testify to what they directly saw or did. The opposing party has the right to challenge those actions or perceptions through cross-examination. The freedom of a witness to testify regarding what she or he heard, however, is significantly more limited due to concerns about the reliability of such evidence. Although testimony that a witness heard a loud noise outside her window would be admissible (if relevant), her testimony that another witness told her that he saw the defendant commit the crime would be barred by what is commonly known as the hearsay rule. Hearsay is defined as "a statement, other than one made by the declarant [witness] while testifying at the trial or hearing, offered in evidence to prove the truth of the matter asserted" (FRE 801(c), 2001). This rule essentially prevents the admission of evidence that relies on the truthfulness of someone who is not present in court and whose veracity and perceptions cannot be challenged. Although many out-of-court statements are generally deemed unreliable, and therefore rendered inadmissible, certain categories of out-of-court statements are made under circumstances that imbue them with a presumption of reliability. Those categories form numerous exceptions to the hearsay rule. For example, one hearsay exception known as the "diagnosis and treatment" exception may permit the forensic nurse to testify to the statements of another made during a medical examination. The reliability of such statements is based on the premise that a person seeking medical assistance would speak truthfully to a medical provider in order to obtain appropriate care.

Certain types of evidence, such as documents, photographs, and physical evidence, must be authenticated prior to presentation in order to establish their reliability. Some items may be considered as self-authenticating, such as certified public documents, but in general, authentication is done by a witness who can attest to the reliability of the item. If the item of evidence is a photograph, for example, the witness will be asked whether the image depicted is a fair and accurate representation of what was viewed by that witness. If physical evidence is collected from a scene, the witness will be asked about the "chain of evidence" to show its reliability. Discussion of physical evidence collection and how to maintain the proper chain of custody can be found in Chapter 16.

Scientific, medical, and other evidence presented by an expert witness is established as reliable when certain requirements for admissibility, as outlined in Supreme Court and state court decisions and rules of evidence, are met. According to FRE 702 "if the scientific . . . knowledge will assist the trier of fact to understand the evidence or to determine a fact in issue, a witness qualified as an expert . . . may testify thereto" (FRE 702, 2001). The current common standards for scientific and other expert evidence are described in the Supreme Court's decisions of *Frye v. United States* (1923) and *Daubert v. Merrell Dow Pharmaceuticals* (1993). These cases make it clear that the judge must act as a "gate-keeper," determining if evidence is reliable and relevant prior to the evidence being presented to the jury. Thus, it is the court that first rules whether any witness is qualified as an expert and may testify on a particular subject. Then, even if the court finds that a witness qualifies as an expert, the judge may determine that a particular subject of the testimony is *not* admissible because it does not meet the criteria for scientific or medical evidence laid out in *Daubert* and FRE 702.

A forensic nurse may be called upon to testify as an expert witness concerning some aspect of technical, scientific, or medical evidence. Forensic testimony may pertain to subjects such as protocols, interpretations of data or medical records, or the administration of tests or treatments. Such testimony falls under the rules of expert witness testimony. Thus, a brief discussion of the development and requirements of the rules regarding expert testimony follows.

The *Frye* Standard. In 1923, the Federal Court of Appeals established the standard for the admissibility of scientific evidence that became the predominant rule for 70 years and still remains in effect in several states. In refusing to admit a polygraph result, the court stated that to be admitted into evidence, a scientific procedure must have gained "general acceptance" in the relevant scientific community (*Frye,* 1923). Critics of the *Frye* standard claimed that this test did not guarantee that evidence was reliable or even that it was the result of good science; *Frye*, they claimed, only required that a significant number of people recognize or use the test and any subsequent results. Questions also were raised about who constituted the relevant scientific community in which there was general acceptance. As technology boomed in the 1980s, the question of what actually makes a technical, scientific, or medical result reliable was revisited.

***Frye-Plus* Standard.** As more complex and varied testing became available in the 1970s and 1980s, some states, particularly California and New York, adopted what is sometimes called the *Frye-Plus* or *"Super-Frye"* standard (*People v. Kelly,* 1976). Under this expanded test, the party offering the evidence is still required to show that the scientific method or standard applied to the evidence is generally accepted in the relevant scientific community. *Frye-Plus* also requires that the party offering the evidence show that the accepted procedures were appropriately followed and that the results are reliable. This standard has been applied primarily for new technologies, such as DNA testing.

***Daubert* Standard.** *Daubert v. Merrell Dow Pharmaceuticals, Inc.* (1993) revolutionized the way courts look at scientific and medical evidence. In *Daubert,* the Supreme Court overturned a lower court ruling that excluded research evidence because it failed to meet the *Frye* standard. The Court held that, although general acceptance in the scientific community was an important factor, other factors should also be considered when determining whether such evidence is reliable. Emphasizing Federal Rule 702 and the judge's role as gatekeeper, the Court presented several factors to weigh in deciding whether to admit scientific evidence:

1. Is the method generally accepted within the relevant scientific community (the *Frye* test)?
2. Has the technique or theory been tested and validated?
3. Have the procedures or technique been reviewed by other scientists in the field or published in a peer-reviewed journal?
4. What is the error rate of the technique or the theory?
5. Are there standards applicable to the theory or techniques applied?

The Supreme Court clearly stated that no one factor is more important than any other, and that all factors do not have to apply for the court to admit the evidence. On the other hand, even if all these factors are met, a judge may still exclude evidence if other issues raise questions about the reliability of the evidence. Some courts have held, for example, that although a procedure may generally be accepted, the specific application in a particular case is not. (Other courts have ruled that the application of procedures to a specific piece of evidence is a matter of weight and not admissibility.)

In 1999, the Supreme Court held that the *Daubert* standard applied to all types of technical expert witness testimony, not just the traditional sciences and medicine (*Kumho Tire Co. v. Carmichael,* 1999). Since the *Daubert* decision, most states have revisited the issue of expert witness testimony and the admission of scientific/medical evidence. Most states have adopted the *Daubert* standard or some modification of that standard for the admissibility of scientific evidence. Some state courts have added factors for consideration by the court in determining relevance and reliability of scientific evidence. Those factors include considerations such as the reputation of the expert and the extent to which a protocol previously has been accepted in the courts.

Competent Evidence

In some situations, even if evidence is determined by the judge to be relevant and reliable, the judge will not allow its use during a legal proceeding. Most relevant and reliable evidence will be found "competent" and admissible; however, there are certain situations, defined by the courts and rules of evidence, in which otherwise admissible evidence may be barred. If a witness is deemed unable to appreciate the duty to testify truthfully or is incapable of perceiving, remembering, or describing the incident in question correctly, that witness will be found incompetent. In some situations the testimony of a proposed witness, although relevant and reliable, may be protected by a legally recognized privilege of the defendant. For example, the defendant in an assault case may have told his doctor that he received his injuries during an ambush of the assaulted party. If this statement were made to the accused's neighbor it would likely be admitted by the judge as an admission by the defendant; however, because the statement was made to his physician as part of his medical treatment, most likely the doctor–patient privilege would apply and the doctor would be barred from testifying about the defendant's statement. Another common situation in which evidence is not competent is when the "exclusionary rule" is applied by the court. The exclusionary rule is applied as a sanction in criminal cases when otherwise relevant evidence was obtained in violation of the accused's constitutional rights. For example, the exclusionary rule will be applied when evidence has been obtained in violation of the search and seizure protections of the defendant guaranteed by the U.S. Constitution (*Black's,* 1999).

Other Evidence Considerations

In addition to the three basic requirements for the admissibility of evidence, the court will consider several other factors to ensure the fairness of a trial. In all cases the court must determine whether the "probative value" of relevant, reliable, and competent evidence is "substantially outweighed by the danger of unfair prejudice, confusion of the issues, or misleading the jury" (FRE 403, 2001). In other words, the judge finds that the impact of the evidence may be so great that it will affect the fact finder in a way that limits his or her ability to reach a reasonable, fair verdict. The court must weigh the probable effect of the evidence against the tendency of that evidence to prove or disprove a fact that is important to a case. If the court determines that the prejudicial impact outweighs the value of the evidence, it will bar that evidence. Not all prejudicial evidence will be excluded. It is axiomatic that evidence presented at trial against a defendant, whether by the prosecutor or plaintiff, will be prejudicial to some extent. Generally, *excludable* prejudicial evidence falls into two categories: evidence that will likely create prejudice in the juror's mind that is unrelated to the case, and evidence that has the risk of having undue impact on a juror and, thus, will be given extra weight during deliberations. The latter situation is sometimes described as evidence that will "inflame the passions" of a juror, which would prevent a cool-headed deliberation of the case against the defendant.

Evidence may also be excluded if it is "cumulative"; that is, if the court finds that the evidence is offered as proof of a fact that has already been supported by sufficient evidence. Such repetitious evidence may be barred because it can waste time, may confuse the jury, or may lead to a juror placing too much weight on a particular fact. The judge also has the discretion to exclude evidence that comes as a surprise to an opponent. The court excludes such "surprise evidence" to ensure a fair trial, especially when the surprise is the result of less than full compliance with applicable discovery rules. Several other areas of relevant testimony that are specifically excluded on the basis of a fair and efficient trial system can be found in the FRE and common law.

OVERVIEW OF CRIMINAL AND CIVIL PROCEDURE

Any trial may be viewed as a search for the legal truth of the issue. The fundamental guideline for legal proceedings is fairness. Thus, the surprise witness as depicted for decades in television shows is rarely seen in a well-conceived trial. Instead, the attorneys, court, and jury function according to well-established procedures and codes of behavior, designed to ensure a fair hearing for both sides.

The following descriptions of the general procedures demonstrate an overview of those processes. Although the general procedures and themes of this discussion should be applicable in most situations, the exact procedures and procedural steps in a case vary among the jurisdictions. The forensic nurse should become familiar with the specific stages of and requirements for case development in the jurisdictions in which he or she practices.

Rules for Proceedings

Evidence pertaining to a trial event must be presented according to applicable rules of evidence and procedure and, in order to prevail, the prosecution or plaintiff must meet the appropriate standard of proof. The standard of proof necessary to prove the ultimate issues in a case varies, depending on whether the legal action is criminal or civil. Generally, however, the standard of proof does not differ based on whether a case is brought in a state or federal court. The same cannot be said, however, about the rules of evidence and court procedure. In order to provide for the orderly and consistent processing of civil and criminal cases in the federal courts, Congress vested authority in the Supreme Court to develop a set of rules for use in the federal courts. In 1938, the Court issued the Federal Rules of Civil Procedure. In 1942, it issued the corresponding Rules of Criminal Procedure. Neither of these sets of rules has remained static since they have been in effect. Both have undergone significant change over the decades as the rules have been tested in court practice and as appellate court judges have considered the application of these rules in the cases brought before them.

Although such rules are consistent among the federal courts, they can vary widely between federal courts and state courts, as well as among the different states' courts. Many states have adopted the federal rules, either in whole or in part, for use in those states' courts. Other states have issued their own sets of rules for practice. It is important for the forensic nurse to become familiar with the rules of procedure as they apply to the jurisdiction in which he or she may practice. Although procedures generally are similar, differences may exist between jurisdictions that are significant enough to create an uncomfortable situation for the expert witness unfamiliar with a certain jurisdiction, for example when dealing with rules that affect the work product or timing for the consultant.

In addition to the federal rules of practice, the federal courts follow the FRE. A quick review of the FRE shows that the language of those rules may be open to interpretation or leave a great deal of discretion to the presiding judge. Some areas of evidence, such as spouse-related privileges, are not addressed at all. Thus, although rules were established for the federal court system, they are flexible rules that still rely on common law decisions for application in specific circumstances.

Because of the design of the federalist system described previously, states are not required to adhere to the FRE. Different rules for different states initially presented problems for people, such as forensic nurses, who might participate in cases within both systems. However, as time passed, many state legislatures sought to codify their own rules of evidence, modeling the state rules after the FRE. Today, most states have rules of evidence similar to the FRE. Like the rules of Civil and Criminal Procedure, the Federal Rules of Evidence are dynamic. For example, recent changes in the FRE incorporated language that reflects current federal evidence admissibility standards outlined in *Daubert v. Merrell Dow Pharmaceuticals* (1993).

The judge is present in the courtroom during all proceedings to ensure that the defendant is given a fair trial. The judge accomplishes this to the best of his or her ability, although no trial is error free. What is important is whether the errors the court makes are "harmless" (i.e., do not significantly affect the outcome of the case). The judge's role is key in making sure that any evidence used by the prosecutor was obtained according to constitutional and state guidelines and that the rules of criminal evidence and procedure are followed in the courtroom.

Regardless of whether a case is initiated in federal or state court, that case must wend its way through the court process. Depending on the volume of a given court's caseload and the resources available in a given jurisdiction, the entire process may take months, or even years, to reach a resolution. Even in the rare situation where the backlog of cases is not an issue, the processing of a single civil or criminal case is a lengthy endeavor. As the following sections show in some detail, there are numerous steps in a case; each step takes time and is necessary to the proper and just resolution of a case.

The Criminal Trial Process

A crime may be defined as an act that violates a duty owed to the community by members of a given society (*Black's*, 1999). Any violation of those laws requires that the offender makes some satisfaction to the public. Crimes are violations of the rules outlined by communities for the purpose of providing its citizens a safe and orderly environment in which to live, function, and relate to each other. Thus, although the act that constitutes a crime may be committed against a particular person (the victim), the crime actually is committed against the society that proscribed that conduct. For example, although the perpetrator of a sexual assault commits the act against a specific person, society has also been harmed and the act is a crime because the community (i.e., the state) enacted a law prohibiting such conduct. Accordingly, a crime is prosecuted by the community, not the particular person victimized by the criminal act. In some instances, the crime may even be prosecuted over the objection of the person or persons who were victimized. Consequently, when local laws are violated, the criminal case is brought by and prosecuted on behalf of the people of the state. When a federal criminal law is the basis of the prosecution, the case is brought on behalf of the people of the United States. Thus, cases have names such as "The United States versus John Doe," or "State of Connecticut versus Mary Smith." The person who prosecutes the case for the community may be designated the United States' Attorney, the state's attorney, district attorney, or other title, depending on the jurisdiction. Figure 7–3 shows the procedures in the criminal justice process.

Commencement of a Case

As stated earlier, every case begins with an event: the criminal act. The first step in the processing of the case takes place when that criminal act is brought to the attention of a member of a law enforcement department or division. This step commonly is called the "filing of a complaint." The complainant, or person who files the complaint, may also be the victim of the criminal act or may be some other individual who witnesses the act or in some way becomes aware of its occurrence.

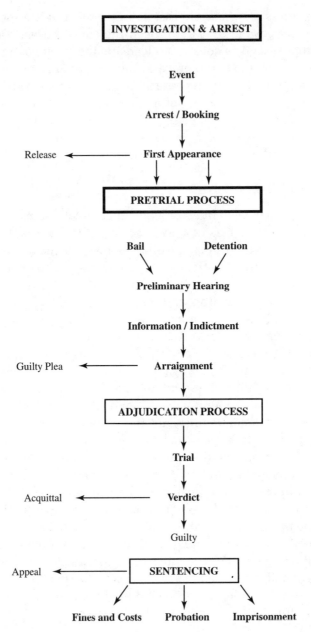

Figure 7–3 The criminal justice process.

Following the receipt of a complaint, the law enforcement department will make a record of such complaint, typically in the form of a report, and will commence an investigation concerning the complaint.

A thorough investigation is one of the most important steps in the successful resolution of a criminal case and the administration of justice. The investigation of a criminal complaint typically involves numerous steps, and space does not allow for a thorough discussion of those procedures. Each step, however, is taken in an effort to discover and to obtain any and all evidence pertaining to the complaint. The victim and any witnesses normally will be asked to provide sworn statements describing their observations or other perceptions about the incident. Investigators often will diagram and photograph any crime scene or scenes, and collect any tangible evidence located during the investigation. Some tangible items of evidence may be submitted for testing or analysis to further determine the helpfulness of that item in the investigation and to the process of proving the crime. Usually at this stage of a case the forensic nurse likely will interface with the law enforcement investigator. The forensic nurse plays a vital role in the collection of evidence in numerous types of criminal investigations. The very nature of forensic work indicates that those investigations likely will concern criminal acts of violence perpetrated upon human victims. Thus, as part of your dual role as a forensic nurse, you will be called upon to simultaneously administer competent and caring health care and collect and preserve evidence of the crime in a manner that is scientifically and legally sound. As discussed in other chapters of this book, the processing of crime scenes and the collection of forensic evidence in examinations performed on patients often are pivotal in the process of solving and proving a crime. Unless all of the important evidence of the crime is collected in a timely manner and preserved properly, the case may not be provable in a court, regardless of the occurrence of the act and regardless of the impact that criminal act may have had upon its victim or society.

The U.S. Constitution and the constitutions of the various states prescribe limitations on the extent and manner in which law enforcement officials are permitted to conduct their investigations. An overview of the search and seizure requirements related to evidence collected by law enforcement may be found in Appendix 2. What is important to understand here, however, is that any evidence that is collected in a manner that violates such constitutional limitations will be barred by the exclusionary rule. Consequently, that evidence will not be usable in the criminal prosecution of the crime. In many instances, not only is the evidence itself rendered useless, but most other evidence collected that is directly linked to any proscribed evidence may be deemed "fruit of the poisonous tree," and will be rendered unusable as well.

Indictment: The Charging Process

The constitutional rights of the accused in a criminal case begin during the investigation stage and are closely protected during the pretrial adjudicative process. Once a suspect is arrested, proper notice must be provided to the accused and the court concerning the charges against the accused and the evidence that supports those charges. In the federal system, a grand jury must be impaneled to determine whether sufficient evidence exists to bring about an indictment. Many states have replaced the grand jury process with a document called an "information," which lists the charges against the accused. In some states a judge may determine whether sufficient evidence exists to support the charges by reviewing the documentation submitted with the information. This document is usually called an affidavit. This determination is known as a finding of probable cause. Generally, probable cause may be found if there exists reasonable grounds to believe that the accused committed the crime charged. The accused is referred to as a "defendant" once he is formally charged and placed under the jurisdiction of a criminal court. In other states, the prosecutor is required to present evidence to a judge to establish that "probable cause" exists. This probable cause hearing must be conducted within a limited number of days after arrest, unless the defendant waives the time limit or waives the hearing itself. At the end of the hearing the judge may decide that the state has an insufficient basis for the criminal charges or that sufficient evidence of probable cause has been shown for the case to go forward. Once the defendant has been formally charged, at some point during the preadjudicative process the defendant must enter a plea of not guilty, guilty, guilty but insane, or *nolo contendre* (no contest). (Of course, based on the Fifth Amendment, the accused does not have to offer a plea. In such cases, the court will offer a not guilty plea for the accused.) If the defendant pleads guilty or *nolo contendre*, this is a conviction and the case proceeds to the sentencing stage. If the defendant pleads not guilty, the case proceeds through the trial process.

Entire treatises exist concerning the pretrial adjudicative process; however, a lengthy discussion about each step and the protections afforded the accused is beyond the scope of this text. The guiding principle behind this process and all proceedings is the assurance that due process rights and other specific state and federal constitutional guarantees are upheld.

Pretrial Activities and Discovery

After charges have been brought, both the prosecution and the defense begin to prepare their cases. During this stage, each side will pursue what it believes to be the most important evidence for case presentation. This may include interviewing witnesses, as well as examining documents and other items of tangible evidence. Because a trial is essentially a formalized process of determining the truth, fairness requires that both sides be provided with notice regarding certain aspects of the other side's case. Failure to comply with these notice requirements, known as disclosure and discovery rules, may result in sanctions ranging from exclusion of the undisclosed evidence to the reversal of the case verdict.

Because of the American concept of a fair trial based on constitutional protections that guarantee the defendant the opportunity to challenge the evidence and confront witnesses, the prosecution is required by rules of procedure to disclose to the defendant a great deal about its case. This rule demands that the prosecutor scrupulously pursue and turn over any potentially exculpatory evidence; that is, any information that may tend to be favorable to the defendant. Central to the requirement of fairness is the rule expounded by the Supreme Court in the landmark case of *Brady v. Maryland* (1963). In *Brady*, the prosecution failed to turn over evidence that it did not use in its case against the defendant. In overturning the guilty verdict, the Court refused to accept the prosecutor's explanations that the unused evidence lacked obvious importance or likely would not have made a difference to the jury deliberations.

The defense attorney's obligation is to zealously defend a client. This obligation must be carried out within the framework of the courts established by the legislature. As discussed in *Taylor v. Illinois* (1988), intentional misconduct on the part of the defense can be punished.

The *Brady* rule is important to the forensic nurse in its application. *Brady* clearly would require that *any* information relating to the prosecution's case that may have a tendency to support the defense must be turned over. For example, a witness's incomplete or contradictory statements would be disclosed to the defendant under *Brady*. *Brady* would also require the disclosure of a reprimand for misconduct of a witness that is unrelated to the case, or a questionable competency test result by an expert. A forensic nurse may find his or her employment record subpoenaed or résumé closely scrutinized pursuant to the *Brady* rule. Similarly, he or she may be questioned about any previous errors or problems related to tests performed by the forensic nurse.

Throughout the time before the trial, motions and other information-gathering processes take place. Once the court has been assured that sufficient time has been allotted for case preparation, a trial date will be set. Activities during this stage may also include the filing of and argument on various motions. These motions, which may be filed by either side, are filed to have the judge determine in advance of trial certain procedural and evidentiary issues. This ensures an orderly and fair presentation of evidence during the trial. Rulings on certain of these motions, such as motions to suppress items of evidence, often may help to resolve a case without the need for a trial. For instance, a defendant may file a motion to suppress her confession, arguing that is was obtained in violation of her constitutional rights. If the judge finds that there was no such violation and allows the confession to be used by the prosecutor, the defendant may decide to plead guilty, believing that results would be inevitable after trial. On the other hand, if all of the prosecution's evidence was obtained as a result of the confession and the judge disallows that confession, under the exclusionary rule all evidence considered fruit of the poisonous tree would also be disallowed. As a result of the evidence exclusion, the prosecution may be left with a case that cannot be proven. Consequently, the prosecution may be forced to drop the case or offer the defendant a chance to plead guilty to a lesser charge.

One of the most important processes during the pretrial process is the negotiated plea. "Plea bargaining" is a crucial step in the criminal trial process. Most cases in the American criminal justice system are resolved by negotiated pleas. Although harshly criticized by some, the negotiated plea often achieves justice without the expense and time of a full trial. Without the plea process the criminal courts would not be able to handle all the cases brought forward. A plea agreement requires that the defendant plead guilty to a particular crime and waive his or her right to appeal the guilty verdict that the judge will enter as a result of the plea. The agreement may be for a lesser crime encompassing the same or similar elements or for fewer crimes than originally charged. Other agreements may be based on the prosecution agreeing to recommend alternate or lesser sentences for the defendant. Prior to accepting a negoiated plea, the judge has an obligation to ensure that the defendant is entering such a plea voluntarily and that he or she understands all implications of pleading guilty to that crime. Because the defendant is unable to appeal a conviction based on a negotiated plea except in rare circumstances, the finality of the resolution also eases the caseload of the appellate courts.

Selection of a Jury

The Sixth Amendment to the U.S. Constitution guarantees trial by an impartial jury of one's peers in most criminal cases. The Supreme Court has stated that the principle purpose of a jury is to employ common sense judgment in its function as fact finder, and that the value of its verdict derives from the "community participation and shared responsibility that result from the group's determination of guilt or innocence" (*Williams v. Florida*, 1970). The guarantee of a jury "of peers" does not necessarily mean that all members of the jury hearing a case will be of the same socioeconomic background, sex, or ethnicity as the accused. This phrase does mean that the pool of persons from which a jury is selected must be representative of the community. There can be no deliberate exclusion of any segment of the population, such as exclusion based on race or sex (*Taylor v. Louisiana*, 1986). Today, jury rosters are usually taken from voter registration lists, registered driver lists, or other public records in an effort to compile a truly random jury pool. However, some people may be excluded from these jury pools by state law. For example, several jurisdictions do not allow police officers to be in the jury pool for criminal cases. Other laws may exempt people in certain groups upon request (e.g., mothers with small children or members of the clergy).

Jury selection is a complex process during which both sides try to choose from the jury pool those people whom they believe will be impartial, unbiased, and free from outside influences. Both sides also hope to choose people who might agree with their version of the facts and what those facts do or do not prove. The actual process of jury selection, called *voir dire*, may be conducted by the attorneys or by the judge. Prior to a more specific questioning process, members of the jury pool go through preliminary questions concerning possible relationships with any of the parties or witnesses in the case, as well as some general questions by the judge concerning their ability to serve. During *voir dire* questions are posed directly to the jurors about topics related to the case that might affect their judgment about the guilt or innocence of the defendant. Lawyers may also ask questions designed to expose prejudices about lifestyles, ethnicity, or other factors apparently less directly related to the case. If a case has received a large amount of publicity, attorneys often ask whether potential jurors have read or heard anything about the case or whether they have preconceived notions about the defendant's guilt or innocence. (It has become popular, especially in high profile cases, for some attorneys to hire psychologists or experts in jury behavior to assist in formulating questions that will result in the "best" mix of persons for the jury.)

The attorneys for each side and the judge eliminate jurors from the pool through the use of challenges. Challenges are of two types: challenges for cause and peremptory challenges. Because the purpose of *voir dire* is to eliminate any potential juror who may not be able to act impartially, any response that may indicate extreme bias or prejudice may lead an attorney to request that the juror be dismissed "for cause." Each attorney has an unlimited number of challenges "for cause." Sometimes, however, answers to questions may cause an attorney to decide that, although no particular bias or other fault is demonstrated, there is some reason he or she does not want that particular person on the jury. For example, counsel may not want a person of a particular age on the jury, or a potential juror's facial expressions during questioning may make the attorney concerned. In such a situation an attorney can exercise a "peremptory challenge"—a request to exclude a person from the jury for no specific cause. Only a limited number of peremptory challenges are available to each attorney. The number permitted may vary depending on the jurisdiction and on the type of case being heard. Although attorneys may exercise peremptory challenges without stating a specific cause, they are never permitted to use peremptory challenges in a way that violates the 14th amendment, particularly with respect to race. If a member of a recognized racial group is excluded by a peremptory challenge, opposing counsel may object, thus requiring the party exercising the challenge to provide a valid, nonracial reason (*Griffin v. Kentucky,* 1987).

The number of people selected to sit on a jury in a criminal case varies among jurisdictions and may differ depending on the seriousness of the crime charged. For example, Connecticut requires a minimum of 6 regular jurors for some criminal trials, but no less than 12 jurors for a murder trial. In addition to the regular jurors, jury selection also will usually include "alternate" jurors. The number of alternates may vary, depending on the size of the jury and the expected length of the trial. Alternate jurors will sit in on the trial and hear all the evidence. When it is time for jury deliberations, however, alternate jurors not needed to make a full, voting panel will be excused and will not participate in either the deliberation or the determination of the verdict.

The jury selection process almost always results in a jury with diverse backgrounds, education, life experience, and familiarity with evidentiary methods and results. This diversity may provide a particular challenge for the forensic nurse who is acting as either a fact or an expert witness. In either role, the forensic nurse must possess an ability to present testimony clearly and to relate nursing training and experience that is an essential part of his or her practice to each member of the jury.

A defendant may choose to have a trial by judge rather than a jury, but it was not until 1930 that the Sixth Amendment was interpreted to allow that choice. To waive the right to a jury requires that the court carefully examine the reasons for that choice and to ensure that the defendant understands what rights are being waived. Often the defendant will waive the right to a jury trial when the question of guilt rests primarily on a legal issue. For example, if the defendant claims that she or he was legally insane when the crime was committed, the defendant may choose to make those legal arguments before a panel of judges rather than a jury. Forensic nurses specializing in this area may find themselves part of competency hearings or similar proceedings before trial or testifying as experts before a panel of judges when the case goes forward.

Opening Statements

Opening statements, in jurisdictions where they are allowed, are presented at the time of trial by both sides in a criminal case. It is during the opening statements that the jury first hears each side's theory of the case. The prosecutor's opening statements will usually outline the elements of the crime charged and the evidence that will be presented to prove the case beyond a reasonable doubt. The roles of supporting factual information and additional witnesses will also be presented. Many prosecutors use a flowchart approach in opening statements, showing the jury how one witness or piece of evidence will lead to another and how the evidence ultimately will lead to the defendant to the exclusion of all others. It is not necessary for the prosecution to provide a motive for a crime in most cases, but the identification of a motive for the criminal act may often be part of the opening statement.

Most frequently the defense will present its opening statement immediately after the prosecution. In some jurisdictions, however, the defendant may defer making an opening statement until after the prosecution rests. In either case, the defense will seek to counter the opening statements of the prosecution by presenting its own theory of the case, pointing out the flaws in the prosecution's case, stressing the lack of evidence to support the criminal charge and, sometimes, by asserting any defenses it will claim later in the trial. If a defendant plans to offer evidence to prove a special, affirmative defense during the trial, that defense and the evidence to support it may also be described. Not all states routinely provide opening statements in criminal cases. Also, these statements may be waived by either or both sides during trial in some jurisdictions. A criminal defendant is never required to make an opening statement.

Even though opening statements can be a powerful tool at trial, they usually are relatively brief. There can be a danger in promising too much or in presenting too detailed an outline for the jury to follow. Then, if during the trial that outline is not followed or if promised items of evidence are excluded by evidentiary rulings, the jury may be left doubting the credibility of the attorney and focusing on the gaps instead of on the evidence that it actually heard.

Case Evidence and the Trial Record

After opening statements, the prosecution begins the presentation of its case in chief. Evidence is presented primarily through the examination of witnesses in a question and answer format. This format permits the evidence to be presented to the jury in a logical sequence. During this process, known as "direct examination," the prosecutor asks witnesses to provide information about what they saw, did, and, to some extent, heard in relation to the case. Witnesses may also be asked to authenticate evidence or "lay a foundation" for the admissibility of certain items of evidence. In addition, witnesses may be asked questions to ensure that evidence was obtained and maintained in a legally sufficient manner. During direct examination the attorney generally asks open-ended, nonleading questions.

When the prosecutor finishes the direct examination of each witness, the defense attorney has the opportunity to ask his or her own questions of that witness during cross-examination. The defense is usually only permitted to ask questions about the information elicited during direct examination or about other closely related information. On cross-examination the defense may also ask questions to test the reliability, accuracy, and bias or credibility of the witness's testimony. The form of the questions during cross-examination can be very different from direct-examination questions because the use of "leading," yes–no questions is permitted. The prosecution and defense may go back and forth for direct and cross several times before the witness is released by the judge.

In its case in chief, the prosecution will have to meet its minimal burden of establishing a *prima facie* case; that is, it must present evidence sufficient to allow a jury reasonably to find that a crime was committed and that the defendant committed that crime. At the conclusion of the prosecution's case in chief, the defense typically will make a motion for a judgment of acquittal. Through this motion the defense asserts that the prosecution has failed to establish a *prima facie* case and asks the court to dismiss the case. By making such a motion, the defendant preserves for a later appeal, if necessary, the issue of whether there existed sufficient evidence to support a guilty verdict. If the motion is granted by the judge, the case ends. If the judge denies the motion, the case proceeds.

When the prosecution completes its case in chief and "rests," the defense then has the opportunity to present its own evidence, if it chooses to do so. The defense may decide to present no evidence, arguing instead that the prosecution has simply failed to meet its burden of proof beyond a reasonable doubt. Alternately, the defense may opt to present evidence that tends to support its theory of the case in order to create reasonable doubt in the jurors' minds. In some cases the defense may present evidence related to a justification of the defendant's actions or an affirmative defense. For example, if the defendant was herself a victim of domestic violence, the defense may offer evidence of previous battering of the defendant by the victim, including hospital records, eyewitness testimony, or an expert witness, to educate the jury on posttraumatic stress disorder. (Refer to Chapter 22 for more information related to this type of expert witness testimony.) Just as the defense is permitted to cross-examine the prosecution witness, the prosecution is permitted to cross-examine all defense witnesses.

The defendant is never required to testify on his or her own behalf. The decision regarding whether the defendant will testify often involves many complex considerations. Although the jury will be instructed by the judge not to draw any inferences from the defendant's decision not to testify, if the defendant does testify the jury is free to consider the credibility of the defendant just as it would any other witness. If the defendant chooses to testify, he or she is subject to cross-examination as with any other witness. After the defense rests its case, the prosecution is given an opportunity to present a final rebuttal case, if necessary to counter evidence offered in the defendant's case. Similar to the restrictions placed on the scope of cross-examination, the scope of the rebuttal case generally is limited to addressing specific facts or issues raised by the defense case.

During both the prosecution's case in chief and the defense's case, each side is permitted to object to evidence being introduced by the other side. Objections play a crucial role in ensuring that only relevant, reliable, and competent evidence is heard by the jury. Chief among the objections raised are those based on relevancy, insufficient foundation, and hearsay. Judges usually do not allow lengthy explanations of objections. A judge may ask the objecting attorney to clarify for the record the basis of the objection in order to make a ruling—whether to sustain the objection, when the judge agrees with the basis, or to overrule it. Objections are an important part of the record of the trial. During the case in chief it is the responsibility of the defense attorney to make all legitimate objections to preserve the issue for appeal. If the defense fails to object, in most cases the defendant loses his or her right to appeal based on an erroneous evidence ruling by the judge. Of course, sometimes objections may be raised as part of a trial strategy to break the rhythm of the opposing attorney, to distract the jury, or even to interrupt the witness. Witnesses who are aware of the possibility of such ploys are better able to minimize their effect.

Closing Arguments

Closing arguments can be an extremely powerful tool during a trial. A closing argument can be the most effective opportunity that either attorney has to "put it all together" for the jury. It is an opportunity not only to summarize the evidence, but also to explain to the jury how that evidence supports an attorney's theory of the case, and provides a final chance to persuade them. Although closing arguments themselves are not considered evidence, the rules for a fair trial extend to closing arguments. During a closing argument, sometimes called the summation, an attorney may not offer personal opinions about the guilt or innocence of the defendant or offer inflammatory remarks. Because these are the last words heard by the jury, the content of the closing argument likely may remain in jurors' minds when they begin deliberations. It has been said that some cases are won or lost based on the closing argument alone. A skilled prosecutor often can weave otherwise tenuous evidence so tightly in summation that no room for doubt remains. Likewise, an adept defense attorney can use arguments to whittle away at even the most solid case to create just enough room for a reasonable doubt to take hold. (Even losing attorneys can deliver memorable closings that take on a life of their own.)

Technology is changing the face of the closing argument, as it has changed the way that demonstrative evidence is used in the courtroom. Today, many closing arguments are accompanied by multimedia presentations that may include recorded statements, photographs, charts, and other evidence presented during the trial. However, these high-tech closing arguments have raised issues concerning prejudice and possible prosecutor misconduct in the courtroom. Such a presentation is the basis of a current appeal in a well-publicized case involving the murder of a young woman in which the audio-recorded statements of the defendant, Michael Skakel, played along with images of the victim. (*Newsday,* 2005)

Jury Instructions and Deliberation

After both sides have rested their cases and final arguments have been made, the judge must turn the case over to the jury for deliberation. Before the jury makes its determination of whether the defendant is guilty or not guilty, however, the judge must provide the jury with appropriate instructions regarding the law that the jury must apply to the evidence. Although most jurisdictions have model jury instructions, in many cases the attorneys suggest specific language to the judge for inclusion in those instructions. Before the judge reads these instructions to the jury, the attorneys have the opportunity to review the instructions and make any objections on the record. In addition to a summary of the law and applicable procedures for consideration of the evidence, jury instructions will also include a detailed explanation of the elements of the crime, the applicable burden of proof, the concept of reasonable doubt, and the factors and burden of proof that must be met for any affirmative defense. The judge will also reiterate the important Constitutional mandate that the defendant is innocent until proven guilty. Many state courts and the federal court allow the judge to provide a written version of the instructions to the jury for use during its deliberations.

During the trial, the jury is regularly reminded by the judge that they are not to discuss the case with each other or with anyone else. Once deliberations begin, however, the exchange of opinions and ideas among the jurors is essential. One member of the jury is chosen to serve as the foreperson—the member who will preside over the group, initiate communication with the judge if questions arise or testimony review is requested, and announce the verdict of the jury. A vote is often taken early on in the process to gauge the diversity of the various opinions in the group at the outset of deliberations. This initial vote rarely results in a binding verdict. Through the sometimes lengthy process of reviewing and weighing the evidence in a logical sequence, the jury often reaches agreement. Several researchers have conducted interviews with numerous juries. These authors have provided fascinating insight into the dynamics of jury deliberation. Researchers often marvel at how a group of people with distinct personalities and diverse histories and life circumstances can find a way to communicate, to put aside prejudices, and to reach a verdict in a case. When a final vote is taken the group decides either that they have reached a verdict or that they are deadlocked. In most jurisdictions, a verdict is reached in a criminal case only when there is unanimous agreement among the members of a jury. However, the Supreme Court has upheld state laws that allow for a conviction on less than a unanimous vote (*Johnson v. Louisiana,* 1972). Whether a unanimous vote is required seems to depend on the type of crime and the number of people on the jury, however. If a verdict is reached, the jury returns to the courtroom to announce the verdict for the trial record. If no verdict can be reached after sufficient deliberation, the judge is informed. Whenever a jury is deadlocked, the judge will confirm that status with the foreperson and will speak to the jury as a whole, reminding the jurors of their duty to consider seriously the opinions of the other members. If after further deliberation no verdict can be reached, the judge will declare a mistrial. When this occurs, several outcomes are possible: there may be a new trial (no double jeopardy attaches because there was no verdict); the prosecutor may attempt to negotiate a plea once again; or, in some cases, the prosecutor may decide not to initiate a new trial.

Recently, a phenomenon called "jury nullification" has been a popular topic in the media and the source of much heated discussion. Jury nullification is the term used when a jury "nullifies" a law by deciding contrary to the proof offered during trial and contrary to the instructions of the court. Although hardly a new phenomenon—a colonial jury found several rebels not guilty of printing inflammatory pamphlets against oppressive British rule prior to the Revolution despite overwhelming evidence—jury nullification was once again debated in the news after the O.J. Simpson verdict. Such nullification may result from perceived injustice in the law, sympathy for the accused, or even retribution for some societal ill unrelated to the specific charge. If a jury, for its own reasons, reaches a verdict that is clearly inconsistent with the evidence presented in a civil case, the judge can disregard or alter that jury verdict in many cases. However, in a criminal case, the U.S. Constitution requires that the judge enter the not guilty verdict of a jury and prohibits any further prosecution of the defendant on criminal charges related to the same facts.

Sentencing

If a person is acquitted, all criminal court proceedings are ended at that time. If a guilty verdict is reached, the court may order the defendant taken into custody or, if allowed by law, may grant release pending sentencing or an appeal. Once the defendant is convicted, the judge must punish the defendant by imposing a sentence. The U.S. Constitution protects against cruel and unusual punishment, which usually means that the punishment must be proportional to the crime committed. The extent to which someone may be punished—whether they must be incarcerated and for how long—is prescribed in the criminal statutes that are violated or in the penal code of the jurisdiction. Most states have sentencing guidelines that establish a range, with a minimum and maximum period of incarceration. This allows the court some discretion when imposing an appropriate sentence within those parameters. Other guidelines, such as the federal sentencing guidelines, are very specific, and provide little leeway for a judge to provide alternate sentencing. The sentence for each specific charge is prescribed and, upon conviction of that charge, the convicted person will be sentenced accordingly. In addition to or in lieu of incarceration, guidelines may also provide for a wide range of alternative sentences, especially in nonviolent cases where rehabilitation of the convicted person may be a more important goal. Depending on the crime, the alternatives may include counseling, treatment programs, supervision by a probation officer, restitution payments, or even community service. In cases in which the death penalty is a possible sentence, the severity and finality of this sentence has led most jurisdictions to require a separate, sentencing phase of the trial. During the sentencing phase the jury decides whether to recommend the ultimate penalty to the court. The crimes for and the conditions in which the death penalty may be imposed must be clearly outlined in applicable state and federal statutes. As one might expect, these statutes and their application are closely scrutinized by the courts.

Most states and the federal system allow victim or family impact statements as part of the sentencing process. These statements provide an opportunity for the victims of a crime or, in some cases, their family members, to convey to the judge the nature and degree of the residual impact of the crime. Victims may describe the physical or emotional scars or the financial hardships they face by virtue of their victimization. This presentencing practice is sometimes very controversial. Victims' advocates value this process as a way for the court to hear the extent of harm upon the victim's or survivors' lives and to consider that impact in sentencing decisions. Opponents of the practice argue that impassioned victim impact statements may lead to longer, harsher sentences and an inequality in the treatment of certain convicted people within the justice system.

Postconviction Activity

Every person is entitled by the U.S. Constitution to an appeal of a guilty verdict. The guarantee of an appeal is one of the most important safeguards in the criminal justice system. The review of cases on appeal helps to prevent and eliminate abuses of power, errors, and other potential due process violations. The right to an appeal and various grounds for an appeal are a matter of federal or state law. The prosecution cannot appeal a case except on a few, specific procedural grounds, such as a dismissal of charges. As discussed earlier, appeals first go to the appellate-level court. Another postconviction safeguard is the writ of *habeas corpus. Habeas corpus* writs are filed after a convicted person exhausts the appeals process. These writs are used to assert claims under certain specific grounds that he or she is being held unlawfully, in violation of the due process protection of the U.S. Constitution. Once a petition is filed, a judge must begin an inquiry into the case within a very limited period of time.

CIVIL LITIGATION

As stated earlier, most criminal laws are enacted to address conduct that society identifies as causing severe harm to the community. Civil law also has evolved to address breaches in the duties owed to another and to hold violators of those duties liable for their conduct. A violation of civil law gives rise to what is called a cause of action or the legal basis for bringing a lawsuit. Many aspects of the civil litigation process are identical or very similar to the criminal justice process. However, additional steps and procedures may also be required according to the federal or state rules of civil procedure. These rules, in part, help to ensure that all stages of a civil trial are conducted fairly and that civil lawsuits brought to court are not frivolous. During a civil trial the court must address several factors including community values, contractual or regulatory duties, conflicting interests, and reasons underlying the litigation process.

Forensic nurses often are asked to participate as consultants or experts in civil lawsuits in areas such as medical malpractice, insurance claims, negligence, and employment. A thorough understanding of the operation of civil procedure in a particular jurisdiction is vital for a forensic nurse to function effectively. An overview of the civil litigation process is shown in Figure 7–4. Although space does not allow a comprehensive study of the complexities of civil litigation here, the following overview should provide a guide for future study and a quick comparison to the processes in the criminal justice system.

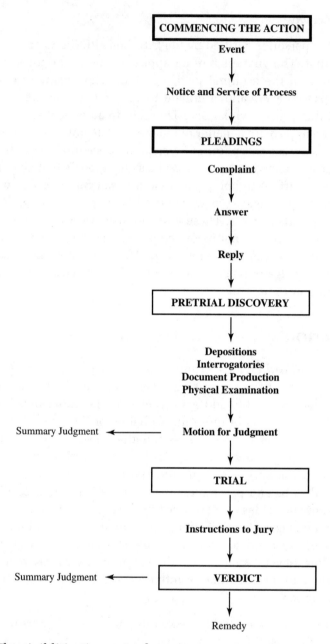

Figure 7–4 The civil litigation procedure.

Initiation of a Lawsuit

A civil case, like a criminal case, usually stems from an event. That event causes one party to believe that another party has harmed them in some way. That harm may be in the form of a personal injury, perhaps from an automobile crash or from a faulty product. The harm may also be in the form of a financial loss, such as from a broken contract or a wrongful job termination. Typically, a person who believes that he or she has been harmed consults an attorney to determine if the person who caused that harm could be found legally liable and whether that harm can be remedied in some way. The type of harm will usually determine the type of remedy sought. For instance, if the harm consists of injuries caused by a defective product, the remedy sought might include monetary damages to cover medical bills and lost wages. Under certain circumstances, such as when a vendor knew about the defect, the remedy may also include punitive damages to punish the vendor's unconscionable conduct.

Once a decision is made to file a lawsuit, the attorney must consider where the lawsuit should be brought. As with the criminal justice system, both state and federal courts exist that may be used to enforce an individual's rights under the law. The selection of the appropriate court or courts in which to bring a case is sometimes one of the most important decisions in a civil case. Various factors such as the available causes of action, the backlog of cases, and potential political implications or pressures may all influence the choice of court. The choice of court does have limits, however. A court must have appropriate jurisdiction over the dispute in question, called subject matter jurisdiction. For example, federal trial courts may only hear particular types of cases as prescribed in certain federal statutes. The most common cases heard in federal court involve a federal question or a dispute where no plaintiff is a citizen of the same state as the defendant and the amount in controversy exceeds the statutory minimum (U.S. Code, Federal Title 28, Sections 1331 and 1332).

Once a court is determined to have appropriate subject matter jurisdiction, it must be determined if that court also has personal jurisdiction over the subject matter (i.e., whether the court has judicial power over the person or property in the lawsuit). The actual place of trial, the "venue," must also be considered. Venue decides which particular court within the chosen jurisdiction is the most reasonable location for a case. Numerous state or federal rules apply to determine whether personal jurisdiction applies and in what venue the trial will take place.

Steps in Civil Litigation

After the proper court has been selected, the plaintiff must begin the civil litigation process. To commence a civil action, the plaintiff must notify the defendant that he or she is being sued. Notice occurs when the plaintiff files a complaint with the court and serves that notice to the defendant. Notice includes a summons issued by the court clerk and a copy of the complaint.

The Federal Rules of Civil Procedure clearly outline the steps in the federal litigation process. Many similarities to the criminal trial process exist, such as the use and purpose of opening and closing arguments and the application of the rules of evidence. In addition, many steps throughout the civil process have been designed to guarantee that the case proceeds appropriately and that ample opportunities are provided for the involved parties to negotiate a settlement between themselves. Because civil cases generally involve disputes between individuals or entities, the case names include the names of both parties. The initiator of the lawsuit is the plaintiff and the person alleged to have caused the harm is named as the defendant. The following are the steps in the process:

1. *Complaint:* The complaint provides the information to the defendant regarding the nature of the plaintiff's complaint. The complaint must be based upon a recognized cause of action. The allegation in the complaint must be sufficiently specific to clearly outline the harm claimed by the plaintiff and to allow the defendant a fair opportunity to provide an appropriate response to the complaint.

2. *Response:* Once the complaint has been filed and served on the defendant, the defendant must provide a response, called an answer or motion. If the defendant fails to respond to the complaint within the specified time period, the plaintiff can ask the court to enter a default judgment in his or her favor. In the response, the defendant may admit to some of the allegations or deny some or all of the claims listed by the plaintiff. If the case is not dismissed after the pleadings, that is after the complaint and the response, the attorneys will begin to prepare the case for trial.

3. *Discovery:* One of the most important steps in the litigation process is discovery. It is through discovery that the defendant and plaintiff obtain information from each other and from witnesses. Although there may always be a voluntary exchange of information, most civil discovery is accomplished in the form of written interrogatories, oral depositions, and examination of documents. If the physical or mental condition of an individual is at issue, there also may be frequent motions for examination. A forensic nurse acting as expert may often be part of the discovery process either by conducting examinations or by responding to inquiries about his or her expert opinions. Further discussion of the expert witness process may be found in Chapter 22.

4. *Pretrial disposition:* Throughout the trial process there are several opportunities for the parties to seek dismissal or rulings on a case. The first of these opportunities comes after discovery. Either party may move for a judgment as a matter of law; that is, a plaintiff or defendant may argue that there is sufficient evidence to support a verdict in their favor without a trial. If the court finds that "no genuine issue of material fact" exists, the trial will not proceed (*Houchens v. American Home Assurance Co.,* 1991). In addition to a judgment as a matter of law, a case may end by default, involuntary dismissal, or voluntary dismissal. Ongoing negotiations throughout the pretrial period may also result in a voluntary settlement between the parties. Because expert information is often necessary to evaluate settlement proposals properly, expert input may continue throughout this process.

5. *Trial:* As with criminal cases, only a small number of civil cases proceed to the trial stage. If a trial does result, the actual trial process will proceed much as that described for criminal trials. The civil trial process includes jury selection, opening statements by both parties, the plaintiff's case in chief, the defendant's case in chief, closing arguments, and instructions to the jury. After the plaintiff rests, the defendant usually moves for a directed verdict claiming that, based on the evidence presented, the plaintiff's claim was not proven. Similarly, a plaintiff will move for a directed verdict after the defendant's case in chief, arguing that the evidence was so overwhelming that the case must be decided in the plaintiff's favor (Federal Rules Civil Procedure: Rule 50(a), 2003.). The plaintiff's motion for a directed verdict is seldom granted. If neither motion is granted, the case will be decided by the jury.

6. *Post-trial:* Within 10 days of a verdict, the losing party in a civil case may move for a judgment notwithstanding the verdict or for a new trial. An appeal can also be filed; however, the appeal must be based on objections that were raised during the pretrial and trial stages of the lawsuit.

The civil litigation process may take many years before a resolution to the case is reached. Today there is a trend toward alternate dispute resolution as a way to arrive at a just settlement in a less complicated and time-consuming way. The plaintiff or defendant will consult regularly with appropriate experts throughout the litigation or mediation process in order to have sufficient basis for an informed decision.

SUMMARY

The forensic nurse can be a more effective expert no matter what his or her specific role by being familiar with the justice system and the rules and procedures of the jurisdiction in which he or she operates. In this way the forensic nurse can avoid spending time on unnecessary and immaterial issues while meeting the challenges of admissibility and expertise in a competent manner.

QUESTIONS FOR DISCUSSION

1. Why are there two types of courts, federal and state, in which trials take place? What factors determine the court in which a case will be heard?
2. The unequal distribution of power between the state and the accused is still a major issue in today's courts, especially among defense attorneys. Identify some of the disparities that many claim affect the fairness of a trial.
3. In a rape case, the victim testifies that the defendant said, "Come with me and do what I say. I'm not kidding. I've been to prison for this before." Do you think this evidence should be admitted? Discuss if this evidence is relevant, reliable, and competent. Is the evidence too prejudicial?
4. What important roles does the discovery process play in a trial?
5. Dr. I.M. DeBest testifies that he has developed a new procedure that can determine the ethnic origin of a blood sample based on a DNA genetic profiling test. Detailed information about the test and other services can be found on his website. Can Dr. DeBest testify in a statutory rape case concerning the ethnic origin of a sample that "matches" the suspect in a *Frye* state? In a *Daubert* jurisdiction?

REFERENCES

Best, A. (2000). *Evidence* (4th ed.). New York: Aspen Publishing Co.

Louis H. Brown, Estate of Nicole Brown Simpson v. Orenthal James Simpson, No. SC036876, Superior Court, State of California, County of Los Angeles. (1995).

Black's Law Dictonary, 7th Edition (1999). St. Paul: West Publishing.

Brady v. Maryland, 373 U.S. 83 (1963).

Conn. Supreme Court to Hear Skakel's Appeal Next Month. (December 15, 2004). *Newsday* accessed at Newsday.com/news/local. Retrieved on January 6, 2005.

Daubert v. Merrell Dow Pharmaceuticals, 509 U.S. 579 (1993).

Federal Rules of Civil Procedure (2003), revised as of December 1, 2002.

Federal Rules of Evidence, Public Law 93-595, revised December 1, 2003.

Frye v. United States, 54 App. D.C. 46, 293 F.1013 (D.C. Circuit) (1923).

Griffin v. Kentucky, 479 U.S. 314 (1987).

Houchens v. American Home Assurance Co., 927 F. 2d. 163 (4th Circuit) (1991).

Johnson v. Louisiana, 409 U.S. 1085 (1972).

Kumho Tire Co. v. Carmichael, 119 S. Ct. 1167 (1999).

Mosk, J. (1988). *The Common Law and the Judicial Decision-Making Process,* 11 35.

Otter Trail Power Company v. Von Bank, 8 N.W. 2d 599 (1942).

People v. Kelly, 17 Cal 3d 24 (1976).

Taylor v. Illinois 484 U.S. 400 (1988).
Taylor v. Louisiana 419 U.S. 79 (1986).
Williams v. Florida 399 U.S. 78 (1970).

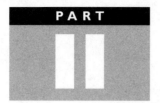

POPULATIONS

CHAPTER

8

Vulnerable Populations

Barbara Moynihan

This chapter will identify and focus on the special needs of those who comprise the population of at-risk or vulnerable groups. The charge to the forensic nurse is to identify and address the unmet and ever-changing complexities inherent in providing services to this population.

CHAPTER FOCUS

Define vulnerable populations

Describe characteristics of these groups

Expand forensic nursing practice interventions to address the present and evolving deficits in the healthcare response to these groups

Address the myriad cultural, legal, and advocacy issues inherent in the development of appropriate interventions specific to this population

Utilize appropriate theoretical foundations specific to the unique needs of at-risk vulnerable populations

Predisposing factors to vulnerability

KEY TERMS

culturally sensitive assessment strategies

disenfranchised/disempowered populations

gender inequities

marginalization

people with disabilities

precursors to vulnerability

The quality of mercy is not strain'd,
It droppeth as the gentle rain from heaven
Upon the place beneath: it is twice blest;
It blesseth him that gives and him that takes.

—William Shakespeare, *The Merchant of Venice,*
  Act IV, Scene I: Portia's Speech

INTRODUCTION

There are many facets to forensic nursing practice that are consistent
with nursing practice in general, but are specific to the specialized
expertise of the forensic nurse. The neediest, the disenfranchised, and
the least powerful comprise a population that may become invisible
within the healthcare system. Table 8–1 lists some of the vulnerable
population groups of special concern to the forensic nurse. These groups
do not represent all vulnerable groups, however. "Vulnerable populations are defined as social groups who have an increased relative risk or
susceptibility to adverse health outcomes" (Flaskerud & Winslow, 1998).
According to the web of causation model of health and illness shown in
Figure 8–1 (Stanhope & Knollmueller, 1997), the interaction among
numerous causal variables creates a potent combination of factors that
predisposes an individual to risk. This model can be used by nurses to
understand the relationships among various factors that contribute to
health status and vulnerability. Based on their skills as nurses and as
forensic experts, forensic nurses have the potential to identify vulnerable populations and to assist with the development of services for the
most disadvantaged. The scope and standards of forensic nursing practice are both broad and comprehensive, and provide an extensive frame
of reference within which the forensic nurse can flourish.

Table 8–1   Vulnerable Population Groups

- Poor/disadvantaged people
- Homeless people
- Pregnant adolescents
- Migrant workers
- Mentally ill individuals
- Substance abusers
- Abused people
- People with communicable disease(s)
- People who have the Hepatitis B virus, STDs, or who are HIV positive

Source: Stanhope, M. & Lancaster, S. (2000). *Community & public health nursing.* St. Louis: Mosby, p. 639.

Risk Factors   **Resource Factors**

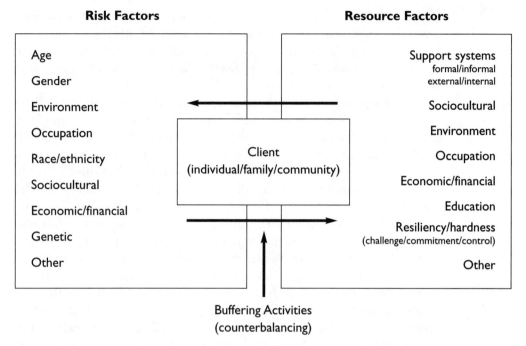

Source: Lundy, K. & Janes, S.. (2000). *Community health nursing* (5th ed.). Sudbury, MA: Jones & Bartlett, p. 579.

Figure 8–1   The web of causation model.

Due to ever-increasing concerns regarding national and international vulnerability and risk, assessment and interventions related to local as well as global populations are essential. Violence is rooted in the social, cultural, and economic fabric of human life. These factors interact with family, community, and other external factors to create a feeling of vulnerability among certain populations. These vulnerable, invisible populations suffer not only from a climate of oppression, which is compounded by a lack of resources, but also from feelings of helplessness and hopelessness. Consider the factors that contribute to an individual seeing himself or herself as invisible, as being isolated, or as excluded from or denied services and resources for a variety of reasons. The reasons for this sense of invisibility have many causes; included among those reasons is not even being recognized as needy.

PREDISPOSING FACTORS TO VULNERABILITY

The vulnerable represent all segments of society and are not a homogeneous group. Vulnerable populations are a subgroup that shares common risks or combinations of risk factors; one that is pervasive is poverty or low socioeconomic status (U.S. Department of Health and Human Services, 1998, 2000). Poverty, which is a growing problem in the United States, has been noted by some as a primary cause of vulnerability (Northam, 1996; Pesznecker, 1984). According to the landmark study by the World Health Organization (2002), poverty is a major factor internationally as well. This study also shows that poverty is linked to all types of violence. Although the topic of violence is discussed in another chapter, it should be noted that the linkages between vulnerability and violence are clear and compelling. Other factors that contribute to risk and vulnerability noted among all countries studied include family dynamics, substance abuse, and a lack of resources. In the United States, more than 40 million people have incomes below the federal poverty level, according to the National Coalition for the Homeless (1998a). In addition, approximately 20.5% of America's children live in poverty (National Coalition, 1998b). Within this context, a lack of understanding on the part of the nurse or other healthcare providers can add to the formidable barriers that already exist and prevent those in need of services from receiving them. The fears, misconceptions, and biases that are communicated by caregivers due to perceived conflicts in values, lifestyles, and so on result in even deeper feelings of oppression and powerlessness already possessed by the client. Vulnerable populations among the poor include people with special needs, the unemployed, the homeless, and the disenfranchised.

There are many factors related to vulnerability and many consequences associated with this status. Health-related issues include limited access to care, higher infant mortality rates, trauma-related injuries and death, substance abuse, and chronic illness. The physically, emotionally, or mentally challenged are at significant risk for being underserved. Not only does vulnerability result in poor health care and access to services, but the risk factors associated with vulnerability often lead to violence. That violence may involve the vulnerable person as either a victim or a perpetrator. Family, school, community, and sociocultural and cultural factors all influence coping skills of young people and their ability to deal with their community. This is another arena in which the forensic nurse, who is able to understand the relationships among social factors as they contribute to vulnerability and violence, may be able to reduce or interrupt the downward cycle that poverty, family stress, and lack of supports create within the vulnerable population.

Populations currently experiencing poor health status are increasing, while those experiencing good health status are decreasing. According to some experts, this disparity in health status created by socioeconomic, racial, and ethnic differences are great, and on the rise in the United States. When elements of racism, poverty, and community converge, greater overall threats to health develop. The health risks within these vulnerable populations were recognized in the objectives identified by the U.S. Department of Health and Human Services document *Healthy People 2010* (2000). The objectives included increasing the composition of racially and culturally appropriate programs that address substance abuse, mental health services, violence, and unintentional injuries, as well as nutrition, exercise, and stress management. By utilizing a theoretical framework of holism and caring, the forensic nurse is well positioned to intervene in addressing the inequities in both health care and social services among vulnerable populations. Identifying the underserved, developing cultural sensitivity, and creating a climate of acceptance and safety contribute to reversing the cycle of vulnerability and risk. Primary prevention, however, may not always be possible; when primary prevention is not feasible, secondary or tertiary prevention may be significant in breaking the cycle.

It is beyond the scope of this chapter to review all populations who are vulnerable or at risk; however, a brief overview of selected populations has been included. Chapters in this text regarding policy, nursing leadership, and other topics are the "threads" that address the comprehensive network of forensic nursing practice as it applies to vulnerable populations.

VULNERABLE POPULATIONS

Vulnerability implies that, when compared with the general population, some people are more sensitive to certain risk factors that can negatively impact their health. Those who are vulnerable are particularly sensitive to risks that originate from economic, physical, social, biological, and genetic factors along with their lifestyle behaviors. Rarely does one factor act in isolation, as illustrated by the web of causation shown earlier. The interaction of multiple risks results in increasing vulnerability to other factors, which also can negatively impact an individual's health (Sebastian & Bushy, 2000). Trauma, violence, chronic illness, natural disasters, and, currently, the possibility of terrorism can all result in increasing vulnerability.

The Homeless

Who are the homeless? There are many definitions used for various reasons. In general, a person is considered to be homeless if he or she lacks a fixed regular address and adequate sleeping arrangements. Homelessness includes people whose primary night-time residence is a supervised publicly or privately operated shelter, an institution that provides a temporary residence (a half-way house), or a public or private place not designated for sleeping (a park bench). This definition addresses those people who are literally homeless (e.g., living under bridges or in shelters), but does not include those who are living with relatives or in substandard housing (Scholler-Jaquish, 2000). Since the 1980s the number of homeless people has surpassed that of the Great Depression. And the face of this new homeless population is more varied than the unemployed male that dominated the Great Depression homeless. This new era of homelessness includes women, children, adolescents, whole families, immigrants, substance abusers, the elderly, the chronically and mentally ill, and war veterans. The causes of homelessness are many. Homelessness in the United States leads to major health problems that fall into three basic categories: health problems that contribute to homelessness, health problems that are a consequence of homelessness, and treatment of health problems that are complicated by homelessness (Institute of Medicine, 1988). The vicious cycle of poverty, isolation, and limited access to resources, including health care, contributes to overwhelming stressors for many homeless people. Chronic stressors, physical and sexual abuse, lack of family supports, poverty, domestic violence, street violence, overcrowding, poor hygiene, and poor nutrition often lead to substance abuse, the development of depression, infant mortality, child abuse, poor parenting, and a myriad of other predictable outcomes of poverty, unemployment, poor education, and homelessness.

Migrant Workers

There are approximately 5 million migrant farm workers in the United States (Migrant Clinicians Network, 2004). Many migrant workers enter this country through the nation's southern border with Mexico. The majority of these workers are men who rarely return to their native country. Because of tougher immigration laws after the September 11th terrorist attacks, higher travel expenses, and tighter restrictions at border crossings, moving between the United States and Mexico is difficult for the farm workers. This is especially true if they are undocumented. If the workers do leave the United States, they may not be able to return. Migrant workers rarely present for health care; when they do, depression and substance abuse are common. Medical problems often are untreated until they become acute and complex (National Farm Workers Health Conference, 1998). A number of factors, including language barriers, work demands, work environment, and fear related to being "undocumented" interfere with timely access to medical care for this population. The difficulties of daily life, with implications for resulting healthcare issues, are illustrated in a variety of opinions expressed by migrant workers presented in Figure 8–2.

Migrant farm workers are at high risk for suicide, as well. The suicide rate for men is four times that of women (Archives of Internal Medicine,

Health and Health Care

"What we have to do is reeducate our people and let them know that we have many rights to live and work and to educate and to have health care. And without health care, we cannot have the other three."

Unidentified Male Farm Worker, California

Work Conditions

"We're used to working. We don't want to be given things, we just want to be respected and to be paid the salaries."

Teresa, California

"Right now, because I'm here today (testifying at hearing on work conditions), I may not have my job. Possibly I may not have my job tomorrow."

Jose, California

Housing

"My slogan is, there must be a way to build houses. I believe we have the right to live in a decent way. We are the labor force. It's like we are foreigners—I am a U.S. citizen.

Margarita, California

"The foremen even charged [the farmworkers] for sleeping under the trees."

Teresa, California

Women

"...Another thing I would like to mention is the way we are treated as women. As women we are discriminated with our coworkers because they see us as insignificant beings. The men think that they are superior."

Maria, California

Children and Youth

"... [the children] go out to the fields. They lay under the trees and there is a residue falling on the children. They are picking grapes, what happens? The sprayers are there with the residue falling on the children."

Irma, Oregon

Source: Stanhope, M. & Lancaster, S. (2000). *Community & public health nursing*. St. Louis: Mosby, p. 703. Citing Galarneau C., ed. (1993). *Under the weather: Farm worker health*. Austin, TX: National Advisory Council on Migrant Health, Bureau of Primary Health Care, USDHHS.

Figure 8–2 Workers' comments on migrant life.

2000). Other health risks include tuberculosis due to poor living conditions, overcrowding, traveling in crowded buses, and malnutrition (Clesielski et al., 1994).

The migrant worker may also be among the "hidden homeless" because once employment ends, housing may become a serious issue. There are a myriad of complex issues to consider when addressing the needs of the migrant worker. These include the needs of families who often accompany the worker to the new location: housing; sanitation; health care for women, infants, and children; education for children; and work-related injuries or diseases. The infant mortality rate among migrant workers' children is 25 times that of the national average. Deaths from tuberculosis, influenza, and pneumonia are 25% higher than the general population and the life expectancy for migrant workers is 49 years compared with a national average of 75 years (Sandhaus, 1998). Successful programs have included mobile clinics, convenient time schedules, cultural sensitivity, and bilingual workers (Lundy & Janes, 2001).

Disenfranchised Populations

Disenfranchisement refers to feelings of separation from the mainstream of society (O'Connor, 1994; Sebastian & Bushey, 1999; DHHS, 1998, 2000). When these feelings occur, the individual or group does not experience an emotional connection with the rest of society. The disenfranchised include the chronically mentally ill, the homeless, immigrants, refugees, and people with HIV/AIDS. Those who are disenfranchised or marginalized may be treated as though they are insignificant; thus, these people begin to believe that this is their status—insignificant. Once they acquire such a belief, the disenfranchised may develop behaviors that further contribute to isolation, a sense of being invisible, and serious healthcare issues.

The Severely Mentally Ill

The severely mentally ill individual is at high risk to join the ranks of the powerless, marginalized, and disenfranchised population. The numbers of homeless individuals residing in public shelters has increased, in part, because some of these individuals do not have the capacity to perform the activities that support independent living. The deinstitutionalization of the mentally ill did not result in the simultaneous development of comprehensive community services in every community; thus, the severely mentally ill person was on his/her own when seeking health care or other related services. Many of these individuals lived in institutions for years and had no idea how to live independently. This lack of knowledge led to many unfortunate situations for the impaired person, including being arrested and becoming homeless. Another consequence for the severely mentally ill individual was the lack of routine health screening and preventive care (Callahan et al., 1995).

Women

Millions of people, particularly women, do not have access to the basic resources necessary to achieve a state of health. Although women live longer than men, they are often less healthy. This difference is often related to poverty. Women represent 70% of the people in the world who live in poverty (Craft, 1997). In spite of this fact, the issue of gender is often overlooked in the prevention of health problems. The magnitude of intimate partner violence, sexual assault, and sexual harassment contributes to the development of both physical and emotional health problems for women who are victims of these offenses. Unwanted pregnancies as well as limited access to health care result in women being at high risk for developing stress-related conditions and even HIV/AIDS. About 26% of women in the United States are members of racial and ethnic minority groups. The life expectancy for minority women is 73.5 years, whereas the life expectancy for white women is 79 years (NCHS, 1996). The problem of women's health was noted in *Healthy People 2010* (DHHS, 2000), which called for a reduction in health disparities between the majority population and special populations in the United States, particularly for people of color (Hamburg, 1998).

Children and Adolescents

Although the number of adults and the elderly living in poverty has decreased in recent times, the number of children living in poverty has significantly increased. Nearly 40% of those living in poverty are younger than 18 years of age, whereas 11% of those living in poverty are older than 65 (DHHS, 1998, 2000). Those living in single parent families are twice as likely to fall into this group, while African American children represent one-third of poor children. Native American children are among the poorest and most likely to live in substandard housing and on reservations (National Center for Health Statistics, 1999; U.S. Bureau of the Census, 1997). Dr. Jocelyn Elders, a former U.S. Surgeon General, stated that many of these children were members of the 5-H Club; they are "hungry, homeless, hugless, hopeless and without health care" (Lundy & Janes, 2001). Disadvantaged adolescents are also at significant risk for developing criminal behaviors, dropping out of school, developing substance abuse behaviors, and becoming parents at an early age (National Center for Health Statistics, 1998; National Rural Health Association, 1994, 1998, 1999).

American Indian and Alaskan Native Populations

American Indians and Alaskan Natives (NI/AN) are people having origins in any of the original peoples of North and South America, including Central America, and who maintain tribal affiliation or community attachment. According to the 2000 U.S. Census, those who identify themselves as only NI/AN constitute 0.9% of the U.S. population, or approximately 2.5 million individuals. The Census Bureau projects modest growth within the next few decades, exceeding 5 million individuals by the year 2065. The greatest concentrations of these native populations are in the West, Southwest, and Midwest, especially in Alaska, Arizona, Montana, New Mexico, Oklahoma, and South Dakota (U.S. Census, 2000). There are 569 federally recognized tribes, and an unknown number of tribes that are not federally recognized. Each tribe has its own culture, beliefs, and practices. NI/AN populations have a unique relationship with the federal government because of historic conflict and subsequent treaties. Federally recognized tribes are entitled to health and educational services provided by the federal government. However, because U.S. Census (2000) statistics show that more than half of these people do not reside on a reservation, native populations have limited or no access to Indian Health Services, an organization charged with serving the health needs of these populations. Geographic isolation, economic factors, and suspicion toward traditional spiritual beliefs are some of the reasons why health among native groups is poorer than other groups. Other factors include cultural barriers, poor housing, and poor sewage disposal.

The relationship between vulnerability and at-risk behaviors is apparent in reviewing some of the information relating to the 10 leading causes of death of youth among the Native American and Alaskan Native populations. According to the Office of Health Ministries (2002), suicide is the second leading cause of death among Native Americans and Alaskan Natives ages 15–24. Automobile accidents are the leading cause of death for Native American children. HIV/AIDS was 1.6 times higher in the Native American/Alaskan adolescents than for non-Hispanic whites; the death rate from AIDS was 4.9 per 100,000 Native Americans compared to 3.32 for whites. Barriers to care include fewer emergency services, ambulances, and life support services; long distances to hospitals; and inadequate and inconsistent health care through Indian Health Services. Another contributing factor is that health care through Indian Health Services is nontransferable. Additional barriers to care for native populations include lack of prevention education and few disease prevention programs, as well as a lack of understanding and respect for Native American culture. Few, if any, health education programs exist for youth.

This population represents a different type of challenge to the culturally naive forensic practitioner. Values clarification, cultural sensitivity, and an understanding of the history of oppression, discrimination, and exploitation specific to this population are critical if intervention is to be both allowed and effective.

Assessment of vulnerable populations must also include the assessment of grief and loss. The Native American population in particular has "lost" a great deal, not only in terms of material goods, but also in terms of identity. This may be a prevailing theme among those who are suffering from a variety of losses and for whom identity has been shattered. The forensic nurse can no longer assume that he or she will not be asked to interact with this underserved population, especially in this time of growing numbers of casinos and increased recognition of native groups by the federal government. It is incumbent on those who are providers of care for Native Americans to develop the knowledge and skills necessary to effectively provide care to those who may present at your facility. The following case study reflects some of the difficulties that may be encountered when providing comprehensive treatment to a Native American teenager.

Case Study

Eric, a 16-year-old Native American, comes to the walk-in clinic that you staff. Your clinic is managed by Indian Health Services; however, Eric does not live in an authorized and recognized reservation. He was involved in an altercation the previous evening and presents with bruises and a cut on his arm that would have required sutures if he presented earlier. Your assessment includes a psychosocial component and you discover that Eric is very depressed, has been abusing alcohol, and his 15-year-old girlfriend is pregnant.

There are many challenges inherent in this situation that require extensive exploration and collaboration in order to meet this young man's needs. Assessment is one of the most critical skills that nurses possess. For forensic nurses, the ability to see through a "forensic lens" enhances completeness and comprehensiveness in order to develop more accurately a realistic treatment plan. Healthcare providers working within systems may encounter limited resources and formidable barriers to comprehensive care.

SUMMARY

It is essential that the forensic nurse listen and try to understand the relationships between lifestyle and vulnerability and the resulting, often predictable, health consequences. Understanding requires knowledge of the client's culture, beliefs, and lifestyle without further alienating an already compromised population (Kudzma, 1999; Leninger, 1997). Nurses, particularly forensic nurses, can play an important role as agents of change, both nationally and globally. Effective delivery of care requires culturally appropriate, knowledge-driven, holistic, and humane practices. Influencing the delivery of care to the most needy populations (the "vulnerable") can begin to break or interrupt the cycle that imprisons the neediest in both the United States and the world. In addition, the power of legislation to address inequities and gaps in services to the most vulnerable cannot be overlooked. The forensic nurse, with his/her knowledge of statutes and the legal process, could not be in a better position to assist with or develop legislation to meet these needs. He or she can take the lead in breaking the barriers that continue to exist, whether within the system or due to a lack of effective legislation that addresses the issues important to the disenfranchised.

This chapter has focused on identifying and addressing vulnerable and at-risk populations. We have defined vulnerability and discussed the relationship between these terms. If issues contributing to vulnerability are not addressed, inevitably at-risk behaviors will develop in direct relationship to the causes of vulnerability, such as poverty, violence, crime, unemployment, and the lack of education, among other factors. Essential considerations for the forensic nurse include rigorous inquiry regarding personal biases and beliefs. If the nurse believes that people in need exploit the system or take advantage of resources, or if he or she utilizes a "we" and "them" attitude, the cycle of hopelessness will continue. We must adhere to the forensic nursing standards of practice (American Nurses Association [ANA], 2001), which include assessment, diagnosis, outcome identification, planning, implementation, and evaluation. Professional performance that includes quality of care, performance appraisal, education, collegiality, collaboration, research, and resource utilization is essential. In addition, consistent with collaborative practice are mutual trust and mutual respect for cultural diversity, shared planning, and so forth (ANA).

Florence Nightingale described nursing as an "art that requires as exclusive a devotion and as hard a preparation as any painter's or sculpture's work" (1969/1859). This could not be truer than in the practice of forensic nursing in general, and with vulnerable populations in particular. In forensic nursing we have the privilege of utilizing one or more theoretical frameworks that have been developed by nursing professionals. For example, Barbara Dossey's theory of holism (2000), Betty Neuman's systems model (1972), and Jean Watson's theory of caring (1995) are available as tools and references to guide forensic nursing practice. Promoting a healing and caring environment is essential in all areas of nursing practice, regardless of the behavior that precedes entry into the forensic nursing practice arena; this is especially true with the vulnerable.

During the 21st century the forensic nurse should be the standard bearer for excellence in nursing practice, as well as an agent for change in the treatment of those who comprise the neediest of populations who present for care.

QUESTIONS FOR DISCUSSION

1. Who are vulnerable populations?
2. What are the health risks specific to selected at-risk groups?
3. What is the role of poverty in increasing the risk of vulnerability?
4. What are the links between various types of vulnerability?
5. What groups are the most vulnerable?
6. How can the forensic nurse influence the resources and treatment of vulnerable populations?

REFERENCES

American Nurses Association. (2001). *Scope and standards of forensic nursing practice.* Washington, DC: American Nurses Publishing.

Archives of Internal Medicine. (2000). Depression, coronary heart disease and death in males.

Belcher, J. R., Scholler-Jaquish, A., & Drummond, M. (1991). Three stages of homelessness: A conceptual model for social work & healthcare. *Health Social Work, 16*(2), 87–93.

Callahan, J. J. et al. (1995). Health/Substance abuse treatment in managed care. The Massachusetts Medicaid experience. *Health Affairs, 4*(3), 173.

Clesielski et al. (1994). The incidence of tuberculosis among North Carolina migrant farm workers, 1991. *Public Health, 84*(11), 1836.

Craft, N. (1997). Women's health: A global issue. *British Medical Journal, 315*(7116), 1154.

Dossey, B., Keegan, L., & Guzzetta, C. (2000). *Holistic nursing: A handbook for practice (3rd ed.).* Gaithersburg, MD: Aspen.

Elders, J. (1997). *Health United States.* Washington, DC: U.S. Government Printing Office. As cited in Lundy, K. & Janes, S. (2001). *Community health nursing.* Sudbury, MA: Jones & Bartlett, p. 583.

Flaskerud, J. H. & Winslow, B. J. (1998). Conceptualizing vulnerable populations health related research. *Nursing Research, 47*(2), 69.

Hamburg, M. (1998). Eliminating racial and ethnic disparities in health: A response to the presidential initiative on race. *Public Health Report, 113*(July/August), 372.

Institute of Medicine. (1988). *Homelessness, health and human needs.* Washington, DC: National Academy Press.

Kudzma, E. (1999). Culturally competent drug administration. *American Journal of Nursing, 8,* 46–52.

Leninger, M. (1997). Transcultural nursing research to transform nursing education and practice: 40 years. *Nursing Research.*

Lundy, K. & Janes, S. (2001). *Community health nursing* (5th ed.). Sudbury, MA: Jones & Bartlett.

Migrant Clinicians Network. Retrieved June 1, 2004, from www.migrantclinician.org.

National Center for Health Statistics. (1996, 1998, 1999). *Health United States.* Hyattsville, MD: U.S. Public Health Service.

National Coalition for the Homeless. (1998a). *How many people experience homelessness? Fact sheet #3.* Washington, DC: Author.

National Coalition for the Homeless. (1998b). *Why are people homeless? Fact sheet #1.* Washington, DC: Author.

National Farm Workers Health Conference. (1998). National Advisory Council on Migrant Health, May 13–17. Houston, Texas.

National Rural Health Association (1994). A shared vision: Building bridges for rural health access: Conference proceedings. Kansas City, MO: Author.

National Rural Health Association (1998). Bringing resources to bear on the changing care system: Conference proceedings for 2nd annual rural minority health conference. Kansas City, MO: Author.

National Rural Health Association (1999). A national guide for rural minority health. Kansas City, MO: Author.

Neuman, B. & Young, R. S. (1972). A model for teaching total person approach to patient problems. *Nursing Research, 21,* 264–269.

Nightingale, F. (1969/1859). *Notes on nursing: What it is and what it is not.* New York: Dover.

Northham, S. (1996). Access to health promotion, protection and disease prevention among impoverished individuals, *Public Health Nursing, 12*(5), 353.

O'Connor, F. (1994). A vulnerability stress framework for evaluation interventions in schizophrenia. *The Journal of Nursing Scholarship, 26,* 231–237.

Pesznecker, B. (1984). The poor population at risk. *Public Nursing, 4*(1), 237.

Presbyterian Congregation of the United States Health Ministries U.S.A., 2004. *DC USA News.* Available at www.wfn.org. Accessed May 24, 2005.

Prevention Institute (2001)

Sandhaus, S. (1998). Migrant health: A harvest of poverty. *American Journal of Nursing, 98*(9), 52–54.

Sebastian, J. G. & Bushy, A. (2000). *Special populations in the community.* Gaithersburg, MD: Aspen.

Stanhope, M. & Lancaster, S. (2000). *Community & public health nursing.* St. Louis: Mosby.

U.S. Bureau of the Census. (1997). *Population profile of the United States.* Washington, DC: Government Printing Office.

U.S. Bureau of the Census. (2000). Population profile of the United States. Washington, DC: Government Printing Office.

U.S. Department of Health and Human Services. (1998). *Update to the recommendation of the National Advisory Council on Migrant Health.* Austin, TX: National Migrant Resource Program.

U.S. Department of Health and Human Services. (2000). *Healthy people 2010 (Conference ed.).* Washington, DC: U.S. Government Printing Office.

Watson, J. (1995). *The philosophy and science of caring.* (pp. 9–10). Boulder, CO: Colorado Associated University Press.

World Health Organization. (2002). World Report on Violence and Health.

CHAPTER 9

Sexual Offenders: Who Are They and Why Do They Commit Sexual Abuse?

David A. D'Amora
Ted Brandhurst
Randall Wallace

Forensic nurses are critical collaborators in the management of situations involving sexual deviancy. A clear understanding of the dynamics underlying the thinking and behavior of sexual offenders is critical to providing holistic, caring interventions to both current and potential victims and offenders. Without such understanding, preventive measures designed to protect vulnerable populations from becoming victims or offenders cannot be realized. Forensic nurses, armed with an informed basis for understanding the genetic and environmental complexities that come together to result in an act of sexual deviancy, are key players in proposing effective intervention strategies.

CHAPTER FOCUS

What is sexual abuse?
Informed consent
Theories of sexual offender behaviors
   Psychodynamic model
   Psychosocial model
   Addiction theory
   Family systems model
   Sociopolitical (feminist) theory
   Biological theory
   Social learning theory

Behavioral theories
Cognitive behavioral model
Theory integration
Sexual offense typologies
Typology of rapists
Crossover
Etiological considerations for adult sex offenders

KEY TERMS

age of consent
attachment theory
blockage
coercion
crossover
differential association
disinhibition
Electra complex
emotional congruence
informed decision
mental incompetence
modeling
Oedipal complex
pedophilia
role diffusion
role reversal
sexual abuse
triangulation
typology
volition

WHAT IS SEXUAL ABUSE?

Although the fine points of what constitutes sexually abusive behavior may vary from state to state, country to country, and culture to culture, sexually abusive behavior can be defined as any sexual interaction between person(s) of any age that is perpetrated: 1) against the victim's will; 2) without consent; or 3) in an aggressive, exploitative, manipulative, or threatening manner (Ryan, 1997). Another definition of sexually abusive behavior posited by the National Task Force on Juvenile Sexual Offending (1993) states that such behavior occurs without consent, without equality, or as a result of coercion.

Consent

Central to any definition of sexually abusive behavior is the concept of consent. Just as the constituents of sexually abusive behavior may be defined differently in various milieus, consent usually is composed of several key elements (see Table 9–1).

There must be an understanding of the nature of the sexual act that is proposed (e.g., vaginal, oral, or anal sex, or even sadomasochistic acts). There must also be a knowledge of societal standards for what is proposed (e.g., incest, cultural expectations, and taboos). An awareness of potential consequences and alternatives (e.g., health concerns, pregnancy) must be present. There is an assumption that agreement or disagreement will be respected equally (e.g., one party's right to say "no" to the sex act at any point). It is a voluntary decision to engage in a particular sex act; there is an assumption that all parties in a consensual sex act are not having sex against their will. The act of volition assumes that there is no coercion by alcohol, drugs, intimidation, or force. Mental competence assumes that the individual is capable of making an informed decision about engaging in a sexual act. People with severe mental illness or developmental disabilities who may not emotionally or intellectually be able to make informed consent fall into this category.

Finally, age and sexual maturity must be appropriate. The age of consent to engage in sexual acts varies widely. In the United States, the age for all consensual sexual acts can range from 16 in Connecticut to 18 in California. There is a further age delineation in a number of states for sexual acts depending on whether they are heterosexual or homosexual. For instance, in the state of New Hampshire the age of consent for heterosexual acts is 16, whereas the age for homosexual consent is 18. In countries such as Mexico, the legal age of consent for heterosexual acts is 12, but for homosexual acts the age is 18. In Saudi Arabia all sexual acts outside of marriage are considered illegal regardless of the age or sex of the persons engaging in them. In countries such as Armenia, the age of consent for heterosexual sex is 16 whereas homosexual acts at any age are illegal.

Table 9–1   Elements of Consent

Understanding the nature of the act
Knowledge of societal standards
Awareness of potential consequences
Assumption of respected agreement/disagreement
Mental competence
Age and sexual maturity appropriateness

THEORIES OF SEXUAL OFFENDING BEHAVIORS

Psychodynamic Theories

Psychodynamic theories describe sexually abusive behavior as a direct reflection of a form of character disorder. Sigmund Freud's psychodynamic theory of the human psyche is divided into three categories (id, ego, and superego) that he believed are in a constant battle in the mind for domination. The ego is the sense of consciousness created by the interaction between the id and the superego; the superego serves as the conscience and modulator of the id; and the id is buried deep in the unconscious mind, with its primitive sexual and atavistic urges operative in each human. According to this theory, a person's mental health is determined by how well he or she reconciles these opposing forces.

Using Freud's model, psychodynamic clinicians suggest that sexual offenders may have very weak consciences (superegos) that allow the overpowering sexual drives (ids) to drive their actions. Initially Freud (1923) discussed reported cases of childhood sexual abuse in a lecture to the Society for Psychiatry and Neurology of Vienna in April 1896 entitled *The Seduction Theory*. He abandoned this position the next year after strong resistance from his peers and his personal belief that the many instances of childhood sexual abuse he encountered were more likely to be fabrications of his patients. From this revised stance, Freud initiated his theories of the Oedipal and Electra complexes to try to reconcile himself to the times and cultural expectations of Victorian Austria. His development of an elaborate schema of defense mechanisms and complexes looked at sexual abuse of children in a context of "intra psyche" as opposed to "extra psyche" modes. Freud also expanded the idea of the unconscious (those mental processes that are buried deep within the mind and accessible only through psychoanalysis) and described numerous defense mechanisms to protect the ego.

The defense mechanisms delineated by Freud are still used to explain behavior in clinical circles. These are mechanisms of denial (this is not really happening, it doesn't really exist), displacement (this is happening outside of me, someone else is responsible), and projection (uncomfortable feelings are placed upon someone else).

The psychodynamic model places great emphasis on the mother–son relationship, suggesting that the mother–son relationship is qualitatively different in sexual offenders than in nonoffenders. The "seductive mother" is one who, though she does not have a sexual relationship with her son, treats him as her spouse or lover. The conflict that arises in the son from this type of mothering can lead him into sexual deviancy later in life due to a variety of feelings of anxiety and inadequacy, both sexual and interpersonal, that interact with aggression directed at the victim as a substitute object for the mother, thus producing a sexual assault.

Psychodynamic theories have been influential with respect to discourse on sexual offending, but not with respect to treatment or prevention due to a lack of empirical support.

Psychosocial Model

Finkelhor (1984) proposes a psychosocial model of child sexual abuse. This model proposes primary factors occurring as *preconditions* (see Table 9–2).

Finkelhor maintains that four conditions must be present before child sexual abuse can occur:

1. There must be *motivation* for the offender to abuse from some internal reason, such as projecting emotional needs onto the child victim or the perpetrator's deprivation of sexual gratification.
2. *Internal inhibitions* are not present or are diminished through the use of alcohol or drugs, by stress, by rationalizations, through the lowering of societal sexual taboos, through subculture norms, or by mental disorders.
3. *External inhibitions* must be lacking or weakened. Examples can involve poor parental/caretaker supervision, isolation, or overcrowding.
4. The *child's resistance* must be overcome. The offender may accomplish this by trickery or manipulation, by using a child's emotional instability, or by garnering the trust of the child. Threats, physical power, and authority roles also can be part of the process to undermine a victim's resistance to sexual abuse (Jackson et al., 1991).

Addictions Theory

In addictions theory, the origins of sexual deviancy are found in dysfunctional family patterns and have many similarities with chemical dependancy and gambling behaviors. Patrick Carnes, PhD, defines sexual addiction as a process where "the addict substitutes a sick relationship to an event or process for a healthy relationship" (2001, p. 14). He goes on to state,

> Sexual addiction can be understood by comparing it to other types of addictions. Individuals addicted to alcohol or other drugs, for example,

Table 9–2   Finkelhor's Preconditions for Sexual Abuse

Motivation
Overcoming internal inhibition
Overcoming external impediments
Undermining or overcoming a child's resistance

develop a relationship with their "chemical(s) of choice"—a relationship that takes precedence over any and all other aspects of their lives. Chemically addicted individuals find that they need drugs merely to feel normal.

In sexual addiction, a parallel situation exists. Sex—like food or drugs in other addictions—provides the "high" and addicts become dependent on this sexual high to feel normal. They substitute unhealthy relationships for healthy ones. They choose temporary pleasure rather than the deeper qualities of "normal" intimate relationships. Sexual addiction follows the same progressive nature of other addictions. Sexual addicts struggle to control their behaviors, and experience despair over their constant failure to do so. Their loss of self-esteem grows, fueling the need to escape even further into their addictive behaviors. A sense of powerlessness pervades the lives of addicts. (Carnes, 2001)

Carnes (2001) has developed an addictive systems model of sexual deviancy that defines sexual deviancy as the result of messages that the individuals tell themselves and how these are acted upon. This model posits the idea of "core beliefs," which are derived from the person's experiences in life. According to Carnes (pp. 112–115), the common core beliefs of the sexual addict are:

- I am basically a bad, unworthy person.
- No one would love me as I am.
- My needs aren't going to be met if I have to depend on others.
- Sex is my most important need.

The sexual addict takes these core beliefs and reshapes them into distorted thinking patterns. Some of the distorted thoughts often seen in sex offenders may be:

- Since I can't get sex through regular means, I'll make people have sex with me.
- She really wanted me and really didn't mean it when she said no.
- She got me to have sex with her because she needed a man.
- She's just too uptight about sex and has sexual hang-ups.

Distortions such as those listed can provide justification for an offender's deviant sexual behavior (Carnes, 2001, p. 17).

Carnes's addiction cycle has four components:

1. *Preoccupation:* This is characterized by obsessive/compulsive sexual thoughts and fantasies.
2. *Ritualization:* To further sexual stimulation, the sexual addict will often engage in rituals that lead up to sexually acting out, such as

cruising, using sexual toys, or wearing women's undergarments to heighten the sexual experience.

3. *Compulsivity:* This is the level at which preoccupation and ritualization become unmanageable and the sexual addict commits a deviant sexual act.

4. *Despair:* At this stage guilt, regret, or hopelessness sets in (Carnes, 2001, pp. 19–20).

As the addictive cycle continues, the sexual addict becomes more and more out of control. His or her obsession with deviant sex may take a toll on his or her family as more and more of his or her time is devoted to deviant addiction. He or she may lose his or her job because of time spent cruising for sex partners or an ever-deepening interest in pornography and strip clubs. The addictive cycle feeds on itself and the sex addict continues a downward spiral. Carnes (2001) states that the sexual addict will go through three stages of this downward spiral if not treated. The first stage is marked by compulsive masturbation, promiscuity, pornography, and use of prostitutes. The second stage is punctuated by exhibitionism, voyeurism, and indecent phone calls. The third and most problematic stage may include child molestation, incest, or rape. Although there is a strong element of compulsivity in many sex offenders' behaviors, most researchers and clinicians in the field of sex abuse treatment and research do not find the global explanations of addictions theory applicable to the adjudicated sex offender.

Family Systems Model

In addition to the sexual addiction system, Carnes (2001) has adapted the circumplex marital and family systems model (Olson, 1989) to describe the effects of family on sexually abusive persons. Olson and Craddock (1980) contend that 16 types of families can be described by their relative positions on 2 intersecting continua. The first continuum concerns dependency issues and has the extremes of chaotic family structure and rigid family structure. The second continuum deals with intimacy issues, with the extremes being a disengaged family structure and an enmeshed family structure.

The chaotic family system can be described as having no accountability for sexual behavior, discrepancies between values and behavior, parental sexual unmanageability and inconsistencies, and consequences. Frequently, role reversals around sexual behavior are apparent. The chaotic family system does not have any clearly defined rules or expectations and the children often are dealt with as though they are authoritatively equal with the parents. Moralistic black and white standards, extreme efforts to control child sexual behavior, punishment for sexual behavior, and unreachable expectations about sexuality are common elements in the rigid family system. As a result of the extreme structure and high expectations, the child is unable to develop his or her own system of self-regulation. The child may respond to the authoritarian parent through rebellious direct acting out behavior.

On the other continuum, the disengaged family structure can be described as having elements of abandonment, having tension and distance around sexual matters, lacking in physical or sexual closeness, and evading sexual issues. The disengaged system views sex as something to be discovered by the individual and not to be discussed. The child in the disengaged family is likely to feel alone and without support.

The opposite of the disengaged family system is the enmeshed family structure. In this family system, a lack of boundaries is evident. The enmeshed family can also be described as having anxiety about a family member's sexual behavior reflecting on the family, secrecy preserved at all costs from outsiders, covert and overt sexual abuse, and limited sexual privacy. Children in the enmeshed system do not develop a self-identity. They tend to develop a communal identity with few boundaries drawn clearly. According to Carnes (2001), most sexual addicts come from chaotically enmeshed families.

Sociopolitical (or Feminist) Theories

Sociopolitical theorists view rape as a pseudo-sexual act that is predominantly motivated by male sociopolitical dominance. Sex role stereotypical beliefs, adversarial sexual beliefs, and acceptance of interpersonal violence are critical factors. Women and children in such environments are seen as property or as an extension of the male to do with as he chooses. There is a growing body of research that indicates acceptance of rape myths and the mythology of machismo contribute greatly to rape behavior. Interpersonal violence is a critical factor.

Biological Theories

These theories posit that genetic, hormonal, chromosomal, or neurological causes create sexual violence. Sociobiological theory in particular suggests that males in general have learned throughout time to become more aggressive and dominant toward women in particular. This would be due to successful reproduction and passing on the male's genetic material. The more aggressive males continued to pass on those genes while at the same time learning from prior generations. Prehistoric women were monogamous by nature—they needed men to assist them during and after childbirth. Without the assistance of men, the mortality rate for women and children would be substantially higher. The more sexually aggressive males mated much more frequently than passive males, and therefore those genes kept evolving. In many respects the human sexual drive and behavior is very similar to that of other mammals. Though our brains have advanced throughout time, our inherent drive to reproduce has not. This theory is put forward as a way to partially account for rape, but fails to address child molestation. Supporters of this theory point to the fact that males commit most sexual crimes. However, there is little research to support these premises, and such a theory does not account for an individual's control over cognitive processes.

The biomedical model suggests that sexual offenders produce more testosterone than nonoffenders, and is similar to the sociobiological theory. Sexual deviancy is viewed as a response to overproduction of testosterone in the testes. The removal of the testes either surgically or chemically reduces or eliminates testosterone. Numerous studies suggest significant reductions in recidivism rates in those who have been castrated. There is a possibility that some type of genetic, hormonal, chromosomal, or neurological process is responsible for sexually aberrant behavior.

Social Learning Theory

Social learning theory looks at the concepts of differential association, reinforcement, and modeling. It suggests that an offender has somehow learned the sexual deviancy from his or her environment. This theory also incorporates "modeling," the idea that the offender learned the behavior from watching someone else behave in a similar fashion, or even by his or her own sexual abuse. Studies have suggested that a number of offenders have been sexually abused themselves in the past, and proponents of this theory view that fact as credible evidence to support this theory. However, there are many sexual offenders who report they have never been sexually abused, and never witnessed sexual abuse in the past. Many offenders do appear to be continually learning and advancing in their sexual deviancy. They learn how to obtain victims more effectively, learn how far they can go, learn what deviant sexual behaviors arouse them, and learn how to avoid or escape detection.

There are a number of "subtheories" including the dynamics of post-traumatic stress disorder, attachment theory, and so forth. Many sex offenders, both adult and juvenile, appear to share the same symptomology: low self-esteem, poor self-perception, depression, isolation from their peers, and difficulty achieving and maintaining intimate relationships. Social cognitive research results suggest that rapists misinterpret the interpersonal cues from women (e.g., negative mood) and overperceive hostility and seductiveness (e.g., friendliness versus seductiveness). Rapists may hold greater adversarial beliefs leading to the belief that women accept and even enjoy male domination.

Behavioral Theories

Behavioral theories suggest that sexual deviance results from classical conditioning, possibly from either sexual assault or covert seduction during childhood, or negative modeling. An example of classical behavioral theory would be the experiment of Pavlov and his dog. Pavlov paired the introduction of meat powder with the ringing of a bell. Soon, just the ringing of the bell was enough to get the animal to salivate. However, these theories do not explain the cognitive progression necessary to behave inappropriately, and human beings have a significantly more complex thinking process than animals.

Cognitive-Behavioral Theories

The proponents of the cognitive-behavioral model state that for a sexual assault to occur, the offender must go through a progression of cognitive distortions and behavioral stages that involve the accumulation of unique behaviors and characteristics and must be defended internally or externally by the offender. According to Nichols and Molinder (1984), a cognitive progression of criminal thinking occurs even before the sexual offense is committed (see Table 9–3).

This cognitive progression may take a matter of a few days or several years to develop. Closely related to the cognitive progression is a behavioral progression (Nichols & Molinder, 1984), during which the offender hunts for his or her victim(s). This hunt may include cruising, stalking, or manipulating a situation. The second stage of the behavioral progression is the offender's "playing" with the victim. This "playing" may include any

Table 9–3 Cognitive Progression of Criminal Thinking

The idea to commit the sexual assault.

The distorted view that most of society is unjust and uncaring and that he or she is a victim and this is an unjust system.

Justifications, excuses, rationalizations, and distortions "give the permission" to commit the offense.

Fantasies about irresponsible use of power over weaker persons for pleasure.

The plan to "successfully" commit the offense.

The belief that the sexual offense can be accomplished without repercussions and the consequences resulting from this belief.

The immediate decision to commit the offense when the first six steps have been accomplished.

behavior that intensifies the sexual experience for the offender such as verbal abuse, winning a child over with gifts, or playing out a role with the potential victim. The last stage of the behavioral progression is the actual sexual assault, which may also expose the victim to direct physical assault.

Sexually deviant individuals must defend their deviancies in order for the deviancies to be maintained (Nichols & Molinder, 1984). This defending usually takes some combination of forms: 1) deception through dishonesty, 2) deception through distortion, and 3) deception through denial. In deception through dishonesty, the offender attempts to manipulate the truth through a system of omissions of details and additions to the truth. Deception through distortion occurs when the perpetrator attempts to defend his or her behavior by utilizing cognitive distortions and justifications such as "He/she came onto me for sex," "We had a true romance that no one understands," "I was just taking his temperature with an anal thermometer because I thought he had a fever," "She/he had sex before me." Deception through denial occurs when the offender admits to others his or her guilt but attempts to deceive him- or herself about being aroused by sexually deviant desires.

Cognitive-behavioral theories explore how thoughts create or mitigate actions. Offenders set up negative emotional states through negative thinking; to relieve the negative mood states they preoccupy themselves with deviant sexual fantasies. The deviant behaviors are then justified, rationalized, or explained away.

The cognitive-behavioral theories suggest that irrational beliefs and cognitive distortions help to initiate sexual deviancy. Soon after this initial step, the offender becomes conditioned to negative sexual stimuli, with "orgasm" being the reinforcement. These constructs combined (cognitive/behavioral) create persistent patterns on how the offender behaves as well as views the world. The secrecy, among other constructs, soon becomes part of the conditioned response and perpetuates the deviancy. Learning theory is also a significant component of this approach. Children who are sexually abused learn sex through inappropriate means, and if exposed enough, children may internalize this learned behavior. Male sex offenders do appear to view the world differently than "normal" men—they perceive women, children, sex, and arousal qualitatively different. When this occurs after a long period of time, the offender begins to behave accordingly. Many times the male or female sexual offender suffers from chronic low grade depression, has very low self-esteem, has been ridiculed his or her entire life, and so forth. These traits tend to distort the offender's view of the world, and the molester may find comfort and acceptance in the children he or she so desires. Immaturity is a trademark of the child molester. This appears to occur due to the fact that he or she has not advanced emotionally since adolescence.

TOWARD THEORY INTEGRATION

A significant number of commonalities are shared by many adult sex offenders, including early life damage to the ability to develop affectional and/or attachment bonds, negative models of behavior, and/or actual abuse. Further, data suggest that supports for sexually abusive behavior through sex role stereotyping and cultural supports for violence play a role in the creation of sexually abusing behavior. Add to this inappropriate and/or deviant coping mechanisms that develop with accompanying cognitive distortions to "normalize" the behavior in sex offenders' minds, and you have a recipe for sexually abusive behavior. One of the most current integrated or multifactoral theories was developed by Ward and Hudson (1999). They state that every sexual offense has both distal, or historical, factors and proximal, or recent, factors. Additionally, they state that every sexual offense involves five factors:

1. Intimacy deficits
2. Deviant sexual scripts
3. Emotional dysregulation
4. Antisocial cognitions
5. Multiple dysfunctional pathways to the offense

SEXUAL OFFENSE TYPOLOGIES

Typologies categorize offenders into distinct and "understandable" groups or subtypes. Ideally they provide guidance regarding distinct and specific treatment needs and interventions; however, they can limit our thinking, lead to "pigeonholing," and inadvertently lead to overlooking individual needs. Some examples of noteworthy typologies include the following.

Child Molester and Rapist Typology

The first typology for adult male sex offenders was developed by Dr. Nicholas Groth in 1979; the second, known as the FBI typology (developed by Kenneth Lanning), is based upon Dr. Groth's work; and the third (the Knight-Prentky typology) takes Dr. Groth's work and validates the different types statistically. The Groth typology breaks down adult male sex offenders into two categories—the child molester and the rape offender.

Child Molester

Child molesters often utilize persuasion and/or manipulation to perpetrate the sexual abuse. They typically begin their involvement with children by using grooming behavior. Grooming behavior is intended to make the victim or potential victim or victim's guardians feel comfortable with the molester and even interested in interacting with him. In addition, the molester often convinces himself that the child wants to be involved in a sexual relationship with him and that his involvement with the child will meet his adult emotional needs. The molester is usually not interested in hurting the child and wants the child to enjoy the experience. The molester often projects thoughts and feelings he wants the child to have about him onto the child. He interprets the child's positive responses to the grooming and manipulation as acceptance of his behavior and convinces himself that the abusive behavior is not hurtful or damaging.

According to the Groth typology, there are two different types of child molesters, fixated/pedophile and regressed/situational. Pedophilia is a clinical diagnosis that appears in the DSM-IV. A diagnosis of pedophilia is made when an individual who is over the age of 16 has a primary or overarching sexual attraction to prepubescent children. An individual does not have to act on his primary or overarching sexual attraction to prepubescent children in order to be diagnosed as a pedophile. It may be helpful to think of this type of child molester as a fixated child molester. In fact, there may be times when someone is considered to be a fixated molester even though he may not fully meet the complex DSM-IV criteria.

When we describe someone as a fixated child molester, we are describing men who have a primary or overarching sexual attraction to children. These offenders often see their attractions as permanent and report that they have had them for as long as they can remember. Often the interests began when the offenders reached puberty. More often than not, the victims of fixated molesters are young males (however, there are fixated molesters who abuse both males and females, and those who abuse only females). A fixated child molester's offenses tend to be planned and carefully carried out over a period of time. In other words, these offenders do not act impulsively or without forethought. Fixated child molesters engage in a variety of sexually abusive activities with children. Typically, however, the activities do not include intercourse or penetration. Fondling, masturbation, and other kinds of sexual stimulation are the most typical behaviors exhibited by fixated molesters. They focus on sexually stimulating both their victims and themselves; they view their behavior as a way to meet their own emotional and social needs. Fixated child molesters usually perpetrate their abuse without using alcohol or other mood-altering substances.

According to the Groth typology, the second type of child molester is known as a regressed (or situational) child molester. Their primary sexual attraction is to adult females. That is, if you asked them the question about the ideal sexual partner, they would more than likely describe an age-appropriate member of the opposite sex. The regressed or situational offender's sexual involvement with children often develops as a result of responses to external stress and situational difficulties that they experience. In other words, these molesters usually turn to children as a way to cope with the stress they are dealing with in their lives—as a way to feel better about their situations and themselves. Unlike fixated child molesters, regressed molesters may go for months or even years without molesting, depending on their ability to deal with stressors in their lives. In many instances, these individuals replace the conflicted and problematic relationships they are having with adult women by becoming sexually involved with children. They place pseudo-adult status on their victims and then view them as they would their peers.

Unlike the victims of fixated molesters, the victims of regressed/ situational molesters are usually female. Most, though not all, incest offenders fit the description of regressed/situational molesters. In general, regressed/situational molesters' victims may be a little older than those of the fixated molester. In addition, although the sexually abusive behavior may begin prior to the time when the victim enters puberty, it may continue after the victim enters puberty. Also, and unlike the fixated molester, the regressed molester typically is involved in consensual, age-appropriate sexual behavior, or has been at some point in his life. A fixated molester's attention is overwhelmingly focused upon the arousal of the child. A regressed/situational molester's focus is primarily upon their own arousal and release. Regressed/situational molesters are also more likely to use alcohol or other illicit drugs as a part of their offense pattern.

Rapist

> Rape is a violent act, but it also a sexual act, and it is this fact that differentiates it from other crimes. Further, it is illogical to argue, on the one hand, that rape is an extension of normative male sexual behavior and, on the other hand, that rape is not sexual. . . . [R]ape is not less sexual for being violent, nor is it necessarily true that the violent aspect of rape distinguishes it from legally "acceptable" intercourse. . . . It is unfortunate that the rather swift public acceptance of the "rape as violence" model, even among groups who otherwise discount feminist arguments, has unintended implications. . . . [E]mphasizing violence—the victim's experience—is . . . strategic to the continued avoidance of an association between "normal" men and sexual violence. Make no mistake, for some men, rape is sex—in fact, for them, sex is rape. The continued rejection of this possibility, threatening though it may be, is counterproductive to understanding the social causes of sexual violence. (Scully, 1990)

The other major form of sexual assault behavior is rape, in which the victims are usually, *though not exclusively*, postpubescent. Rape is associated with very aggressive, though not necessarily physically violent, behavior on the part of the perpetrator. He attacks, threatens, and uses hostility and/or physical force to intimidate and overpower his victim. Although this type of offender may use physical force, he may also use threats and intimidation as a method of forcing his victim into sexual activity. It is important to understand this because, as we discussed earlier in our discussion of victims, rape behavior often does not result in physical injury. When an individual commits rape, he is interested in overpowering and possessing complete control and dominance over his victim. Victims are often viewed by the rapists as weak and easily dominated. Rapists do not care about the emotions of their victims (as some child molesters do), and their primary interests are self-gratification, dominance, and control. Another difference between child molesters and rapists is that some rapists will victimize an individual once, then move on to others, which is much less likely with child molesters. Finally, rapists engage in penetration or specific sexual acts with their victims, as opposed to the high incidence of fondling that is commonly associated with child molestation.

Groth (1979) identified three different kinds of rapists in his typology:

1. Anger rapists
2. Power rapists
3. Sadistic rapists

Anger rapists, as one would assume, are very angry men. Although they may be angry at women in general, or may react angrily to specific behavior of their victim, they are more often angry about a variety of issues in their lives. They cannot and will not face the difficult issues in their lives directly and in a prosocial manner. Anger rapists tend to use a significant amount of physical force when they subdue their victims—in most cases, far more force than is necessary to perpetrate the abuse. This often leaves victims severely battered and bruised on various areas of their bodies. Anger rapists also tend to be verbally abusive during their assaults, which are short in duration and very explosive in nature.

Anger rapists tend not to plan their specific offenses. Rather, they act impulsively to take advantage of situations that have presented themselves. Victim choice depends solely upon whom anger rapists see as vulnerable and available at the moment they decide they want to offend. Between 25% and 40% of known rapes are committed by men who are considered anger rapists.

The second type of rapist in the Groth typology is the power rapist. Power rapists—like anger rapists—use sexual assault as a way to feel powerful and in control. They do not, however, discharge anger during their offenses and they only use the physical force necessary to perpetrate the offense. If power rapists can gain control through threat and psychological coercion (rather than physical intimidation) they will do so. As a result, the physical injuries usually associated with anger rapists are less common with power rapists. Power rapists tend to make demands and give orders to their victims. They are not, however, as verbally hostile as anger rapists. The offenses themselves may last over a longer period of time than those committed by anger rapists, and may be repetitive in nature. Domestic violence offenders who commit sexual assaults against their partners are often power rapists.

Like anger rapists, power rapists often look for potential victims that seem vulnerable. Unlike anger rapists, however, they consider how much intimidation and force are necessary to gain control. Their preference is to attack potential victims who are both physically vulnerable and relatively easy to intimidate. Power rapists usually plan their offenses and may fantasize about how they are going to "look" and "feel."

Both anger and power rapists may have weapons available when they commit their offenses. Anger rapists are more likely to use them to hurt their victims, while power rapists are more likely to use weapons to threaten their victims and thereby decrease the need to physically overpower them. Between 60% and 70% of known rape offenders fit into the power rapist category.

Sadistic rapists are individuals who eroticize power, anger, or violence. Sadistic rapists engage in very compulsive, sometimes very ritualized sexual assault behavior. Because they have an erotic response to power and control, extreme violence and torture often characterize their assaults. In many cases, victims of sadistic rapists are murdered during the assaults. Unlike all of the other types of sex offenders in Dr. Groth's typology, sadistic rapists often have very significant psychiatric difficulties that may have a direct relationship to the offense behavior. It is fortunate, given the high degree of violence and significant likelihood of victim death, that there are relatively few known sadistic rapists. Estimates are that approximately 2% to 5% of all rapists are sadistic in nature. It is also fortunate that once apprehended, sadistic rapists are usually removed from the community for many, many years, or life.

Clinicians do not know how to treat sadistic rapists. Nothing that the treatment community has tried with this population has reduced the

likelihood that they will offend again. In addition, if they are not apprehended, they are more likely than child molesters or other types of
rapists to continue their brutal assaults.

Noncontact Offenders

The Groth typology does not include perpetrators of noncontact forms
of sexual abuse, such as voyeurs and exhibitionists. These types of
offenders are important to keep in mind, as their recidivism rates are
very high and many noncontact offenders have perpetrated, or go on to
perpetrate, more serious, contact types of offenses. This information
reminds us that there is no "one-size-fits-all" response to sex offenders, and gives us insight into how to use the information we get from
and about individual offenders, in determining the best way to super-
vise them.

Knight and Prentky Typology

Knight (1988) and Prentky, Knight, and Rosenberg, et al. (1989) have
proposed one of the most comprehensive and most validated taxonomic systems to date. This model proposes six types of molesters
(interpersonal, narcissistic, exploitative, muted, sadistic, and nonsadistic aggressive) and four types of rapists (compensatory, exploitative, displaced anger, and sadistic) based upon the degree of physical
injury incurred by the victim and the meaning of the motivation of the
offender. This rape typology further defines nine types that come from
four basic categories (opportunistic, pervasively angry, sexual, and
vindictive).

Types include the overtly sexual, sadistic, antisocial person who
plans the offense; the covert sadist with little antisocial history who
plans the offense; the individual who rapes for sexual gratification,
has little sadism and high social competence, and engages in offense
planning; the individual who rapes for sexual gratification, has little
sadism and low social competence, and engages in planning; the vindictive type who focuses anger on women and has low social competence; and the vindictive type, as above, but with high social
competence. In categorizing child molesters, Knight (1988) determined the following dimensions to be significant: the amount of contact with children, the meaning of contact, and the amount of
physical damage of aggression. Both interpersonal molesters and narcissistic molesters desire high levels of contact with children.
Interpersonal molesters are described as wanting interpersonal contact with others' children for a caring relationship that becomes sexual. Narcissistic molesters appear to be primarily concerned with

personal sexual gratification and seek out children for this purpose. For the remaining four types of molesters, the primary distinction is in the amount of permanent damage done and the motivation for the aggression (Knight, 1988). Exploitative and muted sadistic molesters usually do not do much physical damage to victims. Nonsadistic aggressive and sadistic molesters usually do significant damage to their victims.

Prentky, Knight, and Rosenberg (1989) have placed rapists into four categories based on two dimensions. The first dimension is the degree of physical injury incurred by the victim. The second dimension is the meaning of the aggressive motivation intended by the offender at the time of the victimizing event. In Category One, the compensatory offender is attempting to make up for his or her inadequacies and typically uses a minimal amount of violence. The exploitative offender also uses a minimal amount of violence and is seeking sexual gratification; he or she is using the victim as a sexual object. With the displaced anger offender, the motivation is to release pent up anger. The displaced anger offender may use a range of violence from almost no violence to a violent outburst to release this anger. The sadistic offender is seeking to hurt for the sake of hurting the victim. The sadistic molester causes extreme physical or psychological harm to the victim.

The muted sadistic offender has more control than the sadistic offender and usually uses humiliation and degradation rather than physical damage to the victim.

CROSSOVER

Most offenders have some preference for a particular victim or type of behavior. This might lead one to believe that an offender would be less of a danger to those potential victims who do not match his or her preference. Research has demonstrated, however, that although crossover rates vary among different populations of sex offenders, a significant percentage of offenders engage in more than one type of abuse. In 1987, Abel and colleagues examined crossover behavior in sex offenders and found that nearly 50% of the subjects in the study had engaged in multiple sex offending behaviors. Another study conducted in 1998 (Ahlmeyer, English & Simmons, 1999) reports significant crossover with respect to the gender and age of victims. This research has significant implications regarding the need to restrict access to a very wide range of potential victims (all ages, both genders, etc.) when a sex offender is placed under community supervision.

Table 9–4 Etiological Factors Contributing to the Evolution of the Sexual Offender

Exposure to violence, aggressive role models
Cultural/societal influences
Substance abuse
Esteem deficits
Psychopathy
Abuse-supportive attitudes
Attachment difficulties
Intimacy deficits
Physiological/hormonal
Deviant sexual arousal
Social competency deficits
Empathy deficits
Emotional regulation difficulties
Coping skills deficits
Sexual victimization
Etiological considerations for juvenile sexual abusers
Child maltreatment
Exposure to pornography
Poor impulse control

ETIOLOGICAL CONSIDERATIONS FOR ADULT SEXUAL OFFENDERS

Table 9–4 identifies factors that are considered to play an etiological role in the development of sexual offenders; however, none of these factors is correlated strongly enough such that the existence of that factor would indicate increased risk.

SUMMARIZING ADULT SEXUAL OFFENDERS

Sexual offenders hurt others through their behavior, have ongoing empathy deficits, have deficits in emotional expression, have cognitive distortions/thinking errors that make it easier to behave in an abusive fashion, commit more offenses than those they are apprehended for, and are a heterogeneous group with a need for a variety of interventions. They do not all commit their offense for the same reasons or to try and meet the same types of needs. They pose varying degrees of risk and dangerousness and have widely varied rates of recidivism, although the overall average recidivism rate tends to remain below 20%.

QUESTIONS FOR DISCUSSION

1. What criteria determine an instance of sexual abuse?
2. Discuss the most significant elements of the concept of informed consent.
3. How can a knowledge of the dynamics of sexual abuse be used to propose strategies aimed at prevention?
4. Who are the most vulnerable potential victims/offenders in the case of sexual abuse?
5. Propose some measures that might be useful in the prevention of sexual abuse.
6. Describe the role of the forensic nurse in relation to the current management of sexual abuse.
7. Discuss the potential for collaboration between forensic nurses, other healthcare professionals, and the criminal justice system in the management of sexual abuse.

REFERENCES

Abel, G. G., Becker, J. V., Cunningham-Rathner, J., Mittlemann, M., Murphy, W. D., & Rouleau, J. L. (1987). Multiple paraphilic diagnoses among sex offenders. *Bulletin of the American Academy of Psychiatry and the Law, 16,* 153–168.

Ahlmeyer, S., English, K., & Simmons, D. (1999). *The impact of polygraphy on admissions of crossover offending behavior in adult sexual offenders.* Presentation at the Association for the Treatment of Sexual Abusers 18th Annual Research and Treatment Conference, Lake Buena Vista, FL.

Carnes, P. (2001). *Out of the shadows: Understanding sexual addiction.* Center City, MN: Hazelden Publishing.

Finkelhor, David. (1984). *Child sexual abuse.* New York: The Free Press.

Freud, S. (1923). *The ego and the id.* London: Hogarth Press.

Groth, A. N. (1979). *Men who rape: The psychology of the offender.* New York: Plenum Press.

Heil, P., Ahlmeyer, S., & Simmons, D. (1988). Crossover sexual offenses. *Sexual abuse: A journal of research and treatment, 15*(4), 221–236.

Jackson, J. W., Karlson, H. C., Tzeng, O. C. S. (1991). *Theories of child abuse and neglect: differential perspectives, summaries, and evaluations.* New York: Praeger Publishers. U.S. Department of Health.

Knight, R. A. (1988). A taxonomic analysis of child molesters. In Robert A. Prentky & Vernon L. Quinsey (Eds.), *Human sexual aggression: Current perspectives.* New York: New York Academy of Sciences.

Knight, R. A., Carter, D. L. & Prentky, R. A. (1989). A system for the classification of child molesters. *Journal of Interpersonal Violence, 4,* 3–23.

Knight, R. A. & Prentky, R. A. (1987). The developmental antecedents and adult adaptations of rapists' subtypes. *Criminal Justice and Behavior, 14,* 403–426.

Knight, R. A. & Prentky, R. A. (1990). Classifying sexual offenders: The development and corroboration of taxonomic models. In William L. Marshall & Howard E. Barbaree (Eds.), Handbook of sexual assault: Issues, theories & treatment of the offender. NY: Kluwer Academic/Plenum Publishers.

Knight, R. A., Prentky, R. A. & Cerce, D. D. (1994). The development, reliability, and validity of an inventory for the multidimensional assessment of sex and aggression. *Criminal Justice and Behavior, 21,* 72–94.

Knight, R. A. & Prentky, R. A. (1990). Classifying sexual offenders: The development and corroboration of taxonomic models. In W. L. Marshall, D. R. Laws, and H. E. Barbaree (Eds.), *Handbook of sexual assault: Issues, theories, and treatment of the offender* (pp. 23–52). New York: Kluwer Academic Plenum Publishers.

Knight, R. A., Rosenberg, R., & Schneider, B. A. (1985). Classification of sexual offenders: Perspectives, methods, and validation. In Ann W. Burgess (Ed.), *Rape and sexual assault. A research handbook.* New York: Garland Publishing.

Laws, D. R., Hudson, S., & Ward, T. (2000). *Remaking relapse prevention with sex offenders: A sourcebook.* Thousand Oaks, CA: Sage Publications.

Marshall, W. L., Laws, D. R., & Barbaree, H. E. (Eds.). (1990). *Handbook of sexual assault: issues, theories and treatment of the offender.* New York: Kluwer Academic Plenum Publishers.

National Task Force on Juvenile Sexual Offending. (1993). Final Report. University of Colorado Health Sciences Center, Denver, CO.

Nichols, H. R. & Molinder, L. (1984). Multiphasic Sex Inventory. Tacoma, WA: 437 Bowes Drive, Tacoma, WA 98466. Published by authors.

Olson, D. H. & Craddock, A. E. (1980). Circumplex model of marital and family systems: Application to Australian families. *Australian Journal of Sex, Marriage and Family.*

Olson, D. H. (1996). *Clinical assessment & treatment interventions using the Circumplex Model.* (Chapter 5, pp. 59–80). In F. W. Kaslow (Ed.). *Handbook of relational diagnosis and dysfunctional family patterns.* New York: John Wiley and Sons.

Olson, D. H. (1989). *Circumplex model of family systems VIII: Family assessment and intervention.* In D. H. Olson, C. S. Russell, & D. H. Sprenkle (Eds.), *Circumplex model: Systemic assessment and treatment of families.* New York: Haworth Press.

Prentky, R. A., Knight, R. A., Rosenberg, R., & Lee, A. (1989). A path analytic approach to the validation of a taxonomic system for classifying child molesters. *Journal of Quantitative Criminology, 6,* 231–257.

Rosenberg, R. & R. A. Knight (1988). Determining male sexual offenders subtypes using cluster analysis. *Journal of Quantitative Criminology, 4,* 383–409.

Ryan, G. (1997). *Juvenile sexual offending: Causes, consequences and correction.* New York: John Wiley and Sons.

Schwartz, B. & Cellini, H. (1995). *The sex offender.* Kingston, NJ: Civic Research Institute.

Scully, D. (1990). *Understanding sexual violence.* (pp. 142–143). New York: Routledge.

Ward, T., Laws, D. R., & Hudson, S. M. (Eds.). (2003). *The sex offender: sexual deviance: issues and controversies.* Thousand Oaks, CA: Sage Publications.

Ward, T. & Hudson, S. M. (1998). The construction and development of theory in the sexual offending area: A metatheoretical framework. *Sexual Abuse: Journal of Research and Treatment, 10,* 47–63.

Forensic Implications of Intimate Partner Violence

Daniel J. Sheridan
Catherine R. Nash
Shadonna L. Hawkins
Jennifer L. Makely
Jacquelyn C. Campbell

Intimate partner violence has become one of the primary areas of interest for forensic nursing. Early screening, identification, and treatment of intimate partner violence patients can help break often serious and deadly cycles of violence. The scope of practice in the area of intimate partner violence has also grown with awareness of the many aspects of this problem. The forensic nurse who works with victims of domestic violence must be well equipped to recognize and document any injuries. In addition, the forensic nurse must maintain appropriate relationships with representatives of various community services to best serve the needs of this population.

CHAPTER FOCUS

Development of hospital-based domestic violence programs
Screening tools for domestic violence
Identifying injuries and wounds
Written documentation
Photographic documentation

KEY TERMS

abrasions
abuse assessment screen
avulsions
contusions

cuts/incisions
domestic violence
ecchymosis
lacerations
partner violence screen
pattern of injury
patterned injuries
petechiae
strangulation

DEVELOPMENT OF HOSPITAL-BASED DOMESTIC VIOLENCE PROGRAMS

In the late 1970s and early 1980s, nurses conducted some of the earliest and now classic research that identified battering against women by intimate partners as a major health and public health problem (Drake, 1982; Parker & Schumacher, 1977). As early as 1975, during the foundational years of the battered women's advocacy movement, Betty Cavanaugh, an emergency department nurse at the Hennepin County Medical Center (located in Minneapolis), created the Women's Advocacy Program (Jackson, 1992; Sheridan, 1998a). Approximately 30 years later the program still exists as the Battered Women and Men's Advocacy Services.

Susan Hadley, a community-based women's advocate, is credited with developing the first comprehensive nationally recognized model hospital-based domestic violence service program (Hadley, 1992; Hadley et al., 1995). In early 1986, Hadley (1992) registered WomanKind, Inc., Support Services for Battered Women as a tax-exempt nonprofit corporation in Minnesota. She then convinced administrators at Fairview Southdale Hospital (located in the greater Minneapolis area) to allow WomanKind staff and volunteers to provide victim advocacy to abused patients and domestic violence education to the healthcare staff. WomanKind, Inc. eventually merged into the Fairview Health System as a separate department, and its staff continues to provide a variety of advocacy and educational services at numerous Fairview Health System hospitals (Hadley et al., 1995).

On July 1, 1986, the primary author of this chapter created the Family Violence Program (FVP) at Chicago's Rush-Presbyterian St. Luke's Medical Center (Sheridan & Taylor, 1993). The FVP, as its name implies, was designed to provide specialized advanced practice nursing services to survivors of all forms of family violence. Within a few weeks of its inception, the FVP inherited the training, administrative, and fiscal responsibility for the medical center's fledgling volunteer-based Rape Victim Advocacy Program. In addition to victim advocacy and domestic violence training of health professionals, the nurses and social workers employed in the FVP (primarily from grant funding) provided direct patient care assessments, nursing, and/or social work care, including thorough written and photographic documentation. It did not take long before hundreds of patients had been served. Within a few months of providing services, the FVP staff began to be subpoenaed to testify in a variety of criminal and civil cases that resulted from the reported abuse.

In 1991, the primary author created a similar nurse-coordinated Domestic Violence Intervention Team at Oregon Health Sciences University Hospital in Portland, which focused primarily on assessment, interventions, and documentation of intimate partner and elder abuse patients who presented anywhere within the medical center's in-patient system. Again, it did not take long before hundreds of patients had been served and the program staff was being called into a variety of courts.

Nationally, hospital-based family violence programs were providing forensic nursing services to survivors of child abuse/neglect, intimate partner violence, and elder abuse years before such services were identified as forensic nursing. The International Association of Forensic Nurses (IAFN) was not created until 1992. Its creation gave a name to the type of nursing being practiced by innovative nurses all over the country who provided increasingly specialized care to a wide variety of patients who had been victimized in criminal acts.

During the early 1990s the number of hospital-based domestic violence programs slowly increased. In 1994, Susan Dersch, a nurse-advocate, created the Assisting Women with Advocacy, Resources, and Education (AWARE) program at Barnes and Jewish Hospital in St. Louis (Sheridan, 1998a). The AWARE program is unique compared to most hospital-based family violence programs in that it is *not* focused on *nor* housed in an emergency department. Rather, the AWARE program recognizes domestic violence as an issue that primarily affects the health of all women who present throughout the healthcare system. Although the AWARE program collaborates closely with the emergency department, the majority of its referrals are from routine screening for abuse that is conducted by staff throughout the Barnes and Jewish Hospital system.

In recent years the number of hospital-based domestic and family violence programs has grown exponentially. Many of the programs are advocacy based, staff education-focused, and managed via a wide variety of partnerships with community-based domestic violence service providers. Other domestic violence healthcare-based programs are being developed as natural extensions of the rapidly growing number of sexual assault nurse examiner programs. The Family Violence Prevention Fund is collecting data on existing hospital-based family violence programs and offers a treasure of health system–related materials (many free and some for nominal cost) on its website (www.endabuse.com).

SCREENING TOOLS FOR DOMESTIC VIOLENCE

There are several published, reliable, and valid intimate partner violence screening tools used in clinical healthcare settings. Among the best known are varying-length versions of the Abuse Assessment Screen (AAS) and the three-question Partner Violence Screen (PVS).

Helton (1986) developed the first version of the Abuse Assessment Screen as a nine-question screen that was published by the March of Dimes (see Figure 10–1). In 1988, the Nursing Research Consortium on Violence and Abuse (NRCVA) modified the original AAS to a six-question screen (see Figure 10–2) for use in clinical and clinical research

---

1. Do you know where you would go or who could help you if you were abused or worried about abuse?

   Yes _____   No _____

   If yes, where _____

2. Are you in a relationship with a man who physically hurts you?

   Yes _____   No _____   Sometimes _____

3. Does he threaten you with abuse?

   Yes _____   No _____   Sometimes _____

4. Has the man you are with hit, slapped, kicked, or otherwise physically hurt you?

   Yes _____   No _____   Sometimes _____

5. If yes, has he hit you since you've been pregnant?

   Yes _____   No _____   Not Applicable _____

6. If yes, did the abuse increase since you've been pregnant?

   Yes _____   No _____   Not Applicable _____

7. Have you ever received medical treatment for any abuse injuries?

   Yes _____   No _____   Not Applicable _____

8. If you have been abused, remembering the last time he hurt you, mark the places on the body map where he hit you.

9. Were you pregnant at the time?

   Yes _____   No _____   Not Applicable _____

Figure 10–1   Abuse Assessment Screen—Original Version (Helton, 1986)

settings. This version of the AAS asks about three nonphysical forms of domestic abuse: 1) experiencing fear during arguments with a partner; 2) feeling like the partner is trying to emotionally hurt the woman; and 3) feeling like the partner is trying to control the woman. The six-question AAS version has been used very effectively in numerous clinical settings by the primary author. However, using a six-question screen raised concerns about staff time. Therefore, the NRCVA developed a three-question version of the AAS that was used in a large prospective study that screened for battering during pregnancy in a population of about 700 women (McFarlane et al., 1992; Parker & McFarlane, 1991) that established baseline reliability and validity (see Figure 10–3). The three-question AAS received further reliability and validity when used in larger study (N = 1,203) (Parker et al., 1993). A two-question version of the AAS also has been developed, tested, and shown to have reliability and validity (McFarlane et al., 1995) (see Figure 10–4).

Violence is very common in today's world and it can overlap into our homes. Because violence affects so many people, I now routinely ask all my patients (clients) a few questions about violence in their lives.

All couples argue now and again, even the best of couples.

1. When you and your partner argue are you ever afraid of him (her)?
2. When you and your partner verbally argue, do you think he (she) tries to emotionally hurt/abuse you?
3. Does your partner try to control you? Where you go? Who you see? How much money you can have?
4. Has your partner (or anyone) ever slapped you, pushed you, hit you, kicked you, or otherwise physically hurt you?
5. Since you have been pregnant (when you were pregnant), has your partner ever slapped you, pushed you, hit you, kicked you, or otherwise physically hurt you?
6. Has your partner ever forced you into sex when you did not want to participate?

With any yes, say thank you for sharing. Can you give me an example? Can you tell me more about the last time it happened?

Adapted from the Nursing Research Consortium on Violence and Abuse (NRCVA), Abuse Assessment Screen. McFarlane, J., Parker, B., Soeken, K. & Bullock, L. (1992).

Figure 10–2   Abuse Assessment Screen—NRCVA Version (1988)

1. Within the last year, have you been hit, slapped,   YES   NO
   kicked, or otherwise physically hurt by someone?

   If yes, by whom? _____

   Total number of times._____

2. Since you've been pregnant, have you been hit,   YES   NO
   slapped, kicked, or otherwise physically hurt by
   someone?

   If yes, by whom? _____

   Total number of times._____

MARK THE AREA OF INJURY ON THE BODY MAP. SCORE
EACH INCIDENT ACCORDING TO THE FOLLOWING SCALE: SCORE

1 = Threats of abuse including use of a weapon.   _____

2 = Slapping, pushing; no injuries and/or lasting pain.   _____

3 = Punching, kicking, bruises, cuts, and/or pain.   _____

4 = Beating up, severe contusions, burns, and broken bones. _____

5 = Head injury, internal injury, permanent injury.   _____

6 = Use of a weapon, injury from a weapon.   _____

(If any of the descriptions for the higher number apply, use the
higher number.)

3. Within the last year, has anyone forced you   YES   NO
   to have sexual activities?

   If yes, by whom? _____

   Total number of times._____

Figure 10–3 Abuse Assessment Screen—Three-Question Version (McFarlane et al., 1992)

1. Have you ever been hit, slapped, kicked, or otherwise physically
   hurt by your male partner?
2. Have you ever been forced to have sexual activities?

Figure 10–4 Abuse Assessment Screen—Two-Question Version (McFarlane, Greenberg, et al., 1995)

1. Have you been hit, kicked, punched, or otherwise hurt by someone within the past year? If so, by whom?
2. Do you feel safe in your current relationship?
3. Is there a partner from a previous relationship who is making you
   feel unsafe now?

Figure 10–5   Partner Violence Screen (Feldhaus et al., 1997)

The Partner Violence Screen (PVS) (Feldhaus et al., 1997) uses one item from the AAS (being hit, kicked, punched, or otherwise hurt by someone) (see Figure 10–5). The PVS also asks if a former partner is making the woman feel unsafe. From clinical experience, many women are being abused (or at risk of being abused) by current and former intimate partners.

McFarlane et al. (2001) added two questions about withholding services or care to people with physical disabilities to the two-question AAS (see Figure 10–6) to create the Abuse Assessment Screen—Disability (AAS-D), which was tested on over 500 women at public and private specialty clinics. The AAS-D detected a 9.8% prevalence rate of abuse, with the perpetrator of physical or sexual abuse being most often an intimate partner.

Many emergency departments have tried to reduce their screening process to one question on their intake forms. No published studies have found a one-question screen to be a reliable and valid IPV screening tool. A one-item screening question for IPV that has *not* been particularly clinically useful is, "Do you feel safe in your home?" Patients may not feel safe in their homes for any number of reasons, including living in a high crime neighborhood.

INTIMATE PARTNER VIOLENCE-RELATED HOMICIDE

Early screening, identification, and treatment of intimate partner violence patients can help break often serious and deadly cycles of violence. Intimate partner violence-related homicide is identified as the leading cause of death in the United States among African American females between the ages of 15 and 45 and as the seventh leading cause overall in premature deaths of young women (Campbell et al., 2003b).

Campbell states:

> In 70 to 80 percent of intimate partner homicides, despite which partner was killed, the man physically abused the woman before the murder. Thus, one of the primary ways to decrease intimate partner homicide is to identify and intervene promptly with abused women at risk. (2003a, p. 18)

1. Within the last year, have you ever been hit, slapped,   YES   NO
   kicked, pushed, shoved, or otherwise physically hurt
   by someone?

If YES, who? (Circle all that apply.)

Intimate partner	Care provider	Health professional	Family member	Other

Please describe: _____

2. Within the last year, has anyone forced you to have   YES   NO
   sexual activities?

If YES, who? (Circle all that apply.)

Intimate partner	Care provider	Health professional	Family member	Other

Please describe: _____

3. Within the last year, has anyone prevented you from   YES   NO
   using a wheelchair, cane, respirator, or other
   assistive device?

If YES, who? (Circle all that apply.)

Intimate partner	Care provider	Health professional	Family member	Other

Please describe: _____

4. Within the last year, has anyone you depend on   YES   NO
   refused to help you with an important personal need,
   such as taking your medicine, getting to the bathroom,
   getting out of bed, bathing, getting dressed, or getting
   food or drink?

If YES, who? (Circle all that apply.)

Intimate partner	Care provider	Health professional	Family member	Other

Please describe: _____

Figure 10–6 Abuse Assessment Screen—Disabled Four-Question Version (McFarlane et al., 2001)

In response, a recent study spanning 11 cities was completed to identify risk factors pertaining to intimate partner homicide, specifically femicide, the homicide of women (Campbell et al., 2003b). The study was completed using control design methodology. Data was collected from two main sources: femicide cases (dead women) and abuse victims that had similar profiles to the deceased. The data were analyzed from various disciplinary vantage points including domestic violence advocates, police enforcement, and medical examiners. Common themes throughout data analysis were identified as risk factors.

Risk factors that were categorized as putting a female at high risk for domestic violence homicide include:

1. A perpetrator's access to a gun with previous threats of weapon use
2. A stepchild of the perpetrator living in the home
3. Estrangement of the victim from the perpetrator (Campbell et al., 2003b)

In addition, the researchers found that a past history of stalking, forced sex, and abuse during pregnancy increased risk for femicide. The leading socioeconomic factor linked to increased risk of domestic homicide was the abuser's lack of employment (Campbell et al., 2003a, 2003b).

Various intimate partner violence, dangerousness, and harassment tools were used in Campbell's study, including the Danger Assessment (DA) and select items from the HARASS (Harassment in Abusive Relationships: A Self-Report Scale) tool. All of the items on the DA (see Figure 10–7) and the HARASS (see Figure 10–8) are positively correlated with increased risk of homicide. Therefore, whenever one has a positive screen for intimate partner abuse, the patient should be asked to complete the DA and the HARASS. Both tools are self-report scales and can be completed by the patient while the forensic nurse is completing other tasks in or outside the patient's room. The DA will produce better results if completed in conjunction with a calendar where the woman can mark the dates or approximate dates of abusive episodes. The calendar serves as a memory trigger. The data from the DA and the HARASS can guide the forensic nurse in discharge and/or admission to the hospital for safety planning. In addition, when abused women answer the questions on the DA and the HARASS, it lowers their ability to minimize the seriousness of the abuse in the relationship.

Several risk factors have been associated with increased risk of homicides (murders) of women and men in violent relationships. We cannot predict what will happen in your case, but we would like you to be aware of the danger of homicide in situations of abuse and for you to see how many of the risk factors apply to your situation.

Using the calendar, please mark the approximate dates during the past year when you were abused by your partner or ex-partner. Write on that date how bad the incident was according to the following scale:
1. Slapping, pushing; no injuries and/or lasting pain
2. Punching, kicking; bruises, cuts, and/or continuing pain
3. "Beating up"; severe contusions, burns, broken bones
4. Threat to use weapon; head injury, internal injury, permanent injury
5. Use of weapon; wounds from weapon

(If **any** of the descriptions for the higher number apply, use the higher number.)

Mark **Yes** or **No** for each of the following. ("He" refers to your husband, partner, ex-husband, ex-partner, or whoever is currently physically hurting you.)
____ 1. Has the physical violence increased in severity or frequency over the past year?
____ 2. Does he own a gun?
____ 3. Have you left him after living together during the past year?
    3a. (If have *never* lived with him, check here___)
____ 4. Is he unemployed?
____ 5. Has he ever used a weapon against you or threatened you with a lethal weapon? (If yes, was the weapon a gun?____)
____ 6. Does he threaten to kill you?
____ 7. Has he avoided being arrested for domestic violence?
____ 8. Do you have a child that is not his?
____ 9. Has he ever forced you to have sex when you did not wish to do so?
____ 10. Does he ever try to choke you?
____ 11. Does he use illegal drugs? By drugs, I mean "uppers" or amphetamines, speed, angel dust, cocaine, "crack," street drugs, or mixtures.
____ 12. Is he an alcoholic or problem drinker?
____ 13. Does he control most or all of your daily activities? For instance: does he tell you who you can be friends with, when you can see your family, how much money you can use, or when you can take the car? (If he tries, but you do not let him, check here: ____)
____ 14. Is he violently and constantly jealous of you? (For instance, does he say "If I can't have you, no one can.")
____ 15. Have you ever been beaten by him while you were pregnant? (If you have never been pregnant by him, check here: ____)
____ 16. Have you ever threatened or tried to commit suicide?
____ 17. Has he ever threatened or tried to commit suicide?
____ 18. Does he threaten to harm your children?
____ 19. Do you believe he is capable of killing you?
____ 20. Does he follow or spy on you, leave threatening notes or messages on answering machine, destroy your property, or call you when you don't want him to?

_____   Total "Yes" Answers

Thank you. Please talk to your nurse, advocate, or counselor about what the Danger Assessment means in terms of your situation

Source: Jacquelyn C. Campbell, Ph.D., R.N., Copyright, 2003

Figure 10–7 Danger Assessment

IDENTIFYING INJURIES AND WOUNDS

Great importance is placed on accurately identifying and documenting injuries. Many healthcare providers consistently misuse medical forensic terms, and this can have a profound effect on the legal outcome of an assault. The following sections present important terms and their appropriate use as determined by several authors and leaders in the field of forensic medical science and authors of medical dictionaries (Brockmeyer & Sheridan, 1998; DiMaio & DiMaio, 2001; Miller & Keane, 1978; Sheridan, 2001; Venes & Thomas, 2001).

Injury Patterns

Patterned injuries present identifiable markings that allow a provider to discern (with reasonable certainty) that they were caused by a specific or unknown object, and/or by a specific mechanism of injury. Examples of such include fingertip-*like* contusions from being grabbed, cord-*like* contusions and abrasions from being whipped with a corded object, and fingernail scratch-*like* abrasions around the neck from being strangled. Note the appropriate use of the word *like* to describe what the provider identifies as the most likely cause of these patterned injuries.

Injuries in various stages of healing are referred to as a pattern of injury. The term can be used in describing both cutaneous and orthopedic injuries. It should be noted that in other forensic science circles this term may be used to mean "patterned injuries."

Abrasions

Often called scrapes by the lay public, abrasions to the skin are superficial injuries that are caused by the friction or rubbing of the skin against a rough surface or object. The rougher the surface, the more severe the abrasion will be. An important point to remember is that abrasions, especially abrasions that have not been thoroughly cleaned, can be an excellent source of trace physical evidence. Care should be taken to collect any material found in or around the wound and surrounding clothing that may have come from the surface or object that was scraped, prior to cleaning and dressing the wound. The clothing should also be secured and labeled as evidence.

Avulsions

Avulsions refer to skin or other tissue that has been completely torn away by blunt and/or shearing force energies. Frequently occurring over bony prominences, forearms, and hands, blunt and/or shearing force energies can result in partial avulsions (often called skin tears).

H arassment in
A busive
R elationships:
A
S elf-report
S cale

Many women are harassed in relationships with their abusive partners, especially if the women are trying to end the relationship. You may be experiencing harassment. This instrument is designed to measure harassment of women who are in abusive relationships or who are in the process of leaving abusive relationships. By completing this questionnaire, you may better understand harassment in your life. If you have any questions, please talk with the service provider who gave you this tool.

Harassment is defined as: *a persistent pattern of behavior by an intimate partner that is intended to bother, annoy, trap, emotionally wear down, threaten, frighten, terrify, and/or coerce a woman with the overall intent to control her choices and behavior about leaving an abusive relationship.*

There are no right or wrong answers. Do not put your name on the form. The instrument takes about 10 minutes to complete.

For each item, circle the number that best describes how often the behavior occurred. Next, rate how distressing the behavior is to you. If the behavior has never occurred, circle 0 (NEVER) and go to the next questions. If the question does not apply to you, circle NA (NOT APPLICABLE). If you are still in the relationship please circle MY PARTNER. If you have left the relationship, please circle MY FORMER PARTNER.

0 = Never
1 = Rarely
2 = Occasionally
3 = Frequently
4 = Very Frequently
NA = Not applicable
How often does it occur?

0 = Not at all distressing
1 = Slightly distressing
2 = Moderately distressing
3 = Very distressing
4 = Extremely distressing
NA = Not applicable
How distressing is this behavior to you?

THE BEHAVIOR

MY PARTNER   MY FORMER PARTNER (circle one)

The Behavior	How often does it occur?						How distressing is this behavior to you?					
1. Frightens people close to me	0	1	2	3	4	NA	0	1	2	3	4	NA
2. Pretends to be someone else in order to get to me	0	1	2	3	4	NA	0	1	2	3	4	NA
3. Comes to my home when I don't want him there	0	1	2	3	4	NA	0	1	2	3	4	NA
4. Threatens to kill me if I leave or stay away from him	0	1	2	3	4	NA	0	1	2	3	4	NA
5. Threatens to harm the kids if I leave or stay away from him	0	1	2	3	4	NA	0	1	2	3	4	NA
6. Takes things that belong to me so I have to see him to get them back	0	1	2	3	4	NA	0	1	2	3	4	NA
7. Tries getting me fired from my job	0	1	2	3	4	NA	0	1	2	3	4	NA

8. Ignores court orders to stay away from me	0	1	2	3	4	NA	0	1	2	3	4	NA
9. Keeps showing up wherever I am	0	1	2	3	4	NA	0	1	2	3	4	NA
10. Bothers me at work when I don't want to talk to him	0	1	2	3	4	NA	0	1	2	3	4	NA
11. Uses the kids as pawns to get me physically close to him	0	1	2	3	4	NA	0	1	2	3	4	NA
12. Shows up without warning	0	1	2	3	4	NA	0	1	2	3	4	NA
13. Messes with my property (For example: sells my stuff, breaks my furniture, damages my car, steals my things)	0	1	2	3	4	NA	0	1	2	3	4	NA
14. Scares me with a weapon	0	1	2	3	4	NA	0	1	2	3	4	NA
15. Breaks into my home	0	1	2	3	4	NA	0	1	2	3	4	NA
16. Threatens to kill me if I leave or stay away from him	0	1	2	3	4	NA	0	1	2	3	4	NA
17. Threatens to harm our pet	0	1	2	3	4	NA	0	1	2	3	4	NA
18. Calls me on the telephone and hangs up	0	1	2	3	4	NA	0	1	2	3	4	NA
19. Reports me to the authorities for taking drugs when I don't	0	1	2	3	4	NA	0	1	2	3	4	NA

Additional harassing behaviors not listed above:

20. _____	0	1	2	3	4	NA	0	1	2	3	4	NA
21. _____	0	1	2	3	4	NA	0	1	2	3	4	NA

Please answer a few additional questions:

_____ Your age in years

Check the statement that best describes you:

☐ Married, living with an abusive partner
☐ Single, living with an abusive partner
☐ Married, living apart from an abusive partner
☐ Single, living apart from an abusive partner.

How long were you in the above relationship? _____

Are you still in the relationship? ☐ Yes ☐ No

If you have left the relationship, how long have you been out? _____

What is your approximate annual income? _____

How many years of school have you completed? _____

Check the statement that best describes you:

☐ Asian/Pacific Islander
☐ Black/African American
☐ Caucasian/White
☐ Hispanic
☐ Native American/American Indian
☐ Other _____

Figure 10–8 HARASS Scale

Bruise/Contusion

Created by either a blunt or compression force trauma, bruises/contusions are wounds resulting in discoloration in the skin or other organs caused by the breaking of blood vessels. The terms bruise and contusion can be used synonymously. Both contusions and cuts (defined in a later section) are frequently seen along the upper and outer aspects of the upper extremities in defensive posturing when attempting to protect oneself during an assault.

There have been several research studies to assess the accuracy of "dating" bruises. The findings have been consistent—there is *no* scientific basis to accurately date bruises either by looking at photographs of injuries or by viewing the injuries directly (Bariciak et al., 2003; Langlois & Gresham, 1991; Wilson, 1977). Forensic health professionals caution all health professionals to not date injuries by their general appearance (DiMaio & DiMaio, 2001; Sheridan, 2001, 2003). However, in general, bruises go through a relatively predictable color changing process (from red to black and blue, to bluish-green, to greenish-brown, to brownish-yellow, to yellow, to light yellow, and then to fade), but the time between each stage varies from person to person (Sheridan, 2003). The pigmentation of the victim's skin can also make it difficult to document, either through photographs or visually. The forensic nurse may be able to determine if the bruise is from relatively recent trauma or from older trauma. In addition, the forensic nurse may be able to testify if the age of the bruise is consistent or not consistent with the history provided.

Ecchymosis

Ecchymosis is a frequently misused term often incorrectly used as a synonym for a bruise/contusion that is caused by trauma. Ecchymosis refers to subcutaneous, hemorrhagic blotching under the skin often caused by a medical/hematological condition or indirectly caused by trauma. Ecchymotic lesions are usually nonpainful and nonindurated (not hard or firm) in nature. However, it would be forensically accurate to describe a spread of discoloration from a directly traumatized area as ecchymosis. For example, a person who is punched to the mid-forehead right above the nose will almost certainly develop bilateral, peri-orbital ecchymoses (swelling and discoloration to both eyes). The trauma was to the forehead and the blood seeped or leaked downward into the orbital area. In contrast, if a person was punched directly to one eye with resulting swelling, pain, and discoloration to the point of impact, that injury would be most accurately called a bruise/contusion. The color changes related to the resolution of ecchymotic lesions will parallel the color changes of bruising but the etiology of the bleeding under the skin or other body organs are different.

Laceration

The word *laceration* is probably the most mistakenly used term when providers are describing wounds. Laceration refers to the tearing or splitting of tissue from blunt and/or shearing injuries. Lacerations are often to the skin; however, it is not uncommon to receive a laceration to the liver from a blunt or squeezing force trauma. Unlike cuts to the skin from sharp injuries, lacerated wounds typically have a jagged edge or edges and occur most often over bony prominences. A bruise or contusion is also often present embedded around the torn or ruptured tissue.

Cuts/Incisions

Unlike lacerations, cuts or incisions typically have a smooth edge to them and are caused by a sharp instrument or object. The depth of cuts/incisions is also consistent, whereas for lacerations they may be varying. It should be noted that when a provider is in doubt as to whether an injury is a laceration or cut, the term *wound* should be used with an accompanying description.

Petechiae

These tiny, nonelevated, purplish hemorrhagic spots are frequently seen in the face and eyes of victims of strangulation (either manual, ligature, or mechanical). Other medical conditions, such as severe vomiting, severe coughing, severe sneezing, strenuous bowel movements, and platelet deficiency can also cause them. Women giving vaginal birth may develop facial petechiae from pushing, and children have developed impressive facial petechiae from severe screaming.

Traumatic Alopecia

Often overlooked, traumatic hair loss (alopecia) can occur when the victim is pulled or dragged by his or her hair. This alopecia is painful and can be difficult to photograph. If hair pulling has been reported, the forensic nurse may be able to run a comb through the patient's hair to secure large numbers of pulled hairs as evidence to support traumatic alopecia.

Slap Injuries

Slap injuries usually initially present as raised, reddened, painful welts to the skin. As the swelling subsides there are often patterned linear parallel bruises outlining the edges of the perpetrator's fingers. If hit hard enough to the head, a punch or slap can rupture a victim's eardrums. This can sometimes be the only presenting sign of injury from a slap.

Strangulation

Manual and ligature strangulation is a frequent injury inflicted by perpetrators of intimate partner violence onto their partners. Physical findings range from ligature-induced patterned bruising and/or abrasion, to fingernail scratch-like abrasions to the neck, to petechiae of the face or eyes. However, most victims of strangulation present with no physical signs (Strack, McClane, & Hawley, 2001). The danger lies in healthcare providers underappreciating the health risks associated with strangulation and its delayed effect on one's breathing. Even without signs of dyspnea, a victim of strangulation should at a minimum be hospitalized and frequently assessed for 24 hours with continuous pulse-oximetry (Kuriloff & Pincus, 1989). A study found that strangulation is an assault that occurs late in an abusive relationship, thereby placing the victim at increased risk of significant injury or death (Wilbur et al., 2001). Long-term symptoms from repeated strangulations include neck and throat injury, neurological disorders, and psychological disorders (Smith, Mills, & Taliaferro, 2001).

Firearm Injuries

Victims of firearms injuries are frequently seen by healthcare providers in an acute emergency setting. In addition to life-saving measures, efforts should be made to secure and save clothing and to carefully document the location and size of the wounds. Protocols for the collection of evidence should be present in every healthcare facility that may come into contact with victims of violence. Individual pieces of clothing should be placed in labeled paper bags to dry. Bullet fragments should each be placed in separate containers. No attempt should be made with multiple openings to ascertain whether a bullet wound is entrance or exit. Studies have shown that physicians are rarely correct (Randall, 1993).

Bite Marks

Bite marks can occur almost anywhere among victims of domestic violence, but are often seen in sexual areas, especially the breast (Vale & Noguchi, 1983). The unique characteristics of these patterned injuries provide opportune evidence and may be able to be matched to the perpetrator by forensic odontologists if documented appropriately. Again, protocols should be in place at the facility to help make the process easier. Close-up photographs should be taken using a right-angle ruler developed by the American Board of Forensic Odontology (Sheridan, 2001). Cotton tip applicators, premoistened with sterile water, can also be rubbed over the bitten area to secure DNA evidence from the assailant's saliva.

Sexual Assault

Typically overlooked in intimate partner abuse, nearly half of all cases of domestic violence involve forced sexual assault (Campbell, 1989, 1998). Traditionally, if the sexual assault has occurred within 72 hours, a rape exam for the collection and documentation of evidence should be offered. As collection and DNA analysis techniques continue to improve, this 72-hour rule is being challenged. For example, the Maryland State Police crime lab is now recommending collection of sexual assault kits 120 hours post reported sexual assault.

WRITTEN DOCUMENTATION

When documenting histories of intimate partner violence, the forensic nurse should try to be as verbatim as possible with the stated details of the actual reported assault. The nurse should not sanitize statements made by the patient even if the statements include curse words, or write a progress note that reads as if the patient were using accurate medical terms when, in fact, the patient was using slang to describe body parts. The patient's demeanor should also be documented. As with sexual assault patients, patients experiencing intimate partner violence will present for care with a wide variance of emotions. It is critical the forensic nurse encourage the provider (nurse practitioner, physician, or physician's assistant) to list as one of the discharge or admission diagnoses something like "Reported Domestic Violence" or "Reported Adult Maltreatment Syndrome." If the provider only lists S/P Assault, medical records coders would not know to use the appropriate ICD-9-CM code Adult Maltreatment Syndrome (995.80). Failing to use an appropriate code for intimate partner violence could present problems during site visits by the Joint Commission on Accreditation for Healthcare Organizations. As part of chart audits for compliance with documentation of abuse, if a site surveyor asks the hospital to produce records on 15 intimate partner violence patients, it will be difficult to tease out domestic violence assaults from the scores of nonintimate violence assaults seen by the emergency department and/or clinics.

PHOTOGRAPHIC DOCUMENTATION

Forensic photographs are critical pieces of medical documentation of all forms of family and interpersonal violence and can be used as evidence in a criminal or civil case. Forensic photography implies that the photograph may be used in a legal proceeding (Besant-Matthews & Smock, 2001). A photograph gives visual evidence of an observed or treated wound that the healthcare provider assessed on the day of the exam. In addition, a photograph documents injuries or conditions before and after medical treatment and shows detail of a wound or injury that may have been overlooked by a visual inspection. In conjunction with the written medical documentation, the forensic photograph may be able to substantiate a victim's story or, in some cases, exonerate a suspect. When on the witness stand, the forensic nurse needs to become comfortable saying the injuries depicted in the photographs are true and accurate likenesses of the wounds seen and treated on the day of care. A complete overview of forensic photography can be found in Chapter 17. The following discussion reviews some of the important aspects of photography to consider when documenting the effects of partner violence.

Before forensic photographs can be taken, a signed consent for forensic photography must be obtained in most medical settings. Every patient can choose whether to have photographs taken. If the patient is unconscious and the injuries are secondary to a potentially litigious situation, take the picture and get consent later (Pasqualone, 1996). However, in cases when the patient is deceased, victims have no control of whether photographs will be taken; law enforcement and medical professionals make this decision. If the patient decides that photographs should be taken, the healthcare provider should explain the reasons why the photographs are being taken, as well as the risks and benefits, and also ask if the photographs can be used for educational purposes.

The gold standard for forensic photography is the 35 mm camera. One of the major advantages to using a 35 mm camera is that negatives are made and if reprints are necessary they can be obtained easily. However, one of the major disadvantages of the 35 mm camera is that it is not instant. The film has to be developed through a photo lab and may take from an hour to a few days to be developed. If using 35 mm print film, the photographer should use 12-exposure film, ISO 400. If 24- or 36-exposure film is used, there is a tendency either to "waste film" by photographing people and objects not related to the patient or to include two or more patients on one roll of film. One patient/victim per roll of film is the forensic standard (Sheridan, 2001). Disposable cameras and inexpensive fixed lens cameras are of little forensic value. The lens in these cameras will not produce in-focus images closer than 4 feet from the object being photographed.

Every emergency department should be equipped with an instant camera system (Pasqualone, 1996). Even though the 35 mm camera is the gold standard, a Polaroid or digital camera may also be used. An advantage to using the Polaroid camera is that the photograph takes only a few minutes to develop. However, unlike the 35 mm camera, the Polaroid does not have negatives, cannot be easily copied, and over time tends to fade and lose detail.

Digital cameras have been growing in popularity. One advantage to utilizing the digital camera is that the picture is "instant" unlike the Polaroid or 35 mm camera, and reprints can be made easily once the pictures are transferred from the camera to a computer or burned to a CD.

There are a variety of cameras to use when taking forensic photographs. No matter what system best fits one's professional forensic needs, it is important to know the advantages and disadvantages of all systems and to know your hospital's and legal jurisdiction's policy. Once you have decided which camera you will use, various factors must be taken into account when taking a forensic photograph.

One important factor is the lighting. According to Besant-Matthews and Smock (2001), a general principle is to mimic or add to existing light or create your own lighting according to your preference and the kind of subject. Another important factor is background. It is important to view the area to be photographed to identify anything that may need to be altered so the focus is not taken away from what you are photographing. The lens is also an important factor. Some lenses have a focal length that allows you to clearly see detail as close as 2 feet, whereas with a higher powered lens may photograph objects as close as $1^1/_2$–2 inches away with great detail. In cases where trace evidence may be in a "dirty" wound, it becomes important to show detail in the photograph. Fluorescent lighting, which gives off green light not visible to the eye, can produce an artificial greening effect to bruises, which may suggest the bruise being photographed is older than it actually is.

Scales and technique are also important factors when taking a forensic photograph. A scale should be used in at least one of the photographs of every individual injury. If the scale covers a part of the body, another photograph of the injured area should be taken without using the scale. The scale gives an exact measurement or size to the wound. A scale could be a standard color ruler, a coin, or an ABFO scale.

In forensic photography, the sequence or technique of taking the photograph is also important. According to Pasqualone (1996), the first photo should be a full body photo of the patient in order to establish the documented injuries were found on this patient. The second photograph should be mid-distance, and the third should be a close-up shot. A minimum of two close-up photographs should be taken of each injury, one with a scale to show injury size and another without to show that the scale did not obscure information (Pasqualone). This photographic principle is often referred to as the "rule of thirds" (Sheridan, 2001).

Once your photographs are completed, it is important to place identifying information such as patient name, patient hospital number, patient date of birth, name of photographer, case number (if indicated), and most importantly, the date and time the photo was taken. Photographs of injuries taken at differing points in time on the same day may look markedly different. A series of photographs should be taken over time to demonstrate progression of injury. This is often refereed to as serial photography.

Forensic nurses should never label photographs by writing with pen or a marker on either the back or front of the image. The authors recommend using mailing gum labels such as the Avery standard 5163 Shipping 2″ × 4″ label or the 5263 Shipping 2″ × 4″ label on the back of the picture. Depending on focal distance, it may be necessary to write the body part depicted in the photograph. Once the photographs have been properly labeled, it is important to follow your agency's chain of confidentiality and/or chain of custody policy to make sure the photographs are secured properly.

SUMMARY

Assessing for domestic violence with a reliable and valid intimate partner violence (IPV) screen is now considered a nursing standard of care. With any positive finding of abuse the forensic nurse should have immediate access to the Danger Assessment and HARASS tools to further explore for risk of domestic homicide. Written and photographic documentation must be accurate, thorough, and unbiased. The forensic nurse needs to have excellent command of all basic forensic terms and knowledge. This includes being able to discriminate between a cut and a laceration, a bruise and ecchymosis, etc. Intimate partner violence is a major public health problem. Forensic nurses can and should be key members of multidisciplinary coordinated community responses whose focus is to break the cycle of domestic violence through the development and utilization of specific and comprehensive assessment tools as described herein, as well as to focus on prevention and early identification of risk.

QUESTIONS FOR DISCUSSION

1. What are the factors that place women at high risk for domestic violence? In what ways might this categorization assist the forensic nurse in assessment of a client's risk? In what ways might this hinder the identification of those at risk?
2. Which assessment tools are useful in identifying the risk of partner violence?
3. What roadblocks may be encountered when working with a client who does not fit the common conception of the victim of domestic violence? What strategies may be useful to overcome some of these problems?

REFERENCES

Bariciak, E. D., Plint, A. C., Gaboury, I., & Bennett, S. B. (2003). Dating of bruises in children: An assessment of physician accuracy. *Pediatrics, 112*(4), 804–807.

Besant-Matthews, P. E. & Smock, W. S. (2001). Forensic photography in the emergency department. In J. S. Olshaker, M. C. Jackson, & W. S. Smock (Eds.), *Forensic emergency medicine* (pp. 257–282). Philadelphia: Lippincott Williams & Wilkins.

Brockmeyer, D. M. & Sheridan, D. J. (1998). Domestic violence: A practical guide to the use of forensic evaluation in clinical examination and documentation of injuries. In J. C. Campbell (Ed.), *Empowering survivors of abuse* (pp. 214–226). Thousand Oaks, CA: Sage Publications.

Campbell, J. C. (1989). Women's response to sexual abuse in intimate relationships. *Women's Health Care International, 8*, 335–347.

Campbell, J. C. (1998). Making the health care system an empowerment zone for battered women: Health consequences, policy recommendations, introductions, and overview. In J. C. Campbell (Ed.), *Empowering survivors of abuse: health care for battered women and their children* (pp. 3–22). Thousand Oaks, CA: Sage Publications.

Campbell, J. C., & Humphreys, J. (2003). Family violence and nursing practice. Philadelphia, PA: Lippincott, Williams & Wilkin.

Campbell, J. C., Webster, D., Koziol-McLain, J., Block, C. R., Campbell, D., Curry, M. A., et al. (2003a). Assessing risk factors for intimate partner homicide. *NIJ Journal, 250*, 14–19.

Campbell, J. C., Webster, D., Koziol-McLain, J., Block, C., Campbell, D., Curry, A., et al. (2003b). Risk factors for femicide in abusive relationships: Results from a multi-site case control study. *American Journal of Public Health, 93*(7), 1089–1097.

DiMaio, V. J. & DiMaio, D. (2001). *Forensic Pathology* (2nd ed.). Boca Raton, FL: CRC Press.

Drake, V. K. (1982). Battered women: A health care problem in disguise. *Image, 14*(2), 40–47.

Feldhaus, K. M., Koziol-McLain, J., Amsbury, H. L., Norton, I. M., Lowenstein, S. R., & Abbott, J. T. (1997). Accuracy of 3 brief screening questions for detecting partner violence in the emergency department. *Journal of the American Medical Association, 277*(17), 1357–1361.

Hadley, S. M. (1992). Working with battered women in the emergency department: A model program. *Journal of Emergency Nursing, 18*(1), 18–23.

Hadley, S., Short, L., Lesin, N., & Zook, E. (1995). WomanKind: An innovative model of health care response to domestic abuse. *Women's Health Issues, 5*(4), 189–198.

Helton, A. (1986). *Protocol of Care for the Battered Woman.* Houston, TX: Houston Chapter of the March of Dimes.

Jackson, H. C. (1992). The Hennepin County Medical Center's Women's Advocacy Program: Sixteen years of service. *Journal of Emergency Nursing, 18*(1), 27A–30A.

Kuriloff, D. B. & Pincus, R. L. (1989). Delayed airway obstruction and neck abscess following manual strangulation injury. *Ann Otol Rhinol Laryngol, 98*, 824–827.

Langlois, N. E. I. & Gresham, G. A. (1991). The ageing of bruises: A review and study of the colour. *Forensic Science International, 50,* 227–238.

McFarlane, J., Greenberg, L., Weltge, A., & Watson, M. (1995). Identification of abuse in emergency departments: Effectiveness of a two-question screening tool. *Journal of Emergency Nursing, 21*(5), 391–394.

McFarlane, J., Hughes, R. B., Nosek, M. A., Groff, J. Y., Swedland, N., & Mullen, P. D. (2001). Abuse Assessment Screen-Disability (AAS-D): Measuring frequency, type, and perpetrator of abuse toward women with physical difficulties. *Journal of Women's Health and Gender-Based Medicine, 10*(9), 861–866.

McFarlane, J., Parker, B., Soeken, K., & Bullock, L. (1992). Assessing for abuse during pregnancy. *Journal of the American Medical Association, 267*(3), 3176–3178.

Miller, B. F. & Keane, C. B. (1978). *Encyclopedia and dictionary of medicine, nursing, and allied health* (2nd ed.). Philadelphia: WB Saunders.

Parker, B., & McFarlane, J. (1991). Identifying and Helping Battered Pregnant Women. *Public Health Nursing, 17*(6), 443–451.

Parker, B., McFarlane, J., Soeker, K., Torres, S., & Campbell, D. (1993). Physical and emotional abuse in pregnancy: A comparison of adult and teenage women. *Nursing Research,* May June *42*(3): 172–178.

Parker, B. & Schumacher, D. N. (1977). The battered wife syndrome and violence in the nuclear family of origin: A controlled pilot study. *American Journal of Public Health, 67*(8), 760–761.

Pasqualone, G. (1996). Forensic RNs as photographers: Documentation in the ED. *Journal of Psychosocial Nursing, 34*(10), 47–51.

Randall, T. (1993). Clinician's forensic interpretations of fatal gunshot wounds often miss the mark. *Journal of the American Medical Association, 269*(16), 2058–2061.

Sheridan, D. J. (1998a). Heath care-based programs for domestic violence survivors. In J. C. Campbell (Ed.), *Empowering survivors of abuse: Health care for battered women and their children* (pp. 23–31). Thousand Oaks, CA: Sage Publications.

Sheridan, D. J. (1998b). *Measuring harassment of abused women: A nursing concern.* Unpublished doctoral dissertation. Portland, OR: Oregon Health Services University.

Sheridan, D. J. (2001). Treating survivors of intimate partner abuse. In J. S. Olshaker, M. C. Jackson, & W. S. Smock (Eds.), *Forensic emergency medicine* (pp. 203–228). Philadelphia: Lippincott Williams & Wilkins.

Sheridan, D. J. (2003). Forensic identification and documentation of patients experiencing intimate partner violence. *Clinics in Family Practice, 5*(1), 113–143.

Sheridan, D. J. & Taylor, W. K. (1993). Developing hospital-based domestic violence programs, protocols, policies, and procedures. *AWHONN's Clinical Issues in Perinatal and Women's Health Nursing, 4*(3), 471–482.

Smith, D. J., Mills, T., & Taliaferro, E. H. (2001). Frequency and relationship of reported symptomology in victims of intimate partner violence: The effect of multiple strangulation attacks. *Journal of Emergency Medicine, 21*(3), 323–329.

Strack, G. B., McClane, G. E., & Hawley, D. (2001). A review of 300 attempted strangulation cases. Part I: Criminal legal issues. *Journal of Emergency Medicine, 21*(3), 303–309.

Vale, G. L. & Noguchi, T. T. (1983). Anatomical distribution of human bite marks in a series of 67 cases. *Journal of Forensic Science, 28*(1), 61–69.

Venes, D. & Thomas, C. L. (Eds.). (2001). *Taber's cyclopedic medical dictionary* (19th ed.). Philadelphia: Lippincott-Raven.

Wilbur, L., Higley, M., Hatfield, J., Surprenant, Z., Taliaferro, E., Smith, D. J., & Paolo, A. (2001). Survey results of women who have been strangled while in an abusive relationship. *Journal of Emergency Medicine, 21*(3), 297–302.

Wilson, E. F. (1977). Estimation of the age of cutaneous contusions in child abuse. *Pediatrics, 60*, 750–752.

CHAPTER

11

Child and Adolescent Sexual Abuse

Frederick Berrien

The sexual abuse of a child or adolescent is a complex experience that is very different from the sexual assault of an adult. The way children and adolescents experience the abuse depends upon their age and development, the circumstances of the abuse, their relationship to the offender, and the response of their environment to the abuse. This chapter will explain the clinical and forensic approach to children and adolescents who have been sexually abused. The evaluation described in this chapter applies to all prepubescent children who have had sexual contact and to those adolescents who have been involved in abusive sexual relationships. A caring and competent forensic clinical examiner is critical to the appropriate assessment and management of these evaluations.

CHAPTER FOCUS

Epidemiology
Manifestations of sexual abuse
Psychodynamics of sexual abuse
Multidisciplinary issues
Physical evaluation of the child
Medical evaluation of the child
Testing for sexually transmitted infections
Forensic evidence collection
Treatment considerations
   Medical
   Mental health
   Family support
Judicial proceedings

KEY TERMS

child advocacy
colposcopy
consensual sexual activity
guardian ad lidum
nonconsensual sexual activity
nonpredatory
pedophile
power differential
psychodynamics
sexual abuse
sexual assault
statutory rape

From a medical perspective, sexual abuse is any contact involving the breast, genitalia, anus, and inner thighs that is nonconsensual, usually perpetrated by an individual in a position of power or influence over the child. These forms of sexual abuse usually involve a perpetrator who is significantly older than the victim; however, such sexual contact can involve children of similar age. These contacts among children of similar age require an extensive psychological evaluation to determine if such activity is abusive or is generated by other emotional needs.

Participation in pornography or forced exposure to sexually explicit materials is another form of sexual abuse that can cause psychological harm. These forms of sexual abuse require a full investigation and possibly judicial procedures, but rarely require a medical evaluation.

In contrast to sexual assault, sexual abuse is often regarded by the child as a part of a continuum of affectionate interactions with the perpetrator. The perpetrator has usually established emotional ties with the child and, therefore, the child is not necessarily inclined to resist the physical contact. The child is emotionally very vulnerable, often experiencing a complicit role in the sexual abuse and feeling ambivalent about his or her relationship with the perpetrator.

It is important in working with adolescents to distinguish sexual abuse from other types of sexual contact that may be inappropriate and potentially harmful, but not necessarily abusive. Consensual sexual activity among adolescents as young as 13 is not uncommon (Connecticut Department of Public Health, 1996); however, the age difference between the partners should be assessed in the context of their power differential. Consensual sexual relationships among youth with significant age differences are defined by most states as statutory rape. These cases may require investigation; however, a clinical approach should be used by the healthcare clinician. The appropriate approach to these cases is to provide reproductive health and psychological care according to the adolescent's health and developmental status and circumstances of the sexual contact. It is also important to distinguish cases of rape from sexual abuse or consensual sexual relationships. Occasionally adolescents who are discovered by an adult to be engaged in sexual relationships will initially disguise it as a sexual assault. It is important that the clinician give the adolescent the latitude to provide an accurate account of the sexual activity. Evaluation of a rape in an adolescent requires procedures that address forensic and emotional issues which, although similar, are different than those of an abuse victim. See Chapter 18 for details of the rape evaluation.

Children can also offend sexually, usually with younger children. However, it can be difficult to distinguish normal, healthy sexual behaviors that are exploratory and nonpredatory from problematic behavior that requires a clinical evaluation to determine their significance. Friedrick et al. (1998) developed an inventory of childhood sexual behaviors to assist in making this distinction. This inventory has been standardized with several preadolescent populations. In general, sexual acts among children that appear premeditated, involve force or coercion, or involve penetrating or insertive acts should be considered potentially abusive and should be evaluated from the perspective of abuse. Mutual fondling, excessive masturbation, and looking at genitals or breasts are possible indications of stress or other psychological problems that should be evaluated by a child psychologist or pediatric behavioral specialist familiar with sexual development.

EPIDEMIOLOGY

Sexual abuse is an underreported problem with an annual incidence rate of 1.2 cases per 1,000 children, according to U.S. Department of Health and Human Services Administration for Children and Families (2003). These data are based upon confirmed cases of sexual abuse. Many cases of sexual abuse are never reported and many cases are not confirmed by investigation, so these incidence data are regarded as very conservative. Based upon many surveys of adults who have experienced sexual abuse during their childhood, the prevalence of this problem is estimated to be at least 20% for females and conservatively estimated to be 5–10% for males (Finkelhor, 1994). Although sexual abuse rates have declined in the past few years, the decline appears to be leveling off and possibly rising again. The reasons for the changes in case rates are unknown.

Sexual abuse is found in all socioeconomic groups and in all cultures. There appears to be higher incidence among low income populations, which may be a result of limited options for ensuring safe care arrangements for children. Clearly children brought up in households with substance abuse are at greater risk of sexual abuse due to the loss of inhibition and respect for boundaries. Children who are disabled also are found to have a higher incidence of sexual abuse due to vulnerabilities based on mobility and communication limitations. For reasons that remain obscure, it is common to find that children who have been sexually abused have been raised by nonoffending parents who were also sexually abused (Wurtele & Miller-Perrin, 1992).

MANIFESTATIONS OF SEXUAL ABUSE

Sexual abuse is most commonly detected when a child makes a disclosure to a family member, a friend, or a trusted adult. Young children may make a disclosure that is vague, such as statements that express dislike for a person or being in a particular situation. Sensitive follow-up questions then raise the possibility of abuse. With adolescents, the initial disclosure is often to a peer who encourages a report to an adult.

If a child presents with medical symptoms such as genital pain, bleeding, or discharge, questions to parents and children regarding possible genital or anal contact are indicated to determine if abuse may be an underlying cause. Enuresis and encopresis are sometimes associated with sexual abuse and therefore should prompt questions to explore the possibility of sexual abuse.

Changes in behavior and mood are associated with sexual abuse; however, there are many potential causes of these changes. Sexualized behaviors always raise concern about sexual abuse. These behaviors need to be assessed in the context of normal sexual development behavior (Friedrick et al., 1998) and exposures that children have to sexual materials. Children who have been sexually abused may become aggressive, appear depressed, experience eating disorders, have sleep disturbances, or perform poorly in school, so it is important to consider abuse as one of the possible reasons for these problems.

PSYCHODYNAMICS OF SEXUAL ABUSE

Sexual abuse is the result of the interaction among the child, the perpetrator, and the environment. Finkelhor (1984) described four preconditions for sexual abuse to occur. The two preconditions that apply to the perpetrator are motivation and ability to overcome internal inhibitions toward sexual abuse. The third applies to the environment in which external barriers to sexual abuse must be overcome. The last precondition is a child who is unable to resist abuse.

It is clear that the primary factor in sexual abuse is the perpetrator. The motivations of the perpetrator may emanate from a variety of conditions. The true pedophile is a person whose lifelong sexual orientation has involved children; however, the true pedophile accounts for a relatively small number of sexual abuse cases. The more common type of perpetrator is a person who uses children for sexual satisfaction while also having adult sexual relationships. The reasons for their need to have sexual contact with children vary, but usually relate to disordered relationships resulting in deficits in coping abilities, which are compensated with child sexual contact. In some cases these disordered relationships may be a response to the perpetrator's sexual or physical abuse victimization during childhood. For some perpetrators, a lowering of internal inhibitions with alcohol or drugs may permit them to engage with children when they otherwise would not. In essence, the perpetrator's motivation for sexual satisfaction with children comes from a distorted relationship with a child and/or use of psychoactive substances to overcome internal inhibitions.

The environment must permit the contact between child and perpetrator to occur, allowing the perpetrator to carry out the acts without others being aware. This requires that the perpetrator plan the sexual activities in locations or at times when others are not present. In some situations, the perpetrator may distort the perceptions of others present such that the acts are not interpreted as abuse. In some situations the perpetrator will create an environment in which the child perceives the acts as acceptable; for example, the perpetrator may tell the child, "This is what people do when they love each other." As children become aware of the taboos against sexual contact, the perpetrator will resort to coercion or threats. These environmental conditions contribute strongly to the secretive nature of sexual abuse. For example, leaving a preschool child in the care of a sexual offender for predictable periods of times creates an environment that excludes witnesses and permits the offender to distort the sexual contact as special attention; this will be reinforced by rewards such as presents or privileges as long as it remains a secret. For the older child, the abuse may initially appear innocent, but evolves for the child into sexual acts associated with shame or fear that the child will conceal to avoid exposure. In these situations, the environment not only permits the abuse to occur, but also inhibits the child from disclosure.

The child is generally regarded as a passive participant in the sexual abuse. However, if we look more carefully at the position of children in this dynamic with perpetrator and the environment, we recognize that the child has some characteristics that may be protective and others that make the child more susceptible. For example, depending on age, knowledge, and cognitive ability, children are aware that sexual contacts are socially prohibited for children. This is a protective resource for the child. On the other hand, a child's smaller size and strength is usually regarded as characteristics that make them more susceptible. Similarly, the notion that children don't always tell the truth or cannot be believed again leaves children more vulnerable to sexual abuse. In viewing a child's protective and susceptible characteristics, it is recognized that children's participation in sexual abuse is in part determined by these characteristics.

Sexual abuse usually is progressive, with the perpetrator first simply engaging the child during innocent circumstances. The experienced perpetrator will identify the vulnerable child and the proper environment where the circumstances permit a trusting relationship to develop with the child. The child will accept the initial contacts as signs of caring and affection, often not understanding the progression of contact as unusual. For younger children the sexual activities involve fondling, exposure, and masturbation. These sexual acts are usually not painful and may not be regarded by the child as particularly harmful.

Digital penetration of the anus and genital to genital contact are not unusual; however, actual vaginal penetration is not common with prepubescent girls. Nevertheless, children frequently experience these activities as genital penetration, although physical evidence of vaginal penetration is not often found. Frequently the children do not experience pain or discomfort, and in some case may find the sexual contact to be pleasurable. To maintain the secrecy of the abuse, children are often given rewards to reinforce the secrecy or the perpetrator may threaten the child with abandonment or physical harm.

Children will decide to disclose sexual abuse for a variety of reasons. The child may be questioned by a trusted adult who has concerns. A young child may innocently disclose in reference to a discussion about touching. Sometimes the disclosure statements of young children are indirect, such as a general expression of dislike for a specific person or place; follow-up questions may lead to abuse concerns. Older children and adolescents often will want to protect nonoffending parents from knowing about the abuse and choose to disclose to a trusted person outside the immediate family.

Statements of children that suggest sexual abuse must be acknowledged and appropriately explored. In most cases, parents and other inexperienced adults should not ask children detailed questions. Rather, it is the role of adults to support the disclosure, clarify the spontaneous statements of children, and seek out experienced professionals to explore the meaning of children's statements.

Most children do not anticipate the magnitude of distress that such a disclosure will create. The disruption created in a family may lead to a recantation of allegations by children. This is more common with older children who believe that once the abuse has been exposed that it will stop without legal intervention. Unfortunately, families unfamiliar with the magnitude of problems associated with sexual abuse may suppress the allegations with the expectation that the problem can be managed within the family. These approaches to child sexual abuse usually perpetuate the problem, leading to chronic stress, unresolved trust issues, and revictimization.

MULTIDISCIPLINARY ISSUES

Successful investigation and management of sexual abuse cases involves a full understanding of the child, the perpetrator, and the environment. Multiple disciplines are required to assess and understand each of these components to achieve successful outcomes. Successful outcomes include the diagnosis and treatment of the child's medical problems, restoration of the child's mental health, development of appropriate family relationships, protection of the child from further abuse, and prosecution of the perpetrator. To optimize the possibility of successful outcomes, a collaborative relationship among the disciplines is a necessity.

The disciplines required for this work to proceed successfully include health care, child protection services, victim advocacy, law enforcement, and mental health. In addition, the attorneys who are actively involved in the management of these cases, such as the prosecutor and attorney representing the child, are often an essential component of this collaboration. In each community, specific services contribute to the management of child abuse cases; in particular, service providers who specialize in mental health or family relations issues should be a part of this collaboration.

Each discipline has a specific role in the management of sexual abuse; however, the procedures necessary to accomplish their specific roles are often similar and can overlap. This may lead to interference or unnecessary duplication unless care is taken to maximize collaboration. Effective collaboration among the disciplines, including a clear understanding of roles, expectations, and limitations, will avoid conflict and promote efficiency.

Child protection services (CPS) focuses its investigation on what happened to a child and how to prevent it from happening again to that child and others in the family. To accomplish this, the CPS investigation must include an understanding of the family and the circumstances of the sexual abuse. This includes assessing for high risk situations such as substance abuse, domestic violence, and history of prior sexual abuse in the family. Interviews of everyone in the family, particularly other children in the family, are an important part of the CPS investigation. CPS often must present this information to the family and juvenile court system to allow appropriate protection.

Law enforcement's role is to undertake a criminal investigation leading to prosecution. Although the criminal investigation focuses on the alleged perpetrator of the abuse, the evidence available from the child victim is critical to a successful prosecution. Law enforcement usually requires a high standard or quality of evidence to effect a successful prosecution. This requires all interviews of children to be forensically appropriate and properly documented.

At the same time, the medical and mental health status of the child must be assessed, not only for clinical purpose, but also for evidentiary purposes. The details of the medical evaluation are explained in the next section. A specific mental health assessment is necessary to determine the degree to which the child's behavior and cognitive abilities have been affected by the abuse. To fully assess the child's mental status, the child must be viewed within the context of the family and the abuse conditions. CPS usually provides much of this information and uses the mental health assessment in determining the requirements for restoration of healthy relationships within the family.

A major challenge for the investigation is obtaining a credible history from a child whose perception of events and ability to describe them are often different than those of an adult. In addition, children are often under pressure to recant their disclosure of abuse. Because there are rarely witnesses to these events and physical evidence is not frequently found, the statements of the child and an effective investigation of the suspected perpetrator become the paramount components of a forensic investigation.

In the midst of a major family disruption there is a vulnerable child from whom specific and accurate information must be elicited. To obtain this essential information effectively, all of the above disciplines must collaborate. The Children's Advocacy Center (CAC) model has been successfully established in many communities in the United States for the multidisciplinary evaluation of child sexual abuse victims. The core service of the CAC model is the collaborative interview; in this interview, a single trained and experienced member of the team interviews the child in an age-appropriate manner using forensically appropriate techniques to elicit essential details of the abuse. With this approach, the child only gives the story once, the interview is appropriately documented by recording or transcript, and all the appropriate disciplines have an opportunity to obtain necessary information. This approach minimizes the emotional trauma to the child and avoids the chance of conflicting information arising from multiple interviews involving different interviewing techniques.

The CAC model also includes medical and mental health components as well as services for the nonoffending members of the family. Ideally, these services are all located at a single site, providing for the child and family a facility that is secure, child friendly, and familiar. However, if all services are not available at a single site, the cornerstone of the Children's Advocacy Center model is collaboration among all of these disciplines.

Communities that do not have a CAC model may have a multidisciplinary team that provides a structure for collaborative investigation and management similar to the CAC model, but without the single site facility and formalized interviewing process. Generally these community-based teams have a lead agency, which may be the mandated child protection agency, a mental health agency, or another agency involved with family issues.

Another model of multidisciplinary teams is the child protection team, which may be based within an institution such as a school or hospital. These teams are composed of the disciplines involved with child abuse within the institution and may include outside agencies. Generally their purposes are to ensure that cases of abuse are appropriately handled within the institution and to advocate for children and families under their care.

PHYSICAL EVALUATION

The purposes of the medical evaluation are to: 1) identify medical problems that may affect the health of the child or adolescent; 2) identify evidence associated with the sexual abuse; and 3) provide reassurance to the child or adolescent and their family regarding the medical integrity of the child or adolescent.

The type and extent of the examination depends upon the nature of the sexual abuse and the circumstances of the examination. If the complete history of the sexual abuse is known, the determination of the proper examination is clear. For older children and adolescents, the history is clearer and therefore the extent of the sexual abuse better understood. In general, the examination is determined by the interval between the last sexual contact and the proposed examination. (see Table 11–1).

The purpose of the immediate forensic examination is to document evidence of trauma and recover semen for identification of the perpetrator. Therefore, if time has elapsed since the sexual contact such that there is little likelihood of recovery of semen, generally after 72 hours, it is possible to defer the examination to a time and place that best meets the needs of the child.

Whenever possible, a child should be examined by a clinician who is familiar with pediatric and adolescent genital development. This examination should be conducted in a setting that is supportive of the child and nonoffending parents. Staff providing this evaluation should have time and experience that they use to help the child through this new and stressful procedure. In many emergency departments where these children first present, these conditions do not exist; therefore, if the immediate examination is not necessary, the exam can be deferred to a facility where the needs of the child can be better addressed.

The medical evaluation of a child who has been sexually abused starts with a history. The history includes details of the sexual abuse including when it occurred, who was involved, and what parts of the perpetrator's and victim's anatomy were involved. This information may be available through a forensic interview or from adults who accompany the child or adolescent. If this information is not available from either of these sources, focused, nonleading questions should be asked by the examiner with recording of both questions asked and responses of the child or adolescent. Additional details of the abuse involving the con-

Table 11–1 Medical Evaluations

Time Interval Since Last Sexual Contact	Type of Sexual Contact	Type of Evaluation	Timing of Examination
<72 hours	Contact with male genitalia or semen	Complete medical evaluation with evidence collection	Immediate
<72 hours	No contact with male genitalia or semen	Complete medical evaluation	As soon as possible with an experienced examiner
>72 hours	Any sexual contact involving victim's genitalia, mouth, or anus	Comprehensive medical evaluation	As soon as possible with an experienced examiner

text of the abuse should be obtained by trained interviewers (see "Multidisciplinary Issues" earlier in the chapter for a discussion of forensic interviews).

Additional necessary medical history includes symptoms frequently associated with the abuse including anal and vaginal discharge, anal and vaginal bleeding, dysuria, urinary frequency, urinary tract infections, and sore throat. If these symptoms are current and significant, a focused examination should be performed regardless of the other determinates of the examination type. It is also useful to have a history of other injuries involving the genital or anal region because such injuries may result in scars or other findings that could be misinterpreted.

Behavioral symptoms may include phobias, fears, sleep disturbances, changes in eating habits, emotional outbursts, and mood changes. If any of these behavioral symptoms are severe, they should be evaluated as soon as possible by a mental health professional; a mental health evaluation may provide additional forensic information as well as assist the child and family in dealing with the sexual abuse and the secondary symptoms.

A past medical history is important to identify specific genital or anal problems including injuries, constipation, or other causes of bleeding or trauma (see Table 11–2). In addition, major medical problems that may affect the outcome of the examination should be identified.

Proper preparation of the child and adolescent for the examination is essential for a successful assessment. The preparatory phase of the evaluation is time consuming, but necessary to accomplish a complete

Table 11–2   Components of the Medical History

Focused details of the abuse	Behavioral changes
Who was involved?	Specific fears
What parts of the body were involved?	Emotional outbursts
When was last sexual contact?	Mood changes
Genital and anal symptoms	Eating habits
Bleeding	Aggressiveness
Discharge	Sleep patterns
Pain	School performance
Dysuria	Past medical history
Constipation	Injuries
Prior injuries	Chronic or recurrent illnesses
	Surgery
	Allergies

examination with a minimum of fear for the child. The parent or other adult who is present to support the child or adolescent during the examination should be fully informed of the procedures in advance. Older children and adolescents should be given the option of having the procedure without such a support person. The child should be informed in advance regarding the details of the procedure according to their age and ability to understand the information provided. In all cases, the child or adolescent should be told in age-appropriate language that the examination will involve their genitalia and anus, but be reassured that the examination is not expected to cause any pain.

The examination of a child or adolescent includes a general medical examination. This examination will identify conditions such as trauma, which may relate to the sexual abuse. In addition, this part of the examination provides the examiner an opportunity to establish rapport with an anxious child and observe the reaction of the child to a standard examination prior to the more sensitive genital and anal examination. For very young children, particularly those under 3 years of age who may be uncomfortable with any form of examination, the general physical exam may be minimized.

The genital and anal examination on a child or adolescent may include the use of a colposcope or other device that permits the magnification and photo documentation of the findings. These devices are an adjunct to the exam, but are not necessary if the examiner is familiar with the appearance of the genitalia of children and adolescents at various stages of development and the signs of abuse.

Proper positioning and use of exposure techniques are very important to obtain good visualization of a girl's genitalia. An assistant who is familiar with the examination procedure is usually essential for positioning of the child and handling specimens. Young children who are anxious may be examined on their mother's lap, as illustrated in Figure 11–1. Girls whose legs are too short for use of stirrups can assume a frog leg position for good exposure. Older girls and adolescents are usually examined in stirrups. In addition, both males and females may be examined in the knee-chest position (see Figure 11–2) to obtain better exposure of the anus as well as an alternative view of the female genitalia. This position is usually necessary to confirm abnormalities of the hymen.

The technique of exposing girls' genitalia involves labia separation and labial traction. Labial separation is simple separation of the labia majora laterally, usually with the thumb or forefinger of the examiner or assistant (see Figure 11–3). This permits observation of the labia majora, labia minora, clitoral hood, and possibly the hymen. Initially care should be taken to observe for posterior labial agglutination, which is often friable

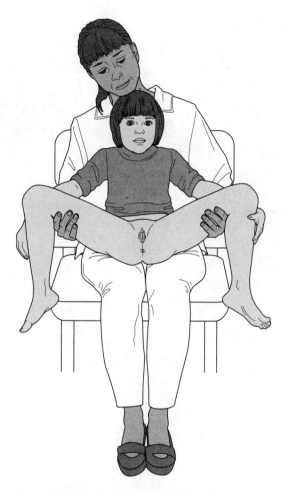

Figure 11–1 Prepubertal child positioned in the lap of accompanying adult for genital and anal examination. *Source:* Reece, R. M., and Ludwig, S. (2001). *Child abuse: Medical diagnosis and management.* Philadelphia: Lippincott, Williams & Wilkins.

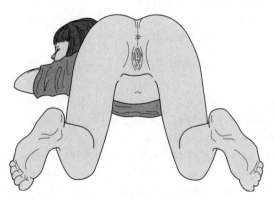

Figure 11–2 Knee-chest position for genital examination of the prepubertal child. *Source:* Reece, R. M., and Ludwig, S. (2001). *Child abuse: Medical diagnosis and management.* Philadelphia: Lippincott, Williams & Wilkins.

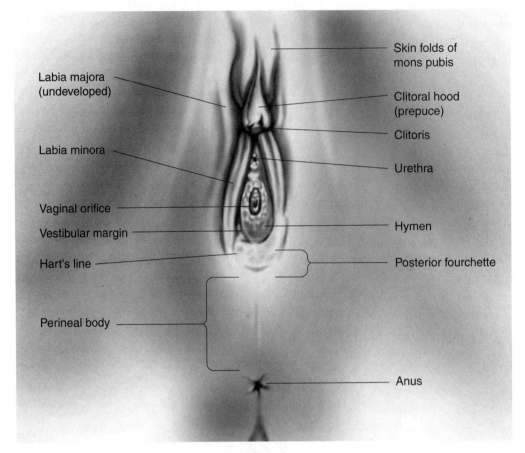

Figure 11–3 The prepubertal vulva. *Source:* Heger, A. and Emans, S. J. (1992). *Evaluation of the sexually abused child: Medical textbook and photographic atlas.* New York: Oxford University Press.

and easily lysed, causing pain. To get better exposure of the inner aspect of the labia majora, vaginal vestibule, and hymen, labial traction is used. This is accomplished by grasping the labia majora with the thumb and forefinger and gently pulling the labia toward the examiner.

The examiner should first identify the major landmarks on the genitalia of girls. These include the clitoral hood and adjacent labia minora. These structures define the anterior and lateral boundaries of the vaginal vestibule. The posterior border of the vaginal vestibule is the posterior commissure (fourchette). Penetrating trauma usually involves the vaginal vestibule and in particular the fossa navicularis, which is the posterior portion of the vaginal vestibule. Using the techniques noted, the hymen is usually easily identified at the proximal end of the vaginal vestibule.

The hymen changes over time (Berenson, 1995 and Berenson, Heger & Andrews, 1991) and its appearance varies with position and technique

(McCann et al., 1990). The hymen may be annular, surrounding the hymeneal opening, or there may be no anterior portion of the hymen, which is described as crescent shaped. The hymen may be redundant and evert into the vestibule, making definition difficult in the lithotomy position. A young girl's redundant hymen may fold and overlie, resulting in unusual appearances. In young girls the hymen may appear to cover the entire hymeneal opening, making observation of the hymeneal border difficult. It is essential that the examiner be familiar with the variety of hymeneal appearances through supervised examinations and access to published atlases that provide examples of normal anatomy.

Speculum examination should not be performed in prepubescent girls and usually is not necessary in young adolescents who have not experienced vaginal penetration. If there appears to be intra-vaginal injury in a prepubescent child or early adolescent, an examination under anesthesia may be indicated with preparation for surgical repair.

The older adolescent or younger adolescent who has experienced vaginal penetration should have a speculum exam whenever possible to observe for injuries to the vagina and for obtaining appropriate specimens.

Genital findings in girls that are consistent with acute sexual contact include abrasions, ecchymoses, and lacerations (see Table 11–3). Abrasions may be small and may be appreciated only with magnification. Lacerations are usually noted in the posterior aspects of the vestibule (fossa navicularis) and hymen; using the face of the clock, they are usually found between 3 and 9 o'clock.

Indications of nonacute trauma are less definitive. It is known that acute injuries heal relatively rapidly, and traumatic defects to the hymen can heal with almost complete restitution of normal appearance in some cases. In general it is accepted that a healed defect, referred to as a notch or cleft, that extends through at least 50% of the hymen is an indicator of prior hymeneal injury (Berenson et al., 2000). Minimal hymeneal rim

Table 11–3 Significant Physical Findings

Acute Sexual Contact	Nonacute Contact
Ecchymoses	Absent hymen
Presence of semen	Deep hymeneal notches
Lacerations	Pregnancy
Abrasions	Minimal hymen
	Anal scars
	Absence of rugal folds

is considered significant by some examiners. A minimal hymeneal rim is defined as less than 1 mm of hymen when compared to a previous exam in which the width of the hymen was greater (APSAC, 1995). It is not common to have successive examinations that permit this comparison. The hymen often has irregularities to its margin or edge resulting in bumps or mounds; these are usually variants of normal, and are considered abnormal only if they are associated with a deep cleft or notch (> 50% of the hymeneal width).

The examination of the genitalia on the male victim of sexual abuse consists of inspection of the penis, scrotum, and adjacent areas. Significant findings include abrasion, contusions, lacerations, bite marks, and other signs of trauma. In the uncircumcised male it is important to examine under the foreskin.

The anal examination consists of an inspection of the anus to observe for signs of trauma or laxity of the anal sphincter. This examination is ideally accomplished in the knee-chest position, holding the position for up to 2 minutes for complete relaxation; however, many children and adolescents become anxious in that position and alternative positions such as lateral decubitus or prone may be used.

Acute signs of anal trauma include lacerations, ecchymoses, and abrasions. Signs of healed anal trauma may include deep fissures or loss of normal rugal folds. It is important to be aware of smooth, pale areas mid-line at the 12 and 6 o'clock positions, which may be slightly depressed; this is considered a normal finding in most cases. Anal dilation up to 2 cm has been found in nonabused children (McCann et al., 1989); therefore, anal dilation must be greater than 2 cm to be considered significant.

TESTING FOR SEXUALLY TRANSMITTED INFECTIONS

Testing for sexually transmitted diseases (STDs) in prepubescent children depends upon a number of risk factors associated with the abuse. When a child has a discharge, bleeding, or other signs of inflammation associated with the abuse, testing is indicated. Testing would also be indicated if the abuse was perpetrated by a person known to have an STD. Because there is increasing likelihood of an STD in postpubescent victims, it is generally agreed that testing for these girls is appropriate in most cases with or without symptoms (Siegel et al., 1995). Many tests are available for chlamydia and gonorrhea. There is concern that nonculture methods such as elisa assays and nucleic acid amplification tests are not sufficiently specific for forensic purposes in children, resulting in a significant rate of false positive results, thereby invalidating the results. However, for clinical purposes these results may be valid; if nonculture techniques are used, all positive results should be repeated with a culture prior to treatment.

Obtaining vaginal specimens in girls requires good technique to avoid contact with the prepubescent hymen, which is very sensitive to pain. The hymeneal opening is usually only a few millimeters wide, so the use of a small calcium alginate applicator rather than the larger cotton applicator can often permit specimen collection from the vagina with minimal trauma. When the child has a crescent-shaped hymen, inserting the applicator against the anterior surface of the vagina, avoiding the urethra, will usually not induce pain. If it is not possible to obtain a vaginal specimen, collection from the vaginal vestibule may be adequate. Care should be taken in obtaining these specimens because the vestibule is a sensitive area as well. Cervical specimens are not necessary in prepubescent girls. In pubescent and adolescent girls, cervical specimens are desired, but a speculum examination may be difficult, in which case a vaginal specimen may be adequate. A wet mount examination of vaginal secretions will identify bacterial vaginosis and trichomonas.

The male victim may need urethral specimens if symptoms or exposure suggest that he could have acquired an STD. Because obtaining these specimens is painful, collection of these specimens should be determined according to clinical indicators and the child's ability to understand and tolerate the procedure.

Serologic testing for HIV, syphilis, and hepatitis C are recommended if the sexual abuse includes potential exposure to those infections. For many families and children, such testing may be reassuring even when the risk of exposure is negligible. These serologic tests should be appropriately timed to ensure that the negative test will not convert at a later point in time. In general, testing for HIV 3 months postexposure should be adequate. However, it is advisable to have baseline testing shortly after the exposure to demonstrate that the child did not acquire the infection prior to the alleged sexual exposure in question.

The most commonly observed STD in young children is genital or venereal warts *(condyloma accuminata)* caused by human papilloma virus (HPV). However, HPV can be transmitted to a child congenitally, by cutaneous contact, or by sexual contact. This virus may be congenitally acquired and remain latent for months or years. Mothers carrying HPV in their genital tract may be asymptomatic. Other mothers may have evidence of HPV with an abnormal Pap smear or symptomatic genital warts. Most congenital genital warts will appear within the first 2 years; however, it is believed that it is possible for the virus to remain latent for many years. HPV can also be transmitted from cutaneous warts to the genitalia, particularly prior to a child being toilet trained. These multiple modes of transmission in addition to sexual transmission create a dilemma for forensic evaluations of HPV infections. For children less than 2 years of age, if investigation does not identify other indicators of sexual abuse, it is acceptable to attribute the infection to congenital acquisition. For children over two years of age it is more likely that the infection is caused by sexual contact. Over 5 years of age it becomes virtually certain that sexual contact is the mode of transmission.

Many STDs require a clinical assessment to determine their significance to sexual abuse. These include chlamydia, herpes, HIV, and hepatitis B and C. Chlamydia is known to be acquired at the time of birth and has the ability to persist without signs of illness for weeks or months. Therefore, the significance of genital chlamydia infections in the first year of life must be evaluated within the context of possible congenital acquisition. Herpes simplex types 1 and 2 can be found on the genitalia as a result of sexual contact or contamination from other sites, such as the mouth. In cases of contamination, the virus may be auto-inocculated from a lesion on the victim or from a lesion on a person providing care for an infant or toddler. Distinguishing between Herpes simplex types is not clinically or forensically significant unless you are comparing viruses between the victim and an alleged perpetrator. Because HIV and hepatitis B and C are transmitted in body fluids, as well as congenitally, it is important to understand all of the possible exposures if testing indicates infection possibly related to sexual contact. Congenital infections of Herpes simplex, syphilis, and gonorrhea are usually diagnosed in the neonatal period or early infancy with very characteristic manifestations. See Table 11–4 for the clinical significance of bacterial vaginosis and trichomonas.

Table 11–4 Significant Sexually Transmitted Infections

Infection	Methods of Infection	Specificity for Sexual Abuse
Gonorrhea	Congenital, sexual	High
Syphilis	Congenital, sexual	High
HIV	Congenital, blood, sexual	Needs clinical assessment
Chlamydia	Congenital, sexual	Needs clinical assessment in first year of life
HPV	Congenital, cutaneous, sexual	Needs clinical assessment
Herpes simplex	Congenital, casual contact, sexual	Needs clinical assessment
Hepatitis B and C	Congenital, blood, sexual	Needs clinical assessment
Trichomonas	Sexual, fomites	Moderate
Bacterial vaginosis	Sexual and other	Low

FORENSIC EVIDENCE COLLECTION

Forensic evidence collection should be considered in all cases seen within 72 hours of the last sexual contact. Because the primary focus of this collection is the recovery of semen, this collection is only necessary to pursue if there has been contact with male genitalia. However, in many cases, children are not aware of the extent of genital contact or are unable to initially disclose complete details. Therefore, when the circumstances indicate the possibility of contact with male genitalia, the collection should be undertaken. The collection procedure for a child and adolescent is a modification of the procedures used with adults (see Chapter 18). The modifications are dictated by the circumstances of the abuse and the need to minimize physical and emotional trauma to children. In most cases, sexual abuse of children and adolescents, in contrast to adults, is not a violent physical assault; sexual abuse involves emotional manipulation combined with dominating power and authority. Therefore, findings associated with resistance or injuries to other areas are not usually found.

It is essential to obtain specimens from the appropriate orifice whenever there is reason to think that the sexual contact involved the mouth, anus, or vagina. The technique for obtaining female genital specimens is similar to that used for STD specimens described in the previous section. Specimens from the labia of girls and intergluteal areas may provide additional evidence. Although fluorescence with the Wood's lamp examination is not very specific for semen, such an examination indicates areas of possible semen contamination. In young children who are anxious about the examination, hair plucking and blood sampling can be deferred until such time as it becomes essential for distinguishing the source of positive evidence. With adolescent victims, the full evidence collection procedure may be indicated depending on the circumstances of the abuse and the physical and emotional maturation of the victim.

A study conducted by Christian and others (2000), showed that bed linens and clothing are the most likely sources of positive evidence. Because most sexual abuse of children does not involve penetration, it is less likely that semen will be detected from the orifices. In this study of 273 completed examinations, positive evidence from the child's body was found only when the exam was completed within 24 hours of the sexual contact.

TREATMENT CONSIDERATIONS

Medical

If a child has experienced serious trauma to the genitalia or anus, surgical repair may be necessary. Proper attention to pain control and risks of infection are a component of management of this type of trauma.

Fortunately, superficial trauma will heal without medical or surgical intervention.

Unless exposure to an STD is evident from history or a physical, STD treatment is usually not provided to prepubescent children due to the relatively low risk of infection. In adolescents, treatment for syphilis, gonorrhea, and chlamydia is often given depending upon the extent and likelihood of significant exposure to STDs and the ability to follow up with the adolescent. This treatment would consist of a cephalosporin such as ceftriaxone and a macrolide such as azithromycin, which have the advantage of requiring only a single dose administered at the time of evaluation. In addition, consideration should be given to administering hepatitis B immunization if the child or adolescent has not completed the series. If trichomonas or bacterial vaginosis is of concern, metronidazole may be prescribed. Routine postexposure prophylaxis for HIV infection is generally not recommended due to the potential side effects of the medications. However, if there is good reason to expect exposure to the virus, immediate consultation with an appropriate infectious disease specialist is indicated to determine the best regimen.

Adolescent girls should be evaluated for pregnancy if there is the possibility of contact with semen. This should include an acute evaluation and follow-up in approximately 2 weeks. If an adolescent is not pregnant and is seen within 72 hours of exposure to semen, emergency contraception is an option.

Mental Health

At the time of disclosure, children must feel supported through a process that they often perceive to be frightening and confusing. Initially, the child needs to understand that disclosure was the correct thing to do. In addition, the investigation needs to be explained in terms and details that prepare, but not overwhelm, the child. Family distress and unfamiliarity with the investigation process may limit family members' ability to provide this support to their child, so the professionals need to ensure that this support is provided. In many communities, sexual assault crisis services are available to support children at this phase of their disclosure and investigation.

The emotional trauma experienced by child and adolescent victims of sexual abuse can have long-lasting effects extending into adulthood. Sexual abuse has been associated with smoking, alcohol and drug abuse, chronic pain, suicide attempts (Felitti et al., 1998), personality disturbance (Wonderlich et al., 2001), depression, and sexual dysfunction (Beitchman et al., 1992). In general, the more violent, threatening, and intrusive the abuse, the greater the emotional trauma; however, at initial evaluation, the full extent of the abuse is often not disclosed. It is essential to have a mental health evaluation that addresses the types of trauma the child has experienced, the behaviors of the child, and the current environment of the child. This evaluation will then determine the type and extent of the treatment required.

Family Support

The nonoffending members of the child's family are usually the greatest source of support for child and adolescent victims. However, the family members are also traumatized by these events and need assistance to deal with their concerns as well as those of the child or adolescent.

Because most abuse involves trusted individuals known to the child and family, everyone involved struggles with the issues of deceit and must re-examine the formation of trusting relationships. One approach is to provide nonoffending parents with an understanding of how sexual abuse evolves and progresses. With this information, families are better prepared to move ahead, develop healthy relationships, and protect their children from additional abuse.

In a situation in which the nonoffending parent had an intimate relationship with the offender, it will be important for the nonoffending parent to address their anger and ambivalence related to the abuse and disclosure. If the victim is an adolescent, the nonoffending parent may question the complicity of the adolescent in the sexual activity. In these situations, immediate work with nonoffending parents and the adolescent separately is particularly important in order to understand the concerns of all involved.

If the sexual abuse is within the family, there will be changes in the life of the family. This may mean that some members of the family may need to leave the household. This could mean interruption in the financial support for the family or added financial burden. If one child has sexually offended against another child within a family, parents will need to cope with their ambivalence toward the child who committed the offense; this may require placing one child out of the home or providing 24-hour surveillance of the children's activities.

For most families, this is the first time they must deal with law enforcement, child protection, and other aspects of the legal system. Families need to know the roles of each of the agencies and become familiar with the individuals involved with the investigation. The apparent redundancy of investigations, slowness of resolution, and failure to achieve expected outcomes are major frustrations for many families.

Sexual abuse appears to be a multigenerational problem in many families. Often the nonoffending mothers and/or fathers of the child victims were victims themselves. Many of these parents have never adequately dealt with their own victimization. This compromises their ability to help their children. These parents should be seeking treatment for themselves.

JUDICIAL PROCEEDINGS

The judicial proceedings for child abuse involve two separate systems, one for the protection of the child and one for the criminal justice system. Both systems are dependent upon the information and evidence collected during the assessment of a child. The two systems may use the information and evidence somewhat differently and impose different standards on the verifiability of this information and evidence.

The judicial system for child protection proceeds in either a family or juvenile court. Compelling, complete, accurate, and verifiable information is necessary to arrive at decisions that reflect the best interests of the child. This information is presented by an attorney who represents the investigating agency (CPS), as well as an attorney who represents the child. The latter may represent the child as a *guardian ad litem*. A judge is usually the individual who makes decisions based on material presented in hearings. In most states these decisions are made on the basis of "the preponderance of the evidence." These decisions affect the immediate life of the child, so they must be accomplished over a short period of time, usually involving weeks and months. Once a child is under the custody of the state for a child abuse problem, there will be periodic hearings until a permanency plan is activated. This plan may include reunification with the child's family of birth or adoption. Although all child protection systems are determined by individual state statutes, the federal government imposes expectations of such systems through regulations accompanying federal funding sources.

The criminal court system depends upon the same information and evidence as applies to the child protection courts, but in this case the information is used to prevent the offender from committing additional abusive acts. The evidence is presented by a prosecuting attorney who must convince a jury or judge "beyond a reasonable doubt" that the offender committed the crime. In general, conviction in the criminal court system requires a higher standard of verifiable evidence than applies in the child protection court. Usually the criminal court proceedings occur months or years after the allegations of abuse are made. In many cases when the evidence is strong, the defendant will agree to a plea arrangement, which eliminates the need for a court trial. The defendant does not contest the evidence and receives a sentence that is less harsh than if convicted in a trial. Because a child's testimony in these trials is often very traumatic, it may be in the best interests of the child not to testify when a plea arrangement can be made.

In either court system it is essential for witnesses to be adequately prepared by the attorney who subpoenas them. This preparation should include a clear understanding of the questions to be asked and the anticipated answers. The attorney should also anticipate the questions that will come from the other parties at the hearing or trial. These questions are often the ones that make the witness most vulnerable to presenting evidence and information in a confusing and contradictory manner. However, a well prepared witness will understand the basic aspects of their testimony and will be able to present the basic testimony concisely and cogently to all parties.

SUMMARY

Sexual abuse is a potentially devastating experience for children, adolescents, and their families. The forensic clinician is an important part of the team of professionals investigating the abuse and assisting the children and families to recover and prevent reoccurrence of abuse. This will be accomplished when the clinician works collaboratively with the team and is sensitive to the needs of the child.

The role of the forensic clinician is to obtain history, make physical observations, document findings, obtain forensic specimens, address medical concerns, assess the significance of evidence, and ensure that the child and family have access to other members of the team. The forensic clinician who is evaluating children must be familiar with child and adolescent physical and emotional development. Each child and adolescent presents with their unique circumstances, which must be evaluated in the context of their baseline development. Correct interpretation of observations and findings depends upon an understanding of the dynamics of physical and emotional development.

The goal of a forensic evaluation is to provide convincing information that will contribute to the safety of an individual child and decrease the risks that the perpetrator of abuse can harm other children. This must be performed in a manner that will minimize trauma to the child or adolescent and provide maximum support for nonoffending family members. This can be accomplished by a well-informed clinician who is comfortable with child and adolescent concerns and has knowledge and experience with the components of the evaluation.

The role of the forensic nurse in the evaluation of child sexual abuse is evolving. With sufficient training and experience, the forensic nurse may be the primary examiner and evaluator of the child. In other situations, the nurse may serve as a consultant to a primary pediatric healthcare provider; in this role the forensic nurse will help to guide the inexperienced examiner through an unfamiliar, complex, and detailed examination. The forensic nurse may also be a resource for nonhealthcare investigators who need the forensic medical expertise to understand and interpret the results of a sexual abuse evaluation.

QUESTIONS FOR DISCUSSION

1. How does sexual abuse of a child or adolescent differ from the sexual assault of an adult?
2. What is the difference between statutory rape, sexual abuse, and sexual assault?
3. What are the special considerations in evaluating an adolescent victim of sexual abuse or rape?
4. How do children and adolescents who are victims of sexual abuse usually present in the health care setting?
5. What is the most effective method of obtaining a full disclosure of sexual abuse from a child?
6. Which disciplines are involved with the management of sexual abuse?
7. What determines the extent of a physical examination in a sexually abused child?
8. What are the components of the sexual abuse examination?
9. What techniques assist visualization of girls' genitalia?
10. What are some actions that can be taken during the examination of a child or adolescent victim of sexual abuse or sexual assault to avoid retraumatization?
11. What are the usual findings in acute and nonacute sexual contact?
12. What determines the need for STD testing?
13. When should forensic evidence collection be performed?
14. What are the judicial proceedings that may follow a physical examination?
15. What factors do you think might account for the recent rise in the reported rates of sexual assault?
16. What conditions in an environment pose a risk for the sexual abuse of a child or adolescent?

REFERENCES

Administration for Children and Families, U.S. Department of Health and Human Services. (2003). *Child maltreatment 2001.* Washington, DC.

American Professional Society on the Abuse of Children. (1995). *APSAC practice guidelines: Descriptive terminology in child sexual abuse medical evaluations.* Charleston, SC.

Beitchman, J. H. et al. (1992). A review of the long-term effects of child sexual abuse. *Child Abuse and Neglect, 16,* 101–118.

Berenson, A. B. (1995). A longitudinal study of hymen morphology in the first three years of life. *Pediatrics, 95,* 490–496.

Berenson, A. B., Heger, A. & Andrews, S. (1991). Appearance of the hymen in newborns. *Pediatrics, 87*(4), 458–465.

Berenson, A. B., et al. (2000). A case-control study of anatomic changes resulting from sexual abuse. *American Journal of Obstetrics and Gynecology 182*(4), 820–834.

Berenson, A. B. & Grady, J. J. (2002). A longitudinal study of hymen development from 3–9 years of age. *The Journal of Pediatrics 140*(5), 600–607.

Christian, C. W. et al. (2000). Forensic evidence findings in prepubertal victims of sexual abuse. *Pediatrics, 106*(1), 100–104.

Connecticut Department of Public Health. (1996). *Voices of Connecticut Youth 1996.* Hartford, CT: Author.

Felitti, V. J. et al. (1998). Relationship of childhood abuse and household dysfunction to many of the leading causes of death in adults. *American Journal of Preventive Medicine, 14*(4), 245–258.

Finkelhor, D. (1984). *Child sexual abuse: New theory and research.* New York: Free Press.

Finkelhor, D. (1994). Current information on the scope and nature of child sexual abuse. In R. Behaman (Ed.), *Sexual abuse of children. The future of children.* Los Altos, CA: David and Lucielle Packard Foundation.

Friedrick, W. N. et al. (1998). Normative sexual behavior in children: A contemporary sample. *Pediatrics, 101,* e9.

Heger, A. and Emans, S. J. (1992). Evaluation of the sexually abused child: Medical textbook and photographic atlas. New York, NY: Oxford University Press.

McCann, J., Voris, J., Simon, M., & Wells, R. (1989). Perianal findings in prepubertal children selected for nonabuse: A descriptive study. *Child Abuse and Neglect, 13,* 179–193.

McCann, J., Wells, R., Simon, M., & Voris, J. (1990). Genital findings in prepubertal girls selected for nonabuse: A descriptive study. *Pediatrics, 86*(3), 428–439.

Siegel, R. M., Schubert, C. J., Myers, P. A., & Shapiro, R. A. (1995). The prevalence of sexually transmitted diseases in children and adolescents evaluated for sexual abuse in Cincinnati. *Pediatrics, 96*(6), 1090–1094.

Wonderlich, S. A. et al. (2001). Sexual trauma and personality. *Journal of Personality Disorders, 15*(6), 496–504.

Wurtele, S. K. & Miller-Perrin, C. L. (1992). *Understanding child sexual abuse.* Lincoln: University of Nebraska Press.

Youth Exposure to Violence, Terrorism, and Sudden Traumatic Death

Paul T. Clements
Joseph T. DeRanieri

Forensic nurses can actively provide support and guidance for youth exposed to interpersonal violence, crime, terrorism, and sudden traumatic death. This chapter explores methods for increased awareness and enhanced assessment, and suggestions for intervention by forensic nurses across levels of prevention, referral, and treatment.

CHAPTER FOCUS

KEY TERMS_____

PTSD
terrorism
violence
youth

INTRODUCTION

It is conceivable that violence and crime occur in all countries and across all cultures. Violence occurs in homes, workplaces, and places where we least expect it to happen. "People from all walks of life are subjected to many forms of violence. Some are victimized by strangers and others by family members and intimate partners. [Sometimes] it is difficult to predict when and where it will occur" (Meadows, 2001, p. vii). It is also difficult to predict the impact that exposure to interpersonal violence, crime, terrorism or sudden traumatic death can have on youth (DeRanieri, Clements, Clarke, Kuhn, & Manno, 2004; Mason & Chandley, 1999; Nader, 1997; Rollins, 1997). The possible sequelae of fear, grief, and intrapsychic pain are personal reactions based on individual development and beliefs, and mitigated by family system and culture. These same sequelae create responses that can be potentially disruptive to the ongoing emotional, behavioral, and interpersonal development and related tasks of everyday life (Clements, Vigil, Manno, Henry, Wilks, Das, et al., 2003).

Youth are at particular risk for traumatic effects because they do not have an established identity and their available repertoire of coping behaviors is limited (Stevenson, 1996; van der Kolk, 1987). Exposure to violence can leave youth with disturbing thoughts and images, numerous unanswered questions, and extreme changes in the family structure and function, and ultimately results in the necessity of relearning the world as a potentially dangerous place (Attig, 2001; Burgess, Hartman, & Clements, 1995; DeRanieri, Clements, & Henry, 2002). Exposure to violence can also simultaneously confound multiple developmental tasks and contribute to increased rates of depression, incapacitating anxiety and intrapsychic distress, and isolation from peers and school. Subsequent attempts at coping and adaptation are frequently complicated and can result in affective and behavioral changes including chronic depression; substance abuse; suicidal ideations, gestures, or attempts; and the potential to commit acts of aggression and interpersonal violence on others (American Psychiatric Association, 2000; Burgess et al., 1995; Doka, 1996; Levin, 1998; van der Kolk, 1989; Vigil & Clements, 2003).

YOUTH AND TRAUMATIC EXPOSURE

Trauma-related stress phenomena in youth have been recognized only in the past few decades (Buka, Stichick, Birdwhistle, & Earls, 2001). For adults, the effects of being exposed to interpersonal violence and witnessing atrocities were first clinically described in the early 1900s, particularly after World War I. Severe anxiety symptoms, such as persistent and frightening recollections, intrusive flashbacks, and constant anxiety, were described as war neuroses or shell shock syndrome (Babington, 1997; Binneveld, 1998). Subsequently these symptoms and related behaviors became more obvious in those who served in military campaigns, such as the Vietnam War. There continues to be concerted exploration of response patterns in veterans of war, including those who have participated in the more recent Gulf War and Iraqi military missions (Shepard, 2001; Southwick, Morgan, & Rosenberg, 2000).

History reveals that many veterans who were involved in combat experience or witnessed multiple deaths sought help because of the constant anxiety and re-experiencing of those war scenes that persisted even several years after they returned home (van der Kolk, Weisaeth, & van der Hart, 1996). In recent studies focusing on youth psychological trauma, it was noted that, although manifested in developmentally different descriptions and behaviors, there are clearly underlying similarities to the adult trauma population. It became evident that traumatic exposure is a crucial etiological factor in the development of a number of serious psychological disorders in youth as well as in adults (Eth & Pynoos, 1985; van der Kolk, 1987, 1988, 1989).

During the past three decades, studies of youth exposure to various forms of violence and other disasters have significantly contributed to our understanding of the mental health effects in youth. Such studies include Terr's (1983) work on the Chowchilla kidnapping involving an entire school bus of summer students over a 27-hour ordeal. This study was seen as groundbreaking because it was one of the first studies to involve primary interviews of traumatized youth versus obtaining descriptions of symptoms via parent interview. Prior to 1980, the assessment of youth-related trauma responses was primarily accomplished through clinical case examination and review of case records. Clinicians most often reported case observations and parent or teacher reports of youth reaction. However, after Terr's utilization of primary interviews and examination studies evolved to include interviews with youth exposed to violence and disasters (Eth and Pynoos, 1985a; Garbarino, Kostelny, & Dubrow, 1991; Garbarino, Dubrow, Kostelny, & Pardo, 1992; Greenberg, 1994; Greenberg & Keane, 1997; Jones, Ribbe, & Cunningham, 1994; Monaco & Gaier, 1987; Terr, Bloch, Michel, Shi,

Reinhardt, & Metayer, 1999). It became clear that interviewing youth directly can be an effective method of assessing their experiences and responses.

Additional foundational studies include Green's (1985) work with youth traumatized by physical abuse, Eth and Pynoos's (1985b) work with youth witnessing a parental death or abuse, and Lyons's (1987) work, which found that some youth who witnessed even a single violent event reported symptoms of diminished concentration in school, sleep disturbances, flashbacks, disordered interpersonal attachment behavior, increased startle response, and hypervigilence. The information gleaned from these studies has identified behavioral states of distress in traumatized youth, including depression, dissociation, aggression, and substance abuse. These disruptions may include displays of avoidance of anything suggestive of the traumatic event, as well as withdrawal from family and peers and a general decrease in activity level since the event. Additionally, agitation; aggressive behaviors toward peers, siblings, and family pets; irritability and emotional outbursts; fights at school; verbal hostility to parents; and other acts of defiance may be noted (Burgess et al., 1995; Clements & Burgess, 2002; O'Campo, Rao, Carlson-Gielen, Royalty, & Wilson, 2000; Osofsky, Wewers, Hann, & Fick, 1993; Rollins, 1997).

An ongoing primary issue is the helplessness of youth at having to watch or listen to the sights and sounds surrounding a violent act and being unprotected from the full emotional impact of the violence (Clements & Benasutti, 2003; Clements, Benasutti, & Henry, in press; Clements & Burgess, 2002). Buka and colleagues' (2001) review of empirical work on the distribution, determinants, and consequences of youth witnessing of community violence indicates that males, ethnic minorities, and urban residents are at increased risk for witnessing violence and have higher rates of post-traumatic stress disorder (PTSD), depression, distress, aggression, and externalizing behaviors.

SCOPE OF THE PROBLEM

As a public health problem, youth exposure to myriad forms of violence is not just manifest in witnessing a traumatic event or dealing with the injury or death of a victim; it is additionally an influencing factor in the ongoing formulation and formalization of a developing personality structure, intrapsychic interpretation of the surrounding environment, and attempts at effective coping and adaptation in the everyday stress found in contemporary society. Such exposure to violence is an especially unique and painful burden for youth to bear because it can violate the very basic tenets of trust in the world, social appropriateness, fairness, and basic beliefs surrounding the sanctity of life (Clements & Burgess, 2002; Vigil & Clements, 2003). The impact of violence crosses all cultures, races, and both genders, resulting in youth who must interpret meaning, identify coping mechanisms, and confront realistic fear for the integrity of their minds and bodies (Mason & Chandley, 1999).

"Violence can be defined as the harmful and unlawful use of force or strength. . . . The violent person is commonly understood to be someone who attacks another . . . either with or without the use of weapons" (Mason & Chandley, 1999, p. 6). Youth exposure to violence typically includes seeing or hearing about behavioral acts that have underpinnings of power and control, and which are often exerted by an adult for some form of personal gain and often brutality (Clements & Benasutti, 2003). The Federal Bureau of Investigation Uniform Crime Reports (UCR) (FBI, 2000) provides a nationwide view of crime based on the submission of statistics by law enforcement agencies throughout the country. UCR provides insight into the nature of the barometer of violence in the United States. To best depict total crime data and to provide the most meaningful information, the UCR program collects data on only known offenses and persons arrested by police departments. The selected offenses monitored by the FBI UCR are: 1) murder and non-negligent manslaughter, 2) forcible rape, 3) robbery, 4) aggravated assault, 5) burglary, 6) larceny-theft, 7) motor vehicle theft, and 8) arson. These are serious crimes by nature and/or volume. Additionally, in the nationwide attempt to assess, prevent, and intervene relative to violence, the Centers for Disease Control and Prevention (CDC, 1997), the U.S. Surgeon General (Satcher, 2001), and Healthy People 2010 (U.S. Department of Health and Human Services, 2000) have all declared violence and violence-related deaths to be a significant public health problem in the United States. Confronting violence in the current millennium is also presented as a significant healthcare issue by the American Medical Association (AMA, 2003), the American Nurses Association (ANA, 2001), and the International Association of Forensic Nurses (IAFN, 2004). This nationwide monitoring and promotion of strategies for prevention and intervention supports the need for increased awareness and understanding as it relates to assessment of exposed youth.

EXPOSURE TO VIOLENCE

In cities around the United States, youth are exposed to violence and crime in their neighborhoods and inside their homes; they are witnessing street fights, gang activity, domestic violence, child abuse, drug activity, shootings, stabbings, and other assaults. Exploring this exposure to violence, Groves, Zuckerman, and Marans (1993) provide a descriptive overview of youth who had witnessed such events. This descriptive study found that 1 of every 10 youth attending Boston City Hospital's pediatric primary care clinic had witnessed a shooting or stabbing before the age of 6 years; half of the youth had witnessed this in the home, half on the streets. This same study revealed that a survey of elementary school youth in New Orleans reported over 90% of the sample had witnessed some form of violence, 70% had seen weapons used, and 40% had seen a dead body.

In Los Angeles it was estimated that between 10 and 20% of the homicides committed in that city were witnessed by youth, and in Chicago, in a study of more than 1,000 youth, 74% had witnessed a homicide, shooting, stabbing, or robbery (Groves et al., 1993). Forty-seven percent of these incidents involved family, friends, neighbors, or classmates, and 46% of these youth had personally experienced at least one violent crime as the primary victim (Groves et al.).

Finally, this same study reviewed police accounts of homicides and found that hundreds of youth in urban areas such as Chicago and Detroit witness the homicide of at least one parent each year. Of note, these study statistics did not include the number of youth who witnessed the homicide of an aunt, uncle, brother, sister, or neighbor, which, depending on the nature of the relationship, particularly if the role is that of the youth's primary caretaker, can be quite devastating (Clements & Burgess, 2002).

Exposure to violence can be categorized as direct or indirect. Direct exposure requires a physical proximity that permits experiencing the violence via visual or auditory means or both. Indirect exposure indicates learning of the violence via verbal accounts of family or friends, or from the news media. Indirect exposure precludes being present with the victim at the time of the event, finding the victim alive but mortally wounded, or witnessing the actual death.

Coping and adaptation have been shown to be related to cognitive development and degree of exposure, and to differ with age. Younger youth have a more restricted range of coping skills than older ones, and therefore may have less flexibility and adaptation to traumatic events (Krell & Sherman, 1997; Monaco & Gaier, 1987; Eth & Pynoos, 1985; Schwarzwald, Weisenberg, Solomon, & Waysman, 1994; Spivack & Shure, 1982). One study of 326 children from areas hit by SCUD missiles in the Gulf War found that younger elementary school children (6th graders) were affected more than adolescents (Schwarzwald, et al.). Additionally, a study by North, Smith, and Spitznagel (1994) showed that the degree of exposure and location in proximity to a mass shooting at a playground predicted the intensity of PTSD symptoms 14 months after the event.

Monaco and Gaier's (1987) study of school-aged youth responses to watching the space shuttle *Challenger* explosion determined that traumatic response patterns and coping abilities significantly vary based on age, with the event having a greater impact on the younger child witnesses.

TERRORISM

The September 11, 2001, terrorist attacks resulted in more deaths than any battle on American soil, exceeding the two most devastating battles in American history: Antietam, during the Civil War, which, until 2001, was the greatest loss of life in our history, and the attack on Pearl Harbor (Clements, 2001; DeRanieri et al., 2004). Of note, today's youth have never experienced "war-time America" because all incursions or defensive responses have been deployed on foreign soil. The Oklahoma City bombing and the September 11th attacks have contributed toward understanding the impact and effects of terrorism on contemporary American youth (DeWolfe, 2000; Hopkins & Starr, 2002; Pfefferbaum et al., 1999, 2000). For youth, now faced with understanding ongoing changes in and interpretations of the terror alert colors and the imminent threat of more terrorist acts, this can be a very uncertain and anxiety-provoking time (DeRanieri et al., 2004; U.S. Department of Homeland Security, 2004). Reactions may range from the small child who is afraid to go to sleep at night to the adolescent who must soon register for selective service and possibly face going to war. Youth look to adults for reassurance and to explain the chaos that is happening in the world (Clements, 2001; DeRanieri et al., 2004).

Although the intrapsychic impact on youth of the September 11, 2001, attacks are not yet clear, findings from the Oklahoma City bombing indicate that youth who lost a friend or relative were more likely to report immediate symptoms of PTSD than nonbereaved youth. Trauma-related arousal and fear that manifested within seven weeks after the bombing were noted to be significant predictors of a diagnosis of PTSD (Pfefferbaum et al., 1999). Of note, two years after the bombing, 16% of youth who lived approximately 100 miles away from Oklahoma City reported significant PTSD symptoms related to the event (Pfefferbaum et al., 2000). This is an important finding because these youth were not directly exposed to the trauma of the bombing and were not related to people who had been killed or injured. Of additional note, PTSD symptomology was also predicted by the amount of media exposure and indirect interpersonal exposure (such as having a friend who knew someone who was killed or injured). Based on this research from Oklahoma City, it is predicted that PTSD may develop in children exposed to media coverage or who had a friend or family member that was killed or injured (Pfefferbaum et al., 2000). Due to the nature of the September 11th attacks and the high media visibility, it is additionally predicted that there will be very high rates of PTSD in children who lost a family member or witnessed the plane crashes and after effects.

IMPLICATION OF YOUTH EXPOSURE TO VIOLENCE

Violence never occurs in a positive light. It is often sudden and unexpected, and is still traumatic even when anticipated within a cycle of repetitive abuse. Violence is the purposeful infliction of pain and suffering on one person by another; it is an act of human design. The victim may suffer for hours in severe emotional or physical trauma, or may die. Regardless of the mode, manner, and timing of the violence, for youth, the pain and suffering begins with exposure to the act or the results, and subsequent attempts to understand such violation (Henry-Jenkins, 1993; Redmund, 1996; Rynearson, 1995; Rynearson & McCreery, 1993). Clearly, after such exposure, a diagnosis of post-traumatic stress disorder must be considered, particularly when manifested by significantly disruptive emotional and behavioral symptoms in exposed youth (American Psychiatric Association, 2000).

For youth, exposure to violence can be particularly traumatic in light of the expected developmental tasks and inherent challenges. These include: functioning with an inherent and general lack of autonomy, ongoing development of a strong identification with the permanence of family and friends, and evolving attempts to understand societal norms of behavior, especially describing and defining actions within the context of "right" and "wrong." Violence directly confounds and violates all of these developmental issues in one traumatic event. This can create highly problematic intrapsychic conflicts for exposed youth, who may subsequently express and display trauma-related symptoms and behaviors.

Developmental tasks, including moral reasoning, peer relationships, and interaction with the environment and culture, expand remarkably during youth, particularly as youth move from the protection of family, neighborhood, and friends to the wider world (Clunn, 1991). Youth is a decisive period for relationships with others. Problem solving and interpretation of events and situations are based on perceptions (Erickson, 1993; Erickson & Coles, 2000; Piaget, 1969, 1977; Wong, Hockenberry-Eaton, Winkelstein, Schwartz, & Wilson, 2000). Significant value is placed upon maintenance of the family unit, which includes obeying the rules, showing respect for authority, and maintaining the social order by demonstrating correct behavior (Kohlberg, 1966, 1975, 1979).

As youth develop a firm sense of stereotypical male or female behaviors, exposure to violence may create confusion about what are deemed to be appropriate gender roles. Additionally important in this period of development are an evolving decrease in the objectivity of moral reasoning and an increase in the subjectivity of the same. This leads youth to become increasingly able to evaluate motivations as a factor in judging right or wrong. Additionally there is a greater understanding by youth regarding the thoughts and feelings of others, and of how their own actions may have an impact on their surroundings. Youth also continue to explore and understand the moral tenets of truthfulness and honesty (Erickson, 1993; Freud, 1923; Gilligan, 1983; Piaget, 1977; Stoudemire, 1998).

Youth explore how to compete and cooperate with others; it is a critical timeframe for "learning the rules" (Erickson, 1993). Youth learn how to control their instinctual impulses while dealing with their environment, particularly as they move toward functioning in a more autonomous fashion. Youth who have difficulty completing these developmental tasks will eventually demonstrate difficulty with impulse control, and will exhibit a diminished capacity to sublimate their energies into task completion (Erickson; Marcus, 1997).

During formulation and formalization of a moral code and understanding the rules of family and society, the overt violation created by violence and sudden traumatic death can present a significant threat to the normal path of growth and development. It can confound a youth's ability to understand societal norms of interpersonal safety and respect for value of life. The critical foundation for personal mastery can be disrupted and can lead to confusion and misunderstanding about appropriate personal and interpersonal roles and expectations (Eth & Pynoos, 1985a; Gil, 1991; Rando, 1996; Stevenson, 1996; Sunderland, 1995; Terr, 1991; van der Kolk, 1987).

IMPACT OF YOUTH EXPOSURE TO VIOLENCE

The effects of violence are not limited to the target and the offender. Family members and friends are also affected by the trauma of exposure, whether they are an eyewitness or traumatized from learning about the details of the violent act. Each violent event creates a uniquely complex set of issues for youth, including siblings, friends, neighbors, or acquaintances.

Older youth (typically greater than age 8) understand that death is irreversible and permanent. Therefore, violence activates fears and concerns regarding their own vulnerability and makes them aware that they are not yet old enough to take responsibility for themselves. Furthermore, these youth may feel multidirectional anger, which may be directed at the victim, related to feeling abandoned, and caused by the great pain and sorrow that has accompanied the traumatic event. Youth may also feel angry with themselves for not preventing the event (Clements & Burgess, 2002; Henry-Jenkins, 1993; Rando, 1996; Redmund, 1996). There is also confusion and virtual violation of the senses accompanied by attempts to comprehend that one human could purposefully violate the life of another human, especially when that loved one was their family member. Youth may express their pain and trauma via anger, by becoming withdrawn or depressed, or by developing physical symptoms (Burgess et al., 1995; Rando, 1996; Redmund, 1996).

POST-TRAUMATIC STRESS DISORDER

In the aftermath of violence, youth are at significant risk to develop PTSD with accompanying symptoms that are both disturbing and disruptive to their daily routines and that can impact the trajectory of their growth and development.

According to the fourth edition of the *Diagnostic and Statistical Manual of Mental Disorders* (DSM-IV-TR) post-traumatic stress disorder (PTSD) (Diagnostic Code 309.81) refers to the cluster of symptoms that characteristically occurs after an extremely disturbing life event outside the range of human experience (APA, 2000). Although early literature linked the development of PTSD to brain injury, it is now generally accepted that the etiology is psychogenic, and the condition is classified along the continuum of anxiety disorders; it is perhaps the most extreme state of anxiety that may be experienced.

A diagnosis of PTSD requires a clear implication that the traumatic event would provoke a significant stress response in most individuals (APA, 2000). Currently, the DSM-IV-TR sets forth the following two criteria that must be met for a diagnosis of PTSD: 1) the person experienced, witnessed, or was confronted with an event or events that involved actual or threatened death or serious injury, or a threat to the physical integrity of self or others; and 2) the person's response involved intense fear, helplessness, or horror.

Determining a diagnosis of PTSD requires significant intervention. The DSM-IV-TR requires one month of diagnostic-related traumatic symptomatology to make a diagnosis of PTSD. Unfortunately, youth may not be diagnosed in a timely manner because parents and caregivers may not seek assessment and intervention until the youth is demonstrating maladaptive behaviors or physiological symptoms. It is noteworthy that the DSM-IV-TR acknowledges that these symptoms and behaviors may be manifested differently in youth based upon developmental age and expected tasks and behaviors. This might include agitation, disorganization, and behavioral displays that are reminiscent or symbolic of the traumatic event.

CHAOTIC AFTERMATH

The social barometer of the United States has changed drastically during the last decade. Acts of violence have increased in frequency and have become increasingly interpersonal in nature (FBI, 2003). Such acts are often compounded by the typical dynamic of premeditation or intent of one human to cause harm to another.

Trauma and related behaviors created by violence are intertwined, and the surviving family members may seek assistance within the healthcare system for youth with emergent symptoms such as sleep pattern disturbances, dietary disruption, or significant avoidant or aggressive behavior patterns. They may seek help from or be referred to mental health agencies.

Numerous factors related to violence can complicate the "normal" process for adaptive coping, including the absence of affective response (numbing or dissociation that results in a showing of no emotion), an unwillingness to speak about the violence (avoidance), expression of only positive or negative feelings about the perpetrator or victim, new or increased behaviors of aggression and destructive outbursts, persistent blame or guilt, anxiety and hypervigilence, prolonged dysfunction in school, parentification manifested by increased caregiving to adults and siblings, accident proneness, stealing or other illegal acts, and signs of addictive behavior (illicit drugs, alcohol, and dietary alterations) (Papenbrock & Voss, 1990; Vigil & Clements, 2003).

Within the first hours after traumatic events, a youth may crystallize an altered and restricted view of his or her personal future that will require treatment to reduce the symptom intensity and to potentially integrate the event into the youth's life history (Attig, 2001; Burgess et al., 1995;

Eth & Pynoos, 1994). Factors complicating the "normal" adaptive coping process for exposed youth include suddenness and lack of anticipation, trauma, violence, feelings of horror, thoughts of preventing the event and its unnecessary nature, anger, guilt, self-blame, and shattered assumptions about the world within which they live (Clements & Burgess, 2002; Janoff-Bulman, 1992).

FORENSIC NURSING INTERVENTION

Forensic nursing intervention with exposed youth requires sensitive and accurate assessment. Many youth may be fearful to share information regarding violence, so forensic nurses must approach the assessment interview with a nonreactive and overtly nonjudgmental stance. Although youth may be asked to describe the violent events that have occurred, it is also critical for nurses to assess family strengths and use these to instill some facet of hope for the surviving youth (Clements & Benasutti, 2003; Clements et al., in press; Lynch, 1988).

Congruent with standard nursing assessment, forensic nursing assessment and intervention should revolve around primary, secondary, and tertiary levels of prevention when working with youth exposed to violence. It is important for each family member who has been exposed to violence to understand that he or she will need to approach adaptive coping as both an individual and a member of the family unit. It is typical for youth to attempt to suppress or hide their feelings for fear of "upsetting" their parents while simultaneously parents or other adults will avoid talking about the violence to avoid upsetting the youth. It is important for each family member to express individual thoughts and feelings in their own way and at their own rate, which in turn will help the family with adaptive coping and problem solving as a unit.

Primary Prevention

Congruent with the mission, scope of practice, and current goals set forth by *Healthy People 2010,* the American Medical Association, the American Nursing Association, and the International Association of Forensic Nurses, primary prevention relative to decreasing or preventing youth exposure to violence is of overarching significance. To prevent families from becoming violent or being exposed to high-risk situations for violence, forensic nurses must find opportunities to promote nonviolence in families and society at large. Forensic nurses can assess and promote primary prevention by assessing levels of family stress, stress, communication and problem solving abilities, psychological stress and abuse, and the degree of psychosocial nurturance.

Secondary Prevention

Secondary prevention involves early identification and intervention that prevents any reoccurrence of exposure to violence. Exposure to violence that involves youth requires a report to state child protective service agencies. Families at risk for violence can significantly benefit from referral and collaboration with available mental health agencies, school counselors, parenting workshops, and anger management seminars.

Tertiary Prevention

Tertiary intervention is necessary when exposure is ongoing and apparently unavoidable. When imminent risk for danger to self, others, or property are noted, immediate intervention must occur. Depending on the nature of the risk (disclosure of ongoing abuse, threats of harm, evidence of previous or current injury, etc.), numerous agencies (police, child protective services, etc.) may require reporting and immediate referral for additional assessment, and intervention may be needed (emergency room, primary care provider, crisis intervention agency, mental health assessment services, etc.).

Helpful Hints for Intervention

Families can be very complex, and the relationships within them are typically numerous, different, and sometimes complicated. Thinking about families as a mobile can be a helpful metaphor for assessment and intervention. Many families hang a mobile above their child's crib or just outside on the porch, and they will typically be able to identify with how gentle breezes cause it to spin and move. Families, in essence, are very similar to these mobiles. They come in all different shapes and sizes, the pieces move at different speeds and in various relations and distances from the others, and yet the common struts and wires hold the pieces together as one unit. Typically the gentle breezes of life keep the mobile moving and changing, adding to the excitement, adventure, and beauty of the family. Even when the harsh winds of life's storms blow, some of the pieces may clink and collide, but the mobile remains together and eventually returns to peaceful motion. However, even the most beautiful mobile can be changed if one of its pieces is damaged or destroyed. Exposure to violence creates such damage or destruction. Violence can damage or take away one or more pieces of the mobile, leaving just an open space, yet with a strut still connected to the rest of the mobile—a constant reminder of the damaged or missing piece.

It is important that each piece of the mobile—that is to say, each family member—takes care of him- or herself while also understanding that they will grieve together as a whole family.

The following are helpful hints for exposed youth and their families:

- Youth are often overwhelmed with emotions (anxiety, fear, anger, guilt), as well as practical matters (school, peers, family function and structure). This is often related to the frequently asked question, "Is it normal to be feeling this way?" Because concentration and comprehension may be impaired at this stressful time, forensic nurses should provide information about resources and educational information in writing or printed form when possible. This will allow future access and referral to the information as needed.

- Many youth may struggle with feelings of guilt for not having been able to prevent the violence or the sudden traumatic death. Some youth may blame themselves, believing that the violence was somehow their fault, or some form of cosmic retribution for "being bad" or having done something "wrong." Other youth may have witnessed the event and begin to second guess whether the event could have been prevented by "grabbing the gun" or intervening in other unrealistic and unsafe manners. The forensic nurse can set a platform for adaptive coping and promote reduction of such guilt feelings by reminding the youth that it was not their fault, that any such attempts at intervention would have likely resulted in injury or other severe forms of harm, and that at times, adults make poor decisions (i.e., violent acts) that are not the responsibility of the youth to correct.

- Shock, numbness, and disbelief, or overt denial, are typical reactions to violent events, so a helpful first step is to encourage other family members to talk through their thoughts and feelings. Talking about the event can help validate what has occurred and can facilitate reinvesting in life. Emphasize that telling the story is a helpful way for families to begin adaptation and coping. If family members become upset and cry or get angry, this is all a normal part of the process.

- It is normal for trauma response patterns to vary among family members, even as they respond together as a unit. Trauma responses are not "wrong" or "bad." For example, all boys do not need to cry to be effectively grieving, yet many people believe that not crying during the grief process is unacceptable behavior. Just because some people simply do not allow themselves to show emotion or other behaviors in the presence of others does not mean that they are not coping effectively. This will be mitigated by personality, culture, age, and personal style during coping and adaptation. The forensic nurse who has concerns about a certain behavior, or lack thereof, should inquire further about the individual's and the family's usual coping skills and behaviors. This will clarify the situation and help the forensic nurse promote adaptive coping or identify potentially maladaptive coping approaches that require additional assessment or intervention. Finally, the use of drugs, alcohol, and violence are not a normal part of the adaptive coping process, and anyone displaying such behavior should be referred immediately for additional assessment and possible intervention.

TALKING WITH PRETEEN YOUTH

When talking with preteen youth, forensic nurses should remember the importance of "getting down to their level," both developmentally and physically. With smaller youth, getting on the floor with them as they draw or play will provide eye contact and a sense of importance to the discussion at hand. With larger youth, sitting at a table provides a level field for communication. It is just as important to remember the expected developmental tasks and behaviors of youth. Maximize a youth's ability to explore and understand through play and fantasy (Clements, 2001; Clements & Benasutti, 2003; Clements et al., 2001). For example, drawings or doll play can facilitate exploration and discussion of concerns and confusion. If the forensic nurse asks a youth to draw a picture of what he thinks happened during the violent event or to use dolls to demonstrate the events, it can provide significant insight into his perceptions and fears. Remember, any drawing or doll play is not "right or wrong" or "good or bad," but rather a simple reflection of what the child is thinking and feeling. Avoid trying to psychoanalyze the drawing or the role play, but instead, ask the youth, "So . . . tell me what's happening in the drawing?" or "So what is that doll doing now?" This can provide helpful information regarding fears or concerns that the youth may have (Clements, 2001; Clements & Benasutti, 2003; Clements, et al. 2001, in press).

Remember that youth have varying levels of understanding regarding violence, injury, and death. Some youth may express thoughts and understanding of violence in terms of fantasy and other related belief systems. Other youth may realize that violence is wrong and that the threat of injury and death are real. This can result in more disruption in adaptive coping and in anxiety related to the realization of their vulnerability to such violence and injury.

TALKING WITH TEENAGED YOUTH

Teenaged youth clearly understand the pain and suffering involved with violence. As they are struggling with the task of becoming independent in preparation for adulthood, they may also be aware of the risks and fears associated with the potential for more violence. It is important to discuss the violence with teenaged youth while making sure that normal developmental tasks and behaviors are simultaneously promoted (Clements, 2001). Actually, forensic nurses can use these normal teen behaviors to enhance processing of this information. For example, a teenaged youth's most important peer group is not his or her family, but other teenaged youth. One way to promote conversation and exploration might be to ask a teen, "Have you talked with your friends about this? What is everyone saying and thinking?" This will send a message to the teenaged youth that the forensic nurse acknowledges and understands that talking about this with friends is important, and at the same time the forensic nurse is also concerned about the traumatic events (Clements).

Teenaged youth need to continue other on-task developmental behaviors, such as going to the mall, going to the movies, and "hanging out" at the playground with friends. These are all behaviors that are still as normal as they were before the violence started. If parents have anxiety about keeping closer tabs on their teenaged youth, they can discuss this with the youth and perhaps negotiate some helpful and not too intrusive activities, such as an extra "check in" call home. Explaining to teenaged youth that this is not in response to an increased lack of trust, but is a way of increasing communication and ensuring safety, most teenaged youth, if approached in a realistic and proactive way, may grumble a little, but ultimately understand and agree (Clements, 2001).

SUMMARY

It is normal for youth to be upset after exposure to violent or traumatic acts. Traumatic responses never feel good, but are often a typical part of the process of understanding and coping. It is important for forensic nurses to help promote and teach adaptive methods of coping because these are often reflective of the way in which youth will handle fear, guilt, and intrapsychic pain as they enter adulthood.

QUESTIONS FOR DISCUSSION

1. Why are youth at significant risk for developmental disruption after exposure to violence, terrorism, or sudden traumatic death?
2. Identify and discuss the implications of exposure to violence on youth and their family.
3. Identify how trauma can contribute to maladaptive coping and developmental disruption in youth.
4. Identify and discuss the roles the forensic nurse can take in educating youth and their families regarding trauma and adaptive coping.
5. Identify several different approaches that may be taken when working with youth of varying developmental levels or age groups.

REFERENCES

American Medical Association. (2003). *H-145.986 Violence as a public health issue.* Retrieved March 2, 2004, from http://www.ama-assn.org/apps/pf_online/pf_online?f_n=resultLink&doc=policyfiles/HOD/H-145.986.HTM&s_t=violence&catg=AMA/CnB&catg=AMA/CEJA&catg=AMA/HOD&&nth=1&&st_p=0&nth=14&.

American Nurses Association. (2001). *American Nurses Association demands stricter violence protections for health care workers. Murder of Florida psychiatric nurse prompts profession's call to action.* Retrieved March 2, 2004, from http://nursingworld.org/pressrel/2001/pr0418.htm.

American Psychiatric Association. (2000). *Diagnostic and statistical manual of mental disorders* (4th ed., text rev.). Washington, DC: Author.

Attig, T. (2001). Relearning the world: Always complicated, sometimes more than others. In G. Cox, R. Bendiksen, and R. Stevenson (Eds.), *Complicated grieving and bereavement: Understanding and treating people experiencing loss* (7–22). Amityville, NY: Baywood.

Babington, A. (1997). *Shell shock: A history of the changing attitude to war neurosis.* London: Leo Cooper.

Binneveld, H. (1998). *From shell shock to combat stress: A comparative history of military psychiatry.* Amsterdam: Amsterdam University Press.

Buka, S., Stichick, T., Birdwhistle, I. & Earls, F. (2001). Youth exposure to violence: Prevalence, risks and consequences. *American Journal of Orthopsychiatry, 71*(3), 298–310.

Burgess, A. W., Hartman, C. R., & Clements, P. T. (1995). The biology of memory in childhood trauma victims. *The Journal of Psychosocial Nursing, 33*(3), 16–26.

Centers for Disease Control and Prevention. (1997). Rates of homicide, suicide, and firearm-related death among children: 26 industrialized countries. *Morbidity and Mortality Weekly Report, 46,* 101–105.

Clements, P. T. (2001). Terrorism in America: How do we tell the children? *The Journal of Psychosocial Nursing, 39*(11), 8–10.

Clements, P. T. & Benasutti, K. M. (2003). Mental health aspects of child survivors of abuse and neglect. In E. R. Giardino & A. P. Giardino (Eds.), *Nursing approach to the evaluation of child maltreatment* (pp. 306–329). St. Louis: G.W. Medical.

Clements, P. T., Benasutti, K. M., & Henry, G. C. (2001). Drawing from experience: Utilizing drawings to facilitate communication and understanding with children exposed to sudden traumatic deaths. *The Journal of Psychosocial Nursing, 39*(12), 12–20.

Clements, P. T., Benasutti, K. M., & Henry, G. C. (in press). Drawings in abuse cases. In R. Alexander & A. P. Giardino (Eds.), *Child maltreatment* (3rd ed.). St. Louis: G.W. Medical.

Clements, P. T., & Burgess, A. W. (2002). Children's responses to family member homicide. *Family and Community Health, 25*(1), 1–11.

Clements, P. T., Vigil, G. J., Manno, M. S., Henry, G. C., Wilks, J., Das, S., Kelleywood, R., & Foster, W. (2003). Cultural considerations of loss, grief & bereavement. *Journal of Psychosocial Nursing, 41*(7), 18–26.

Clunn, P. (1991). Sociology and psychosocial theories of child development. In P. Clunn (Ed.), *Child Psychiatric Nursing* (pp. 101–146). St. Louis, MO: Mosby Yearbook.

DeRanieri, J. T., Clements, P. T., Clarke, K., Kuhn, D. W., & Manno, M. S. (2004). War, terrorism and children. *Journal of School Nursing, 20*(2), 17–23.

DeRanieri, J. T., Clements, P. T., & Henry, G. C. (2002). When catastrophe happens: Assessment and intervention after sudden traumatic deaths. *The Journal of Psychosocial Nursing, 40*(4), 30–37.

DeWolfe, D. J. (2000). Field manual for mental health and human services workers in major disasters. Washington, DC: National Mental Health Services Knowledge Exchange Network. http://www.mentalhealth.samhsa.gov/publications/all pubs/ADM90-537/fmrisk.asp. Accessed October 27, 2004.

Doka, K. (1996). *Living with grief after sudden loss: Suicide, homicide, accident, heart attack, stroke.* Washington, DC: Hospice Foundation of America.

Erickson, E. H. (1993). *Childhood and society.* New York: W.W. Norton.

Erickson, E. H. & Coles, R. (2000). *Erik Erickson reader.* New York: W.W. Norton.

Eth, S. & Pynoos, R. (1985a). Interaction of trauma and grief in childhood. In S. Eth & R. Pynoos (Eds.), *Post-traumatic stress disorder in children.* Washington, DC: American Psychiatric Press.

Eth, S. & Pynoos, R. (1985b). Developmental perspective on psychic trauma in childhood. In C. R. Figley (Ed.), *Trauma and its wake* (pp. 36–52). New York: Brunner/Mazel.

Eth, S. & Pynoos, R. (1994). Children who witness the homicide of a parent. *Psychiatry, 57,* 287–306.

Federal Bureau of Investigation. (2000). *Crime in the United States. Uniform Crime Reports.* Retrieved March 1, 2004, from http://www.fbi.gov/ucr/cius_00/contents.pdf.

Federal Bureau of Investigation. (2003). Crime in the United States-2003. *Uniform Crime Reports.* Retrieved June 20, 2005, from http://wwww.fbi.gov/ucr/03cius.htm.

Freud, S. (1923). The ego and the id. *Standard Edition, 7,* 3–66.

Garbarino, J., Dubrow, N., Kostelny, K., & Pardo, C. (1992). *Children in danger: Coping with the consequences of community violence.* San Francisco: Jossey-Bass.

Garbarino, J., Kostelny, K., & Dubrow, N. (1991). What children can tell us about living in danger. *American Psychologist, 36,* 376–383.

Gil, E. (1991). *The healing power of play.* New York: Guilford Press.

Gilligan, C. (1983). In a different voice: Psychological theory and women's development. Cambridge, MA: Harvard University Press.

Green, A. (1985). Children traumatized by physical abuse. In S. Eth & R. Pynoos (Eds.), *Post-traumatic stress disorder in children.* Washington, DC: American Psychiatric Press.

Greenberg, H. (1994). Responses of children and adolescents to a fire in their homes. *Child and Adolescent Social Work Journal, 11*(6), 475–492.

Greenberg, H. & Keane, A. (1997). A social work perspective of childhood trauma after a residential fire. *Social Work in Education, 19*(1), 11–22.

Groves, B., Zuckerman, B., & Marans, S. (1993). Silent victims: Children who witness violence. *Journal of the American Medical Association, 269*(2), 262–265.

Henry-Jenkins, W. (1993). *Just us: Understanding homicide bereavement,* Omaha: Centering Corporation.

Hopkins, G. & Starr, L. (2002). *September 11: Lessons and resources for classroom teachers.* Retrieved March 1, 2004, from http://www.education-world.com/a_lesson/lesson244.shtml.

International Association of Forensic Nurses. (2004). About IAFN. Retrieved March 5, 2004, from http://www.iafn.org/about/default.html.

Janoff-Bulman, R. (1992). *Shattered assumptions: Towards a new psychology of trauma.* New York: The Free Press.

Jones, R., Ribbe, D., & Cunningham, P. (1994). Psychosocial correlates of fire disaster among children and adolescents. *Journal of Traumatic Stress, 7*(1), 117–122.

Kohlberg, L. (1966). A cognitive developmental analysis of children's sex-role concepts and attitudes. In E. MacCoby (Ed.), *The development of sex differences.* Stanford, CA: Stanford University Press.

Kohlberg, L. (1975). The cognitive-developmental approach to moral education. *Phi Delta Kappan, 56,* 670–677.

Kohlberg, L. (Ed.). (1979). *Meaning and measurement of moral development.* Worcester, MA: Clark University Press.

Krell, R. & Sherman, M. (Eds.). (1997). *Medical and psychological effects of concentration camps on Holocaust survivors.* New Brunswick, NJ: The State University of New Jersey.

Levin, B. (1998). Grief counseling [Electronic version]. *American Journal of Nursing, 98*(5), 69–72.

Lynch, V. (1988). Biomedical investigation as a mental health nursing role. In J. Lancaster (Ed.), *Adult psychiatric nursing* (3rd ed.). (pp. 665–668). New York: Medical Examination Publishing Company.

Lyons, J. (1987). Post-traumatic stress disorder in children and adolescents: A review of the literature. In S. Chess & A. Thomas (Eds.), *Annual progress in child psychiatry and development* (pp. 451–457). New York: Brunner Mazel.

Marcus, P. (1997). Personality disorders. In A. Burgess (Ed.), *Psychiatric nursing: Promoting mental health* (pp. 441–460). Stamford, CT: Appleton & Lange.

Mason, T. & Chandley, M. (1999). *Managing violence and aggression: A manual for nurses and health care workers.* Edinburgh: Churchill Livingstone.

Meadows, R. J. (2001). *Understanding violence and victimization* (2nd ed.). Upper Saddle River, NJ: Prentice Hall.

Monaco, N. & Gaier, E. (1987). Developmental level and children's responses to the explosion of the space shuttle *Challenger. Early Childhood Research Quarterly, 2,* 83–95.

Nader, K. (1997). Assessing traumatic experiences in children. In J. Wilson & T. Keane (Eds.), *Assessing psychological trauma and PTSD.* New York: Guilford Press.

North, C., Smith, E., & Spitznagel, E. (1994). Posttraumatic stress disorder in survivors of a mass shooting. *American Journal of Psychiatry, 151,* 82–88.

O'Campo, P., Rao, R., Carlson-Gielen, A., Royalty, W., & Wilson, M. (2000). Injury-producing events among children in low-income communities: The role of community characteristics. *Journal of Urban Health, 77*(1), 34–49.

Osofsky, J. D., Wewers, S., Hann, D. M., & Fick, A. C. (1993). Chronic community violence: What is happening to our children? *Psychiatry, 56,* 36–45.

Papenbrock, P. L. & Voss, R. F. (1990). *Loss: How children and teenagers can cope with death and other kinds of loss.* Redmond, WA: Medic.

Pfefferbaum, B., Nixon, S., Tucker, P., Tivis, R., Moore, V., Gurwitch, R., et al. (1999). Posttraumatic stress response in bereaved children after Oklahoma City bombing. *Journal of the American Academy of Child and Adolescent Psychiatry, 38,* 1372–1379.

Pfefferbaum, B., Seale, T., McDonald, N., Brandt, E., Rainwater, S., Maynard, B., et al. (2000). Posttraumatic stress two years after the Oklahoma City bombing in youths geographically distant from the explosion. *Psychiatry, 63,* 358–370.

Piaget, J. (1969). *The theory of stages in cognitive development.* New York: McGraw-Hill.

Piaget, J. (1977). *The development of thought.* New York: Viking Press.

Pynoos, R. S., & Nader, K. (1993). Issues in the treatment of posttraumatic stress in children and adolescents. In J. P. Wilson and B. Raphael (Eds.), *International handbook of traumatic stress syndromes.* New York: Plenum Press.

Rando, T. (1996). Complications in mourning traumatic death. In K. Doka (Ed.), *Living with grief after sudden loss: Suicide, homicide, accident, heart attack, stroke* (pp. 139–160). Washington, DC: Hospice Foundation of America.

Redmund, L. (1996). Sudden violent death. In K. Doka (Ed.), *Living with grief after sudden loss: Suicide, homicide, accident, heart attack, stroke* (pp. 53–74). Washington, DC: Hospice Foundation of America.

Rollins, J. (1997). Minimizing the impact of community violence on child witnesses. *Critical Care Nursing Clinics of North America, 9*(2), 211–219.

Rynearson, E. K. (1995). Bereavement after homicide: A comparison of treatment seekers and refusers. *British Journal of Psychiatry, 166,* 507–510.

Rynearson, E. K. & McCreery, J. M. (1993). Bereavement after homicide: A synergism of trauma and loss. *American Journal of Psychiatry, 150,* 258–261.

Satcher, D. (2001). *Youth violence: A report of the Surgeon General. Report on community forums—Youth violence and public health.* Retrieved November 1, 2003, from http://www.surgeongeneral.gov/library/youthviolence/forums.asp.

Schwarzwald, J., Weisenberg, M., Solomon, Z., & Waysman, M. (1994). Stress reactions of school-aged children to the bombardment of SCUD missiles: A 1-year follow-up. *Journal of Traumatic Stress, 7*(4), 657–667.

Shepard, B. (2001). *A war of nerves: Soldiers and psychiatrists in the twentieth century.* Cambridge, MA: Harvard University Press.

Southwick, S. M., Morgan, C. A., & Rosenberg, R. (2000). Social sharing of Gulf War experiences: Association with trauma-related psychological symptoms. *The Journal of Nervous and Mental Disorders, 188,* 695–700.

Spivack, G. & Shure, M. (1982). The cognition of social adjustment: Interpersonal cognitive problem-solving thinking. In B. Lahey & A. Kazdin

(Eds.), *Advances in clinical child psychology* (Vol. 5) (pp. 323–372). New York: Plenum Press.

Stevenson, R. (1996). The response of schools and teachers. In K. Doka (Ed.), *Living with grief after sudden loss: Suicide, homicide, accident, heart attack, stroke.* (pp. 201–214). Washington, DC: Hospice Foundation of America.

Stoudemire, A. (1998). *Human behavior: An introduction for medical students* (3rd ed.). Philadelphia: Lippincott Williams & Wilkins.

Sunderland, R. (1995). *Helping children cope with grief: A teachers guide. Picking up the pieces* (2nd ed.). Fort Collins, CO: Services Corporation International.

Terr, L. C. (1979). Children of Chowchilla: A study of psychic trauma. *Psychoanalytic Study of the Child, 34,* 547–623.

Terr, L. C. (1983). Chowchilla revisited: The effects of psychic trauma four years after a school-bus kidnapping. *American Journal of Psychiatry, 140,* 1543–1550.

Terr, L. C. (1991). Childhood traumas: An outline and overview. *American Journal of Psychiatry, 148*(1), 10–20.

Terr, L. C., Bloch, D. A., Michel, B. A., Shi, H., Reinhardt, J. A., & Metayer, S. (1999). Children's symptoms in the wake of *Challenger:* A field study of distant-traumatic effects and an outline of related conditions. *American Journal of Psychiatry, 156*(10), 1536–1544.

U.S. Department of Health and Human Services. (2000). *Healthy People 2010. Injury and violence prevention.* Retrieved March 9, 2004, from http://www.healthypeople.gov/document/html/volume2/15injury.htm.

U.S. Department of Homeland Security. (2004). *Threats & protection advisory system. Homeland security advisory system: Understanding the homeland security advisory system.* Retrieved March 5, 2004, from http://www.dhs.gov/dhspublic/display?theme=29.

van der Kolk, B. A. (1987). *Psychological trauma.* Washington, DC: American Psychiatric Press.

van der Kolk, B. A. (1988). The trauma spectrum: The interaction of biological and social events in the genesis of trauma response. *The Journal of Traumatic Stress, 1,* 274.

van der Kolk, B. A. (1989). The compulsion to repeat the trauma: Re-enactment, repetition, and masochism. *Psychiatric Clinics of North America, 12*(2), 389–405.

van der Kolk, B. A., Weisaeth, L., & van der Hart, O. (1996). History of trauma in psychiatry. In B. A. van der Kolk, A. C. McFarlane, & L. Weisaeth (Eds.), *Traumatic stress: The effects of overwhelming experience on mind, body and society* (pp. 47–74). New York: The Guilford Press.

Vigil, G. J. & Clements, P. T. (2003). Child and adolescent homicide survivors: Complicated grief and altered worldviews. *Journal of Psychosocial Nursing and Mental Health Services, 41*(1), 30–39.

Wolfelt, A. (1996). *Healing the bereaved child: Grief gardening, growth through grief and other touchstones for caregivers.* Fort Collins, CO: Companion Press.

Wolfelt, A. (2001a). *Healing your grieving heart: 100 practical ideas for kids.* Fort Collins, CO: Companion Press.

Wolfelt, A. (2001b). *Healing your grieving heart for teens: 100 practical ideas.* Fort Collins, CO: Companion Press.

Wong, D. L. L., Hockenberry-Eaton, M., Winkelstein, M. L., Schwartz, P., & Wilson, D. (2000). *Essentials of pediatric nursing* (6th ed.). St. Louis, MO: Elsevier Science.

CHAPTER 3

Understanding Arson: Subtypes and Intervention Strategies

Dian Williams

Arson historically has been defined as the willful or malicious burning of, or attempting to burn, a dwelling, vehicle, or personal property. Because the motive for setting a fire is often misunderstood by investigators, valuable information about the criminal intent may be potentially overlooked or dismissed. Forensic nurses who specialize in mental health, domestic violence, emergency room/trauma, correctional or institutional nursing (prisons and detention), family practice, and child abuse, to name a few, interact and assess individuals who may well be active firesetters. Because of their diverse experience, forensic nurses can make a rich contribution to the study of such dangerous conduct and propose effective alternative sentencing and treatments.

CHAPTER FOCUS

Behavior of the arsonist
Demographics of firesetters
National Center for the Analysis of Violent Crime Study
Center for Arson Research Study and Questionnaire
Need for nursing research

KEY TERMS

arson
arson subtypes
assessments
bedwetting
Center for Arson Research study

common diagnoses
conduct disorder
demographic findings
deviance
firesetting research
intervention strategies
juvenile firesetters
methodology
motivation
National Center for the Analysis of Violent Crime Study
questionnaire
research findings
sexual deviance

BEHAVIOR OF THE ARSONIST

The Center for Arson Research has assessed firesetting behavior in children, adolescents, and adults since 1985. Since that time, the Center has interviewed almost a thousand firesetters throughout the United States. As a result of those experiences, researchers have arrived at certain conclusions about firesetting, among them that it is often ignored or misunderstood as a significant behavior, and that lack of understanding has sometimes led to misdiagnoses and/or improper assignment of risk. In this chapter, the terms *firesetting* and *arson* are used interchangeably, although the Center for Arson Research generally uses the word *arson* to denote fires set in the deliberate commission of a crime.

The Study of Arson: An Encapsulated Literature Review

Shortcomings abound in our clinical knowledge of firesetting behavior. There are decided gaps in awareness of specific motivations in those offenders who use fire as a weapon of choice. Emphasis has been placed by some on understanding the ways in which arsonists differ from other criminals while underscoring the view of firesetters as social deviants (Geller, 1992). Research into firesetting behavior has traditionally focused on understanding the motivation of adult male arsonists. Theories of firesetting in children and youth either arose from studies on psychopathic adult males or conversely identified the behavior as either a normal part of childhood or as an act of delinquency.

Arson is defined as a felony index crime in all 50 states. Arson historically has been defined as the willful or malicious burning of, or attempting to burn, a dwelling, vehicle, or personal property. As Inciardi (1996) points out, most jurisdictions now include the use of explosives as a crime of arson. The problem with the prosecution of arson cases, according to Inciardi, lies in proving that there was intent. The state must prove opportunity and intent in order to have a conviction for arson. Because the motive for setting a fire is often misunderstood by investigators, valuable information about the criminal intent may be potentially overlooked or dismissed.

Scientific study of firesetting has fostered theories based, in large part, on bad data, skewed samples, and biased conclusions (Williams, 1999). Early attempts to understand arson led Marc, a French scientist, to decide in 1833 that arsonists were compelled by an irresistible impulse to set fires. He called this condition "pyromania," a term still in popular use as a diagnosis 170 years later (Geller, 1992).

Freud decided to study the meaning of fire in dreams in the early 1930s, leading him to critical decisions about the motivation of arsonists. After analyzing the dream states of several males who dreamed about fire, but were not actual firesetters, Freud wrote a monograph about the behavior and motivation of arsonists. He determined that arsonists were primarily males who were repressed, heterosexually ambivalent, sexually deviant individuals who used fire as a manifestation of sexual power (Freud, 1932). Review of the scientific literature about firesetting reveals that Freud's initial speculations about arsonists are still popular today, despite the paucity of valid research into arsonists as sexual deviants.

A well-known study by Lewis and Yarnell, published in 1951, reinforced Freud's findings of arsonists as sexually deviant misfits. The study focused on the records of 1,145 incarcerated males who were arsonists or had arson "tendencies." Their research concluded that Freud's initial premise was valid and, in fact, devoted over 40 pages of their monograph to the topic of sexual deviance in arsonists. Lewis and Yarnell (1951) determined that their subjects were sexually repressed chronic bedwetters who masturbated at scenes of fires they either set or happened upon and watched. A review of that study by Pisani (1995) found that the conclusions drawn by Lewis and Yarnell were scientifically unsound. Pisani noted that Lewis and Yarnell did not have a control group, did not clearly identify their data sources, and never defined the term "arson tendency." The study by Lewis and Yarnell, notwithstanding its lack of scientific credibility, is still widely cited in the literature.

Other social scientists added to the confusion and sense of misdirection in firesetting research. Magee (1933) believed that arsonists could be divided into two groups: pathological and nonpathological. He stated that pathological arsonists, or pyromaniacs, were adolescent males between the ages of 14 and 16 who set fires without remorse because they were overwhelmed by an irresistible impulse. All other firesetters, according to Magee, set fires for purposes of fraud.

Inciardi (1970) studied 138 white male arsonists on parole and identified six possible motives the subjects had for setting fires. He mixed behavioral descriptions, criminal justice language, and mental status findings to arrive at the motives of revenge, excitement, fraud, vandalism, mental deficit, and creating a red herring. Inciardi bowed to tradition by reinforcing Freud's 1932 monograph in his findings that arsonists had a propensity for sexual perversion, were social outcasts, and had low intelligence. A study conducted by Sakheim, Vigdor, Gordon, and Helprin in 1985 compared 15 juvenile firesetters to 15 juvenile nonfiresetters. They supported Freud's premise that firesetters had poor ego structure and set fires for intense sexual excitement.

Other studies supported the concept of the arsonist as driven by perverse sexual motivation. Schmidberg (1953) theorized that all arsonists were sexually sadistic white males with pathological personalities. He applied this same reasoning to those who set fires as an act of insurance fraud, positing that such behavior is equally as deviant. MacDonald (1977) also found that the arsonist was driven by sexual desires; he claimed that arsonists were men who set fires as an acknowledgement that, without fire, they were impotent. MacDonald also stated that arsonists collected women's undergarments at fire scenes because they were transvestites. Studies such as the ones by Schmidberg and MacDonald reinforced the notion that arson is a crime involving some kind of bizarre sexual perversion. A study by Quinsley, Chaplin, and Unfold (1989) was unable to validate arson as a sexually motivated crime. Williams (2004), in a review of 35 adult male arsonists, was not able to identify a psychosexual link as the motivation for the behavior.

Alternatives to classifying arson as a sexually motivated crime became popular during the 1970s, and social researchers began to criticize earlier studies. Vreeland and Waller (1979) characterized arson studies as lacking scientific validity, designed primarily to support Freud's seminal work. Vreeland and Waller (1979) and Jacobson (1985) noted that they were not able to validate earlier research findings that linked bedwetting, cruelty to animals, and firesetting. Despite their observations, the triad, as it is known, is still referred to in the literature on firesetting behavior. Hellman and Blackman (1966) found a relationship between firesetting and bedwetting whereas a study by Oppel, Harper, and Rider (1968) found that the same rate of bedwetting existed in the general population. Studies by Koles and Jensen (1985) and White (1996) supported the relationship between bedwetting and the incidence of firesetting. The Center for Arson Research abandoned bedwetting as a variable in their assessment tool in 1997, after collecting data on the behavior for 12 years. Their results found no statistically significant relationship between bedwetting and firesetting behavior.

Other researchers began to consider arson as an act of aggression rather than sexual deviance. Vreeland and Waller (1979) posited that arsonists were men who were unable to express their anger to others and instead expressed it against property. A number of other studies supported the concept of arson as an act of anger and aggression. Rasanen, Puumalainen, Janohenen, and Vaisanen (1996) conducted a study of 15 arsonists in Finland and found that 70% of the subjects self-reported destructive behavior and the inability to express anger directly.

As the 1980s wore on, studies into firesetting behavior shifted away from the psychoanalytic perspective into the impact of environment on behavior. That change brought with it more specific sociological studies of firesetting behavior in children and adolescents. Social scientists, such as Gaynor and Hatcher (1987) and Vreeland and Waller (1979), proposed the idea that aggression, constricted emotional disclosure, and firesetting behavior were learned in childhood. Fineman (1980) and Gaynor and Hatcher (1987) proposed that family background, the methods of punishment and reward, and certain environmental conditions predisposed some youth to set fires. Heath, Hardesty, Goldfine, and Walker (1985) studied children who set fires and concluded that firesetters are more likely than nonfiresetters to have severe behavior problems.

Studies on firesetting related specifically to criminological theories, such as social control theory, anomie, and labeling, have not been systematically conducted. Psychogenic theories (e.g., childhood trauma or mental illness) and sociological variables (e.g., poverty and antisocial conduct) remain popular as explanations for firesetting behavior.

FIRESETTER DEMOGRAPHICS

Gender

Most studies on arson focus on male offenders, both as youths and adults; little research has considered female firesetting behavior. Studies of children and youths who set fires permitted a closer look at the demographics of juvenile firesetters. Most firesetters are male, according to Gruber, Heck, and Mintzer (1981); Kolko (1985); and Kosky and Silburn (1984). Wooden and Berkley (1984) suggested that firesetters are disproportionately white, middle-class males, but Pisani (1995) later described this study as suffering from flawed methodology. Williams (2004) found that 90% of a total firesetting population of 150 firesetters between ages 5 and 55 were male. Bourget and Bradford (1989) determined that female firesetters comprise between 10 and 18% of the total population.

Intellect

Studies by Kuhnley, Hendren, and Quinlan (1982) and Showers and Pickrell (1987) did not find differences between firesetters and nonfiresetters in terms of school performance or intellect. Juvenile firesetters are frequently characterized as poor school performers, with histories of truancy, special education placement, and learning problems (Stewart & Culver, 1982; Strachen, 1981).

Family Life

Families with disturbed children may be regarded from the perspective of a disturbed microsystem, according to Williams (1998). Families of juvenile firesetters have been described as deviant, with absent or withholding parents who have poor communication skills and unpredictable patterns of discipline (Kelso & Stewart, 1986; Kolko & Kadzin, 1991; Sakheim & Osborn, 1986). Sakheim, Vigdor, Gordon, and Helprin (1985) compared 30 known juvenile firesetters with 15 nonfiresetters in a residential setting. The authors found that the firesetter group was characterized by histories of maternal rejection, verbal aggression, and sexual excitement at firesetting.

Common Diagnoses

Kolko (1985) noted that juvenile firesetters were often referred to mental health agencies for reasons other than setting fires. Kuhnley et al. (1982) stated that firesetters were often diagnosed with attention deficit hyperactivity disorder. Williams (2004) determined that 70% of the population in a study of 74 firesetters between the ages of 6 and 63 had received diagnoses of attention deficit hyperactivity disorder. Heath et al. (1985) studied the records of 204 children seen at an outpatient clinic and found that a strong association existed between youth who set fires and a diagnosis of conduct disorder.

Forehand, Wierson, Frame, Kempton, and Armistead (1991) studied 36 incarcerated juveniles diagnosed as having a conduct disorder and found a correlation in their histories between firesetting and antisocial behavior patterns. Jacobson (1985) found similar patterns in an earlier study of juveniles who had severe conduct disordered behavior at an early age of onset. Jacobson noted that the youth with firesetting in their histories had more aggressive and antisocial behavior than did their nonfiresetting counterparts. However, a study by Hanson, MacKay-Sorka, and Staley (1994) failed to support other findings in their study of 25 male juvenile firesetters and 25 nonfiresetters. They determined that the only difference in the two groups was firesetting itself.

In general, it is easy to observe that differences exist in the perception of firesetting. Nowhere is that more apparent than in the attempt to determine the motivation for the behavior. Siegal (2003) calls arson a young man's game, and notes that the FBI statistics for 2000 indicate that 46% of all arson arrests occur in the juvenile population. Siegal mentions that adult arsonists may be motivated to set fires because of severe emotional turmoil. Webb, Sakheim, Towns-Miranda, and Wagner (1990) believe that firesetting behavior is a mental health problem that should not be criminalized.

A study of adult arsonists conducted by Sapp, Huff, Gary, and Icove in 1994 correlates, in large part, with ongoing forensic research into motivation for setting fires conducted by the Center for Arson Research, located in Philadelphia. The Sapp study, based on research conducted by the Arson and Bombing Investigative Services Subunit of the National Center for the Analysis of Violent Crime at the FBI Academy (referred to hereafter as NCAVC), analyzed the motivation of a select group of 83 incarcerated serial arsonists, 78 males and 5 females, from two studies. For the purposes of the study, a serial arsonist was defined as an individual who set three or more fires, with a cooling off period between fire events (Sapp, Huff, Gary, Icove, & Horbert, 1994). I believe the NCAVC study presents a thoughtful contribution to research into firesetting behavior in general, while recognizing that their study sample was restricted to incarcerated adults. Much of the remainder of this chapter is devoted to a comparison between findings from the Sapp study and from the Center for Arson Research, along with conclusions from the studies and implications for future forensic research. Findings by Sapp, Huff, Gary, Icove & Horbert are presented first.

THE NATIONAL CENTER FOR THE ANALYSIS OF VIOLENT CRIME STUDY

In general, the violent crime study determined that of the 83 adult subjects, 81% were white, 9.6% were black, 6% were Hispanic, and 1.2% were other. The majority of arsonists in the study were single (65.9%), with five of the sample married at the time of the study. Sapp, Huff, Gary, Icove, and Horbert (1994) determined that their sample had an overall educational level of 10 years. Of the 37 participants who discussed academics, 8 reported good grades, 10 reported that their grades were average and the remaining 19 (51%) had fair to poor grades.

Sapp, Huff, Gary, Icove, and Horbert (1994) also determined that 24 arsonists in the study had a median IQ of 113; only three of the scores were below 90. The sample was generally heterosexual, at 75.4%, while

8.7% claimed to be homosexual and 15.9% claimed to be bisexual. The study also revealed extensive criminal histories in the sample, with 86.6% revealing prior felony arrests; the most felony arrests were for a prior arson (Sapp, Huff, Gary, Icove, and Horbert). The subjects also revealed a significant history of institutional placement; 23 of the participants (27.7%) had spent time in foster care and 45 of the study sample (54.2%) had been in juvenile detention. Thirty-eight of the participants also reported an average of 3.2 commitments to psychiatric facilities, and 21 reported at least one previous suicide attempt (Sapp, Huff, Gary, Icove, and Horbert).

NCAVC Study Firesetting Subtypes

The NCAVC study classified arsonists into six distinct subtypes: vandalism, excitement, revenge, crime concealment, profit, and extremist. Authors of the study defined each of the subtypes according to fire targets and motivation of the arsonist. All subjects for the study were incarcerated adults. Sapp, Huff, Gary, Icove, and Horbert (1994) define the first arson subtype, vandalism arson, as malicious or mischievous firesetting resulting in property damage. The authors identified the most common targets as schools, abandoned property, and vegetation. Sapp and colleagues studied vandalism arsonists and arrived at the following conclusion: The perpetrator of vandalism fires is usually white, male, and unmarried, has a tattoo or birthmark, and has no military history. The vandalism arsonist generally has an eleventh grade education characterized by poor school performance with average or below average intelligence.

Sapp, Huff, Gary, Icove, and Horbert (1994) found that vandalism arsonists enjoyed warm relationships with their mothers and experienced cold and distant relationships with their fathers. They had histories of time spent in youth facilities and adult jails and prisons. They spent time in foster care or in the care of relatives. The sample spent time in mental health facilities and had histories of depression and suicide attempts. They worked steadily as unskilled laborers. They had few friends in school and were unmarried as adults.

The NCAVC study indicated that the typical vandalism arsonist began setting fires in childhood, generally around age 8. His fires were set while alone and were unplanned, impulsive, and opportunistic in nature. He selected trash bins and dumpsters as primary targets but also burned abandoned buildings and flammable vegetation. In the study of vandalism arsonists, the Sapp team found that the arsonists in this subtype set an average of 12 fires, using matches or lighters, and took no action to avoid detection. The vandalism arsonist left the scene immediately after setting his fires and did not return. As a group, vandalism arsonists in the study had no interest in watching the fires or observing fire-fighting activity. The study concluded that vandalism arsonists consume alcohol or drugs before an episode of firesetting, but no more than at any other time. The frequency of fires remained a constant but the severity of the damage appeared to increase, according to Sapp, Huff, Gary, Icove, and Horbert (1994).

The second subtype according to Sapp and colleagues is the excitement arsonist, who is motivated by the desire to seek thrills, attention, and (rarely) sexual gratification. The targets of excitement arsonists range from small fires to occupied dwellings during the middle of the night. The NCAVC group studied four excitement arsonists who were white, unmarried males with an average 11.8 years of education. None had ever served in the military and all four had felony arrest histories. They had unstable work histories and had spent time in juvenile facilities as teens. Three came from middle class families where the father was described as cold and distant and the atmosphere at home was described as troubled. The excitement subtype reported school as a problematic environment but remembered peers positively.

The four subjects set their first fires at age 12 and set an average of 11 fires before arrest. Two of the group used matches while the other two used delayed ignition devices. Their feelings at the time of the fire were fear and excitement. Three of the four remained at the scene, observing and assisting. All returned to the fire scene within a day of the fire. The subjects reported that they would have set fires even if they believed they would be caught. There was no evidence of drug or alcohol use before the firesetting act. The number and consistency of their fires did not change over time (Sapp, Huff, Gary, Icove, and Horbert, 1994).

The third subtype in the NCAVC study is the revenge arsonist. A revenge arsonist sets fires as an act of retaliation. The Sapp group divided revenge arsonists into four subgroups: personal, societal, institutional, and group, based essentially on the target of the arson fire. For our purposes, revenge arsonists are described as a whole and not by NCAVC subgrouping. Sapp, Huff, Gary, Icove, and Horbert (1994) described revenge arsonists as individuals who set fires in retaliation against some wrong, real or imagined. They found that revenge arsonists were more likely to retaliate against an institution than an individual.

The subtype was identified as almost always single white males with an average of 10 years of education and a history of poor school performance. His home life was described as middle class, with both parents present but cold emotionally. This subtype had a history of felony and misdemeanor arrests and spent time in detention facilities and prisons. Sapp, Huff, Gary, Icove, and Horbert (1994) stated that their sample had histories of mental health inpatient admissions. Revenge firesetters in the NCAVC study reported positive relationships with peers but negative experiences in school.

Sapp and colleagues determined that revenge arsonists set an average of 35 fires before conviction and incarceration. The average age of onset for firesetting behavior in revenge arsonists was 15 years. Revenge setters, according to the NCAVC team, set fires primarily in buildings other than residences as well as to vehicles and vegetation. They determined that the fires of the revenge arsonist are targeted, premeditated, and intentional. Sapp noted that revenge arsonists do not have accomplices and do not discuss their fires with anyone.

Revenge arsonists, according to the study, generally use matches to set their fires and do not remove anything from the fire scene. They do nothing to avoid discovery and do not consider the possibility of apprehension. They do not follow their cases in the media and do nothing to attract attention. If interrogated, the revenge arsonist will be questioned an average of five times before an arrest is made. When arrested, he admits his responsibility for the fires and blames his actions on the behavior or actions of others (Sapp, Huff, Gary, Icove, & Horbert, 1994).

Crime concealment arsonists, according to Douglas et al. (1992), set fires to hide an earlier crime activity such as a burglary. Sapp, Huff, Gary, Icove, and Horbert (1994) determined that crime concealment arsonists averaged 11 years of education, and self-described their academic performance as average. The four subjects had extensive felony arrest records. As a group, none of the sample had a history of foster care, while three of the four had mental health histories. All four had stable work histories and came from warm middle-class families. Three of the four families had single fathers as parents while the other family was headed by a single mother. The subjects reported close relationships with peers and positive experiences in school.

Sapp, Huff, Gary, Icove, and Horbert (1994) found that the crime concealment subtype committed an average of five fires each, with two of the four arsonists setting their first fires at age 5 and the other two at age 13. Their fires were set in familiar surroundings to businesses, homes, and vehicles to conceal a theft or to destroy evidence, and three of the four had accomplices. Two deaths resulted from the fires set by this subtype. Following the arson, all the perpetrators left the scene, but each one returned within a day or two to assess the extent of the damage. After the crime, the lives of the arsonists did not change in any manner nor did they follow the progress of the investigations in the media. They made no effort to discuss their crimes with anyone and upon arrest, minimized their responsibility for the event. Two of the subjects used alcohol before their fires and two used drugs. This drug and alcohol use was not unusual for the offenders. Sapp and colleagues found that the severity of their fires increased over time.

The final two subtypes studied by the Sapp team in 1994 were characterized as for-profit and extremist arsonists. Their research determined that for-profit arsonists were individuals who expected to gain financially or in some other way from a deliberately set fire. NCAVC studied four men in this subtype who were professional arsonists. Although the sample size was quite small, the researchers found that all four arsonists were white males who had an average of 9 years of education. They had poor to average academic performance. Three of the four men had a criminal history of misdemeanors and felonies while one had no criminal history. None of the four had histories of foster placement or mental health services. They had stable work histories as skilled/unskilled laborers. Three of the group arose from lower socioeconomic status while one reported middle-class status. They all reported warm relationships with their mothers and mixed relationships with their fathers.

The study found that two of the four set their first fire in early adolescence while the other two were in their early twenties. The four set an average of 11 fires each. Although none of the four contacted the police to confess, when arrested all four accepted responsibility and pled guilty. Sapp, Huff, Gary, Icove, and Horbert (1994) noted that none of the sample remained at the scene of the fire, but two of them watched from a distance and the entire group followed their crimes in the media. Although two of the four used drugs or alcohol before setting fires, their use pattern was not different from any other time.

The extremist arsonist, according to Sapp, Huff, Gary, Icove, and Horbert (1994) often set fires to further some ideological goal or cause. While the NCAVC study teased out this subtype from the others, there is little to differentiate it from inclusion as a subgroup of the revenge subtype.

Although it is generally true that the study of particular incarcerated individuals does not represent the study of a total population, the NCAVC study offers some useful empirical data on a select understudied group, arsonists. This chapter will explore that study by using it to reflect findings in a small group of 74 randomly selected, nonincarcerated individuals with histories of setting fires. This small population is part of a much larger study completed in 2005.

THE CENTER FOR ARSON RESEARCH STUDY

The Center for Arson Research (hereafter referred to as the Center) evaluates firesetters upon request to determine the presence of firesetting behavior, to assess the level of risk for additional firesetting behavior, and to make recommendations for interventions. For the purposes of this work, the Center compiled 74 randomly selected firesetting assessments (part of a larger 300-subject sample) conducted from 2000 through 2003.

The Evaluation Process

Clients of the Center were interviewed using a questionnaire developed by this writer and modified four times since 1985. Forty-nine variables on the questionnaire were used to identify the presence of firesetting behavior, the firesetting subtype, and the degree of risk for continued firesetting, and to suggest recommendations. All interviews occurred in face-to-face meetings, and the questionnaire was utilized as the worksheet during the evaluation process. Results of the information provided by the client were compared with information gathered by other sources, such as psychological and psychiatric evaluations, information from parents/guardians (if applicable), and reports from parole and probation departments. It is my personal experience that firesetters are more truthful about their behavior when they participate in a focused interview and when there are no observers to the data gathering process. The interview style and language were modified to match the maturational and intellectual level of each client. The Center conducts evaluations on individuals starting at age 3 years; there is no cut-off age.

Sample Demographics

Some of the demographics of this study sample are briefly described in this section. As seen in Table 13–1, which shows the breakdown of subjects by age groups, the majority of firesetters studied in this sample group were between the ages of 7 and 17 years.

There were 66 males in the sample, representing 89% of the population under consideration; females comprised the other 11% of the total sample. Thirty-nine of the subjects were white (53%), 28 of the sample were

Table 13–1   Ages and Percentages of Subject Sample for the Years 2000–2003

Age	Number	Percentage of Sample
3–6 years	1	1
7–10 years	19	25
11–13 years	39	39
14–17 years	20	27
18–25 years	6	8
26–33 years	2	2
34+ years	1	1

Table 13–2 Numbers and Percentages of Subjects with Absent Parent(s)

Category	Subject Number	Percentage of Total
Biological parent absent	58	78
Mother absent	28	11
Father absent	35	47
Both parents absent	14	19
One or both deceased	3	4

black (38%), and 7 were Hispanic (9%). Socioeconomic groups were generally lower to lower-middle class, although two of the sample came from upper middle-class backgrounds. One of the more significant and sociologically suggestive findings in this small study was that of the lack of adult permanence in the lives of firesetters. Those data are reflected in Table 13–2, which are representative of consistent findings by the Center over the past 15 years.

The Center for Arson Research Questionnaire

When the Center first began to interview firesetters, it became clear, rather quickly, that recognition of the motivation for setting fires was often a stumbling block for understanding the behavioral dynamic. Because arson is considered a felony, it is a legal term. This term also describes a behavior. Thus, an understanding of motivation often depended upon what discipline explained it. Researchers have confounded the relationship between firesetting and motivation through a lack of consistency in variables and the introduction of disciplinary influences. Much of what people "know" about firesetting and firesetters is based largely upon the acceptance of poor research and the resultant mythology, as discussed previously in this chapter.

The original arson questionnaire at the Center was developed because available instruments at the time did not address variables believed to be important, such as exposure to violence and a family custom of revenge for perceived wrongdoing. Over the course of time, the questionnaire has helped to answer questions related to the motivation of the offender. The questionnaire is also utilized to develop intervention strategies and assists in sentencing recommendations.

Center Firesetting Subtypes

The Center has identified seven specific firesetting subtypes. Our studies suggest that all subtypes share certain similarities while possessing other distinguishing and separate characteristics. The Center subtypes are: curiosity/accidental, delinquent, thought disordered, thrill seeking, cluster/compulsive, revenge, and disordered coping. The attributes ascribed to each subtype are based upon Center research findings of the past 18 years. The cluster/compulsive subtype will not be discussed in this chapter because the random sample of 74 contained no individual who fits the cluster/compulsive profile. Some of the Center subtypes correspond to those identified by NCAVC; other subtypes identified by the Center are unique to that study.

Curiosity/Accidental Firesetters

> Seven-year-old Stevie, his sister, age 5, and their 5-year-old cousin, Gilbert, found a pack of matches in the bathroom. Stevie whispered to them that they could play a "good game of soldiers" and the three of them ran into Stevie's bedroom, where he closed the door. The children's parents were visiting in the family room and believed the children were upstairs watching a video. Stevie tore some pages from a coloring book and piled them up on the floor of the closet "to make an explosion." He used the matches to set the paper on fire and then the children ducked behind the bed to escape "the explosion." The burning papers set clothes hanging in the closet on fire. When the children saw the fire spreading, they became frightened and opened the door to run away. Fortunately, the smoke detector outside of Stevie's room activated and the family was able to escape. The damage estimate for the fire was $86,000.

The first subtype, curiosity/accidental, is found in those youths whom the media often portray as "playing with matches." Children who set an accidental or curiosity fire generally have no intent to cause harm or destruction. Rather, they find an opportunity to set a fire secondary to a lack of adult supervision (even a momentary lack), poor judgment, and the ready availability of matches or lighters. Curiosity firesetters are usually quite young (8 and under) and are often accompanied by other youths in the adventure. Their fires are characterized by a lack of planning, opportunism, and no anticipation of actual danger. Upon interview, curiosity firesetters display both guilt and denial. However, when it becomes clear that their behavior is known, generally curiosity firesetters admit to the firesetting event. Their fires are set close to or in the home, many times in hidden places, such as closets and under beds. Such site selections are related to an intrinsic understanding that firesetting is "wrong" and would not be approved of by adults in charge. Curiosity firesetters may be male or female, although the behavior is male dominated, as it is in all the subtypes.

Firesetters in this subtype benefit from fire safety education of both adult and minor. For example, instruction stresses that in any home where there are young children, matches and lighters should not be available for young hands. This firesetting subtype generally is not at risk for continued firesetting behavior and demonstrates an ability to learn from a mistake. The Center sometimes makes a recommendation for counseling for curiosity firesetters, especially if the youth displays symptoms of post-traumatic stress, such as anxiety that does not diminish over time. Although there were only two curiosity firesetters represented in the random sample, the earlier example illustrates a common theme of this subtype.

Delinquent Firesetters

Ermell is a 13-year-old male who has been in trouble with the law in his small town since he was 9. He has been picked up so often for curfew violations, the police have lost track. Ermell refuses to obey his parents and his father threw him out of the house last year in frustration. Ermell was returned home by the police because he was too young to be out on his own. He is very disrespectful to adults and seldom attends school. He has smoked cigarettes since age 10 and drinks whenever he can find any way to get beer. He accepts no responsibility for his conduct and says that rules are "stupid." He became sexually active last year and says he wears condoms. Two months ago, Ermell and a friend were arrested after they set fires in four cars by pouring gasoline through open windows and throwing in lit matches. Upon interview, Ermell stated, "If people are too dumb to close their car windows, that's what they get. It's pretty funny."

Delinquent firesetters, the second subtype, are distinguished by a number of interesting variables. The NCAVC study, in the description of the vandalism subtype, appears to identify the delinquent firesetter in adult life. The Center has consistently found that delinquent firesetters are noncompliant with rules and social expectations at home and in school. They give themselves adult privileges, such as smoking and drinking, in early adolescence. As a group, delinquent firesetters are disrespectful toward adults, have poor judgment, do not learn easily through consequences, and blame others for their behavior. A total of 31 delinquent firesetters (42%) were represented within the total of 74 randomly selected subjects. Table 13–3 looks at common variables of delinquent firesetters.

The Sapp study of 1994 found that their vandalism subtype, which is compared here to the delinquent firesetter subtype, spent time in foster care and mental health facilities (psychological histories were available on only 26 of their sample). A review of the delinquent sample in the Center study showed that only 5 (31%) spent time in foster care while 21 (68%) had histories of psychiatric interventions. The most common diagnoses of the delinquent sample were oppositional defiant disorder (32%), conduct disorder (43%), and attention deficit hyperactive disorder (71%). Of particular interest is the finding that 61% of the Center

Table 13–3   Variables and Percentages in 24 Delinquent Firesetters

Variable	Number of Subjects	Percentage
Hyperactivity	22	71
Easily led by others	23	74
Remorse for behavior	13	42
Missing parent(s)	24	77
Getting even with others	11	35
Disrespect for authority	23	74
Family discord	25	81
Theft/shoplifting	19	61
Impulsive	23	90

sample was receiving psychotropic mediations, excluding psychostimulants, for behavior control.

The NCAVC study found that their vandalism group began setting fires around the age of 8 years, while the Center study determined the average age at which firesetting began in their sample was 10 years, 7 months. Before firesetting, however, the youth in the Center sample were already engaged in other acting out behavior, such as excessive fighting, theft, and rule breaking. Interestingly, 10 (32%) of the sample revealed that they set fires while alone, 15 (48%) stated that they set fires only with peers, and 6 (19%) reported that they set some fires alone and some fires with friends, depending upon the circumstances. It is clear from evaluations the Center conducted on delinquent firesetters over the past 18 years that this subtype manifests asocial behavior, even if they stop setting fires.

The Center consistently recommends a number of interventions for delinquent firesetters. Among them are: 1) psychoeducational evaluation to rule out the presence of a learning disability that may be contributing to poor school performance and acting out; 2) psychological testing to determine whether a diagnosis of attention deficit hyperactivity disorder has been missed, or conversely, inappropriately applied; 3) community service, if the youth is on a probationary status; 4) a drug and alcohol evaluation and random urine drug screens; 5) an enforced curfew; and 6) family therapy.

Revenge Firesetters

Morris is a 15-year-old arrested for making terroristic threats against his homeroom teacher in his alternative school. He was placed in the school following release from detention for two arson fires, one at his old school and one at a neighborhood store. He was brought up by his parents who did not get along. His father has a history of major mental illness and multiple involuntary psychiatric hospitalizations throughout Morris's life. His father's favorite saying is, "Get the bastards before they get you." Morris reports that he has never had a friend and does not want one because "We come in this world alone and we go out alone." He began setting fires "to get back" at age 13. Morris estimates that he has set 11 fires "so far."

Revenge firesetters are the third subtype presented for consideration. Review of the Center records found that five (7%) of the random sample were revenge setters. Findings with revenge firesetters have consistently pointed to a number of conclusions about this subtype, including the fact that revenge setters tend to view themselves as misunderstood loners. This self-view increases over time and leads to a life of increasing social and personal isolation. The NCAVC study found that revenge setters retaliate against some real or imagined wrong, and the Center study supports this observation. Sapp, Huff, Gary, Icove, and Horbert (1994) describe revenge setters as having a history of arrests, with time spent in detention and prison. They reported positive relationships with peers, but negative school experiences. The federal study sample had mental health histories. Table 13–4 exhibits findings from the Center's client sample.

Sapp and colleagues found the average age at which revenge firesetting begins was 15 years, while the sample in the Center cohort began setting fires on average at age 13 years, 4 months. The small sample size in the Center study does not allow for more than preliminary comments; however, when comparing the revenge firesetter to the delinquent subtype, some additional interesting observations emerge. While 31% of the delinquent sample spent time in foster care, none of the revenge subtype had a history of out-of-home placements. All five of the sample did have a history of mental health services and interventions. Two of the five

Table 13–4 Variables and Percentages of Five Revenge Firesetters

Variable	Number of Subjects	Percentage
Juvenile justice history	2	40
Hyperactivity	3	60
Easily led	3	60
Remorse	3	60
Missing parent(s)	3	60
Getting even	4	80
Disrespect for authority	3	60
Family discord	4	80
Theft/shoplifting	1	20
Impulsive	4	80

were on psychotropic medications at the time of their interviews, while 19 of 31 delinquents were on medication.

The most common diagnoses for the revenge subtype were, as with the delinquent subtype, oppositional defiant disorder (3) and conduct disorder (1); one client was diagnosed with bipolar disorder. All five of the revenge subjects indicated that they set their fires alone. Four of the fire stated they set fires for "revenge" while the other subject stated he set fires "to get even with people who p— me off." Four of the sample report histories of underage drinking and marijuana use and one subject denied any substance abuse.

The Center recommends a number of specific interventions for revenge firesetters, depending upon their ages at the time of the evaluation. The Center further recommends that children and adolescents have an assessment of their cognitive skill development because research shows that revenge setters often have distorted thought processes characterized by rigidity of thinking and a marked lack of trust in others. They "find" facts to support their world views and are quick to blame others for their misfortunes. Revenge setters have enormous difficulty in viewing an issue from more than an ego-centered position.

Additionally, the Center commonly recommends community service and restitution (if the youth or adult is not incarcerated) along with probation. Individual and family therapy is encouraged to interrupt vengeful thinking and response patterns within the system. The Center also argues on behalf of psychological testing to rule out a paranoid thought disorder as well as a review of the appropriateness of any medication that the client may be prescribed. It is appropriate to undertake a substance abuse assessment, especially for those revenge setters with a history of chemical abuse. The Center evaluators note that firesetters in the revenge subtype are difficult to engage and treat. Providers should take seriously any threats that an individual from this subtype might make and should remain aware of personal safety.

Thrill Seekers ("Excitement Arsonists")

Winter is a 21-year-old male evaluated for arson after his conviction for six fires in his community. As a child, Winter was in and out of the emergency room with broken bones and other injuries from high risk behaviors, such as jumping out of trees with a homemade parachute. He wrecked four cars since he began driving and currently has a suspended license. He characterized himself as a "natural born leader; I'm always the guy with the ideas among my friends." He tried to join a police department right after high school but was unable to pass the psychological test, and states, "Now I try to be on the spot to help out. I'm like an informant because I know a lot the cops don't know about what goes on in this town.

They're not as smart as they think." Winter described his fires in this way:"We was [sic] just fooling around with some lighter fluid and things got out of hand." He was unable to explain how he was "just fooling around" on six separate occasions (two to occupied dwellings during the night). Winter displayed no guilt or remorse for his actions and hinted that there "are a lot of things the cops and that fire marshal don't know."

Thrill seekers, the next subtype under discussion, are called excitement arsonists by the NCAVC research group. Seven of the firesetters in the Center study were identified as thrill seekers. This subtype sets fires for two primary reasons: for the "rush" it brings them and for the opportunity to outwit police and fire investigators. This subtype is frequently thought to set fires so they can be identified as "heroes," rushing in to save people from harm. That, however, is not a viable explanation as the motivator for setting fires. Rather, rescue of victims from fires set by the "hero" is another part of the game of being an active, on-site presence. A total of seven (15%) of the sample were found to be thrill seekers. Table 13–5 reviews common variables of thrill seeker arsonists.

The sample of seven reflects a larger study conducted by the Center on thrill seekers. The NCAVC study of 1994 found that the average age for first fires in their excitement (thrill seeker) subtype was 12 years, but the Center study found a somewhat later age onset of 13 years, 9 months. The federal study did not find a history of substance abuse before the arson fires in their sample, while the Center found that five of the seven in their sample used alcohol and/or marijuana before their fires. Substance abuse was not an out-of-the-ordinary pattern for the participants. No members of the Center sample spent time in out-of-home placements, but five of the seven had histories of mental health services. Their most common diagnoses included: attention deficit hyperactivity

Table 13–5 Variables of Seven Thrill Seeker Firesetters

Variable	Number of Subjects	Percentage
Juvenile justice history	6	86
Hyperactivity	5	71
Easily led	4	57
Remorse	3	42
Missing parent(s)	6	86
Getting even	2	28
Disrespect for authority	6	86
Family discord	6	86
Theft/shoplifting	6	86
Impulsive	4	57

disorder (5); dysthymic disorder—depression (1); bipolar disorder (1); and conduct disorder (4). Three of the seven were on psychotropic medications at the time of their evaluations for firesetting. Interestingly, three of the seven were volunteer firefighters at the time of their arrests for arson. Studies have led the Center to recommend strongly that fire departments should conduct personality testing on all applicants to determine high degree risk takers. Five (71%) of the group stated that they set fires with peers while two of the sample (including two of the three volunteer firefighters) stated they sometimes set fires alone and sometimes with friends.

The Center recommends a number of specific interventions for thrill seeker arsonists, including a psychiatric assessment to rule out bipolar disorder. It also recommends substance abuse evaluations and possible treatment intervention. The Center recognizes that appropriate criminal justice punishments are often a consequence for this subtype, who are characterized by poor judgment and an intense attraction to risk taking. Although sometimes a common legal consequence, incarceration or detention does little to extinguish firesetting behavior in thrill seekers.

Thought Disorder Firesetters

> Sam, a 22-year-old male, has heard voices for the past 10 months telling him to do "bad things." He has tried his best to ignore them, but the voices are getting louder. Recently he has begun to hear a male voice telling him to set fires in hospital bathrooms to "get back at the doctors." Sam was recently court committed for harassing customers at a video store for watching "filthy sex about homosexuals."

Only 2 of the 74 arsonists in the random sample were thought of as thought disordered. Such a small number cannot be considered an adequate sample worthy of in-depth discussion in this work; however, a number of observations may be safely made. First, fires set by individuals suffering from a thought disorder are generally secondary to hallucinations and/or delusions. Also, this type of arsonist shows evidence of a lack of adaptive functioning, poor judgment, poor reasoning skills, and impulsive decision making based on paranoid thoughts. When the thought disordered firesetter is compliant and he or she is treated successfully with psychotropic medications, the risk of firesetting behavior decreases significantly. Unfortunately, it is not unusual for individuals with a diagnosis of thought disorder to refuse or discontinue medications. Arsonists who set fires in response to disordered thinking pose a risk to community safety.

Disordered Coping Firesetters

> *Brandon is a 9-year-old boy evaluated for firesetting behavior after he held a lit match up to his little sister's face. He was adopted at age 6 after spending 4 years in the foster care system. Very little is known about Brandon's infancy and toddler years as he was discovered abandoned in a bus station bathroom when he was almost 2 years old. He was moved in and out of various foster homes with some regularity because of "negative" behavior, such as setting fires under his bed, running away, cursing, spitting, and fighting. Brandon admits to sexual abuse in two of his foster placements. Although he receives counseling and wrap-around services, Brandon is doing very poorly in school and at home. At his own count, Brandon believes he has set "maybe 100 fires." His adoptive parents have consulted an attorney about nullifying the adoption.*

The final subtype for discussion, disordered coping, poses a particular challenge for successful discovery and intervention because firesetting is often secret. The firesetting behavior often has its onset in childhood and becomes a primary means of coping with anxiety. The random sample in this study found 27 firesetters (36%) who fit the profile of a disordered coping firesetter. Table 13–6 reveals common variables of disordered coping firesetters.

The NCAVC study did not identify a specific subtype that matched the category of disordered coping firesetters determined by the Center. There is reason to believe that arsonists of this type seldom appear on the radar screen of criminal justice agencies. When disordered coping arsonists are arrested, it is more common to find them charged as sex offenders than as firesetters. The average age of onset for setting fires in this subtype sample was 8 years, 3 months. Six of the 27 had histories of foster care, in com-

Table 13–6 Variables of 27 Disordered Coping Firesetters

Variable	Number of Subjects	Percentage
Juvenile justice history	2	7
Hyperactivity	19	70
Easily led	19	70
Remorse	12	44
Missing parent(s)	21	78
Getting even	9	33
Disrespect for authority	18	67
Family discord	23	85
Theft/shoplifting	16	59
Impulsive	23	85

parison to none in the revenge subtype and 5 in the delinquent subtype. Eighteen (67%) received mental health services, including inpatient hospitalization. Their most common diagnoses included depression (3), dissociative disorder (3), conduct disorder (6), impulse control disorder (5), attention deficit hyperactivity disorder (19), oppositional disorder (2), and pyromania (4). Fifteen of the sample carried multiple Axis I and Axis II diagnoses. Axis I diagnoses refers to primary clinical disorders; Axis II diagnoses codes personality disorders and/or mental retardation.

Twenty of the sample of 27 stated that they set their fires alone, 5 said they set fires only with peers, and 2 mentioned that they set some fires alone and some with peers. The average number of fires set before there was any intervention around the behavior was four. Nine members of the population admitted to a history of substance abuse that they believed did not increase or decrease around a fire event.

The reasons for firesetting behavior in this subtype are a matter of some conjecture. Ongoing study of disordered coping firesetters indicates that this subtype is different in a number of areas than the other identified groups. Disordered coping firesetters report early sadistic fantasy development, and those fantasies become of great importance. A 24-year-old male client stated during his interview, "You don't know what they [fantasies] mean to me. You don't know anything about them. I always did and I always will." Burgess, writing in 1984, described the importance to pedophiles of their child pornography collections. Similarly, disordered coping firesetters appear to have their own important collections. They seem attracted to Nazi memorabilia and sadistic pornography, and many admit to collecting these items since adolescence.

It is clear from this small study and other, larger studies conducted on firesetters that individuals with reported firesetting behavior accrue a multiplicity of diagnoses. Although it seems more common for an individual with a firesetting history to be diagnosed with a disruptive behavior disorder, the importance of that behavior is often lost. Disordered coping firesetters often experience multiple treatment opportunities and never discuss the importance of firesetting to them or the development of sadistic fantasies. Adolescent firesetters in this subtype appear to undergo a transformation in their sadistic fantasy lives as the fantasies convert from sadistic aggression to sexual sadistic aggression.

A number of strategies and interventions appear salient in the attempt to interrupt firesetting behavior in this subtype. An important first step is that of determining a correct diagnosis. As is commonly found in interviews with disordered coping firesetters, although 59% of the sample were receiving psychotropic medications at the time of their evaluation, they continued to have active sadistic fantasies and thoughts about setting fires. This subtype is often seen for behavioral intervention in childhood because they are disruptive at home and in the classroom. Unfortunately, during the assessment for service, many youths or their families are not asked about firesetting behavior. Children and youths who fall into this firesetting category do not volunteer that they set fires and must be directly questioned about the behavior. Therefore, a comprehensive assessment is essential for any youth who is experiencing failure of behavior at home/school.

The Center recommends family therapy and individual counseling with a strong behavioral component for disordered coping firesetters. It is essential that youths who fall into this subtype learn to identify the triggers that elicit sadistic fantasies and to develop positive, alternative responses to anger and anxiety. Ten disordered coping firesetters in the study reported physical abuse and five reported sexual and emotional abuse. There seems to be an association between a history of abuse and firesetting in this subtype. This is in contrast to the revenge setters where two affirmed physical abuse, one reported emotional abuse, and none reported sexual abuse. It is of interest to note that no excitement subtype firesetters in this study reported a history of physical, sexual, or emotional abuse.

CONCLUSIONS OF THE CENTER STUDY: THE NEED FOR NURSING RESEARCH

Firesetting behavior in children, adolescents, and adults has a direct impact on public safety. Heidi (1999), in writing of the public perception about juvenile killers, notes that the media overemphasizes the volume of the event. It may be said that the opposite is true about firesetting: There is a lack of attention to the magnitude of the problem. The evaluation of individuals for firesetting who have asocial conduct should be an important component of any clinical assessment. Too often, firesetting behavior is seen as an isolated act, without meaning or significance. Little attention is paid to the underlying causes of firesetting behaviors. In fact, many times "arson-related" behavior is handled by the criminal justice system with few alternative sentencing recommendations. This underemphasis of the problem of firesetting has led to a lack of funded research into firesetting behavior and decreased emphasis on the value of risk assessment.

There is a compelling need for additional funded research into the motivation and intervention strategies around firesetting behavior. Few longitudinal studies exist that trace the continuation of firesetting into adult life. To date, there have been few contributions to a more comprehensive understanding of firesetting behavior by nurse researchers despite the realization that forensic nurses encounter firesetters daily in their practices. Forensic nurses who specialize in mental health, burn injury, emergency room/trauma, correctional or institutional nursing (prisons and detention), family practice, and child abuse interact and assess individuals who may well be active firesetters. Awareness of the indicators of firesetting behavior and familiarity with assessment tools, such as the Center questionnaire, are the first steps in the development of comprehensive forensic studies of the problem. Nursing research into firesetting behavior would make a rich contribution to the study of such dangerous conduct. Much of the research available on firesetting has little follow-up and suffers from poor methodology. Forensic nurse researchers could offer an advanced understanding of a complex problem because of our unique interactions with individuals in every aspect of health care.

An instrument that would measure the effectiveness of nursing interventions with firesetters and determine the appropriateness of particular strategies could be designed through nursing research. A comparative study that assesses the success of particular nursing interventions with firesetters and a control group of nonfiresetters in a residential treatment setting is an example of a possible focus of forensic nursing research. These studies could lead to the development of guidelines for modalities of treatment for the various firesetter subtypes.

It is clear that specific forensic nursing research in the area of firesetting could be very helpful as a way to further an in-depth understanding of this dangerous behavior.

QUESTIONS FOR DISCUSSION

1. What shortcomings are found in the research on firesetting behavior?
2. What arson subtypes were identified in the Sapp study?
3. How has the research into firesetting affected our understanding of the behavior?
4. What are the firesetting subtypes identified in the Center for Arson Research study?
5. What research efforts do you think should be made to understand firesetting behavior?
6. Discuss some assessment strategies and types of assessment tools that the forensic nurse can use to evaluate the level of risk for additional firesetting behavior and to make recommendations for interventions when working with firesetters.

REFERENCES

Bourget, D. & Bradford, J. M. (1989). Female arsonists: A clinical study. *Bulletin of the American Academy of Psychiatry & the Law, 17*(3), 293–300.

Burgess, A. (1984). *Child pornography and sex rings*. Lexington, MA: DC Heath.

Douglas, J., Burgess, A., & Ressler, R. (1992). Understanding the arsonist: From assessment to confession. In: *Crime Classification Manual.* New York: Lexington Books.

Fineman, K. (1980). Firesetting in childhood and adolescence. *Psychiatric Clinics of North America, 3*, 483–500.

Forehand, R., Wierson, M., Frame, C., Kempton, T., & Armistead, L. (1991). Juvenile firesetting: A unique syndrome or an advanced level of antisocial behavior? *Behavior Research & Therapy, 29*(2), 128–129.

Freud, S. (1932). The acquisition of power over fire. *International Journal of Psychoanalysis, 13*(4), 406–409.

Gaynor, J. & Hatcher, C. (1987). *The psychology of child firesetting: Detection and intervention.* New York: Brunner/Mazel.

Geller, J. (1992). Arson in review: From profit to pathology. *Clinical Forensic Psychiatry, 15*(3), 623–645.

Gruber, A., Heck, E., & Minzer, E. (1981). Children who set fires: Some background and behavioral characteristics. *American Journal of Orthopsychiatry, 51*, 484–488.

Hanson, M., MacKay-Sorka, S., & Staley, S. (1994). Delinquent firesetters: A comparative study of delinquency and firesetting histories. *Canadian Journal of Psychiatry, 39*(4), 230–232.

Heath, G., Hardesty, V., Goldfine, P., & Walker, A. (1985). Childhood firesetting. *Journal of Clinical Psychology, 41*(4), 571–575.

Heidi, K. (1999). *Young killers: The challenge of juvenile homicide.* Thousand Oaks, CA: Sage.

Hellman, D. & Blackman, N. (1966). Enuresis, firesetting & cruelty to animals: A triad predictive of adult crime. *American Journal of Psychiatry*, 122, 1431–1435.

Inciardi, J. (1970). The adult firesetter: A typology. *Criminology, 8*, 145–155.

Inciardi, J. (1996). *Criminal justice* (5th ed.). New York: Harcourt Brace.

Jacobson, R. (1985). The subclassification of child firesetters. *American Journal of Orthopsychiatry, 16*, 84–94.

Kelso, J. & Stewart, M. (1986). Factors which predict the persistence of aggressive conduct disorder. *Journal of Child Psychology and Psychiatry and Allied Disciplines, 27*(1), 77–86.

Koles, M. & Jensen, W. (1985). Comprehensive treatment of chronic firesetting behavior in a severely disordered boy. *Journal of Behavior Therapy and Experimental Psychiatry, 16*(1), 81–85.

Kolko, D. (1985). Juvenile firesetting: A review and methodological critique. *Clinical Psychology Review, 5*, 345–375.

Kolko, D. & Kadzin, A. (1991). Aggression and psychopathology in matchplaying and firesetting children: A replication and extension. *Journal of Clinical Child Psychology, 20*(2), 191–201.

Kosky, R. & Silburn, S. (1984). Children who light fires: A comparison between firesetters and nonfiresetters referred to a child psychiatric outpatient service. *Journal of Child Psychology and Psychiatry, 18*, 251–255.

Kuhnley, E., Hendren, R., & Quinlan, D. (1982). Firesetting by children. *Journal of the American Academy of Child Psychiatry, 21*, 560–563.

Lewis, B. & Yarnell, H. (1951). Pathological firesetting (pyromania). *Nervous & Mental Disease Monographs, 82,* 53–61.

MacDonald, J. (1977). *Bombers and firesetters.* Springfield, IL: Charles Thomas.

Magee, J. (1933). Pathological arson. *Scientific Monthly, 37,* 358–361.

Oppel, W., Harper, P., & Rider, R. (1968). Social, psychological and neurological factors associated with nocturnal enuresis. *Pediatrics, 42,* 627.

Pisani, A. (1995). *Arson research: A critical review of the literature.* Unpublished manuscript.

Quinsley,V., Chaplin, T., & Unfold, D. (1989). Arsonists and sexual arousal to firesetting; Correlations unsupported. *Journal of Behavior Therapy and Experimental Psychiatry, 20,* 203–209.

Rasanen, P., Puumalainen, T., Janohenen, S., & Vaisanen, E. (1996). Firesetting from the viewpoint of an arsonist. *Journal of Psychosocial Nursing and Mental Health Services, 34*(3), 16–21.

Sakheim, G. & Osborn, E. (1986). A psychological profile of juvenile firesetters in residential treatment: A replication study. *Child Welfare, 64*(5), 495–503.

Sakheim, G., Vigdor, M., Gordon, M. & Helprin, L. (1985). A psychological profile of juvenile firesetters in residential treatment. *Child Welfare, 64*(5), 453–476.

Sapp, A., Huff, T., Gary, G., & Icove, D. (1994). *A motive-based offender analysis of serial arsonists.* Washington, DC: National Center for the Analysis of Violent Crime, Federal Bureau of Investigation.

Sapp, A., Huff, T., Gary, G., Icove, D., & Horbert, P. (1994). *A report of essential findings from a study of serial arsonists.* Washington, DC: National Center for the Analysis of Violent Crime, Federal Bureau of Investigation.

Schmidberg, M. (1953). Pathological firesetter. *Journal of Criminal Law, Criminology and Police Science, 44,* 30–37.

Showers, J. & Pickrell, E. (1987). Child firesetters: A study of three populations. *Hospital and Community Psychiatry, 38,* 495–501.

Siegal, L. J. (2003). *Criminology* (8th ed.). Belmont, CA: Wadsworth.

Stewart, M. & Culver, K. (1982). Children who set fires: The clinical picture and a follow-up. *British Journal of Psychiatry, 140,* 357–363.

Strachen, J. (1981). Conspicuous firesetting in children. *British Journal of Psychiatry, 138,* 26–29.

Vreeland, R. & Waller, M. (1979). *The psychology of firesetting: A review and appraisal.* Washington, DC: U.S. Government Printing Office.

Webb, N., Sakheim, G., Towns-Miranda, L., & Wagner, C. (1990). Collaborative treatment of juvenile firestarters: Assessment and outreach. *American Journal of Orthopsychiatry, 60,* 305–310.

White, E. B. (1996). Profiling arsonists and their motives: An update. *Fire Engineering, 149*(3), 80–86.

Williams, D. (1998). *Delinquent and deliberate firesetters in the middle years of childhood and adolescence.* Ann Arbor, MI: UMI Dissertation Services.

Williams, D. (1999). Looking at arson: An overview. *The PAPPC Journal, 59*(2), 16–19.

Williams, D. (2004). *Understanding the arsonist: From assessment to confession.* Tucson, AZ: Lawyers & Judges Publishing.

Wooden, W. & Berkley, M. (1984). *Children and arson: America's middle class nightmare.* New York: Plenum.

Post-traumatic Stress Disorder: An Overview of Theory, Treatment, and Forensic Practice Considerations

Edwin F. Renaud

Post-traumatic stress disorder is an area of significant concern for practitioners in the forensic setting. Forensic nurses may come into contact with traumatized individuals such as rape victims, abused children, and victims of domestic violence. They may also come into contact with offenders who have backgrounds characterized by exposure to violence, neglect, and other severe stressors, the effects of which may go unrecognized due to the patients' criminal behavior. Understanding the nature and origins of PTSD permits the forensic nurse to provide the best care possible to this challenging population.

CHAPTER FOCUS

Defining trauma and PTSD
Risk and resiliency to PTSD
The effects of single incident trauma versus chronic trauma
Treatment and intervention with traumatized patients

KEY TERMS

avoidance symptoms
cognitive behavioral therapy
complex PTSD

cortisol
hyperarousal symptoms
post-traumatic stress disorder
protective factor
re-experiencing symptoms
risk factor
stress response system
trauma

INTRODUCTION

The last 30 years have seen considerable gains in the basic science, theory, and treatment of post-traumatic stress disorder (PTSD). As our understanding of PTSD has improved, mental health providers have begun to consider the impact of traumatic experience on different clinical populations. The forensic population has been no exception.

The organized study of PTSD owes much of its impetus to research on combat veterans. Psychiatric casualties have become an increasingly well-documented aspect of warfare over the last 200 years, with modern accounts dating back to the American Civil War (Dean, 1999). Many people are familiar with the term *shell shock*, which was used to describe the psychological effects of combat during World War I. The underlying belief behind the term *shell shock* was that the concussive force of exploding artillery rounds produced intracranial injury, which resulted in changes in mood and behavior. During and after World War II, psychiatric casualties commanded greater attention as thousands of returning servicemen were diagnosed with psychological conditions related to combat.

The 1980s saw renewed interest in the study of the psychological effects of combat stimulated, in large part by demands from Vietnam veterans who felt that existing mental health services did not adequately understand or address their needs. The study of trauma became a priority for the Department of Veterans Affairs and other federal agencies. The study of psychological and behavioral effects of trauma became a priority for the Department of Veterans Affairs, amongst other federal agencies. The next 20 years yielded a considerably better understanding of the definition, theory, and treatment of PTSD. However, as interest in the study of combat-related trauma grew, it also became clear that combat veterans were not the only population that suffered from trauma-related psychopathology.

As the study of trauma attracted wider attention within the clinical and academic communities, researchers began to look at the experiences of abuse and neglect survivors, victims of crime, and people who had experienced accidents. This led to a greater recognition that psychological trauma was not restricted to combat veterans, and was not limited to single episode or short-term stressors. Indeed, some of the most important contributions to our understanding of PTSD come from the study of adaptation to chronic stress.

More recently, researchers have focused on the stress-related morbidity of police, fire fighters, rescue personnel, and recovery workers assigned to deal with the aftermath of natural disasters or terrorist attacks. One area of special interest could be described as "preventative" trauma research, concerning efforts to predict who may be more vulnerable to suffering traumatic reactions to stress (Roy-Byrne, Russo, Michelson, Zatzick, Pitman, & Berliner, 2004), providing treatment to those who have just undergone stressful events (van Emmerick, Kamphuis, Hulsbocsch, & Emmelkamp, 2002), and understanding more about those individuals who seem resistant to high amounts of stress (Morgan et al., 2002). As the threat of terrorism becomes part of our ongoing collective experience, interest in this branch of the trauma literature is likely to grow.

DEFINING TRAUMA

Practitioners tend to use the terms *trauma* and *PTSD* interchangeably. However, a trauma is an experience, and not necessarily the same experience for different people; post-traumatic stress disorder is a diagnosis. There is considerable variability among individuals in their vulnerability to being traumatized, and further difference among traumatized people as to the specific profile of their symptoms. However, there are broad commonalities to the types of symptoms seen in patients with PTSD. These symptoms fall into three clusters.

The first cluster of symptoms is referred to as *re-experiencing symptoms*. This group of symptoms consists of nightmares, flashbacks, and other unwanted intrusions of the traumatic event into mental awareness. These symptoms may range from persistent intrusive thoughts to full-blown hallucinations. Re-experiencing symptoms is not limited to conscious memory: It may involve symbolic reminders or re-enactments of the traumatic event in dreams or behavior patterns.

The second cluster of PTSD symptoms is known as *avoidance symptoms*. These symptoms consist of feelings, thoughts, or actions meant to diminish contact with people, situations, or other cues that might remind the patient of the traumatic event. Avoidance symptoms can range from an aversion to watching war movies to marked social withdrawal. Because traumatic events often involve the actions of other people, feelings of social estrangement and a reduced capacity for emotional expression are included in this symptom cluster. Avoidance may be more difficult to observe or elicit from the patient if they are more passive, and involved in staying out of sight. Avoidance is sometimes regarded by the patient as an adaptation rather than a "symptom" of PTSD.

The most severe manifestations of avoidance symptom are dissociation and derealization. *Derealization* (sometimes referred to as depersonalization) occurs when the patient experiences events they are participating in as if they were watching them, or are otherwise psychologically detached from the events around them. The patient remains aware of him- or herself in the context of the environment, but that awareness has a quality of being an observer rather than a participant. *Dissociation* is a step beyond derealization, in which the patient experiences him- or herself as being completely disconnected from events, often not having any moment-to-moment awareness of the surroundings while in the dissociative state. Dissociation and derealization symptoms tend to occur episodically, usually under conditions of heightened stress, anxiety, or emotional intensity.

The last cluster of PTSD symptoms is *hyperarousal.* Of all the symptoms of PTSD, hyperarousal is often the most obvious and the most likely to attract attention (positive and negative) from family members, co-workers, and the social environment of the patient. These symptoms include difficulty sleeping, increased irritability, and a globally exaggerated autonomic and subjective response to environmental danger signals. Hyperarousal is characterized by hypervigilance (being chronically on alert for potential sources of danger), claustrophobia, and sensitivity to loud noises. Hyperarousal symptoms are a basic alteration in the perceptual experience of patients with PTSD. They often manifest as heightened sensitivity to potential sources of danger, and a bias towards interpreting neutral environmental stimuli as dangerous. This can result in disproportionately aggressive or fearful responses to their environment, a tendency for interpersonal suspicion and mistrust, and substance abuse in an attempt to diminish their heightened states of fear and anger. Hyperarousal symptoms represent an erosion of the mind's capacity to filter out extraneous information, resulting in an overflow of stimuli that can overwhelm the patient. The aggression, substance abuse, and interpersonal chaos noted in the personal lives of PTSD patients often have their roots in the patients' struggle to cope with the hyperarousal symptoms.

The DSM definition of trauma is descriptive. As with psychiatric diagnosis in general, the DSM-IV definition of trauma does not point to a specific disease process or identify a pathway between organ dysfunction and symptoms. This creates a degree of ambiguity about the meaning of trauma. Having an experience that meets the DSM-IV-TR definition of trauma (criterion A) is not a guarantee of being traumatized (see Exhibit 14–2). It is the experience of symptoms after the stressful

PTSD VERSUS ACUTE STRESS DISORDER

Along with PTSD, the DSM also lists the diagnosis of Acute Stress Disorder (ASD), which is used to describe the symptoms of stress reactions that occur within 1 month after a stressor and resolve within 1 month of onset.

Diagnostic Criteria for 308.3 Acute Stress Disorder

A. The person has been exposed to a traumatic event in which both of the following were present:
   1. the person experienced, witnessed or was confronted with an event or events that involved actual or threatened death or serious injury, or a threat to the physical integrity of self or others.
   2. the person's response involved intense fear, helplessness, or horror

B. Either while experiencing or after experiencing the distressing event, the individual has three (or more) of the following dissociative symptoms:
   1. a subjective sense of numbing, detachment, or absence of emotional responsiveness.
   2. a reduction in awareness of his or her surroundings (e.g., "being in a daze")
   3. derealization
   4. depersonalization
   5. dissociative amnesia (i.e., inability to recall an important aspect of the trauma)

C. The traumatic event is persistently reexperienced in at least one of the following ways: recurrent images, thoughts, dreams, illusions, flashback episodes, or a sense of reliving the experience; or distress on exposure to reminders of the traumatic event.

D. Marked avoidance of the stimuli that arouse recollections of the trauma (e.g., thoughts, feelings, conversations, activities, places, people.

E. Marked symptoms of anxiety or increased arousal (e.g., difficulty sleeping, irritability, poor concentration, hypervigilance, exaggerated startle response, motor restlessness).

F. The disturbance causes clinically significant distress or impairment in social, occupational, or other important areas of functioning or impairs the individual's ability to pursue some necessary task, such as obtaining necessary assistance or mobilizing personal resources by telling family members about the traumatic experience.

G. The disturbance lasts for a minimum of 2 days and a maximum of 4 weeks and occurs within 4 weeks of the traumatic event.

H. The disturbance is not due to the direct physiological effects of a substance (e.g., a drug of abuse, a medication) or a general medical condition, is not better accounted for by Brief Psychotic Disorder, and is not merely an exacerbation of a preexisting Axis I or Axis II disorder.

The key difference between PTSD and ASD is the time frame for the onset and resolution of symptoms. The diagnosis of ASD sets a limit of 1 month for the onset of symptoms, whereas the PTSD diagnosis lists no such time frame for symptom onset. Also the PTSD diagnosis states that symptoms must be present for more than 1 month, whereas the ASD diagnosis states that symptoms must resolve within 1 month. The timeline for ASD leaves a 2-month window for the onset and resolution of trauma-related symptoms. After the 2-month window, the appropriate diagnosis is PTSD.

Exhibit 14–1 DSMIV PTSD Diagnostic Criteria (continued on next page)
Source: American Psychiatric Association.

Exhibit 14–1   (continued)

Diagnostic criteria for 309.81 Post-traumatic Stress Disorder

A. The person has been exposed to a traumatic event in which both of the following were present:
   1. the person experienced, witnessed, or was confronted with an event or events that involved actual or threatened death or serious injury, or a threat to the physical integrity of self or others.
   2. the person's response involved intense fear, helplessness, or horror. **Note:** In children, this may be expressed instead by disorganized or agitated behavior.

B. The traumatic event is persistently reexperienced in one (or more) of the following ways:
   1. recurrent and intrusive distressing recollections of the event, including images, thoughts, or perceptions. **Note:** In young children, repetitive play may occur in which themes or aspects of the trauma are expressed.
   2. recurrent distressing dreams of the event. **Note:** In children, there may be frightening dreams without recognizable content.
   3. acting or feeling as if the traumatic event were recurring (includes a sense of reliving the experience, illusions, hallucinations, and dissociative flashback episodes, including those that occur on awakening or when intoxicated). **Note:** In young children, trauma-specific reenactment may occur.
   4. intense psychological distress at exposure to internal or external cues that symbolize or resemble an aspect of the traumatic event
   5. physiological reactivity on exposure to internal or external cues that symbolize or resemble an aspect of the traumatic event

C. Persistent avoidance of stimuli associated with the trauma and numbing of general responsiveness (not present before the trauma), as indicated by three (or more) of the following:
   1. efforts to avoid thoughts, feelings, or conversations associated with the trauma
   2. efforts to avoid activities, places, or people that arouse recollections of the trauma
   3. inability to recall an important aspect of the trauma
   4. markedly diminished interest or participation in significant activities
   5. feeling of detachment or estrangement from others
   6. restricted range of affect (e.g., unable to have loving feelings)
   7. sense of a foreshortened future (e.g., does not expect to have a career, marriage, children, or a normal life span)

D. Persistent symptoms of increased arousal (not present before the trauma), as indicated by two (or more) of the following:
   1. difficulty falling or staying asleep
   2. irritability or outbursts of anger
   3. difficulty concentrating
   4. hypervigilance
   5. exaggerated startle response

E. Duration of the disturbance (symptoms in Criteria B, C, and D) is more than 1 month.

F. The disturbance causes clinically significant distress or impairment in social, occupational, or other important areas of functioning.

Specify if:
Acute: if duration of symptoms is less than 3 months
Chronic: if duration of symptoms is 3 months or more
Specify if:
With Delayed Onset: if onset of symptoms is at least 6 months after the stressor

event rather than the experience itself that qualifies one for the diagnosis of PTSD. The next logical question might be, what makes a trauma different from a stressful experience?

When a person undergoes a stressful experience that is so severe that it overwhelms their psychological capacity to cope, the result is trauma. This definition, translated through different theoretical languages, is seen repeatedly throughout the trauma literature. All the theoretical models of PTSD discussed in this chapter, whether rooted in a breakdown of psychic structures, cognitive schemas, or functional neurobiology, speak to a breakdown of the mind's capacities to organize experience, and the emotions that go with it, under conditions of extreme stress.

PSYCHOLOGICAL THEORIES OF PTSD

Psychoanalytic Theory

Psychoanalysis has wrestled with the question of trauma since its beginnings. In his 1896 paper entitled *The Neuropsychoses of Defense*, Freud described what came to be known as the seduction theory (Gay, 1988), which proposed that the psychological symptoms associated with "hysteria" (the term used to describe many forms of psychological disturbance at the time) were the result of childhood sexual activity—what would be considered sexual abuse by today's standards. He based this theory on the accounts that a number of his patients had given him over the course of their treatment. The chilly reception that seduction theory received from Freud's colleagues led him to reconsider the relationship of objective experience and subjective interpretation. The result was Freud's insight into the unconscious transformation of thoughts and feelings. This laid the groundwork for psychoanalysis as it has come to be known. Although the rejection of seduction theory inspired Freud's most important theoretical work, it also diminished the value of considering real events in favor of their subjective meaning when trying to understand a patient's symptoms.

Freud most clearly articulates his theory of psychological trauma in his essay *Beyond the Pleasure Principle* (1920). Freud begins by stating that the mind is organized in such a way that it limits the amount of information it takes in from the outside world as a means of protecting itself from the onslaught of overwhelming amounts of stimulation. Freud observes that our senses—hearing, smell, touch, taste, and vision—all detect information within a limited range. (We know, for example, human beings cannot hear sounds at very high or very low frequencies, nor do we see parts of the electromagnetic spectrum beyond the narrow range of "visible light.") Our sense organs give us a limited amount of sensory input compared to the total volume of information available in the environment. This filtering process keeps the information we have within manageable, useful limits.

Freud observes that information coming from within the mind is filtered as well. He states that human behavior is governed by powerful instinctual drives that seek to promote pleasure and diminish pain. These drives create psychological conflict within us because everyday experience is filled with people and things that frustrate the gratification of these drives and impulses. This leads to a clash between our internal drives and the external world. In order to cope with those conflicts, the mind engages in protective maneuvers called defenses. Psychological defenses shape our interpretation of external events in ways that are meant to reduce psychological conflict and subjective distress. The effects of drives and defenses are usually unconscious, which is to say that they take place without our awareness.

The boundary between the mind's sensation of the external world and its sensation of the internal world is called the stimulus barrier. According to Freud, consciousness as we experience it takes place within this stimulus barrier. Our conscious experience of the world consists of both sensations from the environment and the thoughts and feelings produced by the workings of our mind. Conscious experience, according to psychoanalytic theory, is the result of a complex interaction in which external information taken in by the senses is filtered through the stimulus barrier and processed by the workings of psychological defenses and the unconscious mind.

According to psychoanalytic theory, trauma is the result of the stimulus barrier being penetrated and the overwhelming of psychological defenses. When the psychological defenses are overwhelmed, the realities of the external world come into unrestrained conflict with the drives and impulses in the unconscious mind. The mind experiences this as an intrusion, like a splinter beneath the skin. The anxiety produced by the intrusion of external stimuli leads to the renewed engagement of defense mechanisms, which grapple with the intrusive material. It is the unconscious process of attempting to defend against this overpowering information that produces trauma symptoms.

Cognitive Behavioral Theory

Cognitive behavioral theory states that psychopathology is the result of learned errors in thinking, sometimes referred to as cognitive distortions (Beck & Freeman, 1990). These cognitive distortions cause psychopathology by affecting our automatic thoughts about ourselves and the world around us, leading to negative feelings about the self, negative feelings about the present, and the anticipation of negative future experiences. Edna Foa and Barbara Rothbaum (1997), through their work with rape victims, propose a cognitive behavioral model of PTSD and articulate a set of cognitive distortions that contribute to the development of PTSD.

Foa and Rothbaum state that the development of PTSD results from the patient's difficulty processing and integrating the experience of the traumatic event. Normally, when we experience something we are able to process the information and understand it within a framework of expectations and beliefs about ourselves and the world around us. These broad systems of expectations and beliefs are called cognitive schemas. Foa and Rothbaum argue that difficulty processing a traumatic event has to do with the rigidity of one's cognitive schemas. When our assumptions about ourselves and the world around us are powerfully contradicted by the experience of stressful events, our schemas must be revised to accommodate the new information. When our schemas are too rigid, they cannot do this. This results in difficulty processing the experience, which gives rise to specific errors in thinking. This challenge to the rigid structure of the cognitive schema leads to the development of the cognitive distortions that characterize PTSD.

Foa and Rothbaum state that the development of PTSD results from the patient's difficulty processing and integrating the experience of the traumatic event. Normally, when we experience something we are able to process the information and understand it within a framework of expectations and beliefs about ourselves and the world around us. These broad systems of expectations and beliefs are called cognitive schemas. Foa and Rothbaum argue that difficulty processing a traumatic event has to do with the rigidity of one's cognitive schemas. When our assumptions about ourselves and the world around us are powerfully contradicted by the experience of stressful events, our schemas must be revised to accommodate the new information. When our schemas are too rigid, they cannot do this. This results in difficulty processing the experience, which gives rise to specific errors in thinking. It is the challenge to the rigid structure of the cognitive schema that leads to the development of the cognitive distortions which characterize PTSD.

Foa and Rothbaum (1997) propose three primary cognitive distortions associated with PTSD:

1. The trauma victim is completely incompetent.
2. The world is completely dangerous.
3. The trauma victim is to blame for the traumatic event.

The distortion of one's complete incompetence is the belief that one somehow deserved the traumatic event and that the person is damaged beyond repair by the event. The cognitive distortion that the self is incompetent is connected to a similar but distinct distortion of blaming oneself for the traumatic event. Self-blame refers to the idea that the trauma victim feels personally responsible, either by act or omission, for the traumatizing event.

The other cognitive distortion associated with PTSD is that the world is completely dangerous. The individual with PTSD experiences the world as pervasively threatening. He or she is not simply alert for the presence of potential danger, but lives in a state of expectation that danger is everywhere and that he or she must be on guard for it. This could be seen as either resulting from a reinforcement of a pre-existing negative bias or a challenge to previously held positive beliefs about the safety of the world. According to cognitive behavioral theory, these cognitive distortions lead patients to experience themselves as bad, expect the worst from the external environment, and anticipate the worst about the future. This results in the emotional symptoms of anxiety, sadness, isolation, and anger seen in PTSD.

BIOLOGICAL MODELS OF PTSD

Cortisol and the Stress Response System

Research on the biology of PTSD has focused on the interplay of stress response hormones and the biology of the hypothalamic-pituitary-adrenal (HPA) system of the brain. One hormone that has been the topic of considerable interest to trauma researchers is cortisol, a hormone released under conditions of psychological stress, in tandem with other stress response hormones, as part of the body's normal stress response system. The role of cortisol is to rein in the body's stress reaction by suppressing the effects of other hormones (adrenaline and others) involved with propagating and sustaining the body's response to stress. If hormones are like adrenaline, pushing the body's stress response forward, cortisol can be thought of as pulling it back. This push-and-pull serves a protective role against prolonged circulation of stress response hormones in the body, because the chronic circulation of these hormones is damaging to various organs (Sapolsky, 1992). This simultaneous release of cortisol and other stress hormones is thought to be the body's way of containing the stress reaction and returning the body to a normal state as quickly as possible. There is an association between the quantity of cortisol released and the subjective severity of a stressor (Selye, 1956). This association is so well established that certain animal researchers make the deductive leap of asserting the subjective severity of an experimental stressor by the amount of cortisol measured in a subject animal (Yehuda, 1998).

On the basis of animal studies, it was originally thought that people with PTSD would show higher cortisol levels, representing a state of chronic stress; however, the available evidence suggests that people with PTSD release lower levels of cortisol under conditions of stress (Yehuda, Southwick, Mason, & Geller, 1990). The leading hypothesis about the biology of PTSD is that the body's capacity to rein in the stress response system is significantly reduced, resulting in a more easily activated and powerfully expressed stress response (van der Kolk, 1996a), which the body has difficulty returning to a baseline state.

Differences in the Brain Associated with PTSD

Researchers have identified areas of the brain that may be associated with PTSD. One observed difference in the brains of people suffering from PTSD is that Broca's area, which is the part of the brain responsible for translating experience into communicable language, is largely inactive when traumatic memories are being recalled (Rauch et al., 1996). This finding was made during a study using positron emission tomography (PET) scans, a technique for measuring relative activity in different areas of the brain. In this study, patients with PTSD first gave, and were then read, narratives of their traumatic experience. These subjects were then PET-scanned to see which parts of their brains were active when the trauma scripts were read back to them. Some of the areas that showed heightened activity were in the right hemisphere, specifically the amygdala (responsible for the conditioning of fear responses and the affective evaluation of experience), the anterior temporal cortex, and the posterior orbito-frontal cortex. What this study suggests is that, for people with PTSD, there is a reduction of the brain's capacity to translate traumatic memory into language in the context of traumatic reminders. Because language is an important means of organizing experience, deficits in this capacity have major implications for our understanding of traumatic memory.

Another observed difference in the brains of patients with PTSD is volume shrinkage in the hippocampus, which is a structure within the limbic system of the brain that is associated with the categorization of experience and the indexing of memory (Bremner et al., 1995; Stein, Hannah, Koverola, Yehuda, Torchilla, & McClarty, 1994). A number of studies have found that people suffering from PTSD have a lower hippocampal volume than people without PTSD. A twin study conducted by Gilbertson and colleagues (2002) found that small hippocampal volume was associated with greater PTSD symptoms after a stressor. However, in a longitudinal study of trauma survivors, Bonne, Brandes, Gilboa, and their colleagues (2001) found that there was no observed difference in hippocampal volume at 1 week and 6 months after a severe traumatic event. This raises the question of whether reduced hippocampal volume is a risk factor or a result of effects of PTSD over time (Nut & Malizia, 2004).

Memory Formation and Trauma

The role of memory in PTSD has been an area of special interest for trauma researchers, because PTSD can be thought of as a disorder of remembered experience. Reexperiencing, avoidance, and hyperarousal symptoms are all contingent upon the retention of information associated with the traumatic event. Bessle van der Kolk has studied changes in memory storage and retrieval in persons suffering with PTSD. His model of traumatic memory is a useful framework for understanding the effect of stressful experience on memory, and points to a biological model of psychological trauma surprisingly similar to those put forth in the psychological literature.

In normal memory coding, information from the senses is routed to the thalamus, where the information is partially integrated. Sensory information is then passed on to the amygdala, where it is assigned emotional significance, and to the prefrontal cortex. From the amygdala information is passed on to the brain stem, which controls arousal and the autonomic response to the information. The amygdala also passes information to the hippocampus, which plays a significant role in memory formation. See Figure 14–1 for a schematic of this process.

According to van der Kolk (1995), stress has a moderating effect on the strength and integration of the coding of memory. Moderate to high levels of stress are thought to promote memory formation, making memories associated with stressful events more easily remembered. This is a survival enhancing adaptation, which improves personal survival by encouraging the memory of things and events that are dangerous. Anatomically, this function is associated with the hippocampus and the amygdala, which are component structures of the limbic system of the brain. The amygdala is the structure within the limbic system that assigns emotional significance and priority to incoming sensory information from the thalamus, essentially mediating psychological arousal. Once sensory information has been given priority and emotional significance by the amygdala, it moves to the hippocampus. The hippocampus has been linked to memory formation in the brain, and is believed to be responsible for encoding the various sensory components of memory (van der Kolk, 1996a). Extreme stress has been found to disrupt hippocampal functioning, fragmenting the encoding of memory in a way that renders it less integrated, creating distorted patterns of recollection. These patterns can range in sensory modality (sight, smell, image, emotion) on a continuum of consciousness and recollection (van der Kolk, 1996b; van der Kolk & Fischer, 1995). (See Figure 14–2 for a visual representation of this system.) If the psychological definition of trauma is the overwhelming of psychological

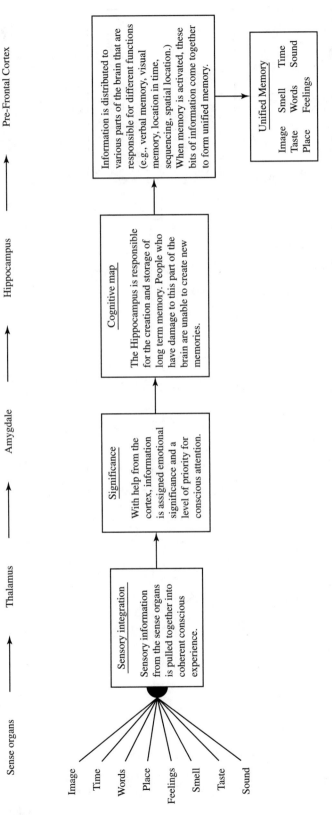

Figure 14–1 Simplified theoretical model for the normal biological organization of conscious memory and experience. *Source:* Adapted from van der Kolk (1996b).

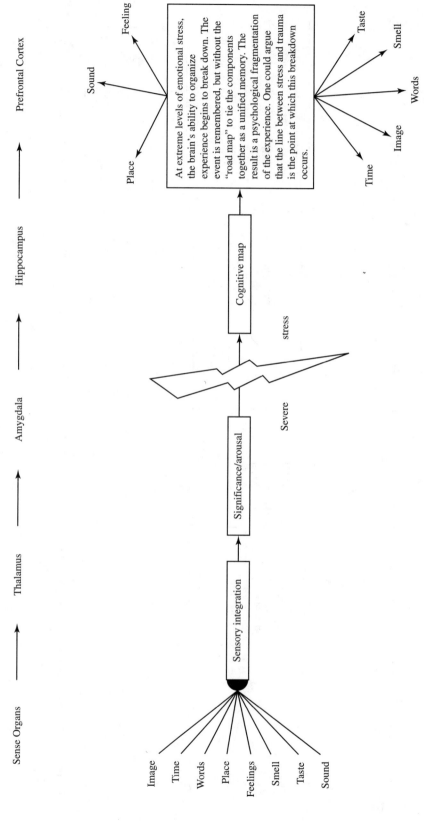

Figure 14–2 Simplified theoretical model for the disruption of organization of conscious memory and experience. *Source:* Adapted from van der Kolk (1996b).

defenses, then the biological equivalent of this seems to be the fragmentation of remembered experience in the context of stimulus overload.

In his studies van der Kolk observes how fragmented memory may be less available to parts of the brain that mediate verbal memory and reasoning, giving rise to feelings that are experienced intensely, but in nonverbal ways. This deprives the traumatized person of one of the primary tools for organizing and relating experience to others. Verbal reasoning and moderation is only one mechanism for the mediation of emotional states, however. If experience is fragmented in memory encoding, this also calls into question how accessible these experiences may be to the executive functions of the cortex, which exert both verbal and nonverbal modulating influence on affect and behavior. The fragmentation of experience has implications for the development of the capacity for regulating emotional states. If traumas are remembered in a way that makes them less connected to the functions of the brain that moderate intense emotional states, the result is diminished capacity to regulate the emotional states associated with the trauma. Those experiences that require the greatest regulatory powers are encoded in a way that works against those regulatory powers being engaged.

Coping strength is an individual trait that is subject to a considerable number of environmental and endogenous factors. What is traumatic for one person may not be traumatic for another. Individual coping may also vary depending on the type of stressor encountered. An individual may be more resilient to the stress associated with an automobile accident than an assault, for example. Although there is a great deal of individual difference in what may be traumatizing, certain risk factors have been shown to make one more vulnerable, or resistant, to the development of PTSD.

VULNERABILITY AND RESILIENCE TO PTSD

One of the most puzzling questions about PTSD is why some people go on to develop the disorder after a stressful event and others do not. The National Comorbidity Survey, a study of the incidence of mental illness in the U.S. population, found that more than 50% of women and 60% of men in the general population experience a stressful event that meets the DSM definition of trauma at some point in their lives (Kessler, Sonnega, Bromet, Hughes, & Nelson, 1995). Yet the lifetime prevalence of PTSD in the general population is roughly 8%. Using the most conservative estimates, this data indicates that less than 20% of people who experience a stressor great enough to meet the definition of trauma go on to have symptoms of PTSD. What makes some people more vulnerable to becoming traumatized than others? What allows most people to survive stressful events without being traumatized?

The term *risk factor* is often used to describe pre-existing characteristics that make a person more vulnerable to developing a particular disorder. The term *protective factor* refers to qualities that pre-date the onset of a disorder and diminish the likelihood of developing pathology. Because of the highly individual nature of vulnerability to being traumatized, researchers have shown interest in the risk and protective factors associated with the development of PTSD. One of the findings of this research is that risk factors and protective factors appear to be at work both before and after the traumatizing stressor.

There have been two major efforts to systematically review the findings of the trauma literature and identify the most common risk factors and protective factors for PTSD. Brewin, Andrews, and Valentine (2000) conducted a meta-analysis (an analysis of multiple research reports to look for commonalities in the literature) of 77 studies on the risk factors and protective factors for the development of PTSD. They found that the most powerful risk factors for developing PTSD that were present before the traumatic event were childhood abuse, a personal history of psychiatric illness, and a family history of psychiatric illness. The risk factors that most strongly predicted the development of PTSD after a traumatic event were a lack of social support, the severity of the trauma itself, and the occurrence of subsequent stressful events. Another meta-analysis of 68 studies conducted by Ozer, Best, Lipsey, and Weiss (2003) found generally similar results; specifically, they found that prior trauma history, prior psychological adjustment, and family psychiatric history were important pre-trauma risk factors for developing PTSD. Consistent with earlier findings, perceived threat of death during the traumatic event (an aspect of trauma severity) and post-trauma social support played an important role in the risk for developing PTSD after the trauma. Ozer and her colleagues also found that the experience of dissociative symptoms and the intensity of emotions experienced by the victim in the immediate wake of the trauma were also predictive of later development of PTSD.

The Subjective versus the Objective Meaning of a Stressor

Freud made the point that the subjective interpretation of an external event—its individual psychological meaning to the patient—should be of greater concern to the clinician than the objective truth of what actually happened, which is essentially unknowable. Whatever may have actually happened to the patient, they reacted to it in a way that causes them pain and it is the pain they experience that brings them to the clinician's door. Because the reaction to an event is what causes symptoms, it is the person's basis for reaction (its subjective meaning) that is of greatest concern. This view has been criticized for failing to acknowledge that some events may be so stressful that they are traumatizing by their very nature. This criticism fails to take into account the variety and strength of the human capacity for adaptation. The epidemiological evidence of the National Comorbidity Survey (Kessler et al., 1995) makes it clear that the interplay among stress, coping, and trauma is complex and individual. There is no evidence that *any* single stressful event, no matter how severe it may seem, invariably makes a person doomed to develop PTSD. Although risk may increase, it is important to remember that risk is not destiny.

Yet among those patients who go on to develop PTSD, certain events appear to be more common, and some stressful events appear to be more traumatizing than others. The National Comorbidity Survey found that being raped was more likely to lead to developing PTSD than any other stressor, for both sexes (Kessler et al., 1995). Other traumas that were found to be more likely to produce PTSD were combat exposure, physical abuse, and being threatened with a weapon. Although it is crucial to recognize the individual nature of coping, we should not ignore the evidence that certain experiences are characteristically more difficult to cope with and are more likely to result in developing PTSD. Another factor that plays a significant role in the development of PTSD is the cumulative effect of stressors over time. Later stressors are themselves a risk factor for developing PTSD after an initial trauma. This suggests that the effects of stress can be cumulative over time. Several studies have shown that there is a dose-effect relationship between stress and the likelihood of developing PTSD. This effect has been demonstrated with torture victims (Mollica, 1998), combat veterans (Zaidi & Foy, 1994), and victims of child abuse (Edwards, Holden, Felitti, & Anda, 2003).

Certain individual qualities have been found to have a positive influence on the effects of severe stress. Active coping, sociability, and internal locus of control have been associated with better outcomes for those exposed to trauma. A study of 10 Vietnam veterans who had survived heavy combat without developing PTSD (Hendin & Haas, 1984) revealed that they shared the ability to communicate with others, an ability to solicit and use social support, and an active, internalized sense of responsibility for their own destiny. This suggests that these characteristics contribute to resiliency from trauma.

Discussing what constitutes a risk factor versus a protective factor for PTSD forces us to take a look at the nature of trauma and hold competing, seemingly contradictory ideas in mind. On the one hand experiences like rape seem more likely to produce PTSD, and certain aspects of personal history seem to make a person more vulnerable. On the other hand, there is no evidence that any single stressful event will automatically result in the development of PTSD, and there appear to be aspects of social support and later stress over time that affect the risk for developing PTSD. No formula, algorithm, or recipe exists to determine who will go on to develop PTSD. What the literature on risk and protective factors tells us is that adaptation to trauma is complex, ongoing, and individual. Although it is important to understand that the development of PTSD is not random and that certain conditions make its occurrence more likely, having a risk factor does not mean one will develop the disorder. Many patients with one or more risk factors for PTSD (or any other illness for that matter) do not go on to develop the disorder. Understanding risk factors helps identify vulnerable populations and target interventions to those patients who are most likely to require them. By identifying risk factors and protective factors we can better target interventions to those populations at greater risk for developing PTSD and identify aspects of functioning that promote greater adaptation to trauma over time.

The Perpetration of Violence as a Risk Factor for PTSD

Most of the risk factors discussed thus far have had to do with being victimized or otherwise impacted by external sources of stress. One of the complexities of working with a forensic population is that one is confronted with patients who may have been both victims and victimizers. The literature on the psychological effects of committing violence is small in comparison to that on being the victim of violence. Committing acts of violence has been shown to have a negative impact on later psychological functioning and increases vulnerability to the development of PTSD. Much of the research on the commission of violence has been conducted on combat veterans who committed atrocities, and has focused on subsequent violent behavior (Beckham, Feldman, Kirby, Hertzberg, & Moore, 1998). The bulk of the evidence suggests that the commission of atrocities is predictive of increased violent behavior later on. Other studies on the effects of committing acts of violence (Yehuda, Southwick, & Giller, 1992) have been concerned with the effect of committing atrocities on later PTSD symptoms. Their findings suggest that the committing of atrocities worsens PTSD symptoms.

There is also a small but notable body of literature about the posttraumatic effects of violence committed by civilians. MacNair (2002)

Table 14–1 Risks and Protective Factors for PTSD

Pre-trauma Risk Factors	Post-trauma Risk Factors
Physical abuse	Trauma severity/perceived life threat
Sexual abuse	Poor social supports/social isolation
Personal psychiatric history	Subsequent traumatic events
Family psychiatric history	Severity of acute stress symptoms
Prior trauma history	Dissociative symptoms
Pre-trauma Protective Factors	**Post-trauma Protective Factors**
Secure attachment	Positive social support
Positive social supports	Effective use of anger
	Active problem solving
	Internal locus of control

presents evidence that both police officers who are involved in the fatal shootings of suspects and criminals who commit violent crimes are at greater risk for developing PTSD. Using a relatively large sample of convicted felons (1,140), Collins and Bailey (1990) found that as many as 15% of felons who were impulsively violent without any secondary goal ("expressive violence" in Collins and Bailey's terms) experienced PTSD symptoms after their crime. Other researchers have found that murderers whose violence was more reactive in nature were more likely to be traumatized by the act itself (Pollock, 1999). This body of evidence suggests that violence committed based on fear or in a reactive emotional way poses a greater risk for the later development of PTSD. Table 14–1 lists the risk and protective factors for developing PTSD.

PTSD FROM SINGLE INCIDENTS VERSUS CHRONIC STRESS

Because PTSD is the consequence of experience, we are used to thinking about trauma as a discrete event, which is somewhat misleading. From our discussion of the various risks and protective factors for the development of PSTD, we know that traumatic events come in many varieties. Some traumatic events are truly singular occurrences like a plane crash or a terrorist attack—events that the victim will most likely not experience twice. Yet these single events can have enduring impact on health and functioning. On the other hand, some traumas stem from circumstances that are hardly events at all, but are chronic conditions or characteristics of their surrounding environment. Examples would include children growing up in conditions of violent political unrest, victims of chronic sexual abuse, or abused spouses. These patients have traumatic experiences that are qualitatively different from those traumas caused by a single event. There is good evidence to suggest that the mental health effects of these two types of trauma have important differences. Studies by Lenore Terr and Judy Herman exemplify these differences.

Lenore Terr: The Long-Term Consequences of Single-Episode Trauma

In 1976, a group of 26 children on a school bus in Chowchilla, California, were kidnapped and placed in a freight trailer that was buried in the California desert. They remained in the trailer for approximately 36 hours before venturing out and finding that they had been abandoned. The kidnappers were never found and no motive for the kidnapping has ever been determined. The abducted children ranged from 6–12 years of age. Lenore Terr followed the victims of this group abduction and reported her findings in the book *Too Scared to Cry* (1990). Terr's follow-up studies give us an opportunity to understand the effects of short-term trauma on long-term psychological functioning.

In the course of her follow-up studies with the children from the Chowchilla abduction, Terr made several observations. First, there were subtle and progressive alterations of the memories of the traumatic event over time. In some cases this was the effect of misleading consensus—small distortions that through repetitions and discussion with other participants took on the legitimacy of fact. Other instances involved specific memories of the kidnapping that were either distorted or elaborated upon to the point of being factually inconsistent with known aspects of the kidnapping. Terr observed that many of the children had some degree of change in their capacity to regulate fear, anger, and interpersonal connection. Various children were observed to have grown either more irritable, hypervigilant, emotionally detached, or some combination thereof.

Finally, Terr found that the themes of the kidnapping had ways of expressing themselves throughout the child's repertoire of conscious and unconscious behaviors. Many of the children had recurrent dreams and nightmares about the kidnapping. Other children re-enacted various aspects of the kidnapping, either overtly or symbolically in their play. The children who were youngest at the time of the kidnapping seemed to engage in the most nonverbal and symbolically transformed behavior over time, as if they could only work through these issues using the capacities developmentally available to them at the time of the trauma. From a single identified stressor, the kidnapping, these children exhibited variable and enduring changes in psychological functioning.

Judith Herman: Complex PTSD

Judith Herman's (1992) work explores the process of adaptation and coping that takes place with the experience of chronic or repeated conditions of traumatic stress. Chronic situations that produce trauma, Herman observes, tend to be characterized by interpersonal relationships that both bind the victim into specific social roles and isolate them at the same time. Women are particularly vulnerable to being placed in these situations due to the emphasis on social compliance in the rearing of young girls in many cultures. However, these same social conditions could be true for physically abused children, victims of partner violence, or combat infantrymen. More broadly, these social conditions can be seen in the experience of people who are victims of discrimination, who are economically disadvantaged, or who otherwise experience themselves as being socially disenfranchised. In all cases the emphasis of social interactions is skewed toward the needs (sexual, aggressive, economic, survival) of one participant in vast disproportion to the other.

The DSM description of PTSD was strongly influenced by the symptom profile of combat veterans, and is less descriptive of patients whose trauma was of longer duration or rooted in psychosocial developmental stressors. Victims of chronic abuse, neglect, or malignant power inequities develop symptoms that are similar to those described in the DSM-IV, but when these symptoms are provoked in early states of development or over long periods of time, their manifestations are different. Although all patients who suffer from PTSD make attempts at adaptation, what distinguishes the presentation of patients who have suffered under chronic trauma conditions is that these symptoms tend to become incorporated into aspects of personality and patterns of interpersonal relatedness. This has a pernicious effect on interpersonal functioning, particularly mate selection and the capacity to relate to others.

Herman proposes a syndrome called "complex PTSD," which describes the more global effects of chronic stress—effects that fall outside the symptom clusters of PTSD as delineated in the DSM manuals, which tend to best describe single episode trauma reactions. Herman states that the trauma at the root of complex PTSD is not a single event, but a sustained period of being controlled by others in a dictatorial or totalitarian way. This could include being in a relationship characterized by domestic violence, being subject to a cult, or other coercive environments.

Herman describes complex PTSD as a pattern of alterations to several areas of psychosocial functioning:

- *Emotional regulation:* Emotional regulation is the capacity to reign in one's own automatic emotional responses and to comfortably experience a range of emotions between extremes of good and bad. Patients with complex PTSD have difficulty feeling a moderate or slight form of an emotion. This can lead to intense feelings of sadness, rage, or fear that are vastly out of proportion to the events surrounding them.

- *Consciousness:* As already noted, stress responses can produce changes in consciousness, including dissociation, intrusive thoughts, and difficulty with memory. Patients with complex PTSD may present experiencing these changes in consciousness on a persisting aspect of their daily lives. This may include re-experiencing phenomena as described in the PTSD diagnosis, or repeated dissociation or depersonalization experiences.

- *Self-Perception:* Patients with complex PTSD can present with feelings of being inadequate, shamed, or stigmatized. These feelings of being damaged are often accompanied by feelings of being alone or being incapable of being understood.

- *Perception of the perpetrator:* Because the conditions that produce complex PTSD often involve intense interpersonal relations between the abuser and the victim, usually of a coercive sort, patients who develop complex PTSD can have an assortment of ideas about their abusers. Some patients may attribute special powers to their abusers or experience their relationship with them as special in a positive way. They may be preoccupied with the abuser in various ways. The overarching principle is that the patient's concept of the perpetrator takes on meaning beyond a mere object of fear or anger.

- *Relations with others:* Patients with complex PSTD often come from backgrounds where interpersonal relationships were exploitive. With that background, intimacy, trust, and the safety of others is thrown into doubt. Patients with complex PTSD have learned through hard experience that people can be dangerous. This creates difficulty in forming and sustaining positive social relationships and social support.

- *System of meaning:* Of all the aspects of complex PTSD, the patient's system of meaning has the greatest implications for long-term growth and change for the patient. The patient's system of meaning refers to the patient's overarching set of beliefs about the present, his or her self, and the future that serves to promote or diminish hope. This includes religion or other spiritual beliefs. It also encompasses the patient's set of expectations about themselves and the future. An urban youth whose only example of power, economic security, and success is drug dealers may see no benefit to other pathways to goals, such as education or conventional employment. A battered woman who only sees worsening anger and threat by her abuser may see no benefit in trying to leave him.

The symptoms of complex PTSD are not very different from the DSM definition. The changes of affect regulation, relations with others, and consciousness are similar to avoidance symptoms. What makes these symptoms different from the PTSD definition given by the DSM is that it encompasses the developmental and interpersonal consequences of living under conditions of chronic and repeated trauma, in which PTSD symptoms become part of personality functioning. What this illustrates most clearly is that chronic stress, especially in children and adolescents, has developmental consequences that are distinct from short-term or single episode trauma. Observing that many psychiatric patients diagnosed with major personality disorders (borderline personality disorder in particular) often present with histories of major sexual or physical abuse, Herman (1992) suggests that these patients might be more accurately described in a framework that accounts for the long-term effects of trauma as expressed in adult personality functioning. Short-term effect or single episode trauma seem to produce symptoms most consistent with the DSM series definition of PTSD. Long-term trauma seems to produce symptoms that create enduring changes in adaptation and the interpretation of experience, becoming incorporated into more global personality functioning.

PSYCHIATRIC COMORBIDITY AND PTSD

PTSD is often diagnosed in conjunction with other psychiatric conditions, which creates challenges for assessment and treatment. Kulka et al., (1990) reported that among a large sample of combat veterans with PTSD, 98.9% met diagnostic criteria for another psychiatric disorder. Studies with civilian populations have shown similar lifetime proportions of comorbidity, but a slightly different profile of comorbid disorders. The results of the National Comorbidity Survey (Kessler et al., 1995) found that 51.3% of men and 57.6% of women currently diagnosed with PTSD in the general population suffer from some other psychiatric diagnosis. When people who had ever been diagnosed with PTSD in their lifetimes were included in the calculations, those figures rose to 88.3% for men and 79% for women. The diagnoses most commonly associated with PTSD are major depression, anxiety disorders, and substance abuse.

Depression and anxiety are common complaints for patients with PTSD, and may be their initial reason for seeking out mental health treatment instead of the trauma itself. Depression appears to make one more vulnerable to developing PTSD, and PTSD appears to make one more vulnerable to developing depression. One of the confounding issues in the diagnosis of depression and anxiety in conjunction with PTSD is that certain PTSD symptoms resemble both depression and anxiety (Davidson & Foa, 1991). Hyperarousal symptoms and reexperiencing symptoms can easily resemble other anxiety disorders. Avoidance symptoms can resemble depression. The relationship between PTSD and depression is complex (Erickson, Wolfe, King, King, & Sharkansky, 2001). The literature suggests that although depression in patients with PTSD appears to have little difference from depression in clients without PTSD, there is a slightly greater experience of self-blame and lower levels of dependency in the patients with PTSD.

Substance abuse in PTSD can be especially difficult to manage and treat. Patients suffering from PTSD and substance abuse will often describe their use as a means of dampening their PTSD symptoms, and may justify their substance abuse on that basis. CNS depressants such as alcohol, opiates, benzodiazepines, and hallucinogens such as marijuana are fairly common substances of choice for patients with PTSD, as they can reduce the subjective experience of hyperarousal and intrusive symptoms. However, the use of stimulants or more activating drugs like cocaine is not unheard of. Using epidemiological data, McFarlane (1998) offers compelling evidence that the relationship between substance abuse and PTSD is largely unidirectional. The notion of self-medication of psychiatric symptoms is not new in the substance abuse literature, but seems to be particularly valid for PTSD patients.

TREATMENT MODALITIES FOR PTSD

Most studies have found that effective treatment for PTSD consists of combined psychosocially oriented therapy (cognitive behavioral, psychodynamic, or group psychotherapy) and medication treatment. Most of the psychosocial therapies have similar common goals: symptom reduction, the improved psychological organization of the traumatic experience, and reducing the destructive power of memories and feelings associated with the traumatic memory. Their differences lay in how they broadly conceptualize the mechanisms of trauma and by extension the steps needed to provide relief.

Psychodynamic Therapy

Freud described trauma as the intrusion of unfiltered external stimuli into the unconscious mind, and the struggle of the unconscious mind to master that information. This basic premise—that trauma is the result of the mind's struggle with information that it has difficulty managing—was prescient of the findings later made about the nature of traumatic memories, and can be heard echoing in later psychosocial theories of trauma. Contemporary psychodynamic therapy for PTSD also proceeds from this basic concept.

The goal of psychodynamic therapy for PTSD is to promote a greater conscious awareness of the connection between traumatic memories, feelings, and behaviors. Psychodynamic treatment emphasizes understanding the personal meaning of the traumatic event to the patient. Psychodynamic theory, articulated from Freud in the 1920s to Herman's contemporary writings, maintains that the personal meaning of a traumatic event has profound implications for the patient's response. Trauma can reshape our understanding of the world and our place in it, often in the direction of hopelessness, rage, and despair. By exploring the issues of personal meaning in relationship to the trauma, the patient and the therapist work to understand the changes in the patient's framework of meaning brought about by the trauma. It then becomes possible to work with the patient to modify that framework of meaning.

Cognitive Behavior Therapy for PTSD

No form of psychosocial treatment for PTSD enjoys more empirical support than cognitive behavior therapy (CBT). Cognitive behavior therapies have been found to be effective (Marks, Lovell, Noshirvani, Livanov, & Thrasher, 1998), with sustained beneficial effects (Bryant et al., 1998). The cognitive behavioral model of psychopathology holds that emotional symptoms are the consequence of systematic distorted beliefs (cognitive distortions) that interfere with the accurate assessment of current experience and the anticipation of future experience. Foa and Rothbaum (1997) articulate a cognitive model of PTSD which states that trauma results from the overpowering of overly rigid cognitive schemas (generalized belief systems about one's self and the environment) and the failure to readjust those schemas in the wake of traumatic experience. The result is a long-term alteration of the processing of emotion and memory related to the trauma. Cognitive behavioral treatment works by helping the patient identify his or her cognitive distortions and the processes by which they are formed and sustained, and adjusting them to less distorted forms. Cognitive behavior therapy incorporates other techniques as well.

One component of cognitive behavior therapy for PTSD is exposure therapy, which consists of introducing (exposing) the patient to aspects of the traumatic situation in small, controlled doses that the patient can manage. By exposing the patient to these reminders in small doses, the fear response brought on by the reminders is smaller and more manageable. This allows the patient to become less sensitive to the trauma reminders over time. The result is a reduction of the fear response brought about by reminders of the traumatic event.

Another component of cognitive behavior therapy is stress reduction and anxiety management training. This consists of deep breathing exercises, relaxation training, and cognitive restructuring. Deep breathing exercises and relaxation training help patients exert more active control over their anxiety, either through reminders of the trauma or other arousing stimuli. Cognitive restructuring is the process of identifying and correcting cognitive distortions associated with the trauma.

A cognitive therapy for PTSD that has attracted considerable attention in recent years is Eye Movement Desensitization and Reprocessing (EMDR). EMDR treatment consists of guided visual imaging of the traumatic event accompanied by rapid back and forth eye movements. The theory behind EMDR is that the eye movements accompanying the guided imagery facilitate changes in the way the traumatic memory is processed and stored, reducing the level of anxiety and arousal associated with the memories. This technique has been the subject of considerable research interest, with findings showing therapeutic benefit roughly equivalent to other forms of exposure therapy, although some question remains as to the benefit of eye movements (Davidson & Parker, 2001).

Group Therapy

Group therapy can be especially helpful to patients who experience feelings of isolation and social estrangement. Group therapy takes many forms, from structured cognitive behavioral groups to open forum general support groups. Group therapies share in common the presence of a group leader (and a co-leader sometimes) who serves a number of functions depending on the situation. Group leaders help structure the group by establishing its purpose and goals, facilitate interaction between the members, pose questions for the group, provide education, give information, and help the group manage moments of tension. Regardless of the specific group structure or orientation, there are certain common benefits to a group modality.

One of the benefits of group therapy is that it allows the group members to provide mutual support with others who share and understand the patient's issues. Because of the isolating nature of trauma, many patients with PTSD feel that no one understands their experience. Group therapy can reduce the sense of being alone or that "no one understands" by having the patient engage with others who are struggling with similar issues.

Another advantage to group therapy is that it is less interpersonally intense than individual therapy. Some patients, particularly in the early stages of treatment, may have difficulty tolerating the personal focus and interpersonal intensity that come with individual psychotherapy.

Because the group members share time and experience, it may allow for tolerable doses of engagement and participation.

Another benefit to group therapy is that it promotes problem solving. As patients discuss one another's experiences, they benefit from knowledge of other group participants, either in what other group members have found helpful or what they have found to be not helpful. This allows the patients to benefit from others' attempts at problem solving.

Also, institutional settings like prisons can lend themselves to group-oriented treatment, given the generally static population and the generally high patient-to-clinician ratio.

Although group composition can vary, it is generally desirable to have groups composed of roughly similar types of trauma when possible. This helps support group cohesion and mutual support. (Rape victims may have difficulty being supportive of a combat veteran struggling with committing acts of aggression, for example.)

Pharmacotherapy

The use of medication has been found to be helpful in the treatment of PTSD. The only medication currently approved by the FDA specifically for the treatment of PTSD is sertraline (Zoloft). Because of the relatively broad symptom profile (depression, emotional numbing, withdrawal, anxiety, agitation) seen in patients with PTSD, medications are often prescribed empirically to treat specific target symptoms. Although guidelines are available (Alarcon, Glover, Boyer, & Baleen, 2000; Francis, 2003), most practice seen in the community tends to be driven by symptom considerations. (An excellent overview of the pharmacological treatment of PTSD can be found in Friedman [2001].) Certain drug classes are more commonly used for the treatment of PTSD. Briefly reviewed, they are:

- *Antidepressants:* The serotonin selective reuptake inhibitors (SSRIs) (sertraline [Zoloft], paraxatine [Paxil], fluoxetine [Prozac], fluvoxamine [Luvox], and citalopram [Celexia]) in general are considered the first-line medications for the treatment of PTSD. These medications have been found to be effective in treating the depressive and anxiety symptoms found in patients with PTSD. Other medications whose mechanism of action involves the serotonin system, including nefazadone (Serzone), trazodone (Desyrel), and venlafaxine (Effexor), have also been found to be effective in treating PTSD. Older antidepressants, including tricyclics and MAO inhibitors, are less often employed but have documented use.

- *Antiadrenergics:* Part of the body's initial stress response involves the release of hormones that prepare it for physical challenge. As discussed, part of the long-term disruption of the stress response system in patients with PTSD involves the ready activation of the stress response system, with a diminished threshold for its activation and impaired capacity to rein in the magnitude of its response. Based on that reasoning, a small but promising number of studies have been conducted on drugs that act against adrenaline and similar hormones (Friedman, 2001). These medications have been found to be particularly helpful in reducing symptoms of hyperarousal and hypervigilance.
- *Benzodiazapines:* Benzodiazipines are sometimes used for their anxiolytic properties to treat the anxiety symptoms described by patients with PTSD. Although these medications may provide effective short-term relief, their long-term use has not been well supported by controlled studies. Some studies (Risse, Whitters, Burke, Chen, Scurfield, & Raskind, 1990) have even shown rebound effects after the discontinuation of certain agents.
- *Anticonvulsants:* Anticonvulsants such as Divalproex/Depakote and Carbamazapine/Tegretol are used for their mood-stabilizing properties with patients with PTSD. These are often prescribed to treat symptoms of irritability, mood swings, and agitation. Because these symptoms are the most likely to get the patient into trouble with family, coworkers, and the law, their benefits can be considerable.
- *Antipsychotics:* Antipsychotic medications are sometimes used to help with irritability, impulsivity, and agitation in patients with PTSD, and can be very effective in managing these symptoms. Older antipsychotic (haloperidol [Haldol] and thioridazine [Mellaril]) come with the risk of tardive dyskenesia (TD). Newer antipsychotics such as Risperidone (Risperdal) or Olanzapine (Zyprexa) carry lower risks for TD, but can have other risks such as diabetes (Sernyak, Leslie, Alarcon, Losonczy, & Rosenheck, 2003) and increased risk for stroke (United Kingdom Medicines and Healthcare Products Regulation Agency, 2004). As with treatment with any medication, good patient education and thoughtful risk/benefit assessment is essential.

THE CARE AND ASSESSMENT OF PATIENTS WITH PTSD IN THE FORENSIC SETTING

Assessment in the forensic setting has different areas of emphasis than those in traditional clinical settings. If the nurse is caring for the victim of a crime, evidence collection and ascertaining details of the crime take on greater importance than they would in a more conventional clinical encounter. If the nurse is caring for an inmate or an alleged perpetrator of a crime, questions of malingering, violence potential, and state of mind may take on greater importance. Caring for patients with PTSD in the forensic setting makes special demands of the nurse—demands that change with the type of patient being cared for. This section will cover assessment considerations that are specific to certain types of patients that the forensic nurse is likely to encounter.

Interviewing Techniques

Some interviewing techniques are useful when working with trauma victims in general.

1. *Approach the topic of the trauma with respect and patience.* Patients will often be reluctant to talk about their traumatic experiences with strangers, even healthcare professionals. Practitioners working with trauma victims should establish a rapport before proceeding into the details of the trauma. This could consist of obtaining more general background history first, or providing other forms of care prior to the interview. It is often helpful to clearly frame questions about the trauma within the helping context (e.g., "I need to ask you some questions about what happened so I can know how to help you"). Do not demand, cajole, or otherwise coerce the victim to talk about the trauma, or to talk about the trauma more than they feel ready to at the time. Forcing emotional displays from the patient or demanding that patients "confront" or "deal with" their trauma in a manner of our choosing rather than theirs has no proven benefit and is poor treatment. This may include accepting the patient's limited ability to remember the details of the trauma or their being unwilling to talk about it. All the following recommendations should be taken with that caveat in mind.

2. *Start with open-ended general questions and follow with more specific and detailed questions.* Begin asking about the traumatic experience using open-ended questions. This allows the patient some obvious control of the interview and is less threatening. It is also more natural to ask about specific details of the trauma against the backdrop of the general information the patient provides. Depending on the rapport and comfort level with the patient, you may choose to ask more detailed questions as the story unfolds or after the patient has completed their account. As the patient gives you their account of the trauma, note areas or details that you wish to know more about and go back to. What questions come to mind? You may find that the patient answers your questions as they continue to describe the

event, but you should keep a mental note of your questions just in case. When the patient has completed their account, you can go back to those areas to fill in the gaps.

3. *Follow the patient's lead whenever possible.* Listen for clues the patient gives you about important aspects of their trauma during the interview. If a particular place, person, time, or situation keeps coming up in the patient's narrative, but is not addressed, ask about it. Observe and note changes in the patient's emotional expression over the course of the account. Conspicuously intense or absent emotion are signals that the material being described is especially troubling to the patient, and may be a sign to slow down or offer additional support. Sometimes the interview will ebb and flow, as the patient will need to move away from the topic of the trauma for a few minutes before returning to it. Patients will sometimes do this as a way of regrouping before moving forward with their account, so this should generally not be discouraged. Because of the emotional intensity of the material, the patient may require time to process a question or think about how to respond. This can lead to moments of silence during the interview. Unless the patient is visibly becoming somnolent or appears to be dissociating, resist the impulse to break the silence or probe further until the patient responds on his or her own.

4. *When possible, help the patient give words to their feelings.* Trauma occurs when coping is overwhelmed. As we have already discussed, one of the changes observed in the brains of patients with PTSD is that the part of the brain responsible for language operates differently in the context of trauma reminders. Words and language are powerful tools for organizing experience. One of the most subjectively disturbing problems trauma victims describe is their difficulty giving words to their emotions and their experience. This can create circumstances where the patient has torturous feelings of fear, sadness, and rage that they cannot give voice to. As the victim describes the aftermath of their trauma, you should also ask about their feelings as well as the facts of the trauma.

Without imposing your words on the victim's experience, it is often helpful to work with the patient to find their own words for the actual events and the feelings associated with the trauma. This helps the patient create an internal account of the trauma and their feelings, which can be communicated to others. This, in turn, helps the victim organize the experience in his or her own mind and "speaks" to the fundamental breakdown that distinguishes stress from trauma. By giving language to the facts and feelings of the trauma, those words can become the currency that the patient exchanges for the help and support of others.

DOCUMENTATION

An essential component of any evaluation is good documentation. The goal of documentation is to clearly communicate to others the findings of the assessment, the interventions performed based on that assessment, and the rationale for those interventions. Nurses working in a forensic setting may be called upon to perform assessments that will become part of legal proceedings or otherwise introduced as evidence. The level of potential scrutiny demands careful attention to detail and an approach to documentation that is mindful of the professional audience who may ultimately read it.

The U.S. Department of Justice, through the National Institute of Justice, has studied medical records used in cases of domestic violence and noted areas that both promote and diminish the usefulness of medical records in legal proceedings. Isaac and Enos (2001) provide several useful recommendations for practitioners performing and documenting assessments of victims of sexual assault or domestic violence:
1. Use a body map to document the location of injuries.
2. Note differences between your observations and the patient's statements; record the reason for the differences.
3. Take photographs of the injuries believed to have been caused by the assault.
4. Write clearly and legibly.
5. Quote the patient directly in the record, using quotation marks.
6. Avoid the use of phrases that introduce doubt about the patient's reliability.
7. Refrain from the use of legal language such as "perpetrator" or "assailant."
8. Document the patient's description of who hurt them by direct quotation; for example, "My husband hit me."
9. Do not state conclusions without supporting evidence.
10. Do not list domestic violence in the diagnosis section. Injuries are diagnosed and treated in medical settings. Domestic violence is an event determined by the court.
11. Document the patient's emotional state during the assessment (sad, angry, quiet) regardless of how it matches what would be "expected" under the circumstances.
12. Note the time of the evaluation and, if possible, the amount of time elapsed between when the injuries occurred and the assessment.

Exhibit 14–2

Specific Patient Populations

Forensic nurses will be called upon to provide care for patients suffering from a wide variety of trauma under equally variable circumstances. To attempt to cover every possible type of trauma is beyond the scope of this chapter. However, the forensic nurse may encounter certain situations more regularly than others. The following sections list certain types of trauma most typically seen in general practice, with facts and practice recommendations specific to them.

Caring for Sexual Assault/Rape Victims

Rape victims may come to the attention of forensic nurses by a number of paths, ranging from acute intervention shortly after the attack to subsequent interventions for counseling or court-related issues. Unfortunately, a comparatively small proportion of rape victims go on to seek medical attention or report their attacks to police. More than 60% of rapes and sexual assaults go unreported to police. Only 59% of rape victims who report their attack receive medical attention. For victims of rape whose assault goes unreported, the likelihood of receiving treatment is worse, only 17% (Rennison, 2002). The likelihood that a rape or sexual assault victim will report their attack appears to have a strong association with the relationship with the victim. Women who are sexually assaulted by a spouse, a dating partner, or an acquaintance are much less likely to report their assault than those assaulted by a stranger. The evidence points to most rapes being perpetrated by people the victim knows, and that the failure to use healthcare services seems closely tied to perpetrator intimacy. This creates the challenge of helping rape victims make use of services in a way that maximizes their safety and is sensitive to the reasons victims choose not to make use of those services. This also has serious implications for the treatment of partner abuse and domestic violence, as the statistical picture suggests that a number of sexual assaults and rapes occur within the context of a relationship. (A more detailed discussion of domestic/partner violence follows shortly.)

Nurses can take several concrete steps to help rape victims when they come for medical attention. The nature of a forensic examination of a rape victim, which involves manipulation of the genital/pelvic area, can trigger considerable anxiety for the victim. As with any medical evaluation, a careful, detailed, and above all, sensitive explanation of all procedures and care should be made to the patient. The person conducting the assessment of the rape/sexual assault victim should be the same sex as the victim. When a same-sex evaluator is not available, it can be helpful to have a person of the same sex accompany the evaluator to provide support to the victim.

Because the initial response to a stressful event is so predictive of later psychological coping and the development of PTSD, it is important to provide as much emotional support to the victim as possible. Listen for and ask about the patient's social supports whenever possible, as social support also has a demonstrated positive effect on post-trauma mental health. Engaging the patient's coping resources, both internal and external, may provide the patient some protective benefit during their initial recovery. Although it is important to gather as much information about the crime as possible, as the patient attempts to organize the experience themselves, information may be provided in an incomplete, sporadic, piecemeal way, which may require time and redirection to facilitate. Again, do not force or demand that the patient talk about the rape more than they are able to.

Follow-up care for rape victims should include referrals for counseling from a mental health professional, support groups, victim advocacy services, and appropriate medical care, including testing for STDs, HIV, and pregnancy as indicated.

Caring for Victims of Domestic Violence

Victims of domestic violence may present for care in the context of being injured by their abuser, through child welfare referrals, or through legal processes related to an incident of abuse coming to the attention of police. The goal of intervention with victims of domestic violence is to ensure the safety of the victim and any dependent children. Victims of domestic violence experience the kind of totalitarian control described by Judy Herman (1992) as producing complex PTSD, and often exhibit symptoms of complex PTSD.

A clinical entity related to domestic violence that has attracted attention in the forensic literature is battered women's syndrome (BWS). First articulated by the psychologist Lenore Walker (1984), battered women's syndrome consists of four basic elements. First, the woman believes that the violence she is subjected to is her fault. Second, the woman is unable to place responsibility for the violence on anyone besides herself. Third, the woman fears for her life or safety and/or that of her children. Finally, the woman feels that her abuser is capable of monitoring her actions at any time. In addition, to be considered to be suffering from battered women's syndrome, the woman must have completed at least two repetitions of what Walker describes as the abuse cycle.

Walker describes abusive relationships as having three distinct phases. The first phase is the tension-building phase, where more subtle forms of aggression and control are exerted by the abuser and tensions within the relationship heighten. The second phase is the abuse phase, when actual violence takes place and the woman is abused. The third phase is the honeymoon phase, when the abuser expresses remorse and regret, the couple reconciles, and there is relative calm. This then leads to the tension-building phase and the repetition of the cycle. This sequence of events is the abuse cycle.

Some authors (Roth & Coles, 1995) have argued that BWS is a subset of PTSD. The characteristics of BWS—the chronic stress, the alterations in the perception of the abuser, the sense of powerlessness, and the feelings of fault for the abuse—are all reminiscent of complex PTSD as described by Judy Herman (1992). Relationships characterized by domestic violence often entail precisely the kind of totalitarian control that, Herman argues, creates the changes in self-perception that foster the continuation of the abuse cycle. Because the trauma associated with domestic violence is tied up with the social roles, expectations, and emotional aspects of being in a relationship, intervention with victims of domestic violence needs to take this into account.

Because domestic violence by definition takes place within a relational context, it is important to learn about the relationship with the abuser. It is important to know and document (using the patient's own words) what types of things the abuser does to maintain control of the victim. The victim should be asked about violence, the threat or use of weapons, control of money or resources, what threats against children or other family members may be made, and any other type of coercive measure taken against the victim. This information is important to understanding the risks posed to the victim and later treatment planning. If the victim feels that she, her children, or others are at immediate risk for being harmed by the abuser, then the first priority is to take action to ensure safety.

Victims of domestic violence are often asked why they remain in the abusive relationship. Several factors often contribute to this decision. The National Violence Against Women Study (Tjaden & Thoenns, 2000) found that a history of childhood abuse was strongly linked to being in an abusive relationship as an adult. The experience of abuse early in life contributes to emotional dynamics of low self-esteem, powerlessness, dependency, and a fear of being alone. Working on these issues constitutes the bulk of the psychological work with this population. In addition to psychological issues, concrete pragmatic considerations such as financial viability and concern for the safety of children also play a considerable role in the victim's decision to stay in these relationships.

Although preserving the safety of the victim of domestic violence logically suggests the victim permanently leaving the abuser, the emotions and distorted attachments associated with the abusive relationship sometimes prevent this from occurring. Victims may allow the abuser, through the abuser's manipulations or their own ambivalence, to return to their homes or otherwise engage with their abuser in ways that make them vulnerable to further violence. Studies have found that women are at their highest risk for being killed by their abusive partner while in the process of leaving them (Brown, 1987). It is important to note that victims of domestic violence are often keenly attuned to the emotional states and current risk posed by their abuser, and can be better gauges of their own risk level than the professional. Separation from the abuser is often a process with gains and setbacks. Although this may be frustrating, it is important to maintain a supportive stance with the patient during these times and support the patient's positive decision making.

One method of helping women who remain in violent relationships is safety planning, by which the patient establishes predetermined courses of action (a place to go, a way of getting out of the home, a stash of money and keys, etc.) as a means of escape when the patient feels acutely at risk. Interventions aimed at leaving the abusive relationship in a more permanent way should be carefully planned unless there is an immediate risk to the patient or dependent children, because such a break is a high-risk time for the patient to be harmed or killed by their abuser. Permanent departure planning should include a specific safe place to go after leaving the abuser; arrangements for child care or school for dependent children; and education about safe houses, legal remedies (protective/no contact orders, family court, protective services, family and child custody laws), longer-term housing resources, financial resources, childcare resources, and support groups.

Caring for Abused Children

Abused children may come to the attention of a forensic nurse through the referral of a child welfare agency, through police intervention in a home, or through the behavior of the children themselves. There is a growing body of evidence that child abuse creates vulnerability to later psychopathology and antisocial behavior. A study of incarcerated adolescent boys found that boys who had been exposed to violence were more likely to see violence as a legitimate way of solving problems and perceive aggressive behavior as positive (Shahinfar, Kupersmidt, & Matza, 2001). Reviewing the literature of the biology of brain development, Allen Schore (2002) argues that childhood abuse impairs the development of those parts of the brain that regulate attachment, affect, and the capacity to modulate stress, all of which create significant vulnerability to PTSD. One could also view these deficits as significant risk factors for impulsivity, substance abuse, and aggressive behavior that would bring a person into the criminal justice system in adolescence or adulthood. Working with abused children poses particular challenges, but has the potential for important effects on later development and social functioning.

Abused children have often been forced to take on adult roles, whether it be caring for themselves or younger siblings, caring for an impaired parent, or exposure to adult sexuality. This affects the way abused children view and relate to adults. Abused children may think of adults as peers rather than authority figures and reject subordinate treatment by adults. This can lead to defiance in the face of limit setting and poor boundaries with adults. Although abused and neglected children may want to be treated like adults, they still have the psychological needs and limitations of children. This can lead to contentious and baffling interactions where the child demands both independence and to be taken care of at the same time. While this tension is true of all children, especially adolescents, it is magnified with this population. One way of facilitating the helping relationship with these children is to show respect for their competencies, avoid power struggles, and allow the child to make choices where appropriate and feasible.

Abused and neglected children can present as guarded or suspicious of adults, especially adults who appear to want something from them (like information about abuse). The child's response can vary when being asked about abuse, especially if the child senses that they are at risk for being removed from their caretakers. Even children who have been horribly abused will sometimes cling to being cared for by their parents in preference to a stranger. On such occasions it is not helpful to challenge or otherwise diminish the importance of the parents to the child. It is better to be respectful of the importance of the parents to the child, while showing concern and emphasizing the child's well-being as the primary goal. Younger children have little or no basis of comparison for what is considered abuse versus their experience of normal treatment by their caretakers. Interviewing may require quite specific, and above all gentle, questions about acts of violence, sexual activity, or neglect.

Caring for Prison Inmates

Prison inmates present a set of unique challenges to the forensic nurse. The confinement, the closed social network of the patient population, and the involuntary nature of treatment can make the care of this patient population daunting. Yet the prison population also has a high concentration of individuals with PTSD compared to the general population. A study by Powell, Holt, and Fondacaro (1997) found that the incidence of PTSD in the inmate population in a rural state prison system was 33%, which is more than double the incidence found in large population studies.

Inmates are at heightened risk for traumatic experiences while being incarcerated. Between 16 and 22% of male inmates are raped while in prison (Struckman-Johnson, Struckman-Johnson, Rucker, Bumby, & Donaldson, 1995, 1996). Reviewing the literature on inmate violence, Drummond (2000) summarizes several factors that make a prisoner more vulnerable to being raped. Those risk factors include youth, small physical size or weakness, having a mental illness or developmental disability, lack of "street sense," lack of gang affiliation, known homosexuality, being a sex offender, being suspected of informing on other inmates, being disliked by staff, and having a history of being sexually assaulted. Very little controlled research has been conducted on the scope of inmate violence, and no official figures for prison rape are currently maintained on any large scale, so it is impossible to precisely quantify the extent of the problem. However, the problem of prison rape has attracted sufficient notice that the Prison Rape Elimination Act of 2003 was recently signed into law. This measure was enacted to more comprehensively study the problem of prison rape and provide a basis for ongoing intervention and policy making.

Inmates struggling with PTSD may be reluctant to acknowledge or discuss their issues for several reasons. Acknowledging being traumatized involves an admission of vulnerability. The risk of being perceived as weak by other inmates is an important consideration in an environment where the image of strength plays such an important role in safety and daily living conditions. This may be particularly true of inmates whose trauma involved being the recipient of abuse, which may cast the patient in a weak or vulnerable light. Another consideration is that PTSD symptoms like hypervigilance and hyperarousal are adaptive in circumstances where aggression plays a pervasive role in social relations.

Despite the obstacles, there is considerable value to providing treatment to inmates with PTSD. Patients with PTSD can experience significant difficulty with substance abuse and anger management. Often these problems contributed to the behaviors that brought the inmate into contact with the criminal justice system in the first place. In addition to addressing the trauma, it is important to address other conditions that contribute to behavior that leads the patient to be in the criminal justice system. Inmates with PTSD may have substance abuse and anger management problems that can aggravate (or be aggravated by) the effects of PTSD. Group treatment can be helpful because it normalizes the experience among the group members, reduces the need for defensive aggression, and builds a support system.

The Question of Malingering

Malingering is a common concern among mental health practitioners in a forensic setting, as inmates or claimants may see an opportunity for diminished sentences, easier inmate conditions, or other advantage. Sparr and Pitman (1999) suggest that nondirective interviewing, attention to personal detail in the relating of PTSD symptoms (biographical versus textbook descriptions), and direct observation of PTSD symptoms during the assessment are useful in discerning genuine versus faked PTSD. Also notable (Resnick, 1997) is a discrepancy between the patient's described capacity for work versus recreational activities (i.e., reporting being too hypervigilant to work with others, but able to go to professional sports games). In a forensic setting, one might extrapolate from this principle into observing for differences in the capacity for activity in one domain of functioning versus another. While any claim of psychological distress by an inmate should be taken seriously, and should be responded to with an appropriate assessment, clinical experience shows that the following aspects of the presentation should be cause for suspicion.

Uniformly Dramatic Description of Symptoms

Like most illnesses or disorders, patients with PTSD tend to describe a profile of symptom severity, with certain symptoms being more prominent than others. The profile of PTSD symptoms encompasses a broad range of mental experience from anxiety to emotional numbing and from agitation to withdrawal. Although patients with PTSD will often present with the full panel of symptoms, there is usually some variability in the relative prominence of those symptoms at different times. Patients who describe uniform, maximum intensity symptoms may be attempting to over-report. The patient who reports having every PTSD symptom at once, especially using DSM jargon ("I'm feeling agitated and emotionally numb"), should be assessed with caution.

Casual, Unhesitating Description of the Traumatic Event

One of the defining characteristics of PTSD is that it represents a breakdown of the capacity to organize experience. This frequently makes the traumatic experience difficult to talk about for the person suffering from PTSD, both for the emotional challenge it poses and the difficulty of integrating the experience well enough to relate it in words. Clinical experience shows that people who suffer from PTSD are often hesitant to discuss their trauma in great detail, and will show reluctance to discuss their traumatic experience with strangers or people they do not trust, regardless of their professional role. Although long-term or otherwise successful treatment for PTSD can reduce this hesitancy, patients who seem conspicuously eager or forthcoming with detailed descriptions of their trauma may be malingering.

A Lack of Subjective Distress When Describing the Symptoms of PTSD or Its Effect on Functioning

PTSD symptoms can be debilitating and extremely difficult to live with on a day-to-day basis. They can exert destructive effects on family, occupational, and social functioning and can be cause for severe subjective distress. Even patients who describe severe avoidance, emotional numbing, or withdrawal symptoms display affect that is conspicuous for its constructed range and intensity. Patients who present without any outward sign of distress, or who seem indifferent when describing the effects of PTSD symptoms on their lives, should arouse suspicion.

PROFESSIONAL PRACTICE CONSIDERATIONS

Feelings Toward the Patient

Forensic patients of any kind can provoke strong feelings in the professionals responsible for their care, and nurses are no exception. Healthcare professionals are often drawn to the field because of their concern for others. Working with forensic patients can pose a challenge because they often come to the forensic setting having been the victim of, or having engaged in, behaviors that are harmful, exploitative, or destructive. A feeling of sympathy and compassion for victims is natural, as is anger, revulsion, and fear for patients who may have committed terrible acts. Awareness and acceptance of one's own feelings for the patient, negative or positive, are essential to maintaining a professional helping stance.

Denial of one's own feelings for the patient can lead to unconscious and subtle forms of interaction with the patient that often cause substandard care and make care more difficult to provide. If one's feelings for the patient are negative, the patient will often sense that they are being treated badly. If one's feelings for the patient are positive, objective assessment becomes more difficult and boundary violations are more likely to occur. It is better to acknowledge one's own feelings for a patient and talk about them with colleagues than to enact those feelings on the unit floor or in the office. Keeping in mind one's role within the larger system and the right of all patients to good care are important in maintaining perspective in working with this challenging population.

Understanding the Role of Trauma Is Not Equivalent to Sympathizing with Criminal Behavior

Working with victims of trauma in a forensic setting can evoke contradictory feelings. On the one hand, you may be working with someone who has been accused of committing terrible acts, yet who may also have been the victim of terrible acts themselves. It can be a struggle to reconcile feelings of empathy for a person who has known terrible suffering with feelings of fear and revulsion for the same person who may have inflicted terrible suffering on others. When working with inmates or the alleged perpetrator of a crime, it is important to remember that understanding the contributions of traumatic experience to the patient's criminal acts is not equivalent to condoning antisocial behavior.

Mental illness does not "justify" a criminal act. The courts consider the role of mental illness in determining the level of culpability and the severity of the punishment for the accused. The necessary conditions for criminal responsibility in the U.S. criminal justice system are the commission of a criminal act and the presence of criminal intent. Although the performance of a criminal act may be comparatively easy to establish, mental illness calls criminal intent into question, and thus criminal responsibility.

One of the most important tasks any forensic healthcare professional performs is translating an understanding of healthcare concepts, issues, and processes to the interdisciplinary forensic team. This is a complex skill that is part teaching, part reframing, and part diplomacy. The criminal justice system is organized around the protection of society through the adjudication and punishment of crimes, whereas healthcare provision is organized around the care and benefit of the patient. When working with trauma survivors or victims of crime, these value sets are broadly aligned, even when the professional becomes a source of information to help "make the case." In investigative or correctional settings, where the survivor or victim may also be a perpetrator, these values may come into conflict. These patients are "the bad guys" after all. This is a fundamental difference in orientation and is a predictable source of tension for the nurse practicing in the forensic setting.

Healthcare professionals provide assessment, care, and treatment. Judges and juries decide the role of mental illness in determining guilt or innocence of a crime. Our role as healthcare professionals is to provide good assessment and good care to our patients, and when obliged provide information to other members of the forensic team (lawyers, judges, juries) to facilitate their work in adjudicating these matters. Fulfilling that role requires that our care be provided in a professional manner and that our assessments are fair, objective, and reliable. By doing so we allow the other participants in the process (colleagues, lawyers, judges, juries) to make arguments, decisions, and judgments with the best information possible.

SUMMARY

Post-traumatic stress disorder is a topic of substantial interest to the field of mental health, the legal system, and society at large. The conditions that create trauma, the interventions that reduce its likelihood, and the treatment of those who suffer from it have broad social implications. It is indisputable in the face of the available empirical data that some people's feelings, thoughts, and behavior are dramatically and negatively altered by the experience of overwhelming stress. The conditions that breed trauma have considerable social components. Violence, substance abuse, and neglect all qualify as large social problems that government and mental health establishments have had mixed results in combating. These issues are also part and parcel of the work the criminal justice system and the forensic sciences engage in every day.

Although mental illnesses such as bipolar disorder and schizophrenia enjoy strong evidence for biologically based etiology and have clear symptom profiles, PTSD is by its nature an acquired mental illness that can have a variable presentation resembling other conditions. The study of trauma brings into bold relief the forensic and legal questions posed by mental illness in general. How do we know another person's mind? To what extent can the hardships of the past explain our present behavior? To what extent do those hardships diminish culpability for our actions? How do we understand the person we are treating now in terms of their past?

Nurses who practice in a forensic setting will encounter patients who have experienced the unimaginable. Sometimes they will be victims, sometimes they will be perpetrators. Too often they will have been both at different times. Patients with PTSD present unique challenges and demand treatment that is mindful of its complexities. Although general information such as that provided in this chapter is a point of departure, it is not a substitute for learning from the patient. Understanding patients with PTSD requires that we stand with them, be they sinner or saint, and bear witness to the darkest aspects of human experience. It is provocative work that demands courage. Working with traumatized patients requires a willingness to help give voice to the unspeakable and to withstand rage from the patient and within ourselves; it also requires the capacity for hope in the face of despair. By doing these things we help the patient begin to make sense of their past experience, define themselves in the present, and develop meaning for the future.

QUESTIONS FOR DISCUSSION

1. What events in your own life have challenged your coping?
2. What strengths and supports can you point to in your own life that have helped you in times of crisis?
3. Is there any similarity between society's response to large national tragedies like the 9/11 attacks and individual responses to trauma?
4. How is a stressful event different from a trauma?
5. Why do some people develop PTSD and others do not?

REFERENCES

Alarcon, D., Glover, S., Boyer, B., & Baleen, R. (2000). Proposing an algorithm for the pharmacological management of posttraumatic stress disorder. *Annals of Clinical Psychiatry, 12*(4), 239–246.

American Psychiatric Association. (2000). *Diagnostic and statistical manual of psychiatric disorders IV—text revision.* Washington, DC: American Psychiatric Press.

Beck, A. T. & Freeman, A. (1990). *Cognitive therapy of personality disorders.* New York: Guilford.

Beckham, J., Feldman, M., Kirby, A., Hertzberg, M., & Moore, S. (1998). Interpersonal violence and its correlates in Vietnam veterans with chronic posttraumatic stress disorder. *Journal of Clinical Psychology, 53*(8), 859–867.

Bonne, O., Brandes, D., Gilboa, A., et al. (2001). Longitudinal MRI study of hippocampal volume in trauma survivors with PTSD. *American Journal of Psychiatry, 158,* 1248–1251.

Bremner, J., Randall, P., Scott, T., Bronen, R., Seibyl, J., et al. (1995). MRI based measures of hippocampal volume in patients with PTSD. *American Journal of Psychiatry, 152,* 973–981.

Brewin, C., Andrews, B., & Valentine, J. (2000). Meta analysis of risk factors for post-traumatic stress disorder in trauma exposed adults. *Journal of Consulting and Clinical Psychology, 68*(5), 748–766.

Brown, A. (1987). *When battered women kill.* New York: Free Press.

Bryant, R., Harvey, A., Dang, S., et al. (1998). Treatment of acute stress disorder: An evaluation of of cognitive behavioral therapy and supportive counseling techniques. *Journal of Consulting and Clinical Psychology, 66,* 862–866.

Collins, J. & Bailey, S. (1990). Traumatic stress disorder and violent behavior. *Journal of Traumatic Stress, 3,* 203–220.

Davidson, J. & Foa, E. (1991). Diagnostic issues in posttraumatic stress disorder: Considerations for the DSM-IV. *Journal of Abnormal Psychology, 100,* 346–355.

Davidson, P. & Parker, K. (2001). Eye movement desensitization and reprocessing (EMDR): A meta analysis. *Journal of Consulting and Clinical Psychology, 69*(2), 305–316.

Dean, E. (1999). *Shook over hell: Post-traumatic stress disorder, Vietnam and the Civil War.* Cambridge: Harvard University Press.

Drummond, R. (2000). Inmate sexual assault: The plague that persists. *The Prison Journal, 80*(4), 407–414.

Edwards, V., Holden, G., Felitti, V., & Anda, R. (2003). Relationship between multiple forms of childhood maltreatment and adult mental health in community respondents: Results from the Adverse Childhood Experiences study. *American Journal of Psychiatry, 160*(8), 1453–1460.

Erickson, D., Wolfe, J., King, D., King, L., & Sharkansky, E. (2001). Posttraumatic stress disorder and depression symptomotology in a sample of Gulf War veterans: A prospective analysis. *Journal of Consulting and Clinical Psychology, 69*(1), 41–49.

Foa, E. & Rothbaum, B. (1997). *Treating the trauma of rape.* New York: Guilford Press.

Francis, J. (2003). Effective treatments for PTSD: Practice guidelines from the International Society for Traumatic Stress Studies. *Bulletin of the Menninger Clinic, 67*(4), 370–370.

Freud, S. (1920). *Beyond the pleasure principle.* London: Vintagu/Ebury.

Friedman, M. (2001). Allostatic versus empirical perspectives on pharmacotherapy for PTSD. In J. Wilson, M. Friedman, & J. Lindy (Eds.), *Treating psychological trauma and PTSD.* New York: Guilford, pp. 94–124.

Gay, P. (1988). *Freud: A life for our time.* New York: W.W. Norton.

Gilbertson, M., Shenton, M., Ciszewski, A., Kasai, K., Lasko, N., Orr, S., et al. (2002). Smaller hippocampal volume predicts pathologic vulnerability to psychological trauma. *Nature Neuroscience, 5*(11), 1242–1247.

Hendin, H. & Haas, A. P. (1984). *Wounds of war: The psychological aftermath of the Vietnam War.* New York: Basic Books.

Herman, J. (1992). *Trauma and recovery.* New York: Basic Books.

Isaac, N. & Enos, P. (2001). *Documenting domestic violence: How health care providers can help victims.* Washington, DC: National Institute of Justice.

Kessler, R., Sonnega, A., Bromet, E., Hughes, M., & Nelson, C. (1995). Posttraumatic stress disorder in the National Comorbidity Survey. *Archives of General Psychiatry, 52,* 1048–1060.

Kulka, R., Schlenger, W., Fairbank, J., Hough, R., Jordan, B., Marmar, C., et al, (1990). *Trauma and the Vietnam War generation.* New York: Brunner/Mazel.

Marks, I., Lovell, K., Noshirvani, H., Livanov, M., & Thrasher, S. (1998). Treatment of post-traumatic stress disorder by exposure and/or cognitive restructuring: A controlled study. *Archives of General Psychiatry, 55,* 317–325.

MacNair, R. (2002). *Perpetration-induced traumatic stress: The psychological consequences of killing.* Westport, CT: Praeger.

McFarlane, A. (1998). Epidemiological evidence about the relationship between PTSD and alcohol abuse: The nature of the association. *Addictive Behavior, 23,* 813–825.

Mollica, R. F. (1998). The dose effect relationship between torture and psychiatric symptoms in Vietnamese ex-political detainees and a comparison group. *The Journal of Nervous and Mental Disease, 186*(9), 543–553.

Morgan, A., Wang, S., Southwick, S., Rassmusson, A., Hazlett, G., Hauger, R., et al. (2002). Plasma neuropeptide-Y concentrations in humans exposed to highly intense and uncontrollable stress. *Biological Psychiatry, 47,* 902–909.

Nut, D. & Malizia, A. (2004). Structural and functional brain changes in posttraumatic stress disorder. *Journal of Clinical Psychiatry, 65*(1), 11–17.

Ozer, E., Best, S., Lipsey, T., & Weiss, D. (2003). Predictors of posttraumatic stress disorder and symptoms in adults: A meta analysis. *Psychological Bulletin, 129*(1), 52–73.

Pollock, P. (1999). When the killer suffers: Post traumatic stress reactions following homicide. *Legal and Criminological Psychology, 4,* 185–202.

Powell, T., Holt, J., & Fondacaro, K. (1997). The prevalence of mental illness among inmates in a rural state. *Journal of Law and Human Behavior, 21,* 427–438.

Rauch, S., van der Kolk, B., Fisler, R., Alpert, N., Orr, S., Savage, C., et al. (1996). A symptom provocation study of posttraumatic stress disorder using positron emission tomography and script-driven imagery. *Archives of General Psychiatry, 53*(5), 380–387.

Rennison, C. (2002). Rape and sexual assault: Reporting to police and medical attention, 1992–2000. *U.S. Department of Justice, Bureau of Justice Statistics, Selected Findings,* NCJ194530. Available at: http://www.ojp.usdoj.gov/bjs/.

Resnick, P. (1997). Malingering of posttraumatic stress disorder. In R. Rogers (Ed.), *Clinical assessment of malingering and deception.* New York: Guilford, pp. 84–103.

Risse, S., Whitters, A., Burke, J., Chen, S., Scurfield, R., & Raskind, M. (1990). Severe withdrawal symptoms after discontinuation of alprazolam in eight patients with combat-induced post-traumatic stress disorder. *Journal of Clinical Psychiatry, 51,* 206–209.

Roth, D. & Coles, E. (1995). Battered woman syndrome: A conceptual analysis of its status vis-à-vis DSM IV mental disorders. *Medicine & Law, 14*(7–8), 641–658.

Roy-Byrne, P., Russo, J., Michelson, E., Zatzick, D., Pitman, R., & Berliner, L. (2004). Risk factors and outcomes in ambulatory assault victims presenting to the acute emergency department setting: Implications for secondary prevention studies in PTSD. *Depression and Anxiety, 19*(2), 77–84.

Sapolsky, R. (1992). *Stress, the aging brain and mechanisms of neuron death.* Cambridge, MA: MIT Press.

Schore, A. (2002). Dysregulation of the right brain: A fundamental mechanism of traumatic attachment and the psychopathogenesis of posttraumatic stress disorder. *Australian and New Zealand Journal of Psychiatry, 36,* 9–30.

Sernyak, M., Leslie, D., Alarcon, R., Losonczy, M., & Rosenheck, R. (2003). Association of diabetes mellitus with use of atypical neuroleptics in the treatment of schizophrenia. *American Journal of Psychiatry, 159*(4), 561–566.

Selye, H. (1956). *The stress of life.* New York: McGraw-Hill.

Shahinfar, A., Kupersmidt, J., & Matza, L. (2001). The relation between exposure to violence and social information processing among incarcerated adolescents. *Journal of Abnormal Psychology, 110*(1), 136–141.

Sparr, L. & Pitman, R. (1999). Forensic assessment of traumatized adults. In P. Saigh & D. Bremner (Eds.), *Posttraumatic stress disorder: A comprehensive text.* Massachusetts: Allyn & Bacon, pp. 284–308.

Stein, M., Hannah, C., Koverola, C., Yehuda, R., Torchilla, M., & McClarty, B. (1994). *Neuroanatomical and neuroendocrine correlates in adulthood to severe sexual abuse in childhood.* Paper presented at the 33rd annual meeting of the American College of Neuropsychopharmacology, San Juan, PR.

Struckman-Johnson, C. J., Struckman-Johnson, D. L., Rucker, L., Bumby, K., & Donaldson, S. (1995). *A survey of inmate and staff perspectives on prisoner sexual assault.* Paper presented at the annual meeting of the midwestern Psychological Association, Chicago.

Struckman-Johnson, C. J., Struckman-Johnson, D. L., Rucker, L., Bumby, K., & Donaldson, S. (1996). Sexual coercion reported by men and women in prison. *Journal of Sex Research, 33*(1), 67–76.

Terr, L. (1990). *Too scared to cry: Psychic trauma in childhood.* Grand Rapids, MI: Harper & Row.

Tjaden, P. & Thoenns, N. (2000). *Extent, nature and consequences of intimate partner violence: Findings from the national violence against women survey.* Washington, DC: U.S. Department of Justice, Office of Justice Programs, National Institute of Justice.

United Kingdom Medicines and Healthcare Products Regulation Agency. (2004). Summary of clinical trial data on cerebrovascular adverse events (CVAEs) in randomized clinical trials of risperidone conducted in patients with dementia. http://medicines.mhra.gov.ok/ourwork/monitorsafequalmed/safetymessages/risperidoneclinicaltrialdata_final.pdf.

van der Kolk, B. & Fisler, R. (1995). Dissociation and the fragmentary nature of traumatic memories: Review and experimental confirmation. *Journal of Traumatic Stress, 8*(4), 505–525.

van der Kolk, B. A. (1996a). The body keeps the score: Approaches to the psychobiology of posttraumatic stress disorder. In van der Kolk, McFarlane, & Weisaeth (Eds.), *Traumatic stress: The effects of overwhelming experience on mind, body and society.* New York: Guilford, pp. 214–241.

van der Kolk, B. A. (1996b). Trauma and memory. In van der Kolk, McFarlane, & Weisaeth (Eds.), *Traumatic stress: The effects of overwhelming experience on mind, body and society.* New York: Guilford, pp. 279–302.

van Emmerick, A., Kamphuis, J., Hulsbocsch, A., & Emmelkamp, P. (2002). Single session debriefing after psychological trauma: A meta analysis. *Lancet, 360*(9335), 766–771.

Walker, L. (1984). *The battered women's syndrome.* New York: Springer.

Yehuda, R. (1998). Neuroendochrinology of trauma and posttraumatic stress disorder. In R. Yehuda (Ed.), *Psychological trauma.* Washington, DC: American Psychiatric Press, pp. 97–131.

Yehuda, R., Southwick, S., & Giller, E. (1992). Exposure to atrocities and severity of chronic posttraumatic stress disorder in Vietnam combat veterans. *American Journal of Psychiatry, 149,* 333–336.

Yehuda, R., Southwick, S., Mason, J., & Giller, E. (1990). Interactions of the hypothalamic-pituitary-adrenal axis and the catecholaminergic system of the stress disorder. In E. L. Giller (Ed.), *Biological assessment and treatment of PTSD.* Washington, DC: American Psychiatric Press, pp. 130–145.

Zaidi, L. & Foy, D. (1994). Childhood abuse experiences and combat-related PTSD. *Journal of Traumatic Stress, 7*(1), 33–42.

PRACTICAL ASPECTS OF FORENSIC NURSING

Death Investigation

Edward T. McDonough

Death investigation is an essential service that involves a focus on the identification of the deceased, determination of the physical condition of the body at an investigative scene, documentation of injuries, gathering and reporting of evidence, estimation of time of death, functioning as a liaison to families, and provision of the final certification as to the cause and manner of death. Increasingly in many jurisdictions, the death investigator is a nonphysician employed by the medical examiner's office. As a representative of this office, the nonphysician death investigator plays a vital role in contributing to the ultimate findings of the medical examiner as to the cause and manner of death, performing many of the duties previously associated with the medical examiner. The death investigator is an evolving role that requires excellent observational, perceptive, and communication skills. A pre-existing knowledge of medical conditions is a most desirable additional asset. Although death investigators traditionally have varied educational backgrounds, the requisite skills make the forensic nurse an ideal candidate to fulfill this role.

CHAPTER FOCUS

KEY TERMS

abrasions
algor mortis
autolysis
cause of death
contusions
coroner
degloving
desiccation
forensic entomologist
forensic pathologist
fracture
homicide
lacerations
livor mortis
maceration
manner of death
medical examiner
mummification
natural death
nosologist
proximate event
putrefaction
rigor mortis
saponification
suicide
toxicology

There is no single uniform death investigation system in the United States. There are at least 50 major jurisdictions, not including the District of Columbia, Puerto Rico, Guam, and all the subjurisdictions such as counties and cities. Further, statutes, law enforcement, and the attendant support structures that evolve around them are all locally generated. The 10th amendment to the U.S. Constitution allows for these individual jurisdictions to exist and operate independently, but it also creates inherent inequity and variation. There is often not a "right way" or a "wrong way" to investigate any particular death, but a "city way" and a "country way"; that is, population centers have greater resources and larger revenue streams available to the governing body, and therefore can offer more services to the citizens than a region with fewer resources. This includes death investigation services. The methods applied to investigating various categories of deaths are well defined, but lack of available local resources may, out of necessity, modify the extent to which particular deaths are scrutinized. For example, a large metropolitan medical examiner's office with sufficient staffing, laboratory facilities, and capabilities may examine firsthand every deceased individual who comes under its jurisdiction. In contrast, some small rural counties may have no medical facilities, and a limited budget for outsourcing only a few autopsy examinations annually.

HISTORY OF DEATH INVESTIGATION

There are many historic seeds, some thousands of years old, that ultimately germinated into the modern practice of death investigation. Identification of a particular death as a suicide was important to early communities who believed that if suicide was not recognized and stopped, the community would be destroyed by the action of the evil spirits thought to be responsible. The counterpart to this community action is seen in the modern epidemiologic approach used to identify and combat infectious diseases.

Some examples of historic medicolegal seeds follow. One is the Hammurabi Code, which was inscribed on stone in approximately 2000 BC and is perhaps the oldest written code of law. When Julius Caesar was assassinated in 44 BC, a Roman medical doctor named Antistius examined the body and noted and reported the presence of 23 wounds. It was his opinion that one stab wound to the chest was the lethal injury. In 1192, when Richard the Lionhearted was kidnapped and held for ransom by Leopold of Austria, the English treasury was unable to cover the ransom. This led to the development of a strategy to make use of corpses as a novel source of income. The title of "crowner" was given to those who acquired custody of a dead criminal's possessions, thus enriching the royal assets. The word coroner (crowner) was originally mentioned in 925 in the "Chart of Privileges." In 1194, the duties of the coroner in England were formally delineated. The local justices provided that three knights and one clerk were elected in every county as "keepers of the pleas of the crown." This coroner position dictated administrative and investigative responsibilities often carried out with the assistance of the local sheriff. One of these duties included holding inquests over the deceased to ascertain the nature of the wounds and provide for the arrest of any individual deemed responsible for their infliction.

In 1250 a Chinese treatise, *Hsi Yuan Lu*, was produced covering such topics as blunt and sharp force injury, drownings, and deaths by fire. This writing addressed questions about whether the person was alive or dead when he went into the water or prior to the fire.

The settlers in early America brought with them the English coroner system. In 1637, records in Maryland discuss the actions of the coroner/sheriff holding inquests. The first recorded autopsy examination was done in 1647 in Massachusetts regarding a case where an individual was killed by a tree limb. Autopsy examinations were still incredibly rare events, but their usefulness was identified in this early time period.

The earliest mention of physicians collaborating with the coroner was in 1860 in Maryland, when the Code of Public General Laws authorized the coroner or his jury to require the attendance of a physician in the investigation of cases of violent death. Shortly after that the legislature authorized the governor to appoint a physician as a sole coroner in Baltimore. In 1877 Maryland adopted a statewide system requiring that a physician known as a medical examiner supplant the coroner. The examiner's responsibilities primarily lay in the investigation of violent deaths. In 1890, a Baltimore city ordinance authorized the Board of Health to appoint two physicians with the title of Medical Examiner and assign them the duty of performing all autopsies requested by the coroner or the state's attorney of the City of Baltimore.

In 1915 New York City adopted a law eliminating the coroner's office and creating a medical examiner system. The medical examiner was authorized to investigate deaths resulting from criminal violence, suicide, sudden unexpected deaths, deaths that were not attended by medical personnel, or the death of an imprisoned person. Dr. Charles Norris was the first Chief Medical Examiner and was given the authority to perform autopsies according to his particular judgment. This established the first essentials of a competent medical examiner system that would investigate a broad spectrum of cases with the authority to perform an autopsy when the public interest demands it.

In 1939 the first statewide medical examiner system was established in Maryland. The medical examiner system, as developed in New York City and throughout Maryland, requires the medical examiner to be a physician. For the most part, this eliminates the death investigator having to be tied to a political party and having to campaign periodically for the office. Running for an elected office might be seen to compromise, to some degree, a coroner's true independence by creating a need to avoid alienating one or more segments of the electorate, such as law enforcement, criminal and civil lawyers, funeral directors, and other potential special interest constituencies including families. However, many elected coroner positions throughout the United States require that the coroner be a physician.

DEATH INVESTIGATOR ROLES

A coroner is an elected or appointed official who may or may not have any medical training, much less subspecialty training in forensic pathology; however, there are many excellent nonphysician death investigators. One advantage to the classic coroner system is the ability to hold mini-trials known as inquests. Here, witnesses can be examined under oath to document and certify evidence associated with a particular deceased in a more formal setting.

A medical examiner is, by definition, a physician. However, the mere fact that the medical examiner is a physician does not in any way guarantee that this person has any training or experience in the field of death investigation. Their inherent knowledge of medicine, dealing with patients and grieving relatives, and understanding of physiology and pharmacology does, however, give them a significant advantage over a lay nonphysician coroner responsible for investigating death.

A forensic pathologist is a physician who has trained in pathology, either in a 3-year anatomic pathology program or a combined 4-year anatomic and clinical pathology program, who then goes on to subspecialty training in an approved medical examiner's office, ultimately sitting for the Forensic Pathology Board examination. It is not uncommon for a forensic pathologist to be triple board certified (anatomic, clinical, and forensic) in pathology.

THE ROLE OF THE MEDICAL EXAMINER

A medical examiner's office may cover an entire state or a single county. Some state systems, such as in Massachusetts and North Carolina, have regional offices apart from the main headquarters because of the geography and large distances that need to be covered. County systems often also contract with surrounding smaller county coroners to perform necessary medicolegal autopsy examinations. A chief medical examiner, who is statutorily responsible for administering the agency, performing the death investigations, keeping records, and providing toxicology services, usually heads such an office. The chief medical examiner may be directly appointed by the governor, appointed by an intermediary body. The office may be a part of a larger state or county agency, such as the Health Department or the Attorney General's office. The duties of the chief medical examiner and his office are dictated by state or county statute, which usually allow the chief medical examiner or his designee to perform investigations and autopsy examinations at their professional discretion.

The purpose of any death investigation system, however it is constructed, is according to statute: to determine the cause and the manner of an individual's death that comes under its jurisdiction. The criteria for which types of deaths must come to the attention of a death investigator were set forth by the New York City Medical Examiner's Office decades ago. Although minor variations occur between jurisdictions, the broad criteria allow a wide net to be cast and therefore decrease the chances of a case that should have been investigated being missed. The generally recognized criteria include deaths caused by trauma (blunt, sharp, chemical, electrical), suicide, accident, or homicide; deaths that are suspicious, impact public health, are in the workplace, or are unattended by medical or hospital personnel; and remains that are to be cremated or buried at sea. Other types of deaths falling within the death investigator's purview include people dying with no physician to sign the death certificate.

THE INVESTIGATION

Initial Scene Observations

The investigation begins when a particular death, meeting the criteria for investigation, is reported to the administrative arm of the death investigation system. Ideally, if the deceased is still at the death scene, the investigator should be dispatched to the scene to gather information and evidence, not to determine that the individual is indeed dead. No state statutes indicate that a physician must pronounce a person dead. The statutes do indicate that a physician must certify the death (i.e., sign a death certificate), usually within 24 hours of becoming aware of it. A person is presumed/declared dead when responsible parties decline to institute emergency procedures and/or transportation to a medical facility. Conditions such as drug or alcohol intoxication and hypothermia can mimic somatic death and there are cases reported where a "dead person" awakened. To avoid these situations, medical control for emergency service personnel should include the documentation of lack of cardiac activity prior to the presumption of an individual's death.

At the scene it is important to establish whether the decedent has been moved or is in the same position as initially discovered. Basic questions can then be ascertained from the police, witnesses, or family members who are also at the scene. How and why was the decedent discovered? What is the identity of the individual? When was the person last reliably known to be alive? What happened just prior to their collapse, if known? What was their condition/behavior in the 24 to 48 hours prior to their death? What are their known medical conditions? The investigator then should make observations about the nature of the environment in which the victim lived. Is it tidy, cluttered, or dirty? Is there anything out of order? What is the temperature of the environment (or what was the temperature of the environment when the first responder arrived?) What is the decedent wearing? What position is the body in?

The investigator should then examine the remains for personal possessions, evidence of identification, and other clues as to their medical condition, such as Medic-Alert bracelets, medications, or medical devices such as insulin pumps or pacemakers. The investigator should also observe any injuries to the body. It is unwise to try and perform a detailed examination under suboptimal conditions such as cramped space, poor lighting, or with inadequate equipment and assistance. If the person who responds to the scene is not the coroner or medical examiner, or the person ultimately responsible for the autopsy examination and/or the death certification, their initial findings should be communicated to the autopsy pathologist. This can now be done by telephone, with video conferencing, or with digital imaging via e-mail or the Internet.

If a crime is suspected, the investigator responding to the scene should correlate further activities with law enforcement and/or evidence technicians so that any potential evidence associated with the body is identified and collected at the scene, or preserved in such a manner that it will not be damaged or destroyed prior to subsequent collection in the autopsy room. The "processing" of the body at the scene is optimal, if permission is given by the investigator and/or the forensic pathologist they represent. The utilization of alternate light sources for the identification and collection of hairs, fibers, and body fluids is done most efficiently prior to wrapping, manipulating, and transporting a body to the medical examiner's laboratory. This should always be done with the full knowledge of the investigator or the responsible coroner or medical examiner, so that any artifacts associated with the identification and collection of evidence left on the body would be known to the pathologist and correctly interpreted. An example of a technique that would create such an artifact would be forming a tent around the body and fumigating the remains with cyanoacrylate (superglue) for the detection, with alternate light sources, of fingerprints.

It is also of great import for the investigator to search the scene, with the knowledge and permission of law enforcement, for medications. A prescription vial label contains a tremendous amount of valuable information including the name of the decedent, the pharmacy where the prescription was filled, the name of the prescribing physician, what was prescribed, the quantity, the instructions, and the date of prescription. This one item is often an invaluable tool with which to start the medical investigation and/or suggest a possible suicide.

Removal of the Body

The appropriate packaging of the remains and the subsequent removal from the scene to the autopsy facility should also be well coordinated. This can be an extremely difficult job depending on location, ranging from simply moving the decedent from a death bed in a hospital or nursing home facility to the funeral cart or transport gurney, to an outdoor location that is potentially dangerous or to a multistory building with no elevator. The state of the remains can be anywhere from recently deceased to badly decomposed and insect infested, to skeletonized. The investigator's observations should be reduced to a written report, transmitted to the forensic pathologist, and kept on file. The accessibility of these reports by outside parties varies from jurisdiction to jurisdiction.

Determination of Death

An investigation into the death of an individual cannot be initiated until a person has actually died. Up until the last two decades the concept of brain death had not been generally accepted. Even after the "Harvard criteria" were established, lawyers in particular were extremely uncomfortable with the thought of removing a normally beating heart from an individual presumed to be brain dead in order to donate it to a recipient. In fact, in one case, criminal defense attorneys attempted to charge the transplant surgeon with the death of an individual who had been declared brain dead as a result of a gunshot wound to the head, and whose family wanted to donate the heart. The attempt, fortunately, was not successful.

Somatic death has, by necessity, been the standard for determining the ultimate demise of a human being. This implies the objective determination that the heart and lungs are no longer functioning. This was done initially by palpation and then subsequently with the utilization of the stethoscope. There are two absolute criteria that any person, regardless of their training or background, can use to determine, even from some distance, that a human being is deceased: decapitation and skeletonization. All other bodies fall somewhere on the spectrum of clearly alive to probably dead.

With the development of the respirator it became possible to supply oxygen with mechanical assistance to the subcranial organs. There are two common mimickers of somatic death in which the mechanical detection of a heartbeat and/or respiration is difficult, if not impossible: hypothermia, particularly from immersion, and intoxication with respiratory depressants such as alcohol, benzodiazepines, and opiates. The utilization of an electrocardiogram machine and/or field defibrillator should be able to demonstrate that the individual is not deceased, and appropriate resuscitation measures can be instituted.

Organ Transplantation

The ability to prolong "life" through mechanical respiration allowed for the advancement of organ transplantation. The heart, lungs, kidneys, and liver can remain oxygenated and perfused for later donation, providing life-saving outcomes throughout the country and the world.

Organ and tissue procurement organizations are, by default, required to interact frequently with members of the medical examiner and coroner systems. It is not an uncommon scenario to encounter an individual with significant head injury or a spontaneous natural disease process such as a ruptured berry aneurysm, where significant trauma and anoxic encephalopathy and brain swelling ultimately lead to brain death. These types of cases come under the jurisdiction of the medical examiner and/or coroner. Most physicians are fully cognizant of the benefits of organ and tissue transplantation. The diagnosis of brain death includes clinical demonstration of loss of the cranial nerves and reflexes such as the corneal reflex, the gag reflex, and calorics. Further, there should be laboratory demonstration that when the patient is removed from the respirator no spontaneous respirations are evident, as demonstrated by an increasing pCO_2 in the blood. Alternative tests such as repeated EEGs or radioactive tagged red cell cerebral blood flow studies are also extremely useful in equivocal cases.

The forensic nurse death investigator, in particular, has the opportunity to act as a liaison between the medical examiner/coroner and the tissue bank, to facilitate the investigation and the determination of the circumstances surrounding the trauma or natural disease processes causing the brain death, to lead the recovery of the organs and tissue by the transplantation team, and to arrange for the examination of the body by the pathologist in the operating room, if necessary. After brain and somatic death have occurred, the medical examiner or coroner can also facilitate recovery of additional tissues, such as corneas, heart valves, skin, bones, and veins, for processing and subsequent transplantation. These tissues are at least life enhancing, if not lifesaving. The importance of collaboration between the medical examiner, coroner, death investigator, and organ and tissue coordinators cannot be overestimated.

CAUSE AND MANNER OF DEATH

The Death Certificate

The primary goal of any death investigation is to allow the medical examiner or coroner to have enough information based on the background data collection to correlate it with the autopsy findings in order to certify a cause and manner of an individual's death. The sole legal requirement to sign a death certificate is to be a licensed physician in the jurisdiction where the body was found dead. This occasionally causes some confusion and difficulties in border towns where an event took place in one jurisdiction and the body has been transported to the closest medical facility, or surreptitiously disposed of in another jurisdiction. The result is a situation in which the certifier may be a significant distance from where the actual event took place, occasionally requiring cross-jurisdictional testimony in criminal and civil actions.

The death certificate itself is modeled after a World Health Organization (WHO) document that includes basic demographic information, an opinion statement regarding the cause of death, and an area to describe the events surrounding the death if it is not natural. There are numerous variations from jurisdiction to jurisdiction based on the types of data that each region wishes to collect. The death certificate is a public document that can be obtained by anyone in a town hall or registry of vital statistics for a small fee, a necessary practice for genealogists.

The "art" of signing a death certificate is usually not taught in medical schools, leaving the casual certifier somewhat bewildered. It is not uncommon for a cause of death to be listed as "cardiorespiratory arrest." This merely indicates that the person's heart and lungs have stopped, which is already evident because the document that is being signed is a death certificate. Theoretically, cardiorespiratory arrest could be put on every death certificate, because that is the final common pathway for all living beings. This practice is often a way of avoiding providing an opinion based on the clinical information present. In some cases this clinical information is understandably extremely limited, thus causing the certifier to fear legal retribution if the opinion is later proven to be incorrect. However, it should be noted that the death certificate clearly states that "the indicated cause of death is an opinion." A professional may render an opinion based on the available information with absolutely no fear of legal consequences. Frequently, amended death certificates, updated regarding the cause or because of correction of clerical errors, can be issued, especially if further data regarding the cause of death comes to light from an autopsy, toxicology, other laboratory tests, or historical information. This information may come days, months, or decades after the initial certification.

A signed death certificate is needed for disposition of the remains according to the family's wishes. Bodies cannot be buried or cremated without it. A cause of death such as "Pending Further Studies," "Pending Laboratory Tests," or "Pending Investigation" are all perfectly legitimate statements to record as the initial cause of death. This preliminary death certificate, containing the other demographic data such as the individual's name, the date and time of their death, and pronouncement, is perfectly legitimate and will allow the funeral home to carry out its duties.

Cause of Death

The cause of death is defined as "that injury or disease process, whether brief or prolonged, that initiates the pathophysiologic downward spiral ultimately ending in death." This means that the certifier, whether a private physician, a medical examiner, or a coroner, should ask him- or herself the question, "What started it all?" In legal terms this concept is known as the "proximate" event. The cause of death box on a death certificate (Figure 15–1) usually has three or four lines labeled A, B, C, and D, separated in fine print by the phrase "due to or as a result of." This ultimately allows for a cause of death statement. For example: "Cardiac tamponade *due to* ruptured left ventricle *due to* subacute myocardial infarction *due to* ischemic heart disease" is a pathophysiologic, accurate cause of death statement. Often, simple one-line cause of death state-

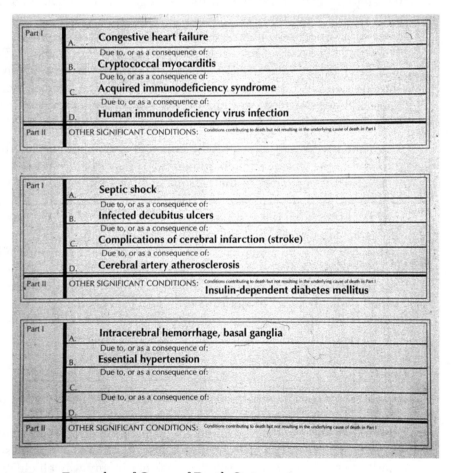

Figure 15–1   Examples of Cause of Death Statements

ments also can be completely accurate, such as "ischemic heart disease" or "atherosclerotic cardiovascular disease."

Certifications for natural death are sometimes more difficult than for traumatic deaths because the person may have multiple comorbid disease processes resulting in chronic individual or multiple organ failures such that the final physiologic event may not be witnessed nor readily evident. However, if it is clearly a natural death, with no evidence of trauma, either chemical or physical, a reasonable cause of death statement can still be crafted.

Traumatic deaths are also often easier to certify because it is not uncommon for the person to succumb to the trauma shortly after it is inflicted. "Gunshot wound of the chest," "Craniocerebral blunt force trauma," or "Heroin toxicity" are all readily apparent by autopsy, toxicology, and investigative data correlation. If there is significant survival in a treatment facility, then the proximate event may be forgotten by the clinicians over time. A common example would be injuries sustained in a motor vehicle accident requiring the person to be hospitalized. Death may ensue from the subsequent effects of the injury, the healing process, and any complications that may stem from either. A typical accurate cause of death statement may be, "Sepsis *due to* pneumonia *due to* blunt force trauma of the chest."

The death investigator may find the proximate event at the beginning of the chart in the emergency department (ED) or ambulance notes that tell what initially happened to the person, such as a fall, assault, or motor vehicle accident. If the person was transferred from another facility, then the ED records from the first facility should be sought. Discussions with the paramedics or EMTs who initially transported the person, as well as the police officers who investigated the initial event, may also help to accurately identify the proximate cause of death. In cases of delayed deaths, blood samples should be sought and recovered from admission so that toxicology can be performed to help provide data as to the presenting state of the individual prior to the initiation of advanced life support and intensive care treatment.

Manner of Death

The other important aspect of signing a death certificate that is often mandated is the manner of death. The manner of death is defined as "the circumstances that surround the cause of death." If an accurate cause of death statement indicates "gunshot wound to the chest" or "multiple blunt force injuries," this does not in any way elucidate the circumstances that surround them. Usually there are only five choices that can be certified: natural, accident, homicide, suicide, and undetermined. Medical examiners and coroners frequently have to certify natural causes of death and therefore, but not exclusively, the manner of death would be natural. Rare exceptions include recent cases in which some individuals were infected and died of "inhalation anthrax." Anthrax is a naturally occurring organism causing a natural disease process; however, the circumstances surrounding contraction of this disease process were clearly intentional and assaultive in nature, leading to a "homicide" manner of death. The argument has also been made for "homicide by heart attack," in which an assailant threatens the victim with a gun and the victim has a cardiac arrhythmia due to the immediate stress of the situation and dies. These are uncommon but documented scenarios.

Usually, medical examiners certify death with a simple one-line phrase indicating the proximate event, or if there is some significant survival between the event and the death, a phrase such as "complications of . . ." or "sequelae of . . ." are adequate. Some pathologists and clinicians feel the need to indicate the significant features of the autopsy report and clinical history on the cause of death statement. If it is sequenced correctly this is not inaccurate, but it is somewhat unnecessary.

Nosologists who work within a strict framework code the individual statements on the death certificate. What is placed on a death certificate may or may not be coded as the certifier had intended, either on paper or in their thought processes. An accidental manner of death is applied to situations where the cause is due to unintended events. These may include reactions to drugs, alcohol, blunt or sharp force, or "semi-natural" situations such as an anaphylactic reaction to a bee sting, peanut butter, or radiologic dyes.

Homicide

Homicide is defined simply as "death at the hands of another individual." It does not imply the true intent of one person to kill another, such as an assassination, but encompasses a wide range of scenarios. For example, the justified shooting of an individual by a police officer is classified as a homicide, even after internal affairs conducts a criminal investigation and the officer is found to be completely within his or her rights and responsibilities to have fired and fatally wounded the individual. The classification of homicide is often used inconsistently—one jurisdiction may call a hit and run fatality of a pedestrian by a person driving a motor vehicle as homicide whereas another may classify it as an accident if the vehicle was not used as a weapon. Similarly, a death caused by a small child playing with a firearm may be called a homicide in one jurisdiction and an accident in another.

Suicide

A suicide usually indicates that the injuries have been caused intentionally by the individual to bring about his or her death. The classic scenario of Russian roulette frequently initiates debate as to whether this is a suicide or an accident. Modification of the word *intentionally* with the concept of volition, indicating a voluntary act that leads to somebody's death, may help clarify the debate, or at least allow consistency among forensic specialists.

Accident

For the manner of death to be certified as accident, the circumstances surrounding the death must be outside of the control of any individual. The most common accident is a motor vehicle death, unless it is determined that the vehicle was being used as a weapon. Other more subtle accidents include deaths from bee stings or unforeseen complications of a surgical procedure.

The determination of the manner of death by a coroner or medical examiner often has no effect on how other organizations interested in that particular death will act. The certification of the death as an accident does not in any way prevent or inhibit the district attorney from filing any range of charges against the person who inflicted the fatal injuries. Also, insurance companies do not automatically accept an accidental manner of death as having fulfilled the particular definition of "accident" in the death benefit policy for the deceased individual.

In other parts of the world death investigation systems may require that the medical certifier not indicate a manner of death. This is often done by the legal authorities that correlate the medical findings with the laws of that country.

Identification

The importance of accurately identifying the deceased is paramount for obvious reasons, as exemplified by the fact that the name is the very first box to be completed on the death certificate. The family will want to have the correct remains returned to them as soon as possible for burial or cremation (Figure 15–2). The identification process is crucial in situations of homicide where the presentation in court must satisfy the legal standards that the deceased individual is who the prosecutors say it is.

Pa. woman mistakenly identified as victim in fatal car accident

HARRISBURG, Pa. (AP) — Funeral arrangements were being made and relatives mourned for Denise Dieter, a 23-year-old law student identified by her stepfather and grandfather as the victim of a car accident.

But as the family gathered in her father's home near Philadelphia on Sept. 15, Dieter walked into her apartment in Harrisburg. Her startled roommate said, "You'd better call your dad."

The crash the day before had obliterated the female victim's face. She had striking similarities to Dieter, who was supposed to have been in the car en route to a picnic but had changed her mind at the last minute.

The victim, Cindy Bowers, was the same height and weight as Dieter. They had the same hair color and were wearing identical hair barrettes. They both had double-pierced ears, were wearing the same earrings and had similar key rings.

"It was really bizarre and weird," Dieter said in a telephone interview.

Ms. Dieter said that when she walked into her Harrisburg apartment that Sunday, her roommate, Jackie Rodriquez, became hysterical and could only blurt out for Ms. Dieter to call her father.

"I thought somebody in my family died," Dieter said.

When Ms. Dieter called her father's home, her stepmother, Patti Dieter, answered.

"I said, 'Hey Patti, What's up?'" Dieter recalled. "She was stunned. She said, 'Denise, they're planning your funeral. Where the hell are you?'

"My father grabbed the phone, he was hysterical. He kept saying, 'Oh my God, oh my God, oh my God.' At this point, I knew they thought I was dead."

Dieter, a second-year student at Widener Law School's Harrisburg campus, had been invited to a picnic to hobnob with lawyers.

"I called and said I wasn't going," she said. "I don't know why."

Figure 15–2   Media report of mistaken identity.

CLINICAL FORENSIC NURSING

The forensic nurse has an important role in an emergency room, operating room, or walk-in clinic: to identify and document injuries in nondeceased patients. As with any type of investigation, appropriate and persistent interviewing is crucial for correlating the injuries with the event. A diagram, 35 mm photography, Polaroids, and digital imaging, with and without rulers, are all valuable for documenting injuries. Also, photographic or digital documentation of injuries should be done over time, either on a daily or every other day basis for a week to 10 days. This is to show the development and possible distribution of injuries, as well as the aging process and the possibility of identifying a pattern within the injuries that was not initially readily apparent. This identification and documentation is important in the event of a subsequent trial, because the victim cannot demonstrate to the jury the nature of the injuries if they have already healed. Utilization of alternate light sources for the identification, preservation, and collection of evidence can also be done by the forensic nurse.

Utilizing this particular area of forensic nursing expertise beyond direct patient care, is somewhat problematic because the only true constituency for this service would be prosecutors. A clinical forensic nurse could be an extension of the medical examiner's office and ideally would be available 24 hours a day for consultation in emergency room and operating room settings. In the new age of HIPAA (Health Insurance Portability and Accountability Act of 1996), the patient, victim, or even perpetrator's permission would be needed to perform this service, or the nurse would need access to a search warrant. The exam would have to be done in a timely fashion because debridement and cleaning of wounds may destroy intimate trace evidence, and treatment and time delay may modify the ability to document the injury in its more "native" state.

Forensic nurses have also made inroads into professionalizing the rape examination by developing the sexual assault nurse examiner (SANE) program. This has developed into an extremely important and valuable service that the nurse can provide, including giving comfort to the victim, explaining in detail the medical procedures and potential complications, and examining the victim for the purpose of documenting injuries and collecting trace evidence. Demonstrating the advantage of using the skills of a forensic nurse to prosecutors and possibly plaintiff's attorneys will be a long, but potentially rewarding journey in the area of forensic nursing.

TIME OF DEATH AND POSTMORTEM CHANGES

There is *no* scientific method for determining the exact time of death outside of a monitored medical setting or an eyewitness. Beyond these modalities, there is nothing about the changes that occur to a human body after death that will in any way be entirely accurate. Only a range should be given based on numerous factors. When the death investigator is asked to give an opinion about the time of death or the time since death, the investigator should establish the two limiting points: when the person was last reliably known to be alive and when the person was found dead. The point at which the person was found dead is relatively easily determined, but the point at which the person was last reliably known to be alive is not that easy. Interviews with family, friends, and coworkers are of course a place to start. The investigator can review personal computers for activity at some particular clock time, such as was done in the investigation into the death of Chondra Levy. Answering machine messages and telephone records are also useful. It is important to recognize that the reliability of any information, particularly regarding when somebody was last known to be alive, must be verified. Witnesses may intentionally mislead the investigator or the witness may be incompetent, due to chemical impairment or brain disease. The time frame that is developed can be a range of minutes, hours, days, weeks, months, or years. Multiple interviews over time may identify witnesses or situations that provide additional information relevant to the times and dates when the person was last seen, thus narrowing the time frame. Even if the time period between last reliably known alive and found dead is a matter of minutes, that is the limit of accuracy.

The three classic pillars used for time of death estimations based solely on examination of the body are rigor mortis, livor mortis, and algor mortis. These are chemical and physical changes that all deceased individuals undergo, but there is such individual and environmental variability and lack of established "testing" criteria that they can be utilized only in the face of appropriate investigative information.

Rigor Mortis

Rigor mortis, or rigidity, is a chemical process within the skeletal muscle cells that causes the cross-linking of the actin and myosin fibers in the muscle cells due to decreased oxygen, lack of ATP production, and the postmortem leakage of calcium from the sarcoplasmic reticulum. This process is manifested by the progressive stiffening of muscles. Rigidity develops in all muscle cells simultaneously at the time of death with the loss of ATP production, although it may be detected in smaller muscle groups before larger ones. These changes, in general, come on over approximately 12 hours, will peak through 24 hours, and will begin to wane through the next 12 hours. This chemical process is accelerated by heat and retarded by cold. In warm environments rigidity can come on more quickly and start to disappear more quickly. There is also "instantaneous" rigor called cadaveric spasm. The theory behind this process is the rapid premortem loss of muscular ATP caused by intensive muscular activity, such as a tonic-clonic seizure, a foot chase, or struggling during drowning. There are numerous reports of an individual holding some object in their hand in full rigor, which, if it were not instantaneous, would not be possible.

There is no "test" for rigidity. It is strictly a qualitative assessment as to the distribution and quantity of the muscle stiffness. The investigator can attempt to manipulate the major joints, particularly the jaw, elbows, and knees, to assess the rigidity. The communication of the quality of the rigor should be descriptive, such as "the jaw is freely moveable, the elbow joint cannot be extended even with great effort, and the knee joint rigidity is easily broken." These types of descriptive phrases are more valuable to the reader than such words as "full rigor" or "partial rigor."

The most important aspect of rigor mortis is the documentation that it is appropriate for the position in which the deceased is found. It is impossible to die, pass out after a night of alcohol, or fall asleep with one's arm straight up in the air perpendicular to the floor (Figure 15–3). If the deceased individual is found in this position, one knows immediately that the body has been moved after the person has been dead long enough for rigidity to form in another position. Often that original position can be easily re-created. The determination that the deceased has been moved is important for police investigators because it indicates an altered death scene. This may have occurred innocently by a first responder, a layperson, emergency medical personnel, or the police.

Livor Mortis

The second postmortem change is livor mortis, or lividity. This is a chemical process that occurs after the heart stops beating and circulation through the arteries and veins can no longer be accomplished. The lack of circulation allows for the blood, particularly in the veins where the vessels are elastic and capillaries have little vascular integrity, to settle and collect in the dependent portion of the body in line with gravity (Figure 15–4). If the deceased is lying on their back the livor would

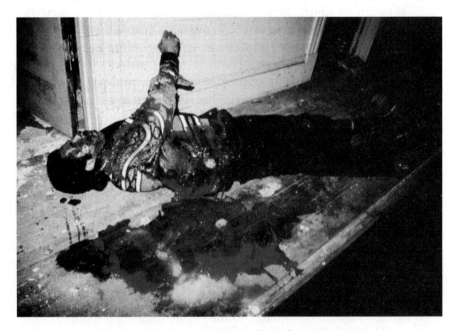

Figure 15–3 Inappropriate Rigor Mortis (rigidity) for a supine position.

accumulate over the posterior aspect of the body. Lividity can come on relatively quickly, depending on the integrity of the cardiovascular system. An elderly person with heart disease may already have compromised circulation, and lividity may even be evident in the perimortem period. In a healthy individual lividity would be detectable in the first couple of hours.

The intravascular blood is liquid, and when pressure is applied to the dependent portion of the body the blood can be squeezed out of the capillary bed and the skin will blanch. After approximately 6 hours the blood will begin to coagulate, and if the skin is compressed and it does not blanch, the livor is said to be fixed. If the position of the body is then changed, a small amount of livor may be detectable in the new dependent portion, but most of it will remain in the original dependent position. Blanched areas in the livor, where the weight of the body compresses the skin and the dermal capillaries are commonly seen over the buttocks, the elbows, and the region of the shoulder blades. It may also be notable in areas of the body that are compressed with clothing, particularly elastic in waistbands or underwear, or objects that the person might be lying on (Figure 15–5).

Using lividity to determine time of death is fraught with tremendous error and must be correlated with the information as to when the person

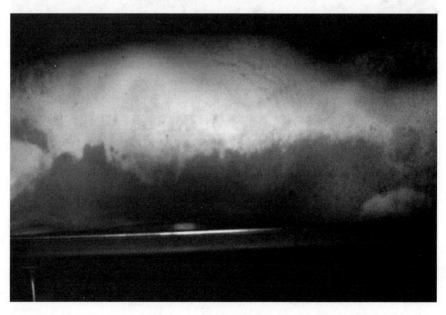

Figure 15–4 Livor mortis evidenced by posterior pooling of blood.

was last reliably known to be alive. Similar to rigidity, lividity is useful in assessing whether the person has been moved after death. An altered death scene is assumed if the person is laying face down and all the livor is noted on their back.

Algor Mortis

Algor mortis is a physical process that uses the physical concept of temperature equilibrium. Mammals and birds are homeotherms, which means they generate their own heat. The maintenance of a relatively constant body temperature is important for maximum operation of enzyme systems that have evolved over hundreds of thousands of years. This is in contradistinction to cold-blooded animals that require an external source of heat to elevate their body temperatures and cellular enzyme systems to an efficient mode. After death the body will cool and ultimately equilibrate to the environmental temperature. Knight, 1995 indicated up to eight models by which measuring body temperature in the early postmortem period might be useful for an estimation of the postmortem interval. Numerous variables must be taken into account: the weight and relative body mass of the individual, the amount of clothing the person is wearing, the humidity of the environment, the temperature of the environment, the temperature of the surface that the deceased is laying on, wind speed,

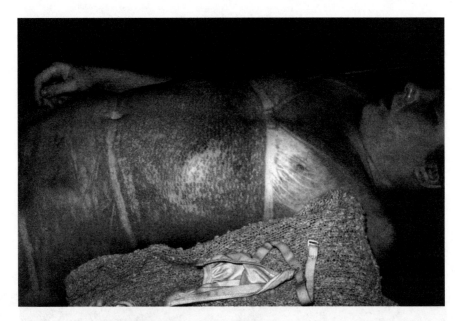

Figure 15–5 Livor mortis showing blanching from undergarments.

and the body temperature that the person had prior to their death. Some of these, such as height and weight, can be measured and incorporated into a nomogram.

One of the models, called the "rule of thumb model," states that the human body in the early postmortem period will cool off 1.5 to 2 degrees Fahrenheit per hour (Figure 15–6). Therefore, a postmortem core (rectal) temperature of 90 degrees would suggest that the person has been dead approximately 6 hours. Once again, because of the numerous variables, only a range should be given, and it should ultimately be correlated with other investigative information. Many death investigation jurisdictions do not even utilize postmortem core body temperatures, and this is often a theoretical discussion.

Entomology

The most scientific estimate of the postmortem interval is achieved through forensic entomology. An entomologist specializes in the study of insects and their life cycles (Figure 15–7). Shortly after a death occurs, insects such as the fly are able to detect chemical molecules that attract them to the remains. The flies will search for a source of liquid food, which is primarily at the natural body openings that are exposed, including the mouth, nose, eyes, ears, and potentially the creases in the neck where fluids might accumulate. If there is a suitable source of food, the flies will then breed and the female will lay hundreds of eggs. These eggs will ultimately hatch into larvae (maggots), which have teeth and will feed on the tissue in the region of their hatching. Bodies that are colonized by flies and other insects will rapidly be consumed, usually start-

---

Temperature-Based Models

Eight Different Models

#1 "Rule of Thumb"

$$\text{P.M.I. (hours)} = \frac{98.6 - \text{rectal temp (F)}}{1.5}$$

Figure 15–6 Estimating time of death from temperature.

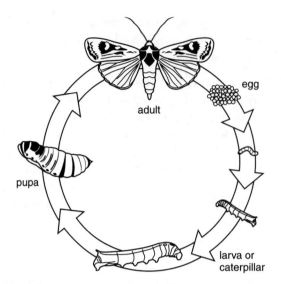

Figure 15–7   Estimating time of death from an insect life-cycle.

ing with the soft tissues of the head and working downward into the chest and abdominal cavities and then ultimately toward the extremities. Ultimately, if the conditions are suitable, complete skeletonization can be accomplished.

Samples of both live and dead insect larvae, as well as adult species, can and should be taken as evidence, preserved in the appropriate media, and sent to a forensic entomologist for evaluation. Information such as where the samples were taken, the general location of the remains (indoors, woods, open parking lot, near a body of water, etc.), and the range of environmental temperatures surrounding the 2- to 3-week period when the remains may have been exposed will greatly enhance the interpretation of the insect evidence.

Bioenvironmental evidence is useful because species of flies grow at a certain rate, and the size of the larvae can be calculated and an estimated minimum postmortem interval can be generated. Remember, this is a minimum postmortem interval and not an exact time of death. There is no way to calculate, other than by history, when exactly the remains had opportunity to be colonized. If the remains were indoors or in an enclosed space for several days prior to being deposited in a site where insects would have access to them, then that would not be known simply by the insect examination.

Identifying, preserving, and collecting insect evidence, whether they be the common fly larvae, beetles, wasps, or bees, can help the consulting forensic entomologist recreate the micro and macro bioenvironmental scene. An opinion can then be offered as to what the minimal postmortem interval is, based on the evidence of insect attraction, reproduction, and maturation. The death investigator should provide as much background information as possible to the entomologist for the most accurate estimation. This should include the location of the remains (e.g., house, car trunk, forest, beach) as well as temperature variations from the closest measuring station to where the remains were located.

The anatomic site of insect collection is also important. The deceased quickly attracts flies, which, requiring liquid for feeding, go to natural body openings, such as the nose, mouth, eyes, and ears, as mentioned earlier. Therefore, these are the locations where eggs are laid and the insect larvae will hatch. Insect larval activity at other atypical areas such as hands, extremities, or torso indicate an alternate, more attractive source of liquid fuel, such as blood from a wound. Photographic and written reports as to the distribution of the insect larvae will be helpful not only in determining the postmortem interval, but also for the possible identification of morbid or fatal injuries. Bioenvironmental evidence may be beneath the body in the soil or around the body in the vegetation. This is particularly true of flying adult insects that may also give information about the micro environmental activity; these should also be collected and appropriately preserved for evaluation.

It is also useful to collect all evident insect species, whether they are associated intimately with the remains, are under the remains, or are flying around the remains. The concept of succession indicates that various types of insects will be attracted to the remains at various stages during this type of decompositional process. Certain species are attracted to the fresh remains, other species are attracted to partly decayed remains, and other species such as beetles are attracted to the decomposers. Some species will actually feed on the insect larvae. Exploring the soil around the remains may also help identify species that have started their final development and have formed pupa casings or are feeding off of the liquid decompositional fluid beneath the body. Collecting a wide variety of specimens will ensure the best information given by the consultant.

The forensic entomologist will use the various combinations of the collected insects associated with the remains to help determine more accurately the postmortem interval. Forensic entomologists Dr. Wayne Lord of the FBI and Dr. Lee Goff of Chaminade University in Hawaii point out that "if you know the players on the field, then you can tell what inning the game is in (Goff, p. 487, 2000)."

Summary

Although there is no scientific method to determine the time of death, the correlation between when the deceased was last reliably known to be alive, when they were found deceased, the other environmental and investigative information such as mail or newspaper deliveries, computer analysis, and witness statements, in conjunction with the early postmortem changes and modalities such as forensic entomology, can be very useful in narrowing down the time of death. This is not necessary in all deaths, but for deaths where it is necessary to confirm or deny an alibi, this information would be crucial.

HUMAN DECOMPOSITION

Autolysis

After death, unless the normal pattern of decay of a deceased entity is inhibited by such processes as freezing or chemical alteration such as embalming, the cells in the tissues will naturally break down. After death, the lack of oxygen to the cells causes the earliest form of postmortem decomposition called autolysis. Autolysis is Greek for "breakdown of self," and is simply due to the lack of oxygen. This is more evident in cells with large quantities of enzymes, such as those within the pancreas and the adrenal glands. Autolytic changes such as softening and loss of histologic structure are evident several hours after death. The most dramatic example of postmortem autolysis is the intrauterine death of a fetus that is retained for 1 to 2 days, if the demise is not infection related. The fetus will begin to "macerate," with development of skin slip; loss of subtle, then more obvious, anatomic features; darkening of the skin that is homogeneous and diffuse; and ultimately loss of anatomic detail and darkening of the internal organs. The most typical etiology of this type of intrauterine death with maceration (autolysis) would be a compromised umbilical cord causing a decreased flow of oxygen to the fetus.

Skin Slip

Skin slip is an autolytic process in which the intercellular bridges, or connections, begin to break down and one layer of skin will literally slip off of or away from the layer beneath with a small amount of applied pressure. This can be seen 24 to 48 hours after death. It can be seen even more quickly in situations such as carbon monoxide poisoning, because the toxicity of the gas causes rapid cellular death, and where there are focal or environmental elevations of temperature. Skin slip is common in areas where there might be pressure, such as the upper back where the shoulder blades protrude, the buttocks, or the hips. This normal postmortem autolytic change can be quite dramatic. A deceased person who appears to be fairly well preserved at a scene may have dramatic evidence of skin slip when ultimately examined at the autopsy room due to the multiple manipulations of the body during the transport from the scene to the autopsy facility.

The presence of skin slip can be useful to the medical examiner. When the cellular connections break down on the hands due to immersion or the process of decay, the thick palmar skin can literally be removed intact as a "glove." This "glove" can then be placed over the gloved hand of the examiner and fingerprints and even palm prints of good quality can be rolled and be useful for identification purposes when facial feature distortion may preclude visual identification.

Putrefaction

The next, and most dramatic, aspect of decomposition is due to a process called putrefaction. This process is a bacterial-mediated progressive form of decay that occurs through the interaction of bacteria with all plant and animal material. This process is seen frequently in the home when milk, vegetables, or other foods begin to "spoil" and are no longer edible.

Both the external and internal surfaces of the body are extensively colonized by bacteria, which are held in check by the normal human immunological systems. After death, when these systems are no longer functioning, the bacteria will break through their normal constraints and utilize the tissues as a "culture medium." Because of the high concentration of bacteria in the intestinal tract, particularly in the colon or large intestine, the putrefactive process is visually observed in the right lower quadrant of the abdomen as a greenish discoloration of the skin. This represents the region of the cecum and the progressive and unrelenting growth of bacteria utilizing the wall of the colon as an area of growth. In "moderate" temperatures this is evident approximately 24 hours after death.

Because putrefaction is a bacterial process, it is extremely sensitive to temperature. Just as food is able to be preserved in the freezer nearly indefinitely or in the refrigerator for at least days, if not weeks, a body in a cold environment may not show evidence of putrefaction for a prolonged period of time. However, even in a morgue refrigerator bodies will eventually decay because cold will only slow down and not kill the bacteria. This is the reason why embalming is important, because the tissues are modified chemically so that the bacteria cannot act upon them, and the remains will be preserved in the short term for whatever funeral arrangements the family has made.

This putrefactive decaying process can be very rapid in warm environments. The bacteria will continue to grow, causing breakdown of the tissues similar to that seen in autolysis where there is loss of subtle and then more dramatic anatomic features, darkening of the skin associated with skin slip, and bloating of the eyelids, lips, abdomen, penis, and scrotum. This is due to the production of gas by the bacteria. This gas can be foul smelling and is often the reason why deceased individuals are eventually discovered. As these gases continue to be produced they can force the liquefying tissues out of the natural body openings (the nose, mouth, and anus). This process is called purging, and can be quite dramatic, particularly if the deceased is face down. It is often initially felt to be related to trauma and must be correlated with the scene and circumstances surrounding the death. It can have a dark purple-red-black color and may be pooling around the head. The bacteria will continue to cause the tissues to decay over a period of weeks.

Mummification

The putrefactive process is in competition with other processes such as mummification. This is not related to the mummification used by Egyptians caring for deceased rulers, where the tissues were actually removed from the body and the remains were wrapped and preserved chemically. Mummification refers simply to the dehydration of tissue. As the putrefactive process continues, the external surfaces of the body may begin to dry out, particularly in a warm, dry environment, to the point where either all of the skin or certain portions of the skin surface, whether it is the face, chest, abdomen, or extremities, will become leathery and so hardened that they cannot be cut with a scalpel. Mummification is often seen in the fingertips and hands where little bacterial activity occurs. This makes the process of fingerprinting the body difficult, if not impossible. The friction ridges may be visible, but because of the wrinkling and the lack of pliability, they cannot be recorded by usual fingerprint techniques. The processes of autolysis, putrefaction, and mummification are often competing, depending on the macro and micro environments.

Saponification

Another postmortem change, saponification, is dependent upon a wet environment. This process results in the hydrolysis of the subcutaneous adipose tissue into a waxy type material (sometimes called grave wax or adipocere) that is akin to soap. Wherever subcutaneous fat is located this process can develop. This process can take weeks to months depending on the environment in which the remains are located. Often the internal structures that are encased by this waxy shell are fairly well preserved and easy to autopsy.

Vegetation Changes

Bioenvironmental evidence, which involves the local vegetation, may give indications and clues that a decaying body is either located at a particular place or had been located there. Broken vegetation or discolored leaves from the gases produced by the bacteria and emitted from the decaying remains may give the first visual signs that there has been a disturbance or alteration in this area. Denser growth provided by the nitrogen nutrients from the decaying remains may also provide evidence that remains have been buried at this particular location. Because of this accelerated growth in the vegetation, infrared photography, particularly from an elevated platform such as a helicopter or unmanned fixed wing drone, may assist in identifying a clandestine grave. Broken plant material should be collected as well as any plant life that is intimately associated with the remains. These might include mosses growing on bones or individual plants that have grown through bones. The plants, including the roots, should be collected, wrapped in newspaper, and placed in a dry place in preparation for submitting to a botanist who understands the local vegetation. Photographs of the location are also crucial. This will assist the botanist in understanding the bioenvironmental locale.

Soil Samples

The soil samples in and around a suspected clandestine grave can also be useful. Decompositional proteins and fatty acids will leech into the soil, which can then be analyzed. Also, the disruption of the stratification of the soil will prove that there has been a disturbance in that area, whether remains are recovered or not. It is always important to remember that "controls" and providing as much information as possible to the consulting forensic scientist will yield the best analysis.

Anthropologic Evidence

The availability for consultation, both at the death scene and in the autopsy facility, with a forensic anthropologist is crucial to the operation of any death investigation system. It is not uncommon for bones to be discovered in a variety of situations such as a family pet bringing one to the house, private or public digging for renovation or construction purposes, or discovery in fill dirt. The forensic anthropologist has to immediately be able to answer the simple question "Are these bony remains human?" If this question can be answered in the negative, then there is no concern for police officials and nothing further need be done, although it is wise to not return the bony remains to the discovering or presenting authority, because the same bone may end up having to be re-evaluated in the near future when it is rediscovered in a second site. If the question is answered in the affirmative, it then needs to be determined, probably by the anthropologist, whether the remains are historic or recent.

The discovery of historic human remains (defined as remains that are old enough that any assailant would no longer still be alive, i.e., 100 years) is not uncommon. Throughout New England and the eastern seaboard are numerous undocumented colonial and Native American gravesites. These are frequently discovered serendipitously. It is important to know that if the remains are identified as Native American then all efforts must be made by the local authorities and any state archaeology group to return the remains to the tribes that were known to have been located historically in that region.

If the remains are identified as human and "recent," then it is likely that they have been buried in a criminal-related manner. It is then imperative that a forensic anthropologist have access to the remains to determine the age at death, the ancestral background (Asian, African, or European), and sex. If the remains are determined to be prepubescent, the determination of age to within 6 months to 1 year is relatively easy because the eruption of teeth and the growth of individual bones and the fusion of epiphyses (growth plates) is fairly constant. It would be impossible by morphology alone to determine the sex of the individual and also difficult to identify the ancestry.

The age of an adult can be determined to a range of approximately 5 years based on bone morphology, epiphyseal and cranial suture closure, and wear on the face of the pubic symphysis. The intact skeleton also makes it very easy to determine the sex primarily by examination of the morphology of the pelvis. The female pelvis is designed for childbirth and has a significantly different shape than the male pelvis. The nature of the muscles also shows smaller and more gracile areas of muscle attachment due to the lack of testosterone, which creates larger muscles, and therefore more robust muscle attachments to bone. Ancestral determinations are more difficult, particularly as interracial marriages and progeny are produced. Stature can be estimated from multiple measurements of the long bones.

The forensic anthropologist is also invaluable in identifying deformities of the skeletal structures that may have been caused by natural disease processes, which would help identify the individual through medical history and/or suggest a cause of death. The identification of subtle blunt and sharp force trauma, including gunshot wounds and their directionality, is also information that the consultant can provide to the forensic pathologist, the death investigators, and law enforcement. The identification of human remains that are completely skeletonized is always an interesting challenge.

IDENTIFICATION OF HUMAN REMAINS

Mass fatality events require the death investigation system to utilize multiple methods so that the correct remains are returned to the grieving families. The anguish and stress inherent in these situations is played out vividly in the media and can add to a family's distress. Examples such as the identification of the victims of the terrorist attacks on the World Trade Center, the Pentagon, and United Flight 93 on September 11, 2001, and more recently the identification of the sons of Saddam Hussein, are dramatic examples of such media coverage. The process of identification is simply a comparison of premortem data with postmortem data. This can be done circumstantially, where the premortem record is somebody's memory, compared with a postmortem personal viewing of the remains and/or a photograph of the deceased. Identification is done frequently at the medical examiner's office, hospital, or funeral home.

Fortunately, most of the people in this country are who they are purported to be, and visual identification is readily acceptable, especially because true positive identification for everyone would be too costly and time consuming. Problems with visual identification as the primary method occurs in the case of identical twins; friends or family that have not seen the deceased for some period of time; trauma that obscures or modifies the identifying features, including treatment such as bandages; and/or a healing process that includes swelling, hematoma formation, and inflammation. The most recognizable features of a person are their eyes and hair. Distortion of these areas complicates the visual identification process. The circumstantial identification would also include appropriate "circumstances" where an individual of known age, race, and sex is compared using anthropomorphic techniques with the deceased individual. For example, an elderly Caucasian male who lived alone has not been seen recently and the remains of an elderly Caucasian male are found in the burned house where he was known to reside, allowing for a circumstantial identification. These are nonscientific methods. In order to positively identify an individual, premortem data such as dental records, fingerprints, direct or indirect DNA samples, or X rays must be sought out and recovered. There may be extremely unique features of a person such as distribution of tattoos, scars, surgical clips, or prostheses that may at least give clues as to the identity of the person during the initial stages of identification, but may also rise to the level of positive identification at some point. The scientific and statistical elimination of all other persons on the planet would be a positive identification.

The investigator, with the assistance of the investigating police department, should seek out all premortem data that is available, whether the situation involves a single individual or a mass fatality situation. These would include age, race, and sex documentation; dental records; previous X rays (Figure 15–8), from either a clinic, a

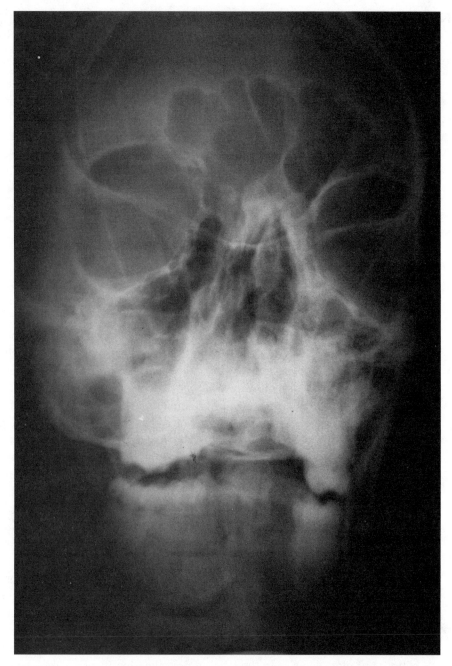

Figure 15–8 X-ray of skull showing unique characteristics (frontal sinuses).

walk-in immediate medical care center, or a hospital; and previous sources of fingerprints such as arrest records, military service, civil service, pistol permits, or immigration records. The premortem data is often assembled when an individual is reported missing, especially when the circumstances suggest that the individual may have been the victim of an assault and is likely to have died. The search for premortem records if no family is readily identifiable can be difficult, but personal records; hospital, medical, or dental bills; interviews with friends; and record searches of hospital or walk-in clinics in the vicinity of the person's home or workplace will generate leads to premortem records that will be helpful in identification.

The postmortem data is available from the autopsy examination. Forensic technicians are often quite skilled in obtaining fingerprints from recently deceased individuals or even badly decomposed individuals. The process of autolysis causes the thick palmar skin to slough off the deeper layers, often intact. The sloughed skin can be placed over the gloved finger of the technician, who can take his or her time to roll fingerprints (Figures 15–9 and 15–10). Desiccated, mummified, or water-logged (washerwoman) fingertips require potential rehydration and/or subcutaneous injection with various fluids to reconstitute and create rollable prints. Prior to any manipulation of the fingerprints a photograph should be taken in case the friction ridges are ruined or are unable to be rolled.

It may be necessary to enlist the services of a consulting dentist to help appropriately document the jaws (Figures 15–11 and 15–12). A consulting dentist is also crucial to help evaluate and interpret dental records in order to make a positive identification. A forensic anthropologist is invaluable, particularly when the remains are badly decomposed or completely skeletonized, to determine the basic age, race, and sex of the individual. Other valuable individual osseous features that might be useful for identification can be documented. Appropriate samples can be taken from the deceased for DNA typing. A simple blood sample is valuable; however, if the remains are in an advanced state of decomposition, bone marrow or teeth where cellular and nuclear material are protected against decay are valuable specimens.

When we see our husband, wife, children, coworkers, or friends, we are comparing the known data (i.e., our memories) with the "unknown data" (i.e., the person that is standing before us at that particular moment). The most identifying features of a human being are their face, including their eyes and eye color, and their hair. If an individual, such as a celebrity, wishes to become somewhat anonymous they either go someplace where they might not be recognized or they put on sunglasses, a hat, and generic clothing. Technically, the process of visual

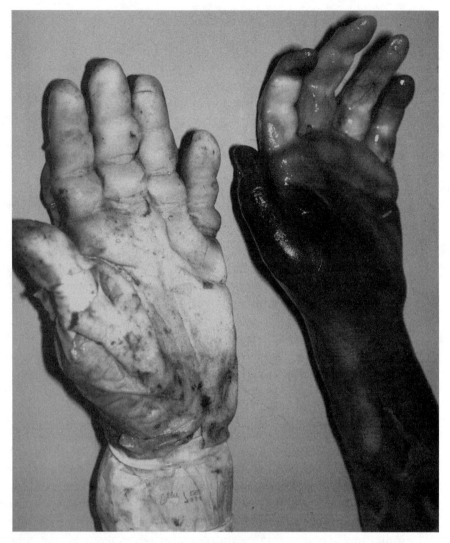

Figure 15–9 Autolyzed glove placed on technicians hand to effectively roll finger-prints.

identification is not a "positive" identification. Even parents or siblings often mistake identical twins for each other. Babies and children, before they have had a chance to develop significant individuating features such as eye color and hair color, can be confused. People that are injured, such that their features are distorted by the trauma, and if they survive, by the treatment (surgical modification, suturing, and bandaging) and/or healing processes (edema, discoloration from bruising), also may not be readily identifiable by even the closest relative or friend. Also, postmortem changes such as putrefaction and insect infestation

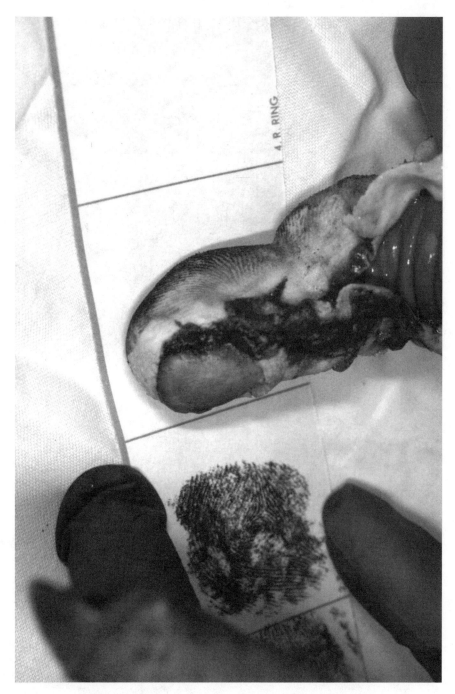

Figure 15–10   Printing de-gloved fingers of deceased.

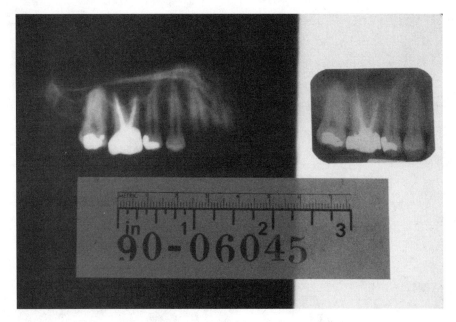

Figure 15–11   Post- and premortem dental x-rays for comparison.

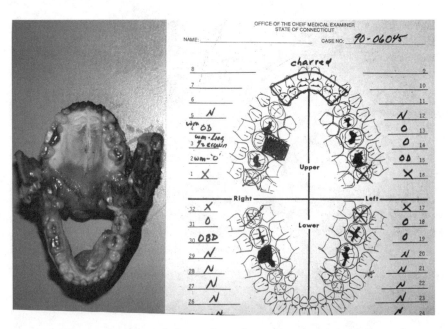

Figure 15–12   Excised jaws and charted teeth as the postmortem record.

can destroy the features that are readily identifiable such as the shape of the nose or facial or head hair.

The vast majority of identifications, either on live people or deceased, are done visually. Somebody looking at an injured person and declaring their name, someone witnessing an event, or a family member viewing a body at a funeral home and signing an identification form are everyday occurrences that are uncomplicated. When they are complicated, or when there is a specific need for more definitive determination such as a civil (paternity) or legal reason, a positive identification must be accomplished.

Tattoos and semipermanent features may not rise to the level of positive identification, but may help investigators establish a strong tentative identification. Because tattoos are handmade and are of specific numbers, at certain anatomic locations, and contain certain details, they can be compared with an artist's tattoo log or family photographs for positive ID.

A positive identification is a statistical comparison and elimination of the possibility of anyone else on the planet being confused with the person in question. This is accomplished by: a) the determination that there is no apparent dissimilarity or discordance, and b) the identification of multiple points of similarity. The more points of similarity, the greater statistical likelihood that one would reach a confidence level that is well beyond even the remotest chance.

The gold standard for positive identification has been fingerprint comparison. The friction ridges on the palmar surfaces of the hands, as well as the feet, are unique, even to identical twins, and for decades have been utilized in positively identifying individual human beings. The advent of molecular biology over the last several decades, starting with simple ABO blood typing, and progressing to identification of different isoenzymes within cells to the nuclear and mitochondrial extraction, even in the most minimal specimen of DNA, has and will continue to revolutionize individuation. The process of comparing pre- and postmortem dental records is also a common practice. However, this and techniques such as pre- and postmortem comparison of any X ray can be accomplished only if a tentative identification has been done. One cannot seek out dental or medical records from their repositories without knowing who you are looking for. This is unlike comparison to large databanks such as the automated fingerprint identification system (AFIS), where an unknown print can be put into the system and compared to those present in the database, and the growing development of DNA databases. The forensic nurse is invaluable in seeking, reviewing, and understanding medical and dental records and understanding where the repositories might be, such as hospitals, walk-in clinics, industrial medical offices, clinics, and private and university-based dental offices.

Another unique method of either assisting or accomplishing a positive identification involves tracking down serial numbers from such items as pacemakers, breast implants, orthopedic prostheses, and hearing aids.

When a body is badly decomposed, burned beyond visual recognition, or the legal system requires a positive identification, the collection and documentation of postmortem data and the collection of premortem data may take a significant period of time as the repositories are searched. If the person is completely unidentified, the first step in identification is to consult local, state, and even national missing person registries. If no missing person reports have been filed, the remains, regardless of the cause of death, may never be identified.

TYPES OF INJURY

Blunt Trauma

Injury or damage to tissue as a result of the application of some quantity and quality of force results in what is called blunt force trauma. The individual's tissue reaction to the magnitude and direction of force can potentially give information about the nature of the event. The force can be applied to the tissue in either of two ways: a moving object can impact the body or vice versa. Identical applications of force with the same direction and magnitude may not result in the same type of injury to different people. An important variable is the quality of the tissue of the individual to which the force is applied. A young individual who has supple, pliable skin and elastic ribs may show no external and little internal injury because the force is easily diffused throughout the tissue without overcoming the tensile or elastic strength of the tissue. In contrast, an elderly person with thin, fragile skin and osteoporosis may suffer significant injury with potentially lethal consequences from the same force that caused minor injury in the young person. Other variables include the normal cyclical interaction of the immune system, causing the same individual to react differently to the same application of force just weeks apart, based on the current capabilities of their immune system that may be affected by stress or diet. Diseases also render the tissue more or less vulnerable. Skin diseases, infection, or cancer all modify the tissues' ability to withstand the application of force.

Blunt force trauma is the most common type of trauma seen in clinical forensic medicine or forensic pathology. Nearly every person, every day, is walking around with some evidence of blunt force trauma, from the tiniest scratch or bruise to injury that would require intensive nursing care. The evidence of the tissues' reaction to the applied force is broken down into four categories: abrasions, contusions, lacerations, and fractures.

Abrasions

Abrasions are injuries of the skin that result in damage of various layers of the epidermis. If the force is applied tangentially then it results in a scratch-type injury. This can be a linear injury or, if the surface is broad, it can be a very wide confluent collection of linear scratches retaining their individuality or coalescing into one large area of denuded epithelium. Close examination of the wound may find tiny triangular-shaped tissue segments whose apical point is directed opposite to the vector of force, or pointing to where the force came from (Figure 15–13). Also, there may be a collection of the abraded epithelium at one edge of the wound (Figure 15–14). This epithelial piling also indicates the direction of force.

Even the most mundane or simple abrasion-type blunt force injury should be documented in detail because a history or witness statement may be confirmed or denied simply on the basis of one nonlethal, relatively "minor" injury. Abrasions can be superficial or deep, with the deeper ones having a much redder base and being more likely to bleed. The quantity of blood from abrasion is relatively minor compared to other types of injuries. After death, if the abrasion is exposed, it may begin to dry out. It may have a dry maroon-brown color or may even blacken. As the injury dries out, the subtleties and potentially even a pattern that it may have had in the fresh state become obscured. After death, force can still be applied to a body and cause injuries. A postmortem abrasion should have no evidence of a "vital reaction" such as erythema or swelling. It often has a dull yellow-tan appearance with no margin of redness. The abrasion is, by definition, the exact point of force on the skin.

Contusions

A contusion, or bruise, is defined simply as blood leaking into tissues after the vessels have been disrupted by the application of force. A contusion can be seen in any tissue, including the skin, brain, lungs, or liver; bone is not included because if there is enough force to break blood vessels within the bone it will cause the fourth type of blunt trauma, a fracture. The amount of energy required to break blood vessels within the skin, in the subcutaneous tissue, or within an organ causing the leaking of red blood cells, is really quite variable, depending on the quantity and quality of the force as well as the elasticity of the tissue.

A contusion or a bruise does not necessarily indicate the exact point of force. If blood vessels are broken, then the blood can dissect

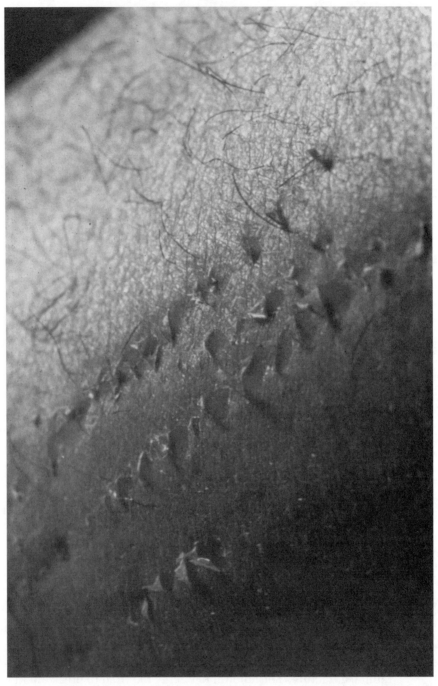

Figure 15–13   Scrape-type abrasion with force directed top right to bottom left.

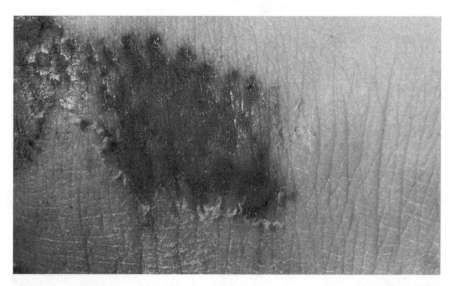

Figure 15–14 Abrasion with piled epithelium indicating downward directionality of injury.

through the tissue planes and be affected by gravity. Individuals that survive blunt trauma and that are in a recumbent position may have significant dissection of the blood that will accumulate in the flanks or even the back. Areas where the tissues are fixed and the tissue planes have ended will also accumulate blood, such as beneath the eyes at the level of the cheekbones. Blood accumulating from a fracture at the base of the skull, behind the ear, does not indicate the point of contact. This is called Battle's sign (Figure 15–15). Similarly, force applied to the head, such as a gunshot wound or other types of blunt trauma that would cause the brain to impact on the thin, delicate orbital roof causing fractures, may allow blood to dissect anteriorly into the upper and lower eyelids. There may be complete confluence of blood in the upper and lower eyelids; this is called "raccoon eyes" or spectacle hemorrhages (Figure 15–16). This can be incomplete, with only a small amount of blood seen in the medial canthus of either the right or left side. A hematoma is an actual collection of blood (the suffix "oma" being Greek for swelling or tumor—e.g., lipoma, carcinoma, sarcoma). The importance of a true hematoma is that it will take longer for the blood to resorb and heal and can actually be used as a postmortem toxicology sample, because it can be collected as a unit.

The documentation and classification of blunt force injuries are important, but it may also be important to give an estimation of the date of an injury. Multiple injuries that appear to have been inflicted

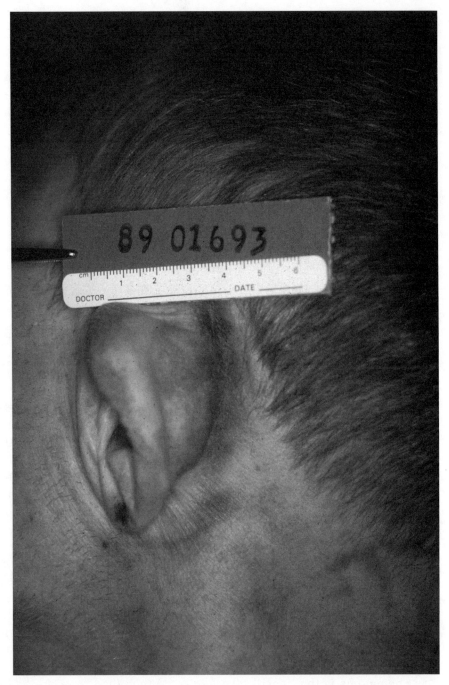

Figure 15–15   Battles sign (blood accumulating behind the ears following a skull fracture).

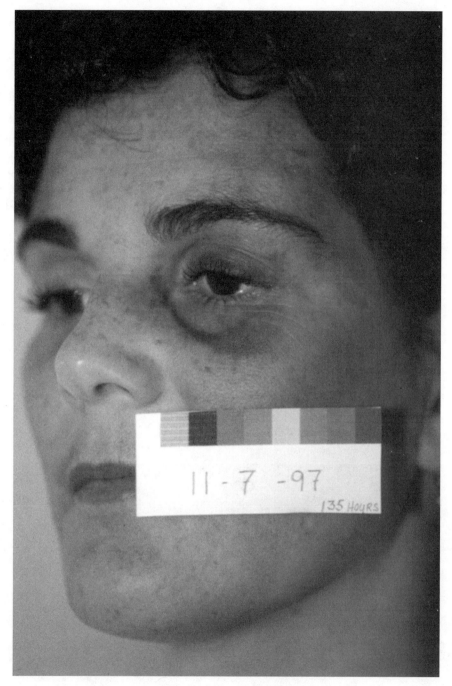

Figure 15–16   Spectacle hemorrhage (blackened/"racoon" eyes).

over time may lead to certain conclusions about the nature of the events. This would be important in an abusive situation, whether it be child abuse, spousal abuse, or elder abuse. The examiner should be extremely wary of rendering an opinion as to the age of a contusion or bruise solely based on its appearance and color changes (Figure 15–17). The color of a bruise is based on the metabolism and breakdown of the hemoglobin pigment within the red cells. The bruise appears to be initially dark purple and then over time, as the hemoglobin breaks down, it turns a series of blue, green, brown, tan, and yellow colors. No good correlation studies provide any reasonable opinion about the age of a particular bruise based on these color changes. Bruises have numerous variables including the actual quantity of blood that constitutes the contusion, and the quality of the inflammatory or healing abilities of that person. The only opinion that should be rendered is that the bruises are of "various ages." This can be confirmed by a microscopic examination of the bruises to identify the quality and quantity of the inflammatory response and the breakdown of the hemoglobin. This spectrum again is quite variable and has significant overlap. In the future, identification of molecular immune mediators histologically should help clarify and increase the specificity of the timing of individual injuries.

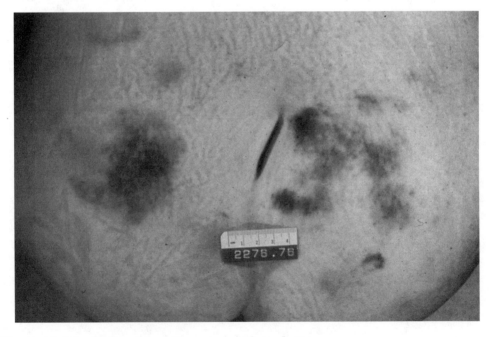

Figure 15–17 Bruises in varying stages of resolution.

Lacerations

A laceration is a tear of tissue. Once again, this can be skin or any internal organ or tissue other than bone. This injury and designation is not to be confused with a cut or incised wound. It is not infrequent to see in medical records the generic reference to "lac" when referring to any external wound noted on the body. It is important that forensic investigators are able to communicate their findings accurately and specifically because it may direct an investigation toward or away from a specific object. When sufficient force is applied to the tissue to overcome the tensile elastic strength of that entire tissue, it will tear (Figure 15–18). The skin should show several basic features including a marginal abrasion, tissue bridging, and possibly undermining. A marginal abrasion occurs because in the milliseconds prior to the tissue actually tearing, the skin is scraped. The dimensions and shape of the marginal abrasion may indicate the nature of the object that came in contact with the skin. A very narrow marginal abrasion suggests that the object had an edge to it (Figure 15–19), and a wide marginal abrasion indicates that the object is broader and flatter (Figure 15–20).

If the force is not sufficient to tear or destroy all of the tissue within its path, then there may be evidence of arteries, veins, nerves, or other elastic fibers that go from one edge of the wound to the other (Figure 15–21). This is a key finding in differentiating blunt force trauma from sharp force trauma. An incised wound or a cut will sever these tissues and there will be no evidence of tissue bridging.

If the force is not perpendicular to the skin then there may be more destruction beneath the skin (undermining) in the direction of the force. One might be able to do a digital or probe type examination noting that it may be several centimeters deeper on one side than the other side. This will aid in the determination of the direction of force and should be documented. Internal organs, such as the liver and lungs, may show lacerations of the parenchyma when there is no damage to the overlying capsule. It is also not uncommon to have very little external evidence of injury, but significant internal injury as the force is transmitted through the more elastic skin and subcutaneous tissue into the less resilient tissue parenchyma.

Like abrasions, lacerations indicate the exact point of force on the skin. For this reason, it is important to examine the depth of the laceration for any trace evidence that may have been deposited there (Figure 15–22). This can be collected and submitted to the police and/or crime lab for possible correlation with the object that impacted the skin. Unless there is complete perforation of the skin and subcutaneous tissue, the lacerations of internal organs should not have any trace evidence or particular pattern that would assist in determining the nature of the event. Because of their superficial nature, abrasions often do not have trace evidence associated with them.

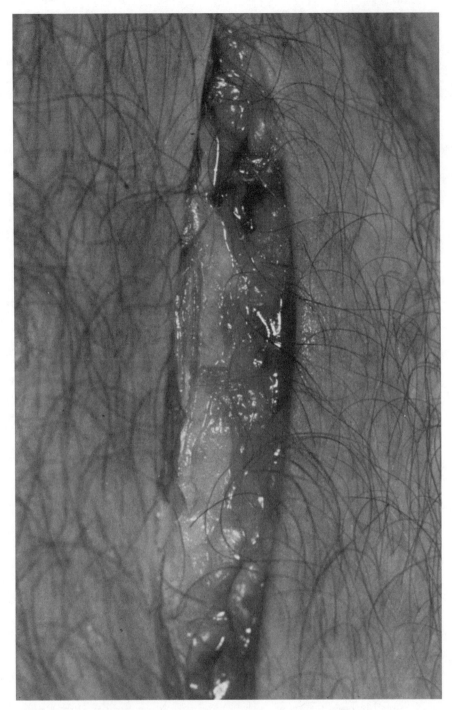

Figure 15–18   Laceration with sharp edges.

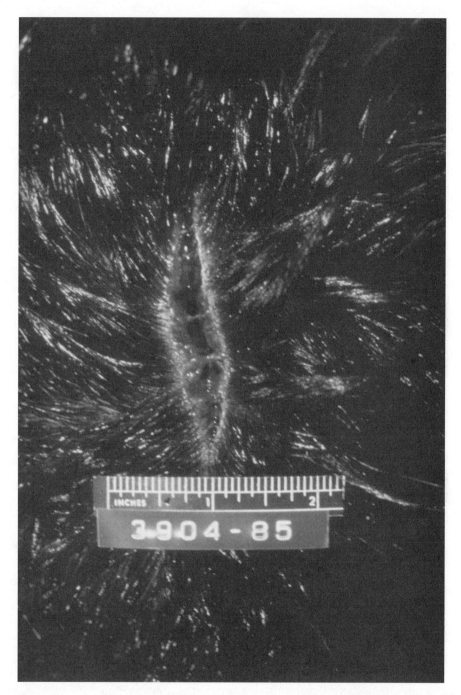

Figure 15–19   Laceration with marginal abrasion and tissue bridging.

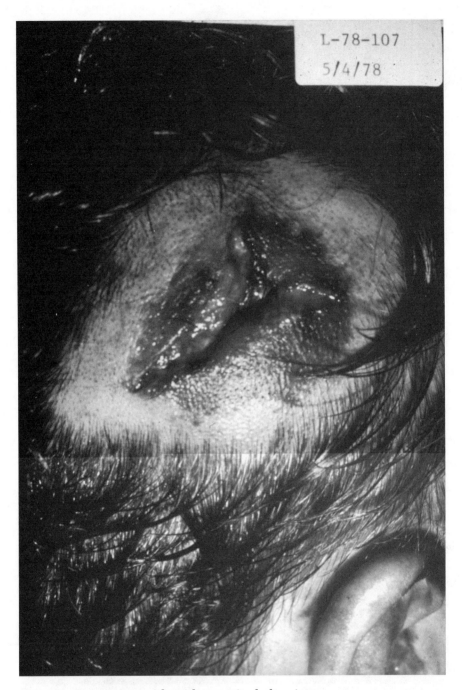

Figure 15–20   Laceration with wide marginal abrasion.

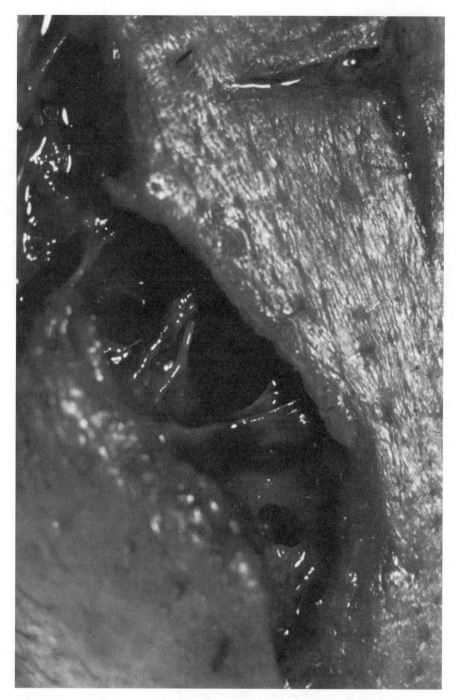

Figure 15–21   Laceration with evidence of structures transversing the wound (tissue bridging).

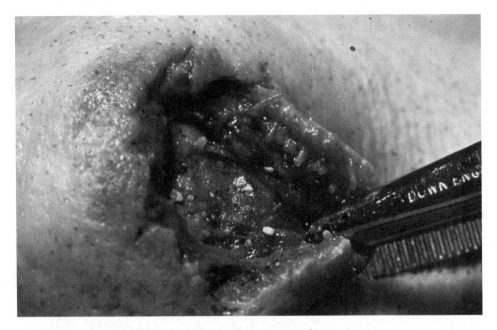

Figure 15–22 Examining a laceration for trace evidence.

Fractures

The final type of blunt force trauma is a fracture. This is any disruption of the normal anatomy of a particular bone. There may be a minor disruption in the cortex or complete disruption of the bone with overlying laceration of the skin, called a compound fracture. A comminuted fracture is shattering of the bone into multiple pieces. A displaced fracture is one where the fractured ends are no longer in alignment. The amount of force necessary to cause a fracture is generally greater than that required to cause an abrasion, contusion, or laceration; however, there are very thin bones that are relatively easy to fracture, such as the orbital roofs and the squamos portion of the temporal bone. Also, there is great relativity in the resistance of individual bones, which can fracture depending on the moment, direction, and magnitude of the force as well as the health of the individual bone. Elderly individuals with osteoporosis or children with congenital abnormalities such as osteogenesis imperfecta are susceptible to fractures.

Pathologic fractures are those that happen spontaneously, usually with no direct application of force, due to the extensive loss of calcium such as in osteoporosis or more commonly due to the infiltration of tumor. Linear fractures, particularly of the skull, can often lead to the original point of impact as they radiate out from its center. Also, similarly to fractures in glass, fracture lines that abruptly end at another fracture line indicate that it came subsequent to the one that it meets.

Depressed skull fractures occasionally can reflect the shape of the object that caused them. Also, as the bone is depressed and then approaches its return to its original position it may "bite" tiny pieces of whatever the object may have been. Close examination of the edges of these types of wounds may yield trace evidence. Bone may also indicate directionality. The lower legs, particularly the tibia, should be examined in any case of pedestrian struck by a motor vehicle. There may be little, if any, injury to the skin or subcutaneous or muscular tissue at the primary strike point (the point where the leading edge of the vehicle, usually the bumper, strikes the person). A triangular-shaped fracture may be seen along the shaft of the bone across its full thickness. The apex, or the point of the triangle, points in the direction of the force, unlike abrasions and lacerations where the apex of the torn tissue points in the opposite direction of the force (Figure 15–23). Once again, directionality may help confirm or deny a particular piece of information that is related to the incident. If the body is badly decomposed or skeletonized, the bones must be completely cleaned and defleshed for the forensic pathologist or forensic anthropologist to examine because subtle injuries may be hidden, such as blunt or sharp force trauma that would help determine the cause of death.

Patterned Injury

A patterned injury is a representation of the shape of the object that caused the injury, whether an abrasion, contusion, or laceration. It is important to recognize patterns and document them because it is not uncommon for the exact shape of the object, or the object itself that impacted with the skin, to be readily and independently apparent (Figures 15–24 and 15–25). Appropriate documentation by Polaroid, 35 mm camera, digital imaging, drawing, and/or tracing may be useful many years later when a specific object may come to the attention of the authorities. Objects found in nature rarely have a pattern that would be reflected in an injury. Man-made objects often have a pattern, and even the simplest object such as a cylindrical pool cue or a baseball bat has several surfaces that can cause an impact. These types of objects, when the long portion of the shaft is impacted on the skin, leave a patterned contusion composed of two parallel linear contusions with sparing at the center (Figure 15–26). This is because when the force is perpendicular to the skin it compresses the blood vessels, forcing the blood laterally, where the increased pressure actually breaks the capillaries causing the contusion. This is similar to that seen with tire tread imprints on the skin. These are patterned contusions formed when the skin in the space

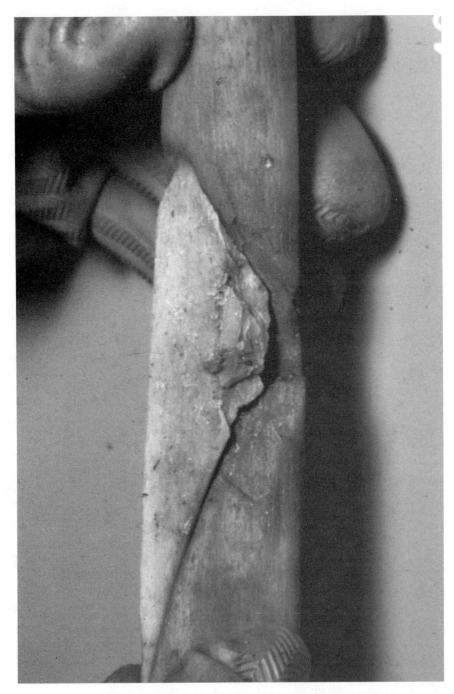

Figure 15–23   Triangular fracture showing left to right force.

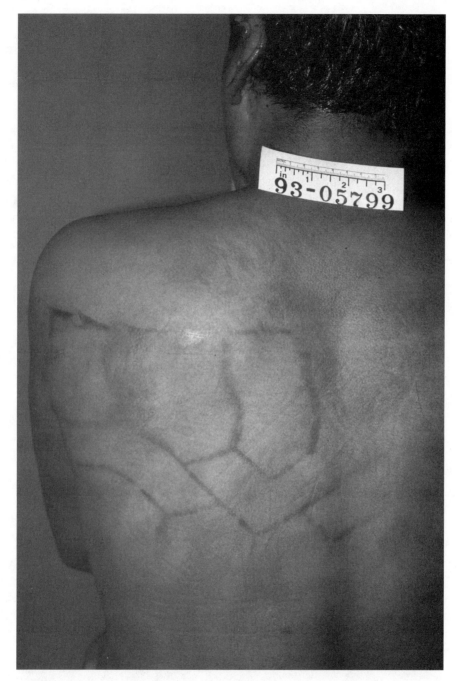

Figure 15–24   Pattern of contusions resulting from tire treads.

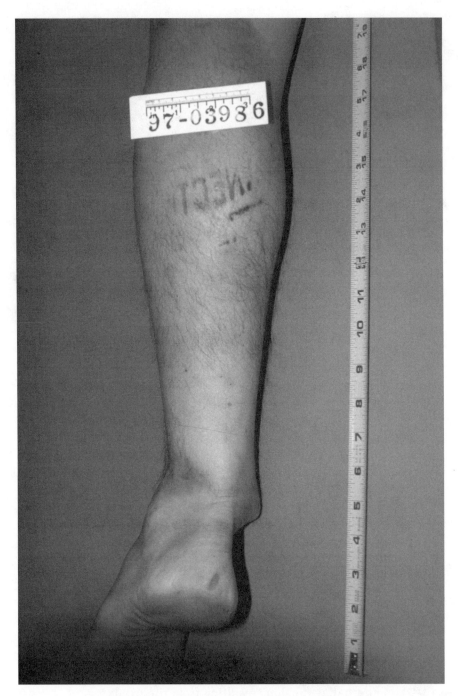

Figure 15–25   Compression abrasion resulting from license plate imprint.

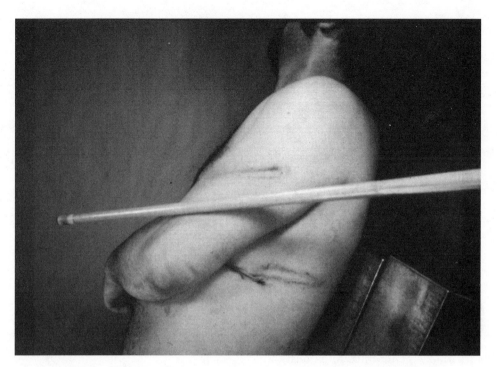

Figure 15–26   Pool cue pattern (linear contusions with sparing at center).

between the actual treads that come in contact with the surface are forced into the grooves, leaving the pattern. The actual point of impact where the tire treads touch is without visible contusion. Patterned abrasions also may be seen in situations where the muzzle of the gun leaves the pattern of its face on the skin of a contact gunshot wound. If the force is perpendicular to the skin the epithelium may actually be crushed instead of scraped, providing a greater opportunity to reflect the shape of the object that caused it (Figure 15–27). Due to the imposition of clothing between the object and the skin the pattern of the weave of the clothing could also be stamped into the epidermis.

Curvilinear lacerations over various surfaces of the body, particularly the head, upon closer examination may indicate a standard hammer. If the hammer impacts directly perpendicularly there should be the suggestion of a circular abrasion or contusion with a central, possibly stellate, laceration, particularly if this involves the scalp that overlies bone. If the injury is crescent-shaped it may have fairly well demarcated edges, from the disc-shaped hammerhead to a crescent-shaped hammerhead edge (Figure 15–28). A blow with a hammer may or may not cause

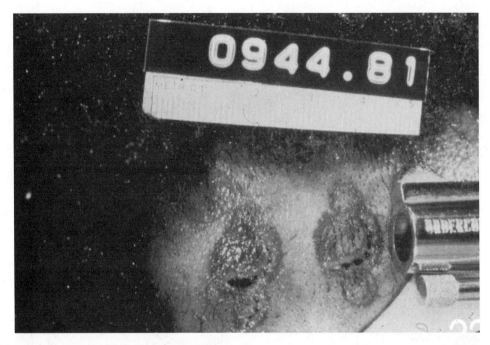

Figure 15–27 Gun muzzle pattern.

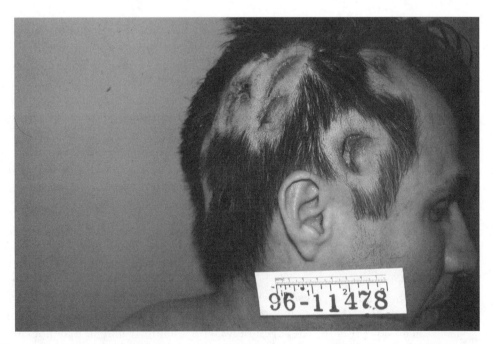

Figure 15–28 Crescent-shaped lacerations consistent with the head of a hammer, as the head is angulated relative to the skin.

a fractured skull, and may not need to fracture the skull in order to be lethal.

One way of documenting the injury is to lay a piece of clear plastic (such as a plastic bag) over the injury and simply trace it (Figure 15–29). In this manner multiple surfaces of the suspect object can be compared to the shape of the injury. Further, a suspect object can be examined by taking a piece of plain white paper, placing it on top of a phone book, and then placing a piece of carbon paper over that. Striking the carbon paper may leave the outline of that portion of the object on the paper, and the shape can then be compared to the injury on the skin. No doubt digital imaging techniques available in crime labs or research facilities might also be able to help elucidate the shape.

Patterns, or constellations of injuries, may also be important in determining what happened to an individual or how they were positioned in the environment during the incident that caused blunt force trauma. Each individual injury may not have a specific shape, but the patterns, or constellations, of the injuries, or the distributions of the injuries over the body surface may reveal what happened to the individual. An example of this would be a group of abrasions that may or may not include contusions or lacerations of the eyebrow lateral to the eye or the cheek, the tip of the nose or the chin. This entire array, or portions of it, is typical in a "fall" type pattern (Figure 15–30). If an individual becomes unconscious for whatever reason, and is unable to protect their head while they fall, the high points on the face will impact with the surface. This can be seen in victims of cardiac dysrhythmias who become unconscious very rapidly.

A motor vehicle driver has multiple opportunities for blunt force trauma. An unbelted driver in a head-on collision may reveal the "driver's triad"—injuries to the face from the windshield, the chest from the steering wheel, and the knees from the bolster or dashboard. These injuries may be subtle, and in a nondeceased individual may be reflected only in complaints of pain in those areas. Subjective focal complaints or the demonstration of point tenderness over the chest may help separate the purported driver from his or her passengers. Also, the tempered (heat-treated) glass of the side windows breaks up into small cube-like fragments that often impact the side of the face. Having "dicing" type injuries predominantly on the left side of the face is generally associated with the driver of the motor vehicle and on the right side of the face with the passenger. It should be noted, however, that unrestrained occupants of the motor vehicle inside "t-bone" collisions go toward the force of impact, so that a driver may have right-sided dicing type injuries by going toward the passenger's side at the area of impact.

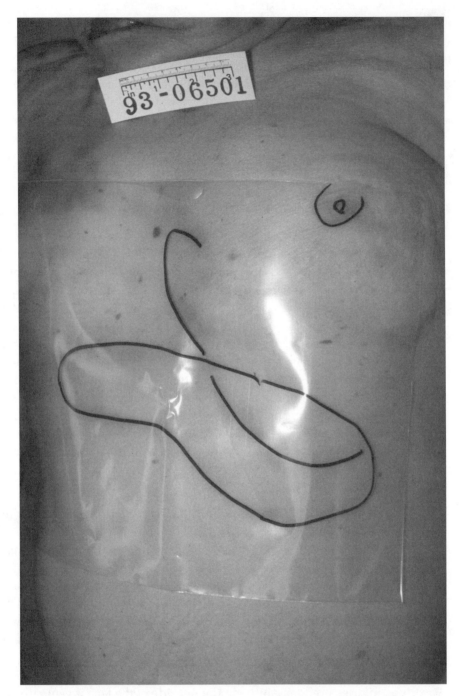

Figure 15–29 Method of tracing injury pattern for later comparison to suspected weapon(s).

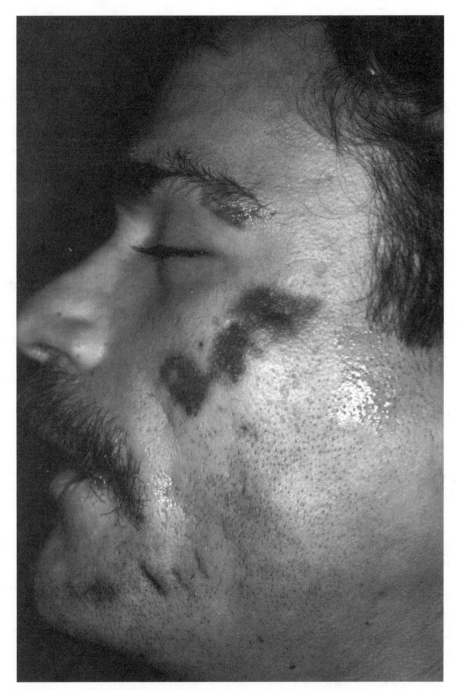

Figure 15–30   Constellation of abrasions consistent with a fall.

Pedestrians also have distributions of injuries that help identify the fact that they indeed have been struck by a motor vehicle and the relative position that they may have been in at the point of impact. Identifying the primary strike point (bumper injury) of the lower legs, whether they are anterior, lateral, or posterior is helpful. Dissecting the tibia for a possible triangular-shaped fracture would also indicate the direction of the force. If the force is enough to cause a fracture, usually only one leg shows the fracture pattern. The gait of a normal human being has the weight distributed over only one leg at a time. It is that weight-bearing leg that has enough resistance to cause the force to go through the bone, resulting in a fracture. The secondary injuries happen when the adult is thrown upward (because they are struck below the center of gravity), and hits the hood of the car and/or windshield, injuring the shoulders, chest, hips, face, and/or head. Tertiary injuries occur when the individual falls onto the surface of the roadway. It is at this point where lethal injuries often take place, when the head strikes the ground and/or the weight of the body distorts the normal position of the cervical spine. Quaternary injury may then occur as the individual lying in the road is subsequently run over by another vehicle. Categorizing each abrasion, contusion, and laceration and placing it in its appropriate temporal relationship may be difficult, if not impossible; however, the general distribution of the injuries can help answer many questions. A deceased individual laying in the middle of the road with no injuries to the lower extremities, the tips of the elbows, or the hips and having bilateral anterior and posterior rib fractures, lacerations of the liver, and fractures of the pelvis indicates that the person was already lying on the ground prior to being run over, meaning that the person had not been struck while being a pedestrian. This type of correlative information may clear an individual of charges that may be brought against him.

Physical Abuse

In abuse situations, the distribution of the injuries as well as the relative age of individual injuries can be correlated with the proffered history of how these injuries took place. Injuries of various ages distributed over the back, the front, the arms and legs, and various sides of the head are entirely inconsistent with a history of the baby "having fallen off the changing table."

SHARP FORCE INJURIES

The other major type of injury is sharp force injuries. There are only two mechanisms by which skin and internal tissues can be affected by sharp objects, cuts (incisions) and stabs (penetrations).

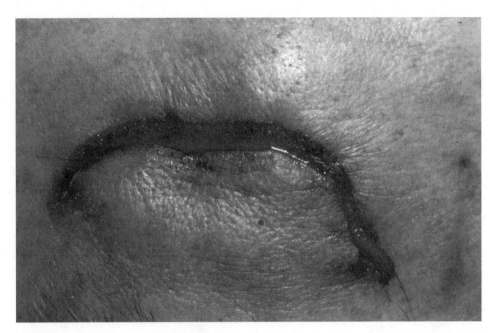

Figure 15–31 Incised wound (longer than deep).

Incised Wounds

Cuts or incised wounds are longer than they are deep. They may be caused by any object with an edge, including paper, a knife, glass, a razor, or the lid of a can (Figure 15–31). Incised wounds may involve only the skin or may involve the subcutaneous tissue and even deep muscle. The depths may be the same or they may be variable throughout the course of the wound. Superficial epithelial cuts at one edge of the wound, called "tails," may suggest the finishing side of the event. It is very difficult, however, to suggest a directionality to a simple incised wound. Whether the force is going from left to right or whether the perpetrator is left-handed or right-handed, or has inflicted the wound from in front or behind, is usually far too speculative to be of any true forensic value.

Penetrating Wounds

A stab, or penetrating wound, is deeper than it is long. A knife, a stick, a pencil, a rod, or any object that can be thrust into the body or onto which the body can be impaled would fall under this category. Classic knife wounds can reveal significant information. Close examination of the wound may show a sharp or V-shaped edge and a blunt or squared edge (Figure 15–32). This reflects the cutting and noncutting edge of a single-edged blade. The vast majority of all knives are single

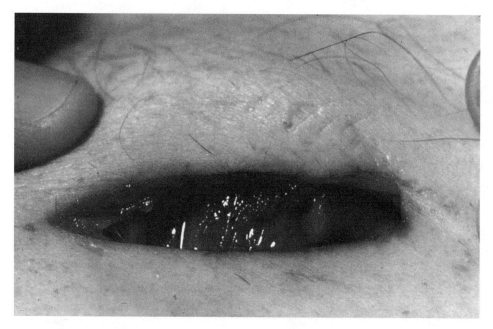

Figure 15–32   Penetrating wound inflicted by a single blade knife.

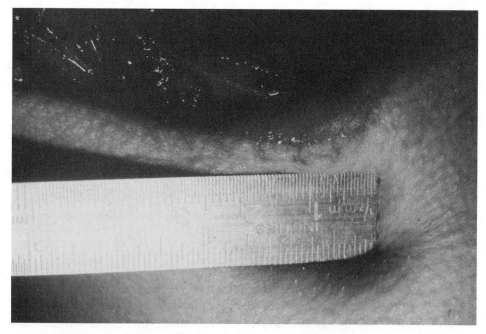

Figure 15–33   Wound inflicted by knife with a serrated blade.

edged. Occasionally a serrated knife upon its entry or exit from the skin may cause tiny periodic curvilinear epithelial abrasions that may be visible with a magnifying glass (Figure 15–33). However, the vast majority of serrated knives cause a simple stab wound with blunt and sharp edges. Two V-shaped edges or corners suggest a double-edged knife (Figure 15–34). The orientation of these blunt and sharp edges should be documented. One way to document them is to describe the orientation of the wound as compared to the face of a clock (e.g., "There is a sharp edge at 3:00 and a corresponding blunt edge at 9:00. The wound measures 3/4″ in length with the blunt squared edge measuring 2 mm").

The true nature and dimensions of the stab wounds may not be evident until the wound is reapproximated into its previous anatomic position. The elastic fibers will cause the wound to gape, particularly if it is vertically oriented. This is less evident if the wound is horizontally oriented because the elastic fibers run around the body in a horizontal fashion. Wounds can be reapproximated with fingertips, clear tape, clear fingerprint lifts, or even cyanoacrylic glue (superglue). At this point, photographs and measurements can be made for documentation.

Examination of the edges of the stab wound for epithelial abrasions may also indicate the relative force of a stab wound in which the handle

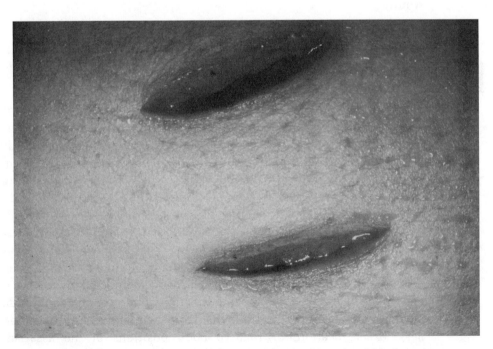

Figure 15–34 Wound inflicted by knife with a double-edged blade.

came into contact with the skin or forced clothing into the skin around the stab wound. The wound track should be documented by following the injury to the internal tissues beneath the skin. Documentation of whether these wounds exhibit hemorrhage is also important because stab wounds that occur after death would be bloodless.

Determining the depth of a stab wound is important, because it may help determine whether the weapon could be a 2-inch knife, a 4-inch knife, or an 8-inch knife. However, documenting the depth of the wound is fraught with great error and should be reported as a range. The very nature of the internal examination during the autopsy is a layer-by-layer stepwise procedure. The end of the stab wound may be on the surface or within an organ. One would then have to reconstruct the dissection process, put in some sort of a probe to the deepest portion of the wound, and measure from the entrance of the skin with a ruler. However, this reconstructive process is not exact; Tissues such as the lungs collapse so that the exact length within the lung as it was originally aerated would be impossible to identify, and organs are moveable, particularly the heart, lungs, and intestines. Also, the abdomen, and to some degree the chest are compressible. A 4-inch blade may easily cause a wound that is 6 inches deep. Solid, relatively moveable organs such as the liver, kidneys, and to some degree the heart, provide the best chance of determining the depth of the wound.

All individuals who have suspected stab wounds should be X rayed because it is possible for the tip of the knife to be broken off within the body. If possible this should be recovered and submitted as evidence for possible physical matching to a suspected weapon.

Stab wounds that are generally perpendicular to the body surface may be more complex than a simple blunt and sharp edge. If the knife or the victim moves, which is entirely possible, then the direction that the blade enters and the direction that the blade leaves are different, forming an A- or butterfly-shaped wound of varying angles (Figure 15–35). Complex stab wounds may also be seen in unusually shaped areas of the body, such as the neck or the axillae, where individual cuts and then ultimately a complex stab wound may be seen as separate injuries but reflect a single event. A knife may be held in various manners and can be directed toward a target in a forehand, backhand, or thrusting motion. The knife can be directed overhand or underhand. The shape, depth, and direction of the wound cannot independently reconstruct the events that happened with regard to handedness, exact location, or relative body positions of the assailant. Penetrating injuries may be caused by weapons other than knives, such as long barbecue-type forks, screwdrivers, or other thin natural or man-

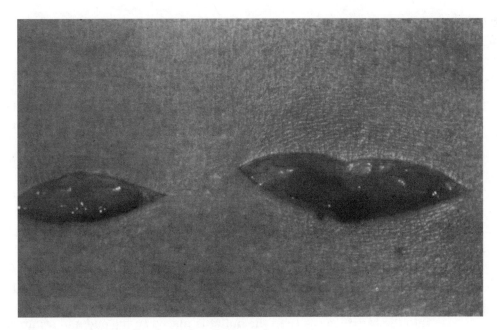

Figure 15–35　Butterfly-shaped stab wound.

made objects. Trace evidence such as paint, hairs, fibers, or parts of the object that caused the injury, may be present within the wound tract. The wound should be explored carefully to identify trace evidence. A Phillips head or flat head screwdriver often shows patterned injuries. The flat head screwdriver has a blunt edge and the Phillips head injuries have cross or star-shaped regular linear abrasions extending from the center of the wound.

When there is sharp force injury it is important to also examine and document other injuries that may be evident on the hands or forearms. Cuts or even other stab wounds in these areas are commonly referred to as defense wounds, implying that the victim was conscious and able to fight back during the attack. These do not in and of themselves guarantee that the person was alive and conscious, but if they weren't that would imply that the assailant caused injuries to these parts of the body intentionally. The identification of individual wounds, particularly in the extremities, may require them to be probed because they may represent direction of force through entry and exit wounds. It may be difficult, if not impossible, to identify the direction of these wounds unless there is an abrasion around one of them. It is certainly possible that defense wounds can be located on the lower extremities because people can defend themselves by kicking. Defense wounds also may be either blunt or sharp force injuries.

GUNS AND GUNSHOT WOUNDS

The Projectile

A lead ball traveling at several hundred feet per second has significantly more energy, and therefore causes more tissue damage, than another propelled object such as one launched from a slingshot. The key to tissue damage is the translation of the energy supplied by the moving object, as represented by $KE = \frac{1}{2}MV^2$, where KE is kinetic energy, M is equal to mass (or weight of the bullet), and V is velocity. Note that if the mass of the bullet is doubled, the kinetic energy is also doubled. However, if the velocity or speed of the bullet is doubled, then the kinetic energy is quadrupled. It is the speed of the bullet that translates into tissue damage. The speed is determined by the quantity of gunpowder that is available to propel the bullet down the barrel of the gun.

A cartridge or round (Figure 15–36) is a brass cylinder with a closed base that has a hollowed out area for a disc-shaped primer cap to be installed (Figure 15–37). The gunpowder granules are then placed loose into the cartridge case and the bullet is placed in the end and crimped, so that it will not fall out. The primer cap contains materials that are high explosives, which are then sent through a small hole called a vent in the cartridge case base that will ignite the gunpowder, producing a tremendous amount of gas that expands, forcing the bullet out of the

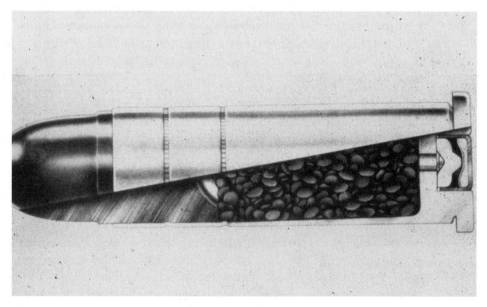

Figure 15–36   Anatomy of a cartridge or round.

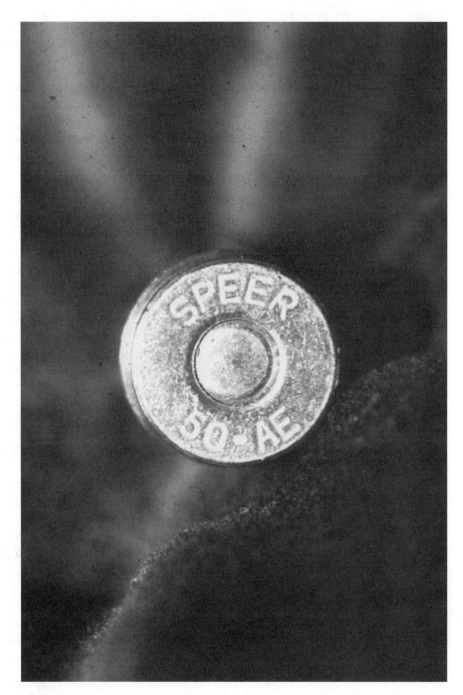

Figure 15–37   Cartridge base with primer cap and head stamp.

cartridge case and down the barrel. These chemical actions are triggered when the hammer of the gun strikes the firing pin, which in turn strikes the primer cap at the base of the cartridge.

The cartridge case may have a small lip at its base. This would be the type of round that would fit into the cylinder of a revolver. The lip allows the cartridge to stay in place and not fall through the open tube of the cylinder. The cartridge case for an auto-loading pistol has no lip, because it sits in a spring-loaded magazine, usually located in the grip of the weapon.

The bullet that is at the end of the cartridge case and propelled down the barrel of the gun toward the target may be made of pure lead or be a lead bullet that is encased completely or partially in copper, silver, or other materials. The diameter of the bullet correlates to the diameter of the barrel of the gun, and the ammunition and weapon are thus classified. The English system uses decimal fractions of an inch for their numerical classifications: .22, .25, .32, .357, .38, .380, .40, .50; the metric system uses millimeters: 7.62, 9, or 10 mm. It has been noted that the diameters of the .357, .38, and .380 are all the same, measuring .357 of an inch. The cartridge for the .357 is usually longer and has more gunpowder, and therefore is more powerful than the .38, although a .38 cartridge can fit into a weapon chambered for a .357.

Lead alloy bullets may be covered with a copper jacket in order to help maintain their shape after impact and to reduce vaporization of the lead. The shape of the bullet may be a simple cylinder, or may have a rounded, or hollowed out tip (hollow point), with numerous other variations. When the hollow point bullet (Figure 15–38) strikes the tissue, the tissue is forced into the central hollowed out area, splaying the soft lead and increasing the leading edge surface area. The bullet will have a mushroom appearance. It is theorized that this deforming and increased surface area makes the bullet less likely to exit from the body. The purpose of the bullet is to transmit all of its kinetic energy into tissue destruction. If a bullet exits the body, then it has not given up all of its energy to the tissue and therefore has wasted its energy. This may be moot with regard to high speed ammunition such as a rifle round, where a tremendous amount of energy is transmitted to the tissues; because of the bullet's speed it would be impossible for the missile to not exit either in whole or in many fragments.

The handling of a recovered bullet, whether from a scene or from tissue, should be done with great care. The barrel of the gun contains grooves cut into the tube in a slight spiral pattern. These grooves help the bullet to dig in and, because of the spiral, impart spin on the bullet. Spinning the bullet along its long axis vastly increases its ability to fly straight, and therefore increases the accuracy of the weapon. This is similar to a baseball that is thrown toward home plate by the pitcher with no spin

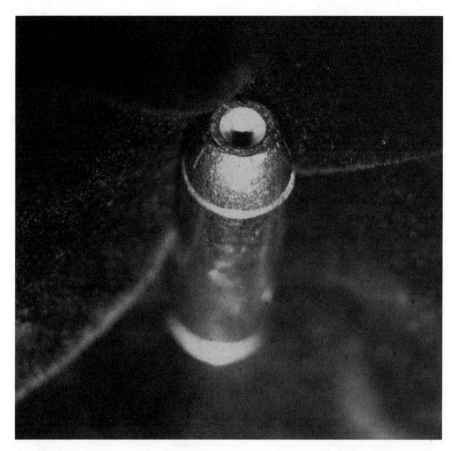

Figure 15–38   Hollow point bullet nose.

on it (a knuckle ball). It is notoriously inaccurate, and left to the vagaries of wind and humidity for its ultimate destination. In order to throw a baseball straight a spin must be imparted to it. The machined markings on the inside of the barrel of the gun have a high point (the true internal diameter) called the "land" and a low point that has been carved out as the groove. The high point will impart a groove, which looks like a slightly angled rectangular impression, into the side of the bullet and/or bullet jacket. The number of high points and the direction of the spiral indicate the general characteristics of the barrel of the gun, for example a right or left twist and five or six lands. The individual characteristics of the machined barrel will leave tiny microscopic striations on the bullet or jacket (Figure 15–39). Test firing a questioned gun and comparing with a bullet recovered from a body or a scene will, using a stereoscopic microscope, essentially be able to match not only the general class characteristics, but also the individual characteristics of that bullet, similar to a fingerprint. These characteristics can change over time to some

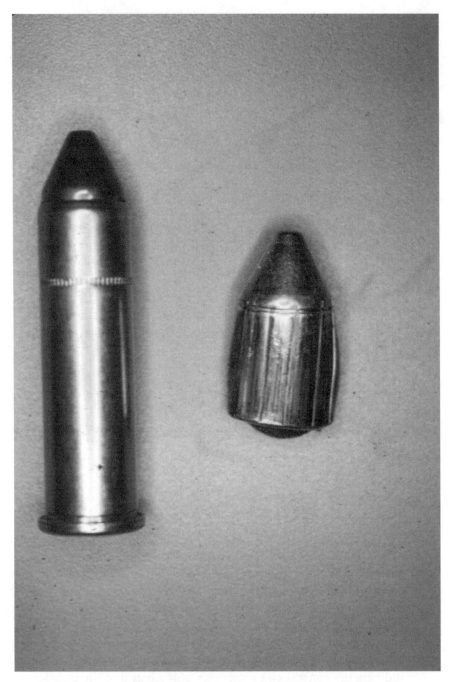

Figure 15–39 Intact round (L) and fired bullet (R) with barrel markings.

degree as the barrel of the gun handles other debris from bullets, gun-powder, and other environmental effects. Rough handling or inappropriate packaging can alter these useful striations. It is often the practice to inscribe a number or initials onto the nose or the base of the bullet for identification or chain of custody purposes; however, appropriate packaging and chain of custody receipts should obviate any problems.

The Weapons

Bullets are expelled from two basic types of weapons: handguns or rifles. Handguns can be held and fired with one hand. They are very concealable and therefore numerous regulations about why and how they can be carried have been codified by federal, state, and local governments. There are two primary types of handguns. The revolver has a revolving cylinder containing several, usually six, cylindrical tubes into which the intact cartridges are placed. These receptacles can be accessed by a single loading area on the side of the gun requiring the cylinder to be rotated each time a cartridge is loaded or an empty cartridge disposed of, a break in the breach between the cylinder, and the posterior part of the frame where all six receptacles are exposed. The cylinder can also swing out from the side of the frame on a hinge where, again, all six receptacles are visible and used cartridge casings can be discarded and new ones inserted. The revolver also has a grip, where the gun is held, and a hammer, which is moved backward and released by the trigger, which then strikes a small cylindrical piece of metal called the firing pin, which in turn strikes the primer, forcing the bullet down the rifled barrel.

The other type of handgun is called the auto-loading pistol, sometimes referred to as a "semi-automatic." This weapon has a magazine that is a rectangular receptacle into which numerous cartridges are stacked, forcing the compression of a spring-loaded platform. This magazine is inserted into the hollow pistol grip. Onto the basic frame, along the horizontal edge, is the barrel, which is attached to a moveable spring-loaded slide. When the slide is pulled backward (racked) the chamber is opened and the hammer is cocked into the ready position. When the slide is released the spring-loaded magazine forces the round into the chamber, and it is peeled off into its proper positioning for firing. The trigger then releases the hammer striking the firing pin and the bullet is propelled down the rifled barrel. Unlike the revolver, after the gunpowder charge is ignited, forcing the bullet down the barrel of the gun, the energy from this ignition causes the slide to compress the spring, eject the used cartridge case, recock the hammer, and allows another cartridge from the spring-loaded magazine to be peeled off into the chamber. The hammer can then be released a second time and the process is repeated until all of the rounds from the spring-loaded magazine in the pistol grip have been expended, leaving the chamber open and exposed. The magazine can be quickly released and a freshly loaded magazine inserted and the process can begin anew. The advantage to the auto-loading pistol is that the magazine often has two to three times more cartridges than a revolver, ejects the used cartridge, and reloads and recocks the weapon, all in the matter of a fraction of a second. This allows for more firepower in a shorter period of time compared to the revolver.

The placing of the hammer into the ready deployment position and its relationship to the trigger or hammer release mechanism is called the action. A single-action mechanism requires manual positioning of the hammer, which also moves the trigger into a shorter release position. This means that the trigger needs to be pulled only a fraction of what it was in the nonready position, and with less pressure. This is often simply done with the thumb of the firing hand or of the free hand; however, in old cowboy movies the person firing the weapon can be seen cocking the weapon manually with the palm of his left hand repeatedly. This is called fanning. Manual cocking of the trigger can also be done on the auto-loading pistol, but fanning is not necessary because after the trigger is released the first time, it is automatically recocked by the slide mechanism from the energy from the fired round. The weapons may also have double-action mechanisms. This indicates that pulling the trigger from its static position toward the release position will also simultaneously pull the hammer back into its ready position until the trigger reaches its hammer release point; thus, the trigger performs a double action of cocking and releasing the hammer.

Regardless of the type of action, each time the shooter wants to fire a bullet the hammer must be cocked and released. A true automatic weapon would be classified as a submachine gun if it is a weapon that can be hand-held, such as a military style rifle, or a machine gun, which is a much larger weapon that usually needs to be operated by a crew or an affixed battery. A true automatic weapon indicates that the trigger only needs to be depressed once and bullets will continually be fired from the weapon until all of the ammunition is gone, or the pressure on the trigger is relieved. Many modern-day military rifles (submachine guns) have several modes of fire. Individual shots can be fired with classic auto-loading features, a burst of three with single trigger depression, or full automatic with a single trigger depression.

Rifles have a similar basic frame and mechanism as an auto-loading pistol with a much longer barrel. They can have magazines that are internal, or external ones that can be changed. These larger magazines take rounds that are also much larger and therefore contain more gunpowder. A group of rounds are held together by a band of metal called a clip, which allows easier manipulation of multiple rounds and assists in the loading of a magazine. Because of the larger ammunition containing more gunpowder, these weapons have a significant amount of energy. In order to increase accuracy they must be held and supported up against the shoulder. The longer steel barrel increases the weight, but also increases the accuracy. Thus much more energy can be imparted at a greater distance without loss of accuracy. Snipers can hit their targets from more than 2 miles away.

The other type of long arm is called a shotgun. Unlike handguns and rifles, the shotgun does not have a rifled barrel. It is a simple smooth bored tube. The cartridge contains a small disc-shaped brass cylindrical base, the bottom of which has a hollowed out area for a primer, similar to the other types of ammunition (Figure 15–40). The remainder of the body of the shotgun shell is paper or plastic, completing a cylinder. Within the cylinder, gunpowder particles are poured into the bottom, where they have access to the vent through which the ignited primer chemicals will react with them. A paper disc wad or a plastic cup is then inserted, which is a material that separates the gunpowder from the missiles. Next, various types of missiles are inserted and the end of the cylinder is closed. The missiles can be hundreds of tiny lead spheres, called birdshot, loaded into a single sphere or cylinder of lead. When

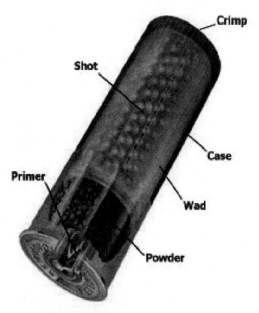

Figure 15–40   Diagram of a shotgun shell.

trying to shoot down a bird, a spray of these pellets is put up into the air, giving multiple opportunities for impacts on the target. Larger spheres, usually numbering nine, are called buckshot, for shooting large animals like buck deer. Numerous missiles can be released from a bullet that is approximately the same size as the .38-caliber bullet and would impact with a single pull of the trigger. When the mass of lead shot exits the barrel of the shotgun, the shot, including the wadding, generally stays in a single unit for several yards. After that the pellets begin to encounter air pressure and start to slow down and peel off from the initial mass. Further away the pellets become individuals and fly toward their target as single missiles.

Analysis of Evidence

Gunshot wounds are merely a compilation and subset of blunt force trauma. However, their importance and implications require them to be analyzed in a different fashion in order to come up with useful opinions and conclusions. When a bullet that is spinning along its long axis impacts the skin, the skin will be indented while the bullet is spinning and forcing its way through the skin prior to overcoming its elasticity. This causes an area of abrasion that ultimately surrounds the circular defect (laceration) caused by the bullet in the skin. This abrasion collar or marginal abrasion around the central defect is the classic feature of an entry gunshot wound (Figure 15–41). Depending on its kinetic energy, the bullet will then travel through tissue, causing lacerations, contusions of tissues, and fractures of any bone that it may impact. The bullet may continue through the body and force its way out of the body, stretching the skin from inside toward out, ultimately causing it to tear, and the bullet continues on its way. This wound is irregular in shape, generally larger than the accompanying entrance wound, and with no marginal abrasion of the skin around the tear. These tears can be stellate or linear and of various sizes. The exit wound may have an abrasion around it if it is shored or supported. As the skin protrudes from the pressure of the bullet going from inside toward the outside, the skin may be forced up against a hard object, such as elastic clothing, a wall, a chair, or the ground. This abrasion may be very similar to that seen around the entry gunshot wound, but more typically because of the nature of the object that it impacts, flat and broad, has a wide irregular marginal abrasion that is dissimilar to the classic entry gunshot wound abrasion collar. Occasionally the exit wound can look very similar to the entry wound, and it can be difficult to tell which is which.

One of the important analyses to be performed on any gunshot wound is the observation and documentation of any gunshot residue. What comes out of the barrel of the gun is the bullet, unburned or partly burned gunpowder particles that become missiles unto themselves, and completely burned gunpowder called smoke or soot. If only the bullet impacts the

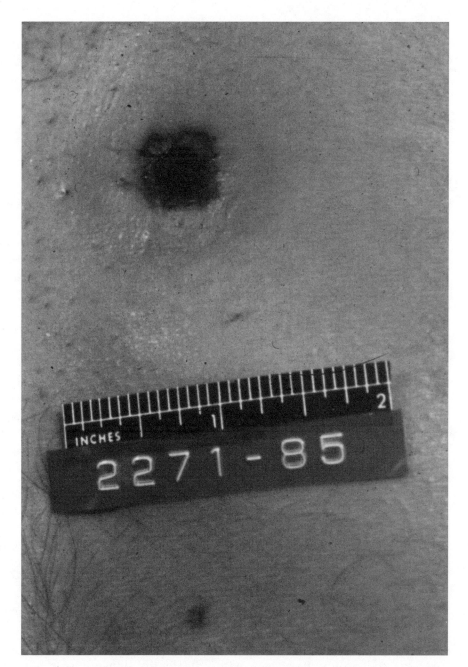

Figure 15–41 Entry wound demonstrating marginal abrasion around the central defect.

skin this would be called a "distant" entry gunshot wound. This range may actually be as close as 3 feet. The absence of gunshot residue around the entry gunshot does not necessarily mean it is a distant gunshot wound if there is intermediary material such as clothing between the end of the barrel and the skin. Gunshot wounds with a classic circular defect, a marginal abrasion, and no visible gunshot residue on the skin surrounding the wound may be gunshot wounds of indeterminate range if it is known that there is clothing, a door, or a window between the gun and the victim based on the scene circumstances. If individual gunpowder particles have struck the skin they may embed into the skin, called powder tattooing, or impact the skin, leaving an abrasion or contusion, called powder stippling. Evidence of the entry gunshot wound with powder stippling or tattooing on the skin surrounding the wound is called a medium or intermediate range gunshot wound.

Individual gunpowder particles can be extracted from the epidermis and retained as evidence. Gunpowder particles come in multitudes of shapes, from true spheres to flattened spheres called flattened ball, to disc-shaped, to flakes, to cylinders. The shape and size of the gunpowder particles allow for variations in the length of time that this nitrocellulose material actually burns, producing the gases within the cartridge casing that expel the bullet. The radius from the center of the wound, or the total diameter of the distribution of these impacts on the skin, should be meticulously recorded and photographed. The radius of the stippling should be measured after the direction of the bullet and its angle to the skin have been determined. The radius or diameter may be different if viewed perpendicular to the skin, as opposed to a tangential entry gunshot wound from the side. A tangential entry gunshot wound will also not be circular; it will be ovoid in shape with an asymmetric marginal abrasion, the larger end being where the bullet first entered. Gunpowder particles generally, although with quite a bit of variation, will travel approximately 2 feet and still have enough energy to impact the skin.

Evidence of an entry gunshot wound, powder particles having impacted the skin, and black material called soot surrounding the entry gunshot wound are all consistent with a close range gunshot wound (Figures 15–42 and 15–43). The range of fire is in the area of less than 6 to 8 inches. The soot is not very dense and will not carry very far. The diameter of the soot should also be documented, and a sample can be collected with a cotton swab for forensic ballistic laboratory analysis. If the muzzle of the gun is in contact with the skin there will be an entry gunshot wound that has thick accumulation of gunpowder particles and soot around its edge or within its depths, depending on how tight the contact is. As the gases penetrate the skin and expand, the skin will be stamped into the muzzle face, leaving a thin, curvilinear patterned abrasion that should mimic the shape of the face of the barrel of the gun. This is called a barrel abrasion or a muzzle stamp. This can be extremely useful in determining which gun may have caused the injury if there is a choice of more than one. If the contact entry gunshot wound

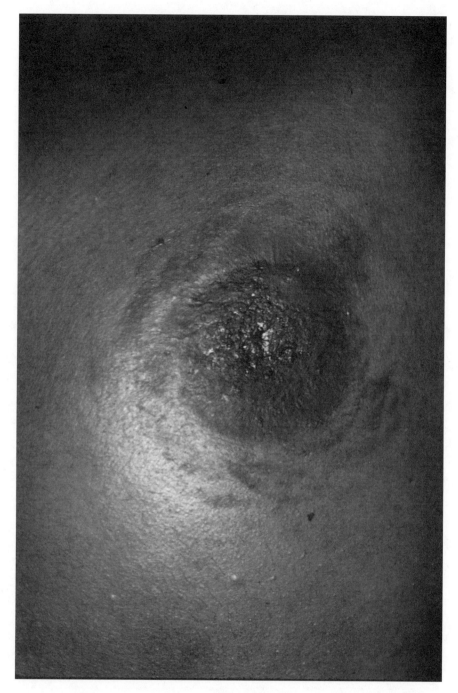

Figure 15–42 Close-range gunshot wound exhibiting gun powder residue.

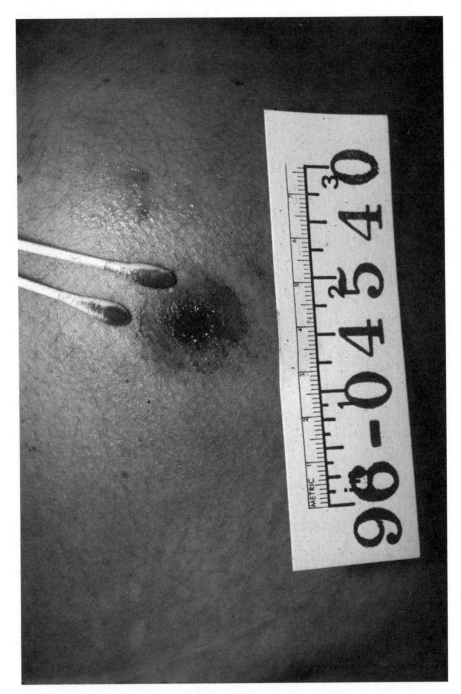

Figure 15–43 Examination of close-range gunshot wound with gun powder residue.

is over bone, commonly over the scalp in suicide situations, the tremendous gases that come out of the barrel of the gun enter between the scalp and the skull, causing a large irregular or stellate tear of the scalp. If the bullet perforates the brain and skull and exits the opposing side, this may be a relatively small wound and flies in the face of the conventional wisdom that the entry wound is smaller than the exit wound. Identification of soot and gunpowder in the depths of the wound easily distinguishes the entry from the exit. After gentle cleaning of the wound to identify the presence of soot or gunpowder particles and the collection of any visible material, the hair surrounding the wound should be shaved so that the features of the wound can be appropriately examined and documented. The hair around the wound, regardless of how bloody or dirty it may be, should be saved for potential laboratory analysis of the gunshot residue. Even if it is not visible on the skin the residue may have adhered to the hairs and would be helpful in estimating the range of fire. Hair around the wounds should always be shaved and never washed until after appropriate evidence collection and wound documentation has been completed.

Radiographic Studies

Any live or deceased person suspected of being a victim of a gunshot wound should always have X rays. This will help locate the bullet as evidence and at least suggest a path and, therefore, the tissue damage. Bullets generally travel in a straight line, although as they lose energy their paths may be deflected by bone. Atypical final locations of bullets can occur; if a bullet enters an artery or a vein, it can be swept either by the action of the heart or gravity into a vessel toward the heart or away from the heart and be located far away from the initial entry wound and suspected tissue path. Trying to locate these bullets can be confounding.

In cases of multiple gunshot wounds it may be difficult to catalog all the entries and exits and the number of bullets. The general rule of thumb is that the number of wounds plus the number of bullets equals an even number. For example, an entry wound with a bullet recovered in the chest is an even number, an entry and an exit wound is an even number, and an entry, exit, re-entry, and bullet recovery is an even number. If the examination and analysis yield an odd number of wounds plus bullets, then an unaccounted for wound or a missing bullet is to blame. The exception to this rule is if a soft lead bullet comes in at a tangential angle and is split, causing a fragment of the bullet to exit and the other fragment to remain in the body. The jacket of a bullet can also be peeled off from the lead core, either by an intermediary target, clothing, or a defective unit, causing two wounds but a single bullet.

ASPHYXIA

Asphyxia essentially means the lack of oxygen to cells. The brain cells are the most sensitive to low oxygen states; therefore, any mechanism that results in decreased oxygen availability to the neurons would be an asphyxial death. Any situation that one could conceive that would prevent oxygen from getting into the blood stream or blood from getting to the brain would lead to an asphyxial death.

Environmental Deficit

External environmental situations that would decrease oxygen not intimately associated with the body include an environment free of oxygen or depleted in oxygen such as an underground manhole that has been sealed for a long time in which the normal bacterial residents have consumed the oxygen and produced carbon dioxide, or an enclosed non-ventilated space such as a vault or refrigerator. Nontoxic gases, such as natural gas or carbon dioxide, that replace oxygen in enclosed environments would also lead to an asphyxial death.

A more localized enclosed space around the body, such as a bag over the head, would rapidly deplete available oxygen. The prevention of oxygen from entering the respiratory tract, such as smothering with some object tightly sealing off the nose and the mouth or a gag forced into the mouth obstructing the posterior pharynx, which also blocks off the nasal pharyngeal passage, would also lead to asphyxia.

Compression

External prevention of respiration can be accomplished by preventing the chest from expanding. A classic scenario concerns a person working underneath a car that slips off the jack, resulting in the undercarriage resting on his chest. This would prevent the expansion of the chest cavity. Another common situation would be in a motor vehicle collision when the integrity of the passenger compartment is significantly compromised and the occupant has some materials pressing on their chest. This might also occur with the seatbelt if the individual is in such a position where they can't release the seatbelt, particularly if the vehicle is inverted. Another human being can also be the cause of chest compression, sometimes called traumatic asphyxia. One or more persons sitting or lying on the chest might inhibit their ability to respire.

Obstruction

Following the oxygen delivery deeper into the respiratory tract demonstrates any number of potential mechanisms whereby oxygen can be prevented from getting from the outside environment into the alveoli.

Materials such as food are not uncommon, particularly if the person's neurological status is compromised by natural disease, such as a stroke, or chemically, such as by alcohol. Chunk-like particles of food, particularly meats, the most common culprit being the hot dog, are prime candidates for this plugging mechanism. An event that would cause swelling of the upper airway, such as an allergic reaction causing edema of the vocal cords and laryngeal soft tissues, and infection or trauma with subsequent hemorrhage and swelling may decrease the amount of oxygen that can flow.

Tumors eventually might close off an airway as well, although this is a much slower mechanism that should be identified long before it becomes a potential upper airway asphyxia mechanism. Conditions such as asthma could cause bronchial constriction in deeper airways and subsequent death.

Chemical Asphyxia

At the cellular level, toxins such as carbon monoxide—which bonds to the hemoglobin molecule 200 to 400 times more avidly than oxygen itself—would cause chemical asphyxia. Cyanide is also a subcellular asphyxiant, preventing the intermitochondrial transport of oxygen.

Hanging

If oxygenated blood is prevented from reaching the brain, an asphyxial death can also occur. The most common mechanism for this would be neck compression via hanging. Oxygen can be prevented from getting into the cells of the brain either by interrupting the arterial flow or, more easily, by interrupting the bilateral venous outflow from the head, thereby disrupting the inflow of blood and oxygen transfer to the neurons. Circumferential bilateral and equal neck pressure will easily compress the veins, which require only approximately 4 pounds of pressure. The arteries, which are deeper and more elastic with thicker walls, require much more pressure to compress. In hanging this occurs as the weight of the body, particularly in the unconscious state, puts relatively rapid and equal pressure on the neck, cutting off the arterial supply as well. This is why no petechial hemorrhages are seen during the ocular examination. Petechial hemorrhages are pinpoint red-purple hemorrhages caused by purely mechanical disruption of the venous flow exiting the head (Figure 15–44). If there is adequate arterial flow, pressure will build up and the small delicate capillaries of the mucosal surfaces will break and be visible. These can even coalesce to be quite large, encompassing much of the sclera. They are readily apparent on the conjunctival surfaces of the globe, beneath the eyelids, and in the skin of the eyelids themselves. Petechial

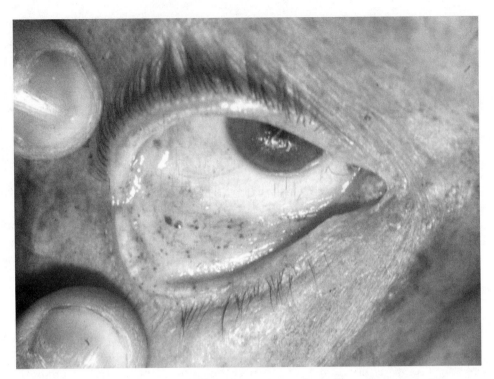

Figure 15–44 Petechial hemorrhages resulting from interference with venous blood flow in asphyxia.

hemorrhages can also be seen on the oral mucosa, although this is often not looked for and is not reflected in previous studies. People that have had their neck compressed, but do not succumb, may have florid petechial hemorrhages seen everywhere on the face.

Petechial hemorrhages seen in true hanging victims should be explained. The most likely reason is that a previous attempt had failed, causing damaged blood vessels that are reacting to the renewed arterial blood flow. Hanging can take place in any position. One does not have to be "swinging from a tree limb." Hanging can be done fully suspended, partially suspended where the person can relieve the neck pressure at any time while conscious, in a seated position, or even lying down. As long as enough bilateral neck pressure is maintained after the person becomes unconscious to prevent blood flow, it will inhibit oxygen transfer to the brain. There should be an identifiable suspension point in the ligature furrow (Figure 15–45), forming an upside down "V."

In assault situations, a ligature can be placed around the neck. This mechanism is a process called garroting (Figure 15–46). This can be done with any object and is usually accomplished from behind. A soft ligature may not leave any marks at all, whereas a narrow or patterned ligature may leave specific injuries that can be identified and docu-

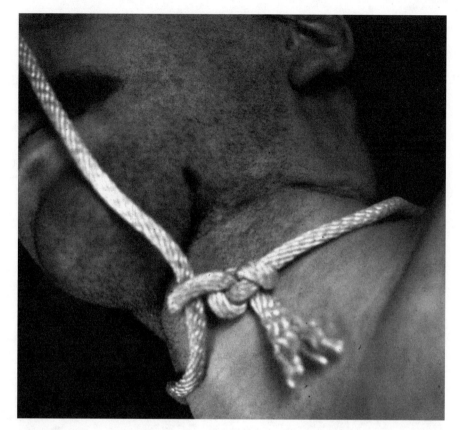

Figure 15–45   Results of hanging: furrow on neck resulting from suspension point in ligature.

mented that would reflect the shape of the object that caused it. The ligature furrow should be horizontal and circumferential around the neck. Because this is a violent encounter, other injuries may also be present, such as abrasions and contusions of the face and potentially the arms. The investigator should also look for injury to the back as the perpetrator may use a knee for leverage, causing a contusion.

Manual Strangulation

Another more dramatic form of external neck compression is manual strangulation. This is a very dynamic event in which the assailant places his or her hands on or around the neck, usually involving significant struggle. During this period shearing forces occur at various levels throughout the neck structures. The hallmarks of manual strangulation include the identification of petechial hemorrhages as the veins are easily compressed but the arteries are not or are interrupted intermittently. Careful examination of the conjunctivae, the eyelids, and the oral mucosa are important in every case, particularly if the deceased is a

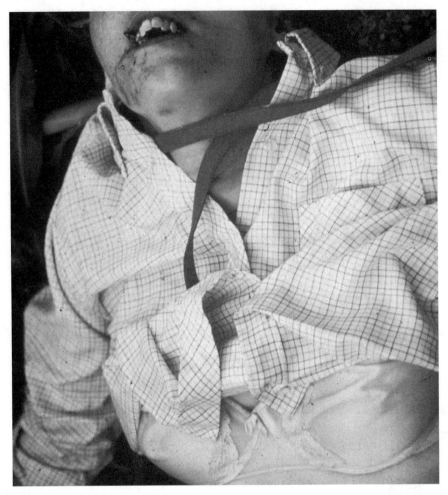

Figure 15–46 Garroting (ligature around neck).

female, if there is disruption of the clothing or she is nude, or if the scene circumstances suggest violence. Careful examination of the skin of the neck may find contusions and abrasions (Figure 15–47), some of which may be small curvilinear abrasions that would represent fingernail marks. Not all "fingernail" abrasions are that of the assailant. During the struggle with the assailant's hands around the victim's neck, attempts to remove the hands may cause the victim to scratch him- or herself. Because of the intimate nature of these types of assaults, whether they are ligature or manual strangulation, it is important to look for trace evidence. Alternate light sources are useful for foreign hairs and fibers, as well as potential semen stains on clothing or skin.

Fingernail scrapings or the complete excision of the fingernails for potential biological material that might link the deceased to the assailant

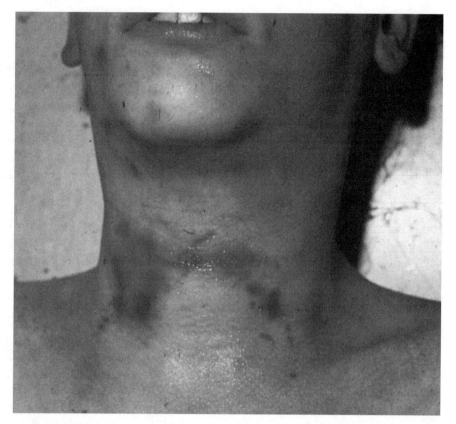

Figure 15–47   Contusions and abrasions on neck resulting from strangulation.

should be taken routinely, and a rape kit should be taken if the deceased is female or known to be a homosexual. This should be done even if the assault does not lead to the individual's death.

The internal examination reveals subtle, usually asymmetric, hemorrhages that may be in multiple layers of the neck structures, which should be dissected meticulously in situ for best results and appropriate interpretation. A prolonged struggle may also lead to massive internal neck hemorrhages. A delicate dissection of the hyoid bone may reveal fracture of the cornu and/or the superior horns of the thyroid cartilage. The presence of fractures in these structures are highly suggestive, if not diagnostic, of a manual strangulation because their location high and deep in the neck structures make it very difficult to apply force that would not be readily apparent from the scene, such as a motor vehicle accident or other type of drastic trauma. However, the absence of hyoid bone fractures does not rule out manual strangulation. If the victim is young then the hyoid bone and thyroid cartilages may be quite elastic, and the hyoid bone may not have ossified and fused and therefore retained its pliability.

Neck compression can also be done with the arms, such as the now discouraged police technique of the "carotid sleeper," where the tip of the neck at the Adam's apple is wedged in the depths of the antecubital fossa as the person wraps their arm around the victim's neck from behind. Utilizing the free arm for pressure and leverage, the upper and lower arm are squeezed onto the neck in a pincher type motion, readily compressing the carotid arteries bilaterally and leading to rapid unconsciousness. If pressure is maintained too long, oxygen depletion, seizure, and/or cardiac dysrhythmia due to stimulation of the carotid body may lead to death. If the anterior aspect of the neck is on the forearm as it is held horizontally across the neck with pressure applied, the larynx may fracture, leading to hemorrhage and swelling and potentially an asphyxial death. This is called the bar hold, which is a very painful experience for the recipient. An inanimate object can also cause neck compression, but instances are very unusual, occurring generally in industrial situations.

Positional Asphyxia

"Positional asphyxia" is a term that is often discussed in police and corrections circles. Sometimes police or corrections officers have to restrain an individual who is out of control due to drugs such as PCP or cocaine, or due to inherent psychoses, for the safety of themselves, people surrounding them, and the officers themselves. This may take four to six people for the necessary restraint, but during the struggle pressure may be applied to the chest cavity for a prolonged period of time, causing the individual to die of traumatic asphyxia, or pressure may be applied to the neck, causing the person to die of asphyxia by neck compression. These are not true positional asphyxias. True positional asphyxia means that the body is in a position where respiration is difficult, if not impossible. True positional asphyxias are difficult to envision and are often complicated by significant alcohol or drug consumption. Lying on their back with their feet touching the surface of the ground while the head, chest, and waist are bent is an example (Figure 15–48). Another example is an individual with a large abdomen who is handcuffed or hogtied, causing inhibition of respiration if they are face down on a hard surface. Lying prone on a surface, such as the back of an automobile where the transmission axle hump is located, can further decrease the ability to expand the chest.

Manner of Death

All types of asphyxial deaths are traumatic except for natural disease processes such as a bacterial infection, asthma, or anaphylaxis. The traumatic mechanisms of asphyxia may be accidental, homicidal, or suicidal. Appropriate scene investigation, including interviews with witnesses, family, and private physicians, as well as scouring the environs for a suicide note, whether written on paper, dictated, or on a home computer, should be accomplished for an appropriate manner of death determination. For

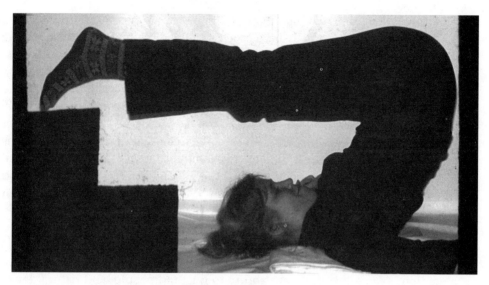

Figure 15–48   Potential positional asphyxia.

example, a young male found hanging in the bedroom, although not fully suspended, may not be a suicide. If the genitals are exposed, pornographic material is present, and there is no previous history of suicidal ideation, attempts, or an apparent suicide message, this may fall under the category of an autoerotic asphyxia, which is an accidental death and not a suicidal death. In these particular situations the discovery that light-headedness enhances the orgasm causes the participant to invent any one of varied and imaginative mechanisms to compress the neck. There should be an escape mechanism so that the pressure can be relieved, preventing the individual from becoming unconscious while the pressure on the neck is maintained and ultimately dying. Occasionally these escape mechanisms will fail, and the deceased can be found in sometimes very unusual situations.

SUMMARY

In order to expand and professionalize the responsibilities of death investigation, more and more jurisdictions are utilizing nonphysician death investigators. This includes the forensic nurse and others, often with college or advanced degrees, with formal or in-house training and hands-on experience in the medical field. With these backgrounds, individuals can develop the experience required to understand the different types of deaths and how to assist the responsible physician for accurate certification.

A forensic nurse is probably the most qualified nonphysician death investigator. The advantage that the nurse death investigator possesses is medical and nursing education that results in a rapid and accurate understanding of the disease processes when reviewing medical records and obtaining pertinent history from treating physicians. The nurse also has a wide background in understanding classes and individual types of prescription medications. Nurses are also uniquely qualified to interact with family members involved in extremely stressful events, such as the violent demise of a loved one. The forensic nurse possesses expert communication skills that can be used effectively with families, loved ones, witnesses, and any other people who might impact the death investigation. Having an understanding of the collaborative nature of the death investigation role enables the nurse to become an effective team member. Even if the nurse has not had any experience in death investigation, the basic procedures, observations, and language can be learned and assimilated readily. In summary, nurses as death investigators are in a unique position to be successful and productive because of their education, experience, inherent ability to relate to people, and natural tenacity to solve problems and to pose and answer questions.

Retired or experienced homicide detectives are another group of professionals well suited to careers in death investigation. They have often participated in police investigations and can learn enough of the medical terminology over time to interact with the treating physicians. People with other types of medical backgrounds such as paramedics, scientists, or other categories of investigative professionals may be suitable as well.

QUESTIONS FOR DISCUSSION

1. Describe the death investigation system in the area in which you reside.
2. What is the primary goal of any death investigation?
3. Describe methods one could use to identify a deceased "John Doe."
4. Describe the sequence of photographs that should be taken at a death scene investigation.
5. What is the best way to determine the time of death of a deceased?
6. What is meant by the chain of custody of collected evidence?
7. What is meant by the term *proximate event*?
8. Describe how two bullets are compared during a ballistics test.
9. Compare the processes of putrefaction and mummification.
10. What are the responsibilities of the death investigator in relation to organ transplantation?
11. What issues might present themselves in a death investigation system that utilizes nonphysician death investigators?

REFERENCES

Byrd, J.H. & Castner, J.L. (Eds.). (2001). *Forensic entomology: The utility of arthropods in legal investigations.* Boca Raton, FL: CRC Press.

Connecticut General Statutes Vol. 6, Titles 17–19a, Revised January 2003.

Courson, S. (October 2, 2001). *The investigative specialty of forensic nursing.* Retrieved February 8, 2003, from http://www.psna.org/c_profdev_forensicnursing.htm.

Dillon, D. (1977). *A history of criminalistics in the United States 1850–1950.* Doctoral Thesis, University of California, Berkeley.

DiMaio, V.J.M. (1999). *Gunshot wounds: Practical aspects of firearms, ballistics, and forensic techniques.* (2nd ed.). Boca Raton, FL: CRC Press.

DiMaio, V.J.M. & DiMaio, D. (2001). *Forensic pathology* (2nd ed.). Boca Raton, FL: CRC Press.

Forensic Timeline. (2002). *Forensic science timeline.* Retrieved February 1, 2003, from http://www.forensicdna.com/Timeline020702.pdf.

Goff, M.L. (2000). *A fly for the prosecution: How insect evidence helps solve crime.* Cambridge, MA: Harvard University Press.

Hanzlick, R.L. (1996). *On the need for more expertise in death investigation (and a national office of death investigation affairs?). Archives of Pathology & Laboratory Medicine, 120,* 782–785.

Hanzlick, R.L. (Ed.). (1997). *Cause of death statements and certification of natural and unnatural deaths.* Northfield, IL: College of American Pathologists.

Hanzlick, R.L. (1997). *Death registration: History, methods, and legal issues. Journal of Forensic Science, 42*(2), 265–269.

History of forensic medicine (October 26, 1996). Retrieved February 1, 2003, from http://140.116.5.4/~chungho/history.htm.

International Association of Forensic Nurses. (1999). *Scope and standards of forensic nursing practice* (3rd ed.). Washington, DC: American Nurses Publishing.

Knight, B. (Ed.). (1995). *The estimation of the time since death in the early postmortem period.* Avon, England: Edward Arnold.

Messite, J. & Stellman, S. (1990). Accuracy of death certificate completion, the need for formalized physician training. *Journal of the American Medical Association, 275,* 794–796.

Saferstein, R. (2001). *Criminalistics: An introduction to forensic science* (7th ed.). Upper Saddle River, NJ: Dave Garza.

Spitz, W.U. (Ed.). (1993). *Spitz and Fisher's medicolegal investigation of death* (3rd ed.). Springfield, IL: Charles C. Thomas.

CHAPTER 6

Evidence Collection and Documentation

Nancy B. Cabelus
Katherine Spangler

Any time two people or objects come in contact with each other there is an exchange of physical evidence. The value of this evidence in forensic investigations may be compromised if the evidence is improperly packaged or if the reliability of the evidence cannot be shown. The forensic nurse must be aware of the proper recognition, documentation, collection, and preservation of evidence in criminal and civil investigations, such as domestic violence, motor vehicle accidents, and other situations involving physical evidence and patterns. This awareness is essential to prevent loss of critical materials and information, which can adversely affect subsequent analysis and proceedings.

CHAPTER FOCUS

Basic theories of evidence
Locard's principle of exchange
The crime scene
Classification of physical evidence
Evidence recognition and collection
Recognition of physical abuse
Evidence documentation
Evidence packaging
Role of the forensic laboratory
Collection of evidence from the deceased patient
Legal considerations

KEY TERMS_____

chain of custody
cross-contamination
documentation
HIPAA regulations
Locard's principle
physical evidence
tangible evidence
trace evidence
transient evidence

INTRODUCTION

Discoveries and developments in forensic science have led to changes within professional nursing practice. Because of these advances, forensic nursing is an evolving discipline that is a blend of two distinct concepts: nursing and forensic science.

The nursing profession interfaces with the law more than ever before, and in a multitude of settings. For example, there is a marked increase in the number of challenges to nursing documentation in both criminal and civil courts. The nurse is no longer automatically granted a high level of trust. She or he must earn that trust among colleagues and other professionals. As forensic nurses face today's challenges in treating victims and perpetrators of violent acts, they must be vigilant in recognizing changes and trends within their field of practice.

This chapter will address evidence recognition, documentation, and collection in the forensic nurse's daily practice. Standards for basic evidence collection techniques, suggested methods of documentation, and issues pertaining to patient privacy and confidentiality also will be discussed.

BASIC THEORIES

Contemporary forensic nursing roles may be largely attributed to the vision exemplified by the earliest founders of our profession. Attention to detail and unwavering dedication were part of the foundations of nursing. Today forensic nurses work in many contemporary roles, but have built upon the nursing theories of the past. By applying critical thinking skills, forensic nurses pay special attention to fine details while never losing sight of the "whole picture." Perhaps if Florence Nightingale crossed paths 100 years ago with Edmond Locard, the elderly woman would have been taken with that young scientist's theory of evidence exchange. If they had an opportunity to discuss their complementary philosophies, the concept of forensic nursing may have started a long time ago.

Florence Nightingale (1820–1910) was the icon of traditional nursing practice during the Victorian era. A critical thinker and a visionary well ahead of her time, Nightingale set the standard for holistic nursing care. Rather than treating the illness, she believed in treating the patient. Although Nightingale addressed the physical needs of the patient, she also integrated spiritual, emotional, and intellectual wellness into the nursing process. In Nightingale's era, the art of nursing practice was enhanced with scientific knowledge acquired through education, theory, and research.

Similarly, contemporary nurses of the 21st century must acquire some knowledge in basic forensic science and the law to treat a forensic patient effectively. Forensic nurses must be aware of current statutes, legal decisions, and mandated professional obligations when treating victims and perpetrators of abuse, neglect, or interpersonal violence. Care plans and charting procedures may need to be updated to document appropriately the standards of care provided by healthcare practitioners. This documentation is always important, but of even greater significance in any case that could potentially interface with a medicolegal investigation.

Locard's Principle of Exchange

Known as the "father of trace evidence," Dr. Edmond Locard (1877–1966) was a pathologist in Lyon, France. For many years Locard conducted scientific investigations and researched the application of analytical methods to criminal investigation. In 1910, Dr. Locard founded the first police laboratory, which was dedicated to the advancement of the forensic sciences. Forensic nurses have followed in Locard's footsteps by understanding the dynamics of trace evidence and the significance of that evidence in medicolegal investigations.

Locard's theory states that whenever there is contact between two objects, there is a mutual exchange of material between those two surfaces. This "theory of evidence exchange" provides a basis for linkage between the victim, the perpetrator, and the scene, as depicted in Figure 16–1. Locard maintained that "no one can act . . . without leaving behind numerous signs of it . . . indications of where he has been or what he has done" (Inman & Rudin, 2001, p. 44).

Thus, the analysis of exchanged or transferred material may show a causal relationship between the victim and the scene, the scene and the perpetrator, or the perpetrator and the victim. This evidence can lead to

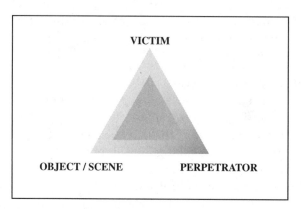

Figure 16–1 Relationship among sources of trace evidence.

the conviction of an offender or, as importantly, show that the person accused is not guilty of an offense.

Profound advances have occurred in the field of forensic science since 1910, including the discovery of deoxyribonucleic acid (DNA) and its application in forensic investigations. In spite of this scientific progress, Locard's principle remains as important now as it was in the early 1900s. Materials that have been exchanged between people or objects may be identified through application of Locard's principle; forensic advances such as DNA analysis allow for greater individualization of that exchanged evidence. (Refer to Chapter 19 for more information on DNA analysis.) Locard's theory of transfer is clearly illustrated by the following homicide case involving the identification of significant transfer evidence.

A CASE STUDY: Locard's Principle Linking a Victim and Suspect

A 10-year-old girl lived in a small Midwest town with her family. She left her school at approximately 3:30 p.m. for a 20-minute walk home, but she never arrived. At 4:30 p.m. her mother became concerned and began looking for her. The mother called the homes of her daughter's friends, but to no avail. She then called the police department. A search of the neighborhood began, but the child was not found.

It was not until 3 days later that the little girl's body was discovered in a wooded area about 6 miles from the school. She was partially clothed and her body was covered with dirt and leaves. Because the ambient temperature was cool, the body was fairly well preserved. A scarf was wrapped tightly around her neck. The girl was naked from the waist down and sexual assault was suspected.

The scene was secured by police officers so that there would be no inadvertent contamination of the scene or of potential evidence. Crime scene personnel processed the scene. During a search of the crime scene, tire impressions were discovered in the moist soil and in close proximity to the body. The tire impressions were photographed and plaster casts were made in order to preserve imprint detail.

A forensic nurse representing the medical examiner's office was dispatched to the scene. The forensic nurse conducted a survey of the body, which included a written description of observations and photographic documentation. This information was provided to the forensic pathologist to assist with the examination and interpretation of the child's injuries and to corroborate findings of the autopsy.

The forensic pathologist used a UV light to perform an external examination of the victim's body. The alternate light source was used to search for further potential evidence that may have been transferred onto the victim's body or the clothing by the perpetrator. Evidence such as semen, other body fluids, chemical residues, and some fibers may fluoresce when exposed to the ultraviolet light. Fine red fibers were found on the clothing that would not have been apparent with the naked eye. Subsequent laboratory evidence of these fibers showed that they had characteristics of a carpet fiber. Samples for comparison were removed by investigators from various locations. The red fiber evidence found on the child's body ultimately linked the victim to the perpetrator; the trunk of the perpetrator's car was lined with carpet having similar red fibers.

The Crime Scene

A crime scene is the location or place where a crime occurs. The scene can be inside or outdoors. A motor vehicle, train, or aircraft can be a crime scene. In the clinical setting, the victim may be the only known crime scene, for example when a sexual assault occurs. Clinicians who treat the victim may not know where the crime occurred, but evidence on the victim's body or clothing could connect that person to the crime scene. For example, if the crime occurred in a wooded area, there may be soil or plant material on the victim's clothing or footwear that would be similar to findings at that scene. It is important for the forensic nurse to understand Locard's theory of evidence transfer and its implications. In this way clinical findings can be interpreted while conducting an examination of the patient.

If there are multiple crime scenes within the scope of the investigation, the locations of interest may be referred to as the primary, secondary, or tertiary crime scenes. For example, in a carjacking incident, the primary crime scene would be where the carjacking occurred, and the secondary scene would be where the vehicle was recovered. In a homicide, a victim may have been abducted from one location, killed in a second place, and left in a third location. Therefore, investigators would ultimately have three crime scenes to process. The vehicle in which the victim was transported would also be considered a crime scene.

Physical evidence, when properly recognized, documented, and preserved, can provide the crucial link between the person and location or object that caused an injury. This is also true in cases of civil litigation, such as motor vehicle accidents and negligence cases. For example, a case of a failed seat belt will be greatly substantiated by identifying the presence of hair and tissue fragments in a shattered windshield, especially if those materials can be related to head injuries of the injured plaintiff.

The Forensic Nursing Role

Forensic nurses who work with evidence collection and documentation require specialized training. The traditional nursing school curriculum does not include education on physical evidence collection procedures or management of forensic evidence after collection. Because of the emphasis on forensic evidence in today's courtroom and with advances in forensic science, especially in the laboratory testing of biological evidence, nursing care plans must be modified to include policies and procedures for both the treatment of the forensic patient and the proper collection of forensic evidence. Because they are excellent communicators, forensic nurses can help to bridge the gap between law enforcement and the physician or other healthcare professionals. In addition, forensic nurses are able to provide better holistic care by applying critical thinking skills when making a nursing diagnosis. Forensic nurses may be called upon to testify in a criminal or civil courtroom because of their interaction with victims, suspects, and members of the legal community. Forensic nurses are readily accepted as credible expert witnesses because of their specialized training.

FORENSIC EVIDENCE

Classification of Physical Evidence

There are many ways to classify and categorize physical evidence. Some forensic experts classify evidence according to the type of action that produced the evidence (e.g., homicide, motor vehicle accident, medical negligence); others concentrate on the type of analyses that will be required (e.g., instrumental analysis, pattern examination, radiography). For the purposes of this chapter, evidence classes that are of greatest concern to the forensic nurse are physical evidence that is identified as tangible, transient, or trace. Tangible evidence is touchable. It may be recognizable on sight, such as a gun, a knife, an article of clothing, or a written document. Multiple gunshot patterns, bloodstains, and other pattern evidence are included in this category. When pattern evidence is encountered, those patterns must be documented in place prior to any alteration. Figure 16–2 shows the proper documentation of multiple gunshot pattern evidence. Note the presence of a scale and proper lighting, which assists in determining the sequence of shots and their relationship to each other on the windshield.

Physical evidence also includes so-called trace evidence, which is any material found in small quantity or size. Trace evidence cannot always be seen by the naked eye, but may be identified with the use of a microscope or alternate light sources; for example, bite mark evidence may include traces of saliva containing DNA. Although not visually apparent, the forensic nurse may recognize the significance of finding DNA evidence in a wound. If collected properly, the foreign DNA sample can potentially be linked to its source. If the nurse were to cleanse a bite mark injury prior to collecting a swabbed sample from the marking, the transferred evidence would be lost. The nurse should also note other characteristics of the bite mark such as size, shape, depth, or pattern of the mark. Use of alternate light systems often aids in locating and recognizing trace evidence.

Evidence that can be washed away, damaged, lost, or destroyed, either intentionally, accidentally, or by environmental factors, is designated transient evidence. Transient evidence is observed when a patient is

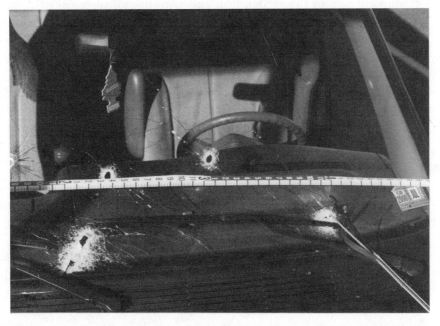

Figure 16–2 A photograph of a motor vehicle with multiple gunshot strikes to the windshield. The photograph depicts the distribution of shots and the scale allows an estimate of the distance among the shots. (Photograph courtesy of the Connecticut State Police, Central District Major Crime Squad.)

treated with injuries having characteristics of bruising, swelling, bleeding, redness, or tenderness. The nurse should carefully document the location and description of those injuries as well as what was palpated upon examination. If possible, these kinds of injuries should also be photographed because they will no longer be visible after they have healed. Photographs should also be taken of the injuries a couple of days after they first occur. This additional documentation will demonstrate any further discoloration of the patient's skin throughout the healing process and any patterned injury that may be seen.

Transient evidence may also be detected through sense of smell, such as an odor of marijuana, alcoholic beverage, or gasoline. Again, this kind of evidence is present only temporarily. It will not be available to show to a court or jury if the case goes to trial in the future. Therefore, the importance of thorough documentation cannot be overemphasized.

Evidence Recognition and Collection

Evidence can be encountered in many situations within the forensic nursing profession. Perhaps the most common or most familiar role in which the forensic nurse must follow prescribed procedures for evidence collection is that of the sexual assault nurse or forensic examiner (SANE/SAFE). The SANE is arguably the most established forensic nursing role in the recognition and handling of physical evidence. As part of their training and education, SANE nurses must demonstrate proficiency in evidence collection and packaging, the ability to properly document their findings in the course of the examination, and also be able to properly initiate the chain of custody. In some parts of the United States, evidence collection procedures for the treatment of victims of sexual assault have been standardized. Forensic nurse examiners may be mandated by law to follow such required protocols. In all cases, any mandated collection kits or protocols have been developed to maintain the proper collection and preservation of evidence. The goal is to limit the potential for challenge of the evidence at a later time.

In clinical practice, the chain of custody usually begins when a healthcare practitioner locates or obtains physical evidence. The documentation process for evidence collection and transfer is facilitated by the use of an evidence custody form. An example of a chain of custody form is shown in Figure 16–3. Any documentation of the evidence should include a description of what the item of evidence is, the date and time it was recovered, and from where it was recovered. A case number or identification code to be used for cross-referencing should also be noted. This initial collection information should also be written on any evidence tags. The person who receives the evidence from the nurse should sign for the evidence, initiating a "paper trail" that

---

Chain of custody flow sheet

Case # or ID Code# H1234

Exhibit #: 1

Description of item: blue T-shirt, size small, torn on right sleeve

Taken from: Kathy Smith

By whom: S. Jones RN **Date/Time:** 1/2/03 4:10am

Transferred to: Off. Coffey My City P.D.

Taken from: Off. Coffey

By whom: Sgt. Bagel **Date/Time:** 1/2/03 6:15am

Transferred to: State Lab

Taken from:

By whom: Date/Time:

Transferred to:

Comments:

Figure 16–3 Chain of custody form.

follows the transfer of evidence. A receipt should also be generated to obtain the signatures of people who have custody of the evidence. As a general rule of thumb, it is always better to write down more information that might be required if you are not sure what to include. Most evidence is presented months or years after collection, so the failure to note appropriate details could result in many hours providing testimony. In some cases, improperly documented evidence or chain of custody may result in the judge ruling the evidence inadmissible during court proceedings.

When providing care to victims or perpetrators of interpersonal violence, the forensic nurse must be aware of what could potentially be physical evidence of a crime. The forensic nurse must consider that when treating a gunshot wound victim, guns, gunshot residue, bullets, bullet projectiles, or fragments may be present on the patient's skin, in the clothing, within applied bandages or dressings, or even on the stretcher on which the patient was transported. Law enforcement officers may arrive at the hospital to collect such evidence. Forensic nurses can better assist the investigative team by recognizing what law enforcement investigators may be looking for.

The forensic nurse should also keep in mind that safety is a very important concern. If weapons are found on a patient, security measures must be taken immediately to protect medical staff and other patients in the facility. Documentation of safety interventions by the nurse who secured the weapons should be noted (e.g., "Handgun, magazine, and 8 bullets turned over to Hospital Security Department"). Because many people are not firearms experts, the nurse should not record information about the weapon that is uncertain (model number or caliber). However, the nurse should document what types of weapons were found (knives, brass knuckles, etc.). If possible, photograph the weapons as shown in Figure 16–4. As always, care should be taken to avoid disrupting other evidence that may be on the weapon's surface.

Victims of motor vehicle accidents, especially pedestrians struck by motor vehicles, may be covered with telling evidence at the time of physical examination. Dirt, debris, glass fragments, and paint samples frequently transfer onto the body or clothing of a victim at the point of impact or in the moments following a crash. Additionally, the forensic nurse can assess for evidence of the driver of the vehicle or where a passenger may have been seated in the vehicle. Types of injuries to evaluate would include abrasions caused by seat belts, shoulder harnesses, or airbags; lacerations to the face or scalp; and contusions to the chest or knees. In car vs. pedestrian accidents, especially hit-and-run incidents,

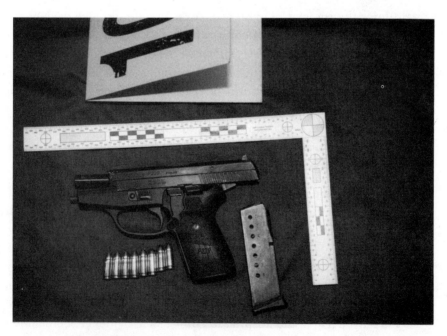

Figure 16–4 Proper photographic documentation of an unloaded, semiautomatic pistol with empty magazine and eight live rounds.

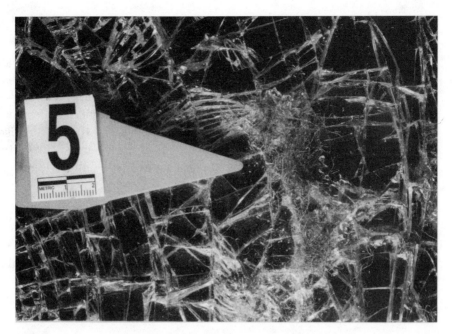

Figure 16–5   A close-up photograph of evidence identified in the search of a motor vehicle involved in an accident. Strands of hair can be seen caught within fractures of the windshield glass.

patterns of injuries caused by impact with vehicle bumpers, side-view mirrors, or tires will often help investigators to match up evidence at the accident scene or to reconstruct the incident. Figure 16–5 depicts an example of hair evidence located on the windshield of a vehicle involved in a hit-and-run accident. The victim's clothing should be carefully handled to preserve stains, rips, and tears in the fabric, as well as trace evidence such as glass, paint, dirt, or debris.

Recognition of Physical Abuse

Victims of physical abuse, domestic violence, or child or elder abuse who seek medical treatment may present with evidence of injuries such as slap marks or grab marks from the hand of their offender, bite marks, burns, contusions, or scars. If an injury appears to have a pattern, the nurse should describe and document the pattern in the patient record. Photodocumentation is very useful to support clinical findings in such cases.

The nurse could ask the patient if he or she was hurt by someone, who did this, or what they were struck with. If the patient is nonverbal or cannot effectively articulate this information, the nurse's job becomes more challenging and difficult. The victim may not be able to answer the nurse's questions for fear of the consequences. The forensic nurse should be aware that the evidence at hand may not be consistent with the story that is being told.

Many times the perpetrator of the abuse is related to the victim in a role such as a caretaker, a relative, or an intimate partner. Sometimes the offender will accompany the victim to the hospital and will stay with the victim during an examination to ensure that the victim does not disclose information or report the offender. Chapters 10 and 11 discuss relationships and abuse in greater detail and may provide additional guidance regarding these considerations when collecting evidence from victims of abuse.

Nurses must be familiar with mandated reporting statutes in their state. In general, nurses are mandated to report cases of abuse or neglect in children, the elderly, and the mentally retarded. Contact with the agencies that protect these populations should be made verbally and also in writing. Most agencies have required documents that must be completed by the clinician. Copies of those documents should be included with the patient record.

Collection of Physical Evidence

Crime scene investigators know what types of basic evidence collection materials are needed to process a crime scene. Such items include paper or plastic bags, paper envelopes, boxes, clean rolled paper, and containers of various sizes. Tools that are useful at the crime scene include tape rulers, a sketchbook, a compass, and a camera. It becomes automatic for the experienced crime scene investigator to arrive at the crime scene prepared to complete the lengthy and meticulous process of gathering evidence.

In the clinical setting, the caregiver may not be as readily prepared to receive a patient who could later be considered a crime scene or source of civil legal dispute. It is important to train medical staff about advances in forensic medicine so that they, too, are ready when a forensic patient is whisked through the hospital doors. In trauma centers, staff may be equipped with prepackaged cut-down sets used to insert intravenous catheters, or tracheal intubation sets used to establish an airway for a trauma patient who is not breathing. Staff members should also be supplied with evidence collection kits filled with collection materials necessary to conveniently and properly preserve evidence that could link the victim to the crime scene or to the suspect.

Preservation of life is the foremost priority when treating a trauma patient. In a stressful and chaotic environment it is easy to overlook forensic evidence that may be inadvertently destroyed or discarded. Evidence of interest to investigators could include the patient's clothing, footwear, hairs or fibers, stains, glass fragments or debris, or any noticeable patterns of injury including cuts, lacerations, abrasions, or bite marks. Prior to packaging evidence, the forensic nurse should refer to the workplace photography policy regarding seized evidence.

Evidence Packaging

In general, physical evidence should be packaged to prevent alteration of the evidence or deleterious change. Some suggestions for packaging commonly encountered physical evidence are listed here. A quick-reference chart listing methods of collection and preservation of various types of evidence may be found in Appendix 2.

Clothing

If possible, the nurse should collect items of clothing and place each item into a separate paper bag to avoid cross-contamination. If articles of clothing are wet, they should be air dried before packaging. If this is not possible, the articles may be temporarily placed into separate plastic bags to avoid leakage or cross-contamination. Then, as soon as possible, transport the items to a place where they can be hung to dry (e.g., drying room or evidence drying cabinet). Failure to completely dry items prior to packaging could result in bacterial or mold growth, contamination, and breakdown of biological evidence.

Patterns of stains, holes, or tears in the clothing fabric should be noted. Effort must be made to preserve such patterns for forensic specialists to examine. A frequent mistake made by first responders and hospital personnel is to cut through the patient's clothing at the site of bullet holes, stab wounds, or tears in the fabric made by a penetrating object. Forensic examiners may be limited in their capability to interpret or reconstruct the incident if the evidence has been altered in such a manner. First responders may not be aware of the value of the evidence that they are destroying or discarding. Although it is acceptable to cut through clothing to enable the administration of first aid, whenever possible defects in the clothing should remain intact. Careful handling of these items by the forensic nurse can help the forensic scientist to successfully complete a laboratory examination.

Footwear

Footwear should be packaged separately from the clothing and each shoe packaged individually. Footwear from both the victim and the perpetrator may be of significance and link each to the crime scene. Soil or debris may have collected within the grooves and ridges of the soles and may match soil at the scene. Footwear sole patterns, stains, or evidence of spatter should be noted. Footprints and shoe impressions should be photographed to scale, as shown in Figure 16–6.

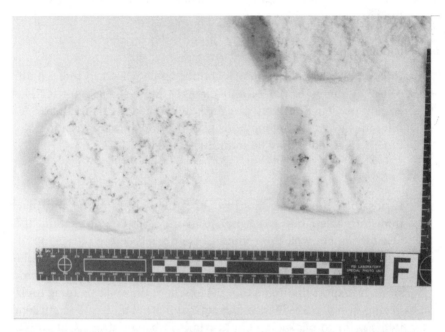

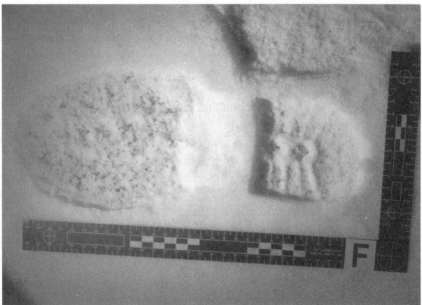

Figure 16–6 A footwear impression in snow photographed with scale using a standard flash (top) and an alternate light source (bottom). Note the additional imprint detail in the photograph taken with alternate light.

Hairs or Fibers

Hairs or fibers found on the victim's body are best preserved when carefully removed. Hair and fiber evidence may be collected by area (e.g., patient's right hand or patient's left hand). When the hair or fiber is removed it should be packaged inside a paper druggist fold and then sealed in a paper envelope. Hair and fiber evidence should not be removed from an article of clothing unless there is concern about damage or loss. Rather, the clothing should be carefully folded and placed in a clean paper bag or in paper wrapping.

Stains or Other Deposits

Dried secretions, samples of dirt, or debris should be swabbed with a sterile swab moistened with sterile water or saline. These swabbings should be air dried before packaging. Some facilities use a simple rack in which swabs can dry before inserting them into paper envelopes. Small, electric, or battery-operated dryers are sometimes used to facilitate the drying process. However, caution should be used to avoid cross-contamination with samples from other specimens or patients when using these devices. It is necessary to clean the drying apparatus after each use to avoid contamination. Also, a dryer with fans may introduce foreign, airborne particles or bacteria onto the collected sample. Avoid using heat lamps or hair dryers because these may alter the physical properties of the sample or degrade the biological material.

Bullets and Projectiles

Bullets or projectiles may contain trace evidence such as fibers, blood, or tissue. The nurse should preserve the projectile by placing it into a clean druggist fold or gauze before sealing it in a clean envelope. The surface of the projectile should be protected from rubbing against hard surfaces or other objects to preserve ballistic markings and detail.

Sharps

Sharp objects such as needles, razor blades, or knives need to be secured in such a way as to prevent injury to others and also to preserve trace evidence on the item. Plastic or glass specimen jars may be used to secure needles, razor blades, or pieces of broken glass. Knives should be secured in cardboard boxes of the appropriate size. Containers that have been designed to store these hazardous objects safely are commercially available.

Evidence collection techniques and choice of collection products can vary among jurisdictions. Training and experience will assist the nurse in determining what to collect, how it should be collected, and how much to collect. It is important for the forensic nurse to be familiar with collection and packaging guidelines specific to the laboratory where the evidence will be tested.

FUNCTION OF THE FORENSIC LABORATORY

Once evidence has been collected it is transferred to the forensic laboratory for analysis. It is important to understand what the laboratory can do when analyzing evidence, but it is also important to understand what the lab cannot do.

Many services within the forensic laboratory are available to police departments, state agencies, and, occasionally, to the private sector. Some of the services available may include, but are not limited to:

- Biological analysis is for the identification and individualization of blood and body fluids. This also includes the fields of immunology, serology, biochemistry, hematology, and molecular biology.
- Chemical analysis is used to identify accelerates that have been collected during arson investigations or other cases in which chemicals have been used in the commission of a crime.
- Fingerprint analysis is available and includes processing for identification of latent prints and fingerprint comparisons from agencies around the world.
- Firearms analysis includes the examination of guns, bullets, and bullet fragments. Tool marks are also examined and compared to tools when encountered during the investigation of a crime. This is a mark that is left when a hard surface comes into contact with a soft surface, leaving telltale marks that may identify the type of tool used.
- Document examination is the analysis of documents, whether in written form or produced by a machine, including typewriters, computers, or copiers. Characteristics of paper and ink may also be included in this process.
- Trace evidence analysis is done using a number of different modalities. It may include the use of a scanning electron microscope or gas chromatograph. The types of trace evidence that may be analyzed are enumerable and may include paint, soil, glass, minerals, fiber, hairs, and plant material.
- Controlled substances/toxicology analysis identifies drugs of abuse and chemicals that may be used in drug-facilitated sexual assaults. Alcohol or drug levels in urine, blood, or other body fluids are also analyzed in toxicology sections.
- Forensic photography utilizes specialized techniques to document and enhance information from crime scenes. Photographic documentation of a note from a crime scene is shown in Figure 16–7.

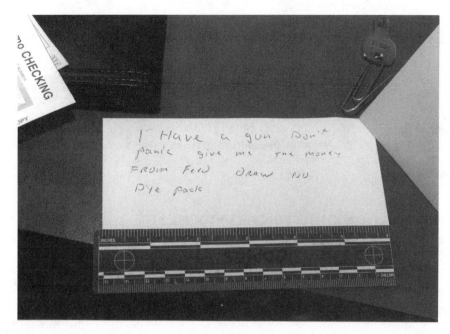

Figure 16–7 A handwritten note that was left at the scene of a bank robbery. As shown in this photograph, evidence should be documented in place prior to collection.

A CASE STUDY: The Importance of the Chain of Custody

In 1973, a young woman parked her vehicle on the upper level of a public parking garage. As she exited her vehicle, she was attacked, chased by her attacker, and stabbed as she entered the descending stairwell. The woman was fatally stabbed through the chest by an unknown assailant. The attacker ran to the victim's vehicle and drove it to a lower level of the garage. While in the victim's vehicle, he noticed that his hand was bleeding and reached into the back seat of the vehicle for a box of tissues. In doing so, he left a bloody fingerprint on the box. The assailant then exited the victim's car, proceeded to his own vehicle, and drove his vehicle out of the garage. He handed his parking stub to a ticket taker and paid for parking. The ticket taker recalled having to wipe the blood from the ticket in order to read the time stamped on it. He watched as the assailant quickly drove away.

A short time later, the victim's body was discovered in the stairwell. Investigators responded to the scene and documented their findings. Items of evidence were seized that included the victim's dress, samples from a bloody trail within the garage, blood from the vehicle, and the tissue box with the bloody fingerprint.

For nearly three decades this case remained unsolved, until one day, when a diligent fingerprint expert entered this bloody fingerprint into the automated fingerprint identification system (AFIS). The AFIS identified a matching print on file, which was confirmed by the examiner. The suspect identified by the fingerprint match still lived in the area of the crime.

Evidence gathered at the scene had been tested by various laboratories over a period of several years. The defense challenged the admissibility of the evidence because of the many years and multiple handling of the evidence. However, the chain of custody had been maintained by extensive photographs of the evidence and documentation in the written records. In addition, the evidence remained securely stored at the police department and laboratory. Evidence preservation, integrity, and documentation by the investigative agency led to successful prosecution of this case that resulted in a 30-year sentence for the perpetrator.

DOCUMENTATION OF PHYSICAL EVIDENCE

Written Records

Nurses who document reports of the treatment of a forensic patient and the collection of physical evidence must adhere to quality charting standards that are typically required for all medical records. Documentation standards are set by licensing statutes, nurse practice acts, the American Nurses Association, and the Joint Commission on Accreditation of Healthcare Organizations (Capuano, Carolan et al., 1999). Errors made by healthcare personnel in the medicolegal documentation of a case could lead to disastrous outcomes in the courtroom. Common problems found in medical charts include the use of sloppy jargon, confusing abbreviations and statements, vague descriptions, and lack of clarity. Failure to report information as stated by the patient, omissions of interventions provided, and late entries in the record could raise legal concerns about the nurse's actions.

Nurses need to communicate the information effectively into the written record by being accurate, comprehensive, and legible. It is important to document the facts as discovered and to avoid personal opinions about the patient or the case.

When charting in the forensic patient's record, the nurse should address the patient's response to treatments given and also describe the recommended plans for follow-up care. Referrals made to protective agencies such as battered women's shelters, sexual assault counseling services, or victims' advocacy groups should be noted.

Other Documentation Methods

In addition to a written description of a patient's injuries, it is often helpful to use drawings and diagrams, sometimes referred to as body charts. For example, if a person sustained multiple stab wounds or

Table 16–1 Considerations for Clinical Photography

- Who will take the photographs? What kind of training does the photographer have?
- What kind of camera will be used? What type of film/equipment will be used?
- What will be photographed?
- Is there a written consent from the patient to be photographed? Or is the consent to photograph included in the "all-inclusive" consent to treat the patient?
- Who will develop/process the film and maintain the chain of custody for the film so it does not end up in the hands of a third party?
- Where do the developed photographs end up? They belong with the medical record, but is there a place to securely store them?
- If using digital photography, where are the disks stored that contain the medicolegal documentation?
- Consider confidentiality and privacy regulations. What steps are taken to ensure that HIPAA standards are maintained? If the photos are subjected to court subpoena, what is the procedure for duplication of the negatives?
- Who pays for the taking of photos and the processing of the film?

bruises, a sketch of the injuries could better depict the location of the injuries than a written description. Rather than describing the injury as being in the "upper left chest" or the "lower portion of the arm" a body chart better clarifies the location, size, or shape of the injury in question.

The use of photography is an excellent way to document findings of forensic evidence while either at the crime scene or treating a clinical patient who has sustained an injury. In clinical environments, it is important to have policies in place regarding use of photography to document injuries relating to trauma as well as domestic violence, sexual assault, or any means of abuse. The authors' recommended guidelines when implementing clinical photo documentation policies are outlined in Table 16–1. Detailed guidelines for forensic photography may be found in Chapter 17.

CASE STUDIES: The Importance of Proper Evidence Collection and Documentation

The following case studies illustrate the importance of evidence collection, documentation, and the integrity of the chain of custody. These cases took place at two different hospitals, a short distance away from each other. Hospital A did not have a forensic nurse on duty. Hospital B personnel had some training in evidence collection.

Hospital A

A 25-year-old female who was 7 months pregnant was having a domestic dispute with her boyfriend. The boyfriend, in a fit of rage, stabbed the woman repeatedly with a knife. Neighbors heard her cries for help as she exited the apartment and ran to the parking lot. Police quickly arrived and ordered the man to drop the knife. The man refused to comply and was shot dead. The female victim was transported to a hospital with wounds to her chest and neck. She was rushed to the operating room where her baby was delivered via Caesarean section. When investigators arrived at the hospital to retrieve the victim's clothing for evidence, the clothing could not be located. Neither the emergency department nor the operating room personnel knew what had happened to the clothing. After several inquiries, it was discovered that the blood-saturated clothing was put into a plastic bag and tossed into the laundry chute. There it became lodged between floors within the hospital. Comingled with hospital linens, this evidence was eventually recovered, but it was cross-contaminated by multiple sources. How would the presence of a forensic nurse on staff have affected the proper collection and preservation of this evidence?

Hospital B

The subject, an intoxicated, adult male, threatened to kill his parents with a knife. The subject's mother ran from the house and called 911. Screaming for help, she told the dispatcher that her son was going to kill her husband. When the first responding officer arrived, he ordered the man, several times, to put down the knife. The man shouted back at the officer and lunged toward him. The officer shot the man in the chest. The wounded man was transported to the local hospital and was rushed to the operating room where he died a short time later. The forensic nurse in this case preserved the clothing and potential trace evidence for police investigators, although the subject's brother was demanding to see the deceased. Detectives photographed the subject's injuries, collected gunshot residue samples, and fingerprinted the subject for the purposes of identification. Once the evidence was collected and documented, hospital staff members addressed the needs of the family. Figure 16–8 shows the decedent's clothing as it was documented before packaging. Quick documentation with a scale in the ER assisted the investigation at a later time.

This case, as police-involved shootings often are, was scrutinized by the general public. Questions frequently arise pertaining to the justification of the shooting. Some of these questions are: Was there reasonable use of deadly force? Was the officer in fear of his life? What was the direction of the shots fired (e.g., front to back vs. back to front)? How close was the officer to the subject? Examination of physical evidence can sometimes answer questions that even eyewitnesses may have difficulty in recollecting or answering.

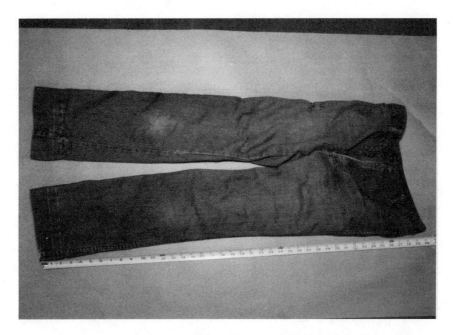

Figure 16–8 An overall view of the clothing removed from the decedent in a police-involved shooting case.

COLLECTION OF EVIDENCE FROM THE DECEASED PATIENT

Identity of the Deceased

At the scene of a homicide or at a death that was not witnessed, investigators will search for evidence to attempt to obtain identity of the deceased. This could include an attempt to locate the next of kin or a picture ID card, such as a driver's license with the name and date of birth of the victim. Investigators at the scene may check through the victim's clothing and inventory the victim's wallet, the contents of pockets in clothing, and any jewelry that the victim may be wearing. Electronic pagers and cellular telephones, frequently found on or within clothing, are also noted and secured by investigators. In some cases, none of the aforementioned items are present. In those instances, identification is made through fingerprint or dental record comparisons or through DNA sampling if known materials are available for comparison purposes.

Trace Evidence from the Decedent

If the victim appears to have been in a struggle or was shot at close range, investigators will secure paper bags over the hands of the deceased to preserve trace evidence that could potentially be destroyed or lost during transport of the body to the morgue. The body is then wrapped in a clean sheet before being placed into a body bag. Again, this is done to preserve trace evidence.

Prior to autopsy, the victim is photographed and trace evidence is collected from the body by the forensic pathologist. Once this is done, the victim can be fingerprinted.

If the victim is transported to a hospital in a resuscitative effort, preservation of trace evidence becomes very difficult. When the victim is pronounced dead, the past practice of the nurse was to provide postmortem care by "cleaning up" the body so that the next of kin could make identification. Forensic nurses now know that the practice of washing away trace evidence is detrimental to an investigation.

The forensic nurse can take some helpful steps that may aid investigators in the preservation of physical evidence. Important points for consideration in preserving physical evidence on the deceased follow. Once these steps are taken, the nurse may either assist family members of the decedent to make identification at the hospital or direct family to the medical examiner's office and to the investigative authorities.

1. If clothing was removed from the body, preserve, document, and package as described in this chapter.
2. Do not wash or attempt to "improve" the appearance of the deceased until a death investigator or forensic nurse has had an opportunity to photograph the victim and remove trace materials.
3. Bag hands to prevent loss of evidence. Gunshot residue samples or other trace samples may need to be collected as soon as possible.
4. Fingerprints may need to be obtained by investigators.
5. Keep dressings, bandages, catheters, and endotracheal tubes intact with the patient.
6. Other items of evidentiary value (weapons, drugs, documents) may need to be turned over to police or death investigators.

EVIDENCE FROM POISONING OR OVERDOSE

Sample Documentation

In cases of suspected poisoning or drug overdose, it is important for the forensic nurse investigator not only to obtain a social and medical history of the deceased, but also to record an inventory of prescription medications found at the scene. Information in a medications inventory should include:

- The name of the patient
- The name of the medication
- The dosage
- Date filled
- Number dispensed
- Number of tablets remaining in the vial

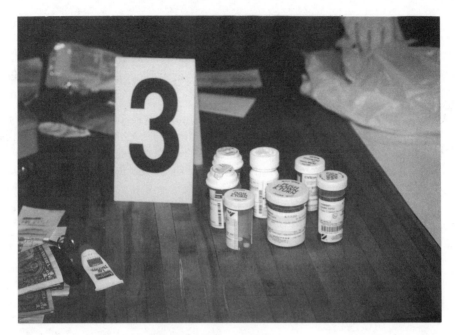

Figure 16–9 Prescription medications located at the scene of a questioned death.

- The physician's name
- The pharmacy that dispensed the order

This information is not only helpful for determining an antidote for a surviving patient, but also assists the forensic pathologist or death investigator in the course of the autopsy and investigative inquiry should the cause of death be an issue. Medications at the scene should be documented in place prior to complete inventory of the materials, as shown in Figure 16–9. It is also important to note the quantity of medication remaining in the containers upon collection.

Poisons can be introduced into the body by ingestion, injection, or inhalation. The elements that may affect the body are many. The forensic nurse must maintain an objective mindset and use critical thinking in analyzing the possibility of poisoning, whether intentional or unintentional.

Sample Collection and Analysis

Determining the element of a poisoning may be done by analyzing any or all of the following:

1. Body fluids, which include blood, gastric contents, urine, breast milk, or fluid in the eye
2. Hair, particularly head hair
3. Tissue, which includes sampling of muscle, brain, and liver

All these tissues may be tested for the identification and quantitation of chemical poison levels. If tissue is collected for testing, the sample must be handled to prevent cross-contamination with other specimens such as blood. Samples should be kept in separate containers for submission to the laboratory (Lee & Harris, 2000).

If administration of poison is intentional and results in a death, the manner of death may be ruled either a suicide or a homicide. If administration of poison is unintentional and results in a death, the manner of death would be accidental. Many deaths of accidental nature are caused by mixed drug intoxication. This means that the individual, though not intending to cause her own death, has taken a mixture of agents such as heroin, alcohol, and painkillers.

Death or injury from poisons may be exacerbated if there are underlying medical conditions such as heart disease or diabetes. Also, a person may be taking prescribed medications that may interact negatively with recreational drugs. Thus, a medical history is important in ascertaining the potential interactions of materials. In addition, when assessing a patient who may have been poisoned, the forensic nurse should understand what types of analyses may be done to detect the possible poisons.

If blood is to be analyzed, the first blood drawn should be saved prior to any other medication being administered in the effort to resuscitate the patient. The type of analysis to be done will dictate what type of tube to collect the sample in and how that tube should be treated (e.g., refrigerated or not). If the forensic nurse is unsure of the analytical process that will be required, she should consult the toxicology laboratory for detailed instructions.

LEGAL CONSIDERATIONS

Collection by Warrant, Court Order, and Consent

During the course of a criminal investigation, known biological samples, including hairs, blood, or buccal swabs, may be requested from the victim or a perpetrator by law enforcement. This collection can be accomplished legally by either written consent or applying to a judge for a search warrant or court order to obtain samples. The results of these tests are to be provided to the law enforcement agency that obtained consent with the authorization of the aforementioned documents. An overview of the legal requirements to collect evidentiary samples from suspects and victims may be found in Appendix 1.

HIPAA

Of late, there has been much confusion in the interpretation of patient confidentiality as outlined by the Health Insurance Portability and Accountability Act (HIPAA) (HIPAA, 2002). Law enforcement officers may have difficulty in obtaining information because healthcare workers do not understand what HIPAA is and what it is not. The following information should help to clarify the impact of HIPAA on the forensic nurse.

All subsets of forensic nursing practice are subject to the standards set forth by HIPAA. HIPAA regulations are categorized into three areas:

1. *Administrative simplification*: Regulations were implemented to create uniform standards and requirements for any health information that is transmitted electronically. This includes health information that may be faxed or e-mailed to another facility. This transfer of information impacts not only the healthcare providers who have physical control over the health information of individuals, but also any person or entity who has received this information for purposes other than providing treatment to an individual. This could include attorneys, courts, police departments, and insurance companies.
2. *Security:* Regulations are outlined for maintaining the security and integrity of medical/health information. Documentation that contains any health information and specific individualizing information must be kept safe and secure while in the possession of the receiving party. This includes protecting information from being viewed by unauthorized individuals, keeping that health information in a secure location, and preventing any possibility of unauthorized duplication.
3. *Privacy:* Regulations exist regarding how that health information may be used, as set forth by the individual whose health information is at issue.

Questions have arisen as to who would fall under the category of healthcare provider. If information is obtained for a purpose other than providing care, does that entity remain under the guidelines as set forth by the HIPAA regulation? It is the authors' opinion that any person or institution that has physical control of health information must follow the HIPAA guidelines as they pertain to privacy and security.

Nurses have always been acutely aware of the fact that confidentiality is of utmost importance when dealing with health information of the patient for whom they are caring. Requirements regarding confidentiality have been an issue of first order from the start of nursing school. Those in healthcare-related professions have been following these requirements for maintaining privacy as part of good nursing practice. However, HIPAA promises more extensive monitoring of confidentiality requirements and stiffer penalties for violators than at any previous time.

Generally, the job of the forensic nurse would be easier if standard forms were utilized for the release of medical information, but HIPAA only sets guidelines. It is each entity's responsibility to follow those standards. The individual or healthcare facility must determine how they will apply those standards. One hospital may accept a standard release form, while another hospital may require its own form to be signed before information can be released. These individual differences can cause the requestor some confusion and delay in obtaining important information. However, time will likely ease the difficulties encountered when preserving the confidentiality, privacy, and security of the information.

The HIPAA mandate, published by the Department of Health and Human Services (HHS), raised great concern as to whether these regulations would adversely affect patient care. In 2002, HHS modified its regulations to improve the implementation of the HIPAA guidelines, modifications that would not affect the quality of patient care. After reviewing public comments, HHS adopted the modifications necessary to ensure that the privacy rule worked as intended. The final rule was adopted in August 2002.

According to the Department of Health and Human Services, the implementation of the HIPAA privacy rule will:

1. give patients more control over their own health information,
2. set boundaries on how the health information is to be released and how it is to be used,
3. establish safeguards so that those in control of the health information are better able to provide protection of the privacy of the patient and of the patient's health information,
4. hold violators of this privacy mandate accountable with resulting civil and criminal penalties,
5. provide a balance when disclosure of health information is needed in order to protect public health,
6. allow patients the ability to make informed decisions as to the care they receive and reimbursement for the care based on how the health information is utilized,
7. advise patients how the health information is to be used and what information is released,
8. possibly limit the information that will be released to the minimum needed for disclosure yet ensure quality of care base upon that information,
9. give the patient the right to examine the records to be released and enable them to get a copy of their own health records,
10. allow the patient to request corrections to the medical records should discrepancies be found that are inconsistent with the actual facts,
11. enable the patient to control the use and disclosure of their own health information (USDHHS, OCR Privacy Brief, 2003).

HIPAA & Evidence Documentation

The use of photographs, videotapes, and digital images has become an important aspect of the forensic nursing practice. These and other methods are used frequently in the documentation process. Caution must be exercised to protect the privacy and confidentiality of the client while ensuring thorough documentation of important materials and patterns. Policies and procedures regarding security of photos, video, and digital images should be in place in any facility that intends to use them as part of their documentation protocol.

The liability issues related to photographs or videotapes of patients are of utmost importance. HIPAA Section 160.103, which relates to the issue of photodocumentation, states:

> Health information means any information whether oral, recorded in any form or medium, 1. that is created or received by a healthcare provider, health plan, public health authority, employer, life insurer, school or university, or health care clearing house. 2. Relates to the past, present or future, physical or mental health or condition of an individual; the provision of health care to an individual; or the past, present or future payment for the provision of healthcare to the individual. (HIPAA, 2002)

Thus, the federal regulations regarding other forms of evidence documentation should be followed to ensure privacy, just as one would follow the handling of other health information. The authorization form for the release of this information must contain specific information. The following information must be provided on an authorization for release of information:

- A description of the information to be disclosed or used. This includes any specific request for the release of x-rays, laboratory findings, history and physical, discharge summary or office notes.
- The identification of the persons or class of persons authorized to make use of the information to be disclosed. The name and address of the physician from whom information is requested. The entity's address should be included in this request.
- The identification of the person or persons making the request. This includes an attorney who represents a client for whom the medical records are requested for the purpose of litigation.
- A description of the reason why the health information is requested. An example of this would be, "for the purpose of litigation."
- An expiration date must be provided on the authorization form. If health information is requested, an end date or time is required for this request. This time could be "the conclusion of the case" or may be a specific date.
- The signature of the individual whose health information is being requested and a date must be provided on the authorization form.
- If the form is signed by an individual other than the person named on the form, such as a personal representative or guardian of the person, the authority of the signer must be documented and must accompany

the authorization form. For example, if the person requesting the information represents the estate of a deceased individual, then the "Letter of Administration" must accompany the request. If the individual is the guardian, then the court documents showing appointment of the guardian must accompany the request.

Other Regulations and Guidelines

In addition to the HIPAA regulations that mandate privacy issues of health information, other regulations impact both the forensic nurse and the forensic patient. For those facilities that are accredited by the Joint Commission on Accreditation of Healthcare Organizations (JCAHO), that organization also provides guidelines to the forensic population (JCAHO, 2003). Specifically, JCAHO states that the goal of the patient assessment function is to determine what kind of care is required to meet the patient's initial needs and his or her needs as they change in response to care. Further, JCAHO points out that it is important to provide a patient with appropriate care at the time the patient is in need of that care, and that care must be provided by a qualified individual (JCAHO, 2003). "Appropriate" care implies that a "forensic" patient must be provided care by a person who is trained to recognize and evaluate the forensic patient's needs. The process of developing and implementing a plan of care in forensic situations clearly includes the recognition and collection of evidence. Thus, only when the caregiver is trained to recognize the needs of the forensic population and act accordingly will the mandate of JCAHO be met.

The American Nurses Association takes this requirement a step further by describing the qualified provider. The Scope and Standards of Forensic Nursing Practice deals specifically with the education of the forensic nurse: "The forensic nurse acquires and maintains current knowledge in forensic nursing practice" (Barber et al., Standard III, 1997). Continuing education in the field of forensic science/forensic nursing is required to meet the changing needs of the forensic patient and to keep pace with the advances made in the field of forensic science. Forensic nurses must not only keep their knowledge current, but also integrate that knowledge in their everyday practice.

THE LEGAL NURSE CONSULTANT

The Code of Ethics and Conduct of the American Association of Legal Nurse Consultants, the Scope of Practice for the Legal Nurse Consultant, and the Standards of Legal Nurse Consulting state that the role of the legal nurse consultant is to evaluate, analyze, and render informed opinions on the delivery of health care and the resulting outcomes (American Association of Legal Nurse Consultants, 1995).

The legal nurse consultant uses both nursing assessment skills and the skills obtained through forensic training. In reviewing a case for possible medical malpractice or personal injury, for example, it is important to understand that the individuals involved in these cases may have suffered some type of injury and that injury may have been caused by one or more individuals. Although this may not be a case that would involve criminal charges, it may end up in the civil court system. Whether at a nursing home, hospital, clinic, physician's office, stand-alone surgical center, rehabilitation center, or any place an individual receives medical care, the medical records are the starting point in an investigation.

SUMMARY

The role of the forensic nurse has evolved as the needs of the populations served have significantly changed. Caring for victims and perpetrators of interpersonal violence has led the field of forensic nursing to meet the challenges of the forensic patient by developing the ability to recognize, document, collect, and preserve evidence. Forensic nurses also must understand the importance of what may seem like insignificant minutiae to an outsider. Whether collecting bite mark evidence in a case of abuse or gathering paint and glass fragments from a victim of a motor vehicle crash, it is the forensic nurse who makes a difference in the collection and documentation of physical evidence. By providing true, holistic care to the forensic patient, Florence Nightingale's legacy—treating the whole patient and not just the injury or symptom—is being carried out within the forensic setting.

Although nurses have protected the privacy of patients as this role has evolved, the forensic nurse is a mandated reporter who frequently interfaces with members of the criminal justice system. It is the responsibility of the forensic nurse to keep abreast of the advances made in the field of forensic science and to stay informed of legal implications pertinent to forensic nursing practice and evidence collection.

QUESTIONS FOR DISCUSSION

1. What types of evidence collection materials would be useful to store in hospital emergency departments and trauma centers?
2. Give examples of how cross-contamination of articles could occur if clinical staff is not aware of proper evidence collection procedures. How could cross-contamination of evidence be detrimental to an investigation?
3. How has HIPAA impacted the forensic nurse's role pertaining to evidence collection and documentation?

4. The newly hired nurse manager of the emergency department asks the forensic nurse specialist on staff to write an evidence collection and documentation policy for the ED. What agencies should the forensic nurse consult with prior to writing the policy? What HIPAA regulations must be included? What patient consent issues should be addressed?

5. A 25-year-old male is admitted to the emergency department with a superficial gunshot wound to the leg following a gang-related altercation. It is discovered upon physical assessment that the patient is armed with a semiautomatic handgun. The police are en route to interview the patient. As the forensic nurse on duty, what steps would you take to ensure safety, document and collect evidence, and initiate the chain of custody?

REFERENCES

American Association of Legal Nurse Consultants. (1995). *Standards of legal nurse consulting practice and professional performance.* Glenview, IL: Author.

Barber, J., Battiste-Otto, F., et al. (1997). *Scope and standards of forensic nursing practice.* Washington, DC: International Association of Forensic Nurses and American Nurses Association.

Capuano, T., Carolan, J., et al. (1999). *Nurse's legal handbook* (4th ed.), Springhouse, PA: Springhouse.

Health Insurance Portability and Accountability Act of 1996, Public Law 104-191. (Revised 2002). 45 CFR Part 160 & Subparts A & E of Part 164. Retrieved April 24, 2004, from www.hhs.gov.

Inman, K. & Rudin, N. (2001). *Principles and practice of criminalistics.* New York: CRC Press.

Joint Commission for Accreditation of Healthcare Organizations. (2003). *Hospital accreditation standards.* Oakbrook Terrace, IL: Joint Commission Resources.

Lee, H.C. & Harris, H. (2000). *Physical evidence in forensic science.* Tucson, AZ: Lawyers & Judges Publishing.

U.S. Department of Health & Human Services, Office for Civil Rights. Summary of the HIPAA Privacy Rule, *OCR Privacy Brief.* Washington, DC: Author. Retrieved April 24, 2004, from www.hhs.gov/ocr/hipaa.

SUGGESTED READINGS

DiMaio, D. & DiMaio, J. (1993). *Forensic pathology.* Boca Raton, FL: CRC Press.

Nightingale, F. (1992). *Notes on nursing: What it is, and what it's not.* Philadelphia: Lippincott.

Reik, T. (1945). *The unknown murderer.* New York: Prentice Hall.

Saferstein, R. (2004). *Criminalistics. An introduction to forensic science* (8th ed.). Upper Saddle River, NJ: Prentice Hall.

U.S. Department of Justice. (1999). *Death investigation: A guide for the scene investigator.* Washington, DC: Author. Available online at www.usdoj.gov.

Concepts of Photography in Forensic Nursing

Kenneth B. Zercie
Paul Penders

Proper documentation is one of the most important aspects of forensic nursing. Proper documentation in many types of cases, such as domestic violence, sexual assault, and child abuse, often should involve a photographic record in addition to other forms of documentation. Knowledge of the basics of photography and the choice of equipment provides the forensic nurse with the necessary tools to enhance records with photographs. Through study and practice the forensic nurse can avoid common photographic errors that can detract from the record or provide grounds for challenges to the photographs in court.

CHAPTER FOCUS

Photographic equipment
The camera, lens, and film
Basic photography
Location and subject matter
Stepwise approach to crime scene photography
Evidence documentation
Digital photography in forensic nursing

KEY TERMS_____

aperture
ASA/ISO
authentication
camera
f-stop
lens
negative
painting with light
photography
Rule of three
shutter speed
supplemental lighting

INTRODUCTION

The use of photographically recorded images has been with us since the 1830s. The first attempts at recording and reproducing a scene resulted in pictures and negatives of limited clarity. However, those attempts did one thing that had never been done before—they captured a moment in time. Artists had been attempting this throughout history in the form of still life paintings. Artists' reproductions, however, were subjective interpretations of what the artists observed. Photography provided the potential for a true and accurate representation of an image. As photographic processes developed the ability to accurately render images, they were recognized as a trustworthy method of recording visually what was actually present. This also permitted the photographer or someone who had personal knowledge of the content of the photograph to present his or her observations to a viewer. The viewers then formed their own unbiased interpretations of the image and its content.

The forensic nurse is faced with the same challenges that any investigator has with respect to photography. He or she must understand the importance of being able to create good quality images of any observations, knowing that those pictures may be used in a court of law as documentation that an injury or event took place. The ability to capture an image using instant imaging, film, video, or digital media is critical for the patient, client, investigator, and judicial system. Proper photographic documentation lets all concerned parties see at a later time and place the forensic nurse's firsthand observations. The use of only verbal descriptions can leave out much detail. Written notes allow for interpretation, even if testimony is given as to what the forensic nurse is trying to communicate. Images that present a true and accurate rendering will facilitate the understanding of others when they supplement written notes and sketches. Images also provide for the possibility that an independent evaluation may be necessary as part of a case or incident. The forensic nurse recording an image does not have to be an expert in the field of photography, but should possess the technical skill and basic knowledge necessary to perform the function well and defend his or her choices in a court of law, if required to do so.

PHOTOGRAPHIC EQUIPMENT

It should be noted that silver-based (film) processes are still the most widely used and give the best possible results with respect to image reproduction. This chapter will deal with the traditional camera, lens, film, procedures, techniques, image composition, and exposure. These principles apply to both film and digital photography. Digital imaging has recently become very popular. The application of digital imaging differs from traditional film mostly by the methodology of capture. The advantages and disadvantages of each technology will also be addressed.

The Camera, Lens, and Film

The camera is the basic component of the photographer's equipment. This section will deal with the 35 mm single lens reflex camera and its application in forensic nursing. Although other types of cameras ("point and shoot" or "instant") and formats (medium, 120 mm roll film and large format, 4″ × 5″ or larger film) of cameras are available, the 35 mm—with its interchangeable lenses, assorted types of electronic flash, size, weight, and film varieties—is still the most practical for forensic use.

Most 35 mm single lens reflex cameras function in a similar fashion (i.e., image viewing is done through the lens). A mirror in the camera body allows the photographer to see exactly what will be recorded on the film. The mirror moves up and out of the way when the film is exposed. The body of the camera is a light-tight box into which film is loaded. Several controls are present on the camera including the shutter button, film advance and rewind cranks, shutter speed, film speed, and exposure. A light meter is also used to determine proper shutter speed and aperture settings, which allow one to properly expose an image onto a piece of film. Manual cameras allow photographers to adjust all of these settings as they see fit for each situation. Many modern cameras have internal computers that will automatically set the camera to take an average exposure of a scene. In most cases these automatic settings will provide acceptable images for basic documentation purposes. The automatic modes are: program, aperture priority, and shutter speed priority.

The camera is designed to allow various types of lenses to be attached to the camera body. The camera lens is essentially a series of lenses that collect light and focus it on the film plane. The aperture (f-stop) of the lens controls the amount of light passing through the lens to the film plane. The aperture works much like the iris of the eye, decreasing in diameter in bright light and opening wider in low light. A focusing ring allows the photographer to bring items into clear view in the viewfinder and thus into focus on the film plane. Another important indicator on most lenses is the depth of field indicator. Pairings of aperture numbers appear on the barrel of the lens. Once the image is in focus the photographer can look at the measurement on the distance scale and determine the area of the object (composition) that is in sharp, acceptable focus.

Film is the memory device used to capture a latent image. The basic silver halide structures of the film emulsion are sensitive to light. As light strikes the emulsion a reaction takes place and the film becomes exposed. After the film is treated with developing, stop, fixing, and wash solutions the image is visible in reversed, tonal presentation. This reversed image is then projected onto treated paper and a standard photographic image results. Films are available in many different types, different speeds (sensitivity to light), black and white, color negative, and positive (slide film) forms. The type of film that should be used in a particular situation depends on lighting conditions, subject matter, and the final product desired (e.g., picture or slide).

BASIC PHOTOGRAPHY

The following factors are necessary to produce a good, clear, sharp image:

- The proper amount of light must reach the film.
- The focus must be accurate.
- The equipment must be steady and free of movement.

The Amount of Light Reaching the Film

The amount of light entering the camera is controlled by the size of the aperture opening, the speed of the shutter, and the speed of the film, identified by its ASA/ISO numbers. The aperture or lens opening controls the amount of light entering the camera. The aperture openings are designed with a mathematical progression, where each succeeding lens opening (f-stop) allows either one-half or twice the amount of light to strike the film than the preceding f-stop. In this context "f" stands for the focal length of the lens when focused at infinity. The f-stops commonly found on most cameras are f-1.4, f-2.0, f-2.8, f-4, f-5.6, f-8, f-11, f-16, f-22, and f-32. These f-stops are referred to as full stops. The lower the number of the f-stop, the larger the iris opening is. If you think of the f-stop numbers as fractions, the concept may be clearer. For example, f-8 (1/8) allows one-half the light of f-5.6 (1/5.6) to fall on the film plane; f-11 (1/11) allows twice as much light as f-16 (1/16), the next highest f-stop.

The shutter speed is the second method used to control the amount of light entering the camera. This control, much like the aperture openings, is designed in a mathematical progression and will either cut in half or double the amount of time the shutter will remain open, allowing light to pass through the aperture to the film. Common shutter speeds of a camera range from several seconds to one-thousandth of a second. Many newer models have even faster shutter speeds. The common shutter speeds are 1, 1/2, 1/4, 1/8, 1/15, 1/30, 1/60, 1/125, 1/250, 1/500, and 1/1000 second. The letter "B" on the shutter dial indicates "bulb." When the shutter is set at "B," it stays open as long as the shutter button remains depressed. This setting is used for taking timed exposures or when using a technique called "painting with light."

The third method that controls film exposure is the film speed. The film speed rating indicates the film's capacity to absorb light. The number ratings are known as ASA (American Standards Association) or ISO (International Organization for Standardization) and are the same throughout the film manufacturing industry. A low ASA number, such as 25 or 64, indicates a low-speed film; that is, the capacity of the film to absorb light is low. This type of film would be ideal for photographing fixed objects, laboratory imaging, or copy work when fine detail is needed. Slower film has the ability to record in greater detail. Medium-speed film would have an ASA rating of 100 or 200. This type of film is ideal for general daylight photography and recording of scenes and evidence. When used with an electronic flash, medium-speed film may also be used in limited distance, low-light situations. High-speed films would have an ASA of 400 or higher. These films are ideal for general law enforcement, low-light situations, and sports and action documentation where the faster film will allow you to use a faster shutter speed to stop action.

The ASA/ISO number of film is extremely important to those who use the camera's built-in light meter. The film speed is the index number the light meter uses to calibrate itself when reading the amount of available light. Automatic cameras also use this number to determine the proper shutter speed, aperture opening, or both, so that proper exposure is possible. With a manual camera the operator must verify the film speed on the film speed indicator normally located on the top of the camera body housing. The ASA/ISO number for each roll of film is printed on the film box and on the canister containing the film itself. With the modern automatic cameras a new method is being employed called DX coding. The camera reads a bar code on the side of the canister and the light meter is automatically calibrated for that type of film. If a camera is not equipped with a light meter (35 mm SLR), a handheld, reflective, or incident meter may assist in determining the proper exposure. The information sheet in the film box can also provide a guide to the proper settings in a given lighting condition. The forensic nurse should be aware that all film is not balanced for daylight photography (sunlight or electronic flash). If such is not the lighting situation, the nurse may need to employ color correction filters. For all general photography and overall documentation, "daylight" type film can usually be used successfully.

There may be occasions when taking photographs that are critical to an investigation present circumstances that will fool the meter. For example, subjects dressed in all white or all black will fool the meter, resulting in either too much or too little exposure. To avoid this situation, the photographer should bracket exposures by altering the f-stops. Bracketing involves taking a picture at the recommended setting and then taking additional photographs one f-stop above and one f-stop below the "proper" exposure. If the indicated exposure was f-16 at 1/125 of a second, bracketed exposures would include another photograph at f-11 (one stop change allows more light in) at 1/125 of a second and another at f-22 (allows less light in) at 1/125 of a second. Similarly, bracketing could also be accomplished by using a constant f-stop and altering the shutter speed, f-16 and 1/60 of a second (one stop more light) and 1/250 of a second (one stop less light) in our example. Both methods will allow for the equivalent of a one-stop change of either half or double the amount of light. The choice of bracketing technique will depend on the conditions, the required shutter speed if handholding, whether the object is in motion, and if using an electronic flash.

Supplemental Lighting

Many images will require the use of electronic flash to supplement or replace the lack of light. Experience has shown that the full-time use of an electronic flash can aid the photographer in establishing repeatable exposures, removing shadows, and balancing the light when artificial lighting is present. Cameras have connectors to mount an electronic flash in a holder called the "hot shoe." Some manual cameras still require a wire connection to the camera's "X sync." Failure to properly seat the unit in the hot shoe or attach the sync cord to the correct terminal will result in an improper exposure. The recommended shutter speed and any speed slower will allow the flash to expose the film. However, at slow shutter speeds movement becomes a consideration.

Some advanced electronic flash units have built-in circuits that measure the distance the light must travel to the subject, allowing only the proper amount of light to be produced. This type of equipment varies the light output and is relatively simple to use. The film speed or ASA/ISO setting must be set on the calculator dial built onto the flash. This will calibrate the metering system, if automatic, or give suggested f-stop for a given distance information, if the camera is manual.

A common technique for indoor photography with a flash is to bounce the light off the ceiling. Generally this will give more even illumination for the subject and avoid harsh bright areas. Avoiding bright spots is important for the proper documentation of wounds and similar evidence. If the ceiling is of normal height and white in color, the flash can be bounced at the ceiling instead of the subject. When the bounce technique is used with a manual flash—camera combination, the camera must be opened two additional f-stops to compensate for the light loss, as the light will have to travel double the distance. Automatic camera and flash combinations will compensate for this light loss. When taking photographs of objects very close to the camera and flash unit, the forensic nurse should consider removing the flash and angling the light toward the object of interest. A clean handkerchief, "kim-wipe," or neutral density filter may also be used to reduce the intensity of the light being produced.

Controlling or Recording Movement

Moving or potentially moving subjects can present difficulty in a forensic setting. Often the forensic nurse may not have sufficient time or inclination to take multiple shots of the subject, for example if the client is a victim of abuse. To avoid blurred photographs due to subject movement or movement by the photographer, it would be advisable to use a shutter speed number that is equal to or faster than the focal length of the lens being used. As an example, when using a 50 mm lens you should not use a shutter speed slower than 1/60th of a second. With a 135 mm medium telephoto lens, you should not use a shutter speed slower then 1/125th of a second. Another factor to consider is the direction of movement of the subject. If the subject moves toward the camera, a shutter speed of at least 1/60th is recommended. However, action moving diagonal to the camera is more difficult to photograph and requires a faster shutter speed of at least 1/250th of a second. This faster time is necessary to give the photographer the ability to stop action and get a sharply focused image.

Focus

You can focus your camera on the subject in several ways. Many manual cameras have manual lenses that require the photographer to rotate a focusing ring on the lens until the subject is in sharp focus in the viewfinder. Others have split image finders that have a vertical line that appears in the viewfinder and splits the subject in two. In split image finders, the focusing ring is rotated until the images come together or the two images become one, at which point the image is in focus.

Modern cameras have many advantages over the manual variety. With the advent of features such as auto-focus, auto-aperture, auto-shutter speed, auto-advance and rewind of film, program modes, and auto-flash synchronization most of the guesswork is gone from traditional photography.

A photographer adjusts for factors that may affect photographic quality by using the various controls on the camera, choosing the proper light environment or flash, and selecting the appropriate film. Ultimately, the skill of the photographer can compensate for some limitations in any of these areas. By planning ahead, the forensic nurse can provide for the various types of photographs that he or she may be required to take. With some practice, today the photographer with limited experience and a good understanding of the owner's manual, types of film, and basic composition principles (what to photograph) should be able to take good quality images suitable for examination, documentation, and presentation in court.

LOCATION AND SUBJECT MATTER

Each of the following areas presents its own set of requirements, equipment, and specialized techniques. As the responsibility to document an item, scene, or individual changes, the conditions under which the images must be taken will also change. For these reasons the forensic nurse photographer must have knowledge of the legal requirements, capability of the equipment, and how best to get the desired results for eventual presentation. Photographs are also used as evidence in court when presented as a true and accurate rendering of what is depicted. This "true and accurate" requirement means you must use photographic techniques appropriate for the situation. Although not all possible environments and their effect on the forensic nurse photographer can be addressed at this time, the following are some common situations that may affect documentation.

Crime and Death Scene Documentation

The scene of an incident creates the most challenging set of problems for the photographer. The photographer has no control over location, time of day, position of evidence, hazards that may be present, weather conditions, or other environmental factors that will affect how you complete your tasks. For example, a death investigator may be required to document an outdoor scene in the middle of winter at the base of a mountain. The primary consideration is to know your responsibility at the scene. This includes how you interface with other investigative groups, such as the police, medical examiners, fire department and other emergency services personnel, and forensic scientists. It is important to remember that you are at the scene as part of a team. As with all teams, there are specific lines of authority and responsibility that should be clear to all involved. Knowledge of these factors will make documentation at the scene faster and easier and will likely facilitate efforts by the forensic nurse to learn supplemental information as part of his or her investigation.

The purpose of scene documentation is to record the location of evidence in its original position and condition before any alterations have taken place. Another use is as a reference for further investigation, deposition, courtroom presentation (both civil and criminal), and to refresh the memory. Photographs should be taken of the entire area of involvement showing spatial relationships of items, perspectives of witnesses, and views as noted by other involved parties at the scene. This initial documentation provides the forensic nurse and others with a firsthand representation of observations. An accurate depiction allows anyone to observe at a remote time and place what was seen and the conditions that existed at the moment you took the photograph. As noted previously, photographs do not stand alone as the only form of documentation: notes, video recordings, and sketches all complement each other and are essential supplements used to record the scene. When these documentation methods are combined during courtroom testimony, the trier of fact will have a clearer understanding of relevant observations. Proper photographic documentation will also help to establish the credibility of the forensic nurse as part of the investigative team.

There is no specific number of photographs to take at any given crime scene. Once an item or person has been moved from the scene or patterns have been cleaned up, the forensic investigator can never recover those images. Therefore, it is necessary to document all aspects of the scene as completely as possible. Film and processing costs are minimal compared to not having the images recorded when asking questions in the future or reviewing a case. The basic definition of a completely photographed scene would be: The photographic documentation of a crime scene from beginning to end overlooking nothing. This is an easy thing to remember, but not always a simple process. Every scene will present its own set of limitations and problems. For example, it may not be necessary to document the entire house in specific detail if an assault took place in only one room. On the other hand, an entire neighborhood may be involved if the scene investigation involves a major traffic accident.

Stepwise Approach to Crime Scene Photography

The investigator often needs to photograph a scene quickly and accurately. Good planning before the incident will provide the forensic nurse with a basic set of procedures that can be modified, as necessary, to meet the specific needs of an individual case. The following are guidelines to follow when conducting photographic documentation at a scene.

1. Arrive at the incident scene as quickly as possible. Check in with the individual in charge.
2. Check your equipment to ensure that it is operational.
3. Upon arrival consult with the first responders and determine if the emergency is still ongoing. Also, identify if anything has been disturbed.
4. If the others are still dealing with the emergency, begin to document the surrounding area and people at the scene, if practical.
5. Once the emergency is under control, determine the scope of the scene and walk through it with the initial responders. Caution should always be taken so as to not destroy evidence (e.g., footprints, tire tracks, etc.). (Polaroid and digital imaging may be useful at this time.)
6. Begin to document your way into the scene. Consideration should be given to using a point of entry not used by any suspects.
7. First photograph items that are perishable or will be lost if not immediately seized.
8. If working at a death scene, photograph the decedent in place before disturbing the body. Photograph both sides of the decedent when moved and the area underneath the body.
9. Photograph a minimum of four overviews of each room and specific areas of involvement and patterns.
10. Take medium close-ups of each item of significant evidence as it relates to its immediate surroundings.
11. Take close-ups of specific items of evidence as found or processed (e.g., latent fingerprints, footprints).
12. Photograph all hallways, stairways, entrances, and exits.
13. Rulers, surveys tapes, and other measuring devices may be necessary to document blood spatter patterns. Number stands or attention devices may be used to supplement the initial images; photograph both with and without the device, if used.
14. Photograph the scene using only existing light as well as with electronic flash.
15. Maintain a comprehensive record of the images taken.
16. Additional photographs may include evidence found outside of the scene, tool marks, tire marks, and witness or victim perspectives. Aerial photographs should also be considered.

Table 17–1 Equipment Recommended for General Scene Photography

- 35 mm camera body
- 28–70 mm zoom general-purpose lens
- 80–200 mm zoom telephoto lens
- 60 mm macro lens with close-up adapter (allows 1-to-1 ratio, life-size image reproduction of an object on the film)
- Electronic flash unit with tilting head
- Remote synchronization cord (camera to flash)
- Assorted film types, scales, flashlight, cards, and cleaning material
- Tripod, camera bag, spare batteries, and instruction manual

17. Review the crime scene diagram, notes, videotape, and instant images prior to seizing evidence and altering the scene further.
18. Have the film processed and printed as soon as possible; review and mark the photographs as required. Preserve the film because it can now be considered evidence.

The type of equipment recommended for general crime scene use is a 35 mm single lens reflex camera body, manual or fully automatic, with exposure control, shutter control, flash synchronization, focus, film ASA adjustment, advance, and film rewind. Camera lenses come in a wide variety of styles and configurations. A zoom lens with macro (close-up) capabilities will cover most of the scene photographer's needs. The flash used should synchronize with the camera and have as much output as possible. A macro lens will be of great help in taking detailed close-up photographs, allowing you to make life-size exposures on the negatives (1-to-1 ratio). Table 17–1 lists photographic equipment recommended for general scene documentation.

A well-designed photographic system configuration is shown in Figure 17–1. Such a configuration will help to ensure repeatable quality once the photographer is familiar with and has tested the equipment in controlled conditions. As a general rule, color negative film is recommended for crime scene use. Film having an ASA of 100, 200, or 400 should give sufficient sensitivity to light, good color rendering, and, when used with electronic flash, is adequate for most outdoor and nighttime photography. Other films to consider are those with higher ASA settings (800, 1600, etc.), for extremely low-light situations. Black and white film may also be advantageous in documenting items like fingerprints, tool marks, imprints, and other impression evidence. Information about special application films may be found in the readings listed at the end of this chapter.

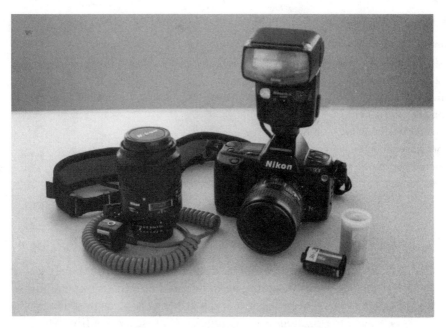

Figure 17-1 A well-designed photographic system includes a standard 35 mm camera, macro and zoom lenses, remote extension cord, electronic flash, and film.

Instant Imaging

The use of instant imaging, such as Polaroid products, allows the photographer to see his or her results before leaving the scene. Instant film is also a good way to quickly document injuries, a body, and other evidence for reference by other investigators and those who have an interest in the case, but should or cannot be in contact with the scene. Instant documentation should be considered as a backup or supplement to those images captured on 35 mm film. The Polaroid Corporation has made several specialized cameras and adapters that are helpful for close-up images. The units shown in Figure 17–2 are the Polaroid Spectra and the Macro 5, both of which are relatively simple to use. Instant images have been admitted as evidence in court even though there is no negative or direct way to produce a copy of the image.

Hospital Situations

The forensic nurse will be familiar with many of the situations in which the hospital is a setting for photographic documentation. Although the protocols of each institution may differ, written permission from the client is usually recommended prior to taking any photographs. Healthcare facilities do not always have clear protocols for the retention of photographs. Prior to taking any images, the photographer should have established a procedure for proper storage of this type of documentation. Certainly client privacy and regulations such as HIPAA are

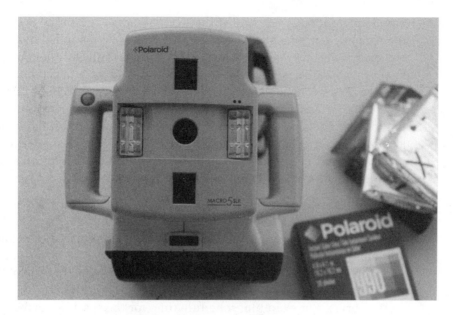

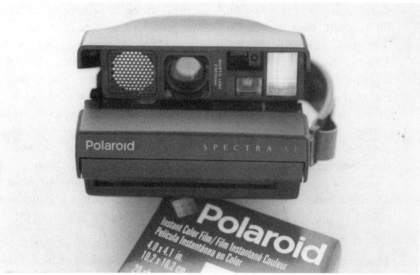

Figure 17–2 Two types of Polaroid cameras. A professional Macro 5 camera is shown in the top photograph. The lower photograph depicts the Spectra camera, a model that is readily available at retail stores.

considerations. In addition, improper storage of photographic records proffered for use as evidence could result in that evidence being barred from admission during trial. Before documenting injuries, the forensic nurse should always explain to the client why each photograph is being taken. It is important to exhibit great sensitivity to the client's physical comfort, emotional state, and need for privacy during this process. These concerns are best addressed if there are no interruptions during the photographic process and if the forensic nurse is familiar with the photographic equipment. The patient should be photographed in a position that creates the least amount of discomfort while still demonstrating the characteristics of the injury. In addition, it may be a good idea for the client to participate in the process, whenever possible. For example, the client can assist in draping and other acts to protect privacy and limit contact to achieve the correct photographic position. Often images taken in this setting are of a patient being treated for child abuse, domestic violence, sexual assault, physical assault, blunt trauma injuries, stab wounds, gunshot injuries, and surgical wounds.

Images of injuries, wounds, and scars should be taken both before and after treatment whenever practical, with the understanding that vital care for the patient always comes first. If images are to be taken after emergency procedures and while the patient is still in the hospital, then arrangements should be made with the treating physician and charge nurse if additional photographs are necessary to document injuries. For example, schedule time for the session during bandage changes to make the patient more comfortable. An overall photograph that shows the injury and the victim must be taken. In this way, the specific contusions, lacerations, and so on can be directly connected to the victim, because the close-up photograph of an injury must be linked to the victim in question. The use of a mirror may facilitate photographing the victim's face along with the injury itself. After documenting their locations, injuries must be photographed close up, with and without a scale. This documentation may be used for subsequent criminal and/or civil purposes. It is therefore important to consider the specific people who may use and access any photographs. To prevent an implication of bias or the melodramatic during court proceedings, the client should never be posed in an unnatural manner or to accentuate the injury for other than a scientific purpose.

The previously described three-shot sequence should be followed by a shot that gives the viewer the perspective of actually seeing the injury as observed at the time of treatment. An additional image is also required: a photograph of the injury or medical procedure using a scale of contrasting color. Examples of various types of scales are shown in Figure 17–3. This scale is critical for pattern interpretation and the comparison with various edged or impact weapons to the injury. Including a scale allows better reproduction of the size and color. A scale also provides the necessary reference so that a life-size (1-to-1 ratio) image can be printed. Whenever possible, a color standard, such as a Macbeth ColorChecker, or the Kodak Gray Card should be photographed under the same conditions as the area of interest (see Figure 17–4). Use of a color standard leads to more accurate

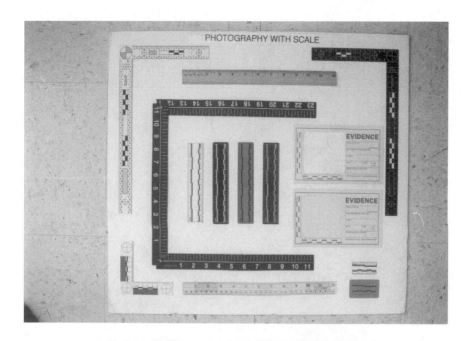

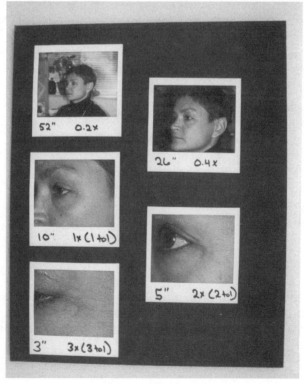

Figure 17–3 Various types of scales available for photographic documentation are shown in the top photograph. The lower photograph shows how the use of scale and contrast facilitates subsequent examinations with enlargement to life-size proportions for direct comparison.

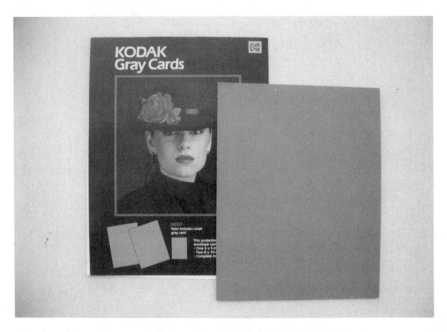

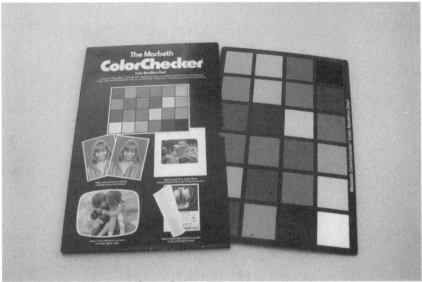

Figure 17-4 Gray (upper photograph) and color (lower photograph) scales provide standards of color and exposure when images are printed. Use of scales is especially important to provide a true and accurate rendering when documenting injuries.

reproduction and a truer rendering in the print. Although it is axiomatic that injuries must be documented before they heal, some injuries, such as bruises and bite marks, will become more apparent with the passage of time. Adequate images for scar evaluation may be difficult to produce with the flat lighting delivered by flash units built into a camera. Taking the time to use proper photographic procedures will give some creditability to the interpretation of bruises and wounds based on the color in the photographs, such as when aging bite marks.

Autopsy

The autopsy room presents several restrictions when documenting a deceased individual. The protocols of the agency and the needs and concerns of the pathologist must be considered. Whenever possible, the images of a deceased should not show background equipment such as tables or tools. A background of an 18% gray tone (standard color for all exposure balancing) provides a suitable backdrop in most instances. Photographs of the decedent should proceed in a logical sequence and should be taken from all angles. Close-up photographs of the face, injuries, clothing, footwear, and any other items of evidence or patterns of interest need to be taken prior to the removal of any garments. As layers of garments are removed, the documentation process should be repeated until the body is completely exposed. Additional images of the decedent should be taken after any blood or debris is removed or cleaned. These photographs will more clearly reveal the extent of injuries and damage.

Depending on the cause of death (homicide, suicide, accidental, natural, or undetermined), it may be advisable to document the body and evidence using an alternate light source. Available alternate light includes not only the commonly used ultraviolet lamp (Woods lamp), but also a laser or variable wavelength forensic light source. This may be done when the decedent is received, as well as before and after clothing and areas of stain are removed. Alternate light may also enhance patterns and injury. Items that fluoresce must be documented before collection to show their location and relationship to the body. Photographs taken using alternate light sources follow the same metering and exposure guidelines as previously discussed. The program mode on automatic cameras is recommended, as is the use of a tripod to stabilize the image during long exposures. A barrier filter the same color as the viewing goggles must be used in front of the lens. Table 17–2 identifies the recommended films, filters, and corresponding wavelengths to be used when photographing fluorescence or luminescence.

Table 17–2   Photographic Filters, Films, and Wavelengths

Color	Wavelength	Viewing/Camera Filter or Equivalent	Film Type
Ultraviolet	360–400 nm	Kodak Wratten Nos. 2A, 2B, 12 Absorption	B&W, Color
Yellow	400–450 nm	Kodak Wratten No. 8 Yellow	B&W, Color
Blue-Green	450–540 nm	Kodak Wratten No. 21, 22 Orange	B&W, Color
Blue	540–700 nm	Kodak Wratten No. 25 Red	B&W, Color
Infrared	700–1100 nm	Kodak Filters Nos. 15, 25, 29, 70, 87, 88A, and 87C	B&W high speed IR ektachrome Infrared

EVIDENCE DOCUMENTATION

Any item of interest in an investigation should be considered as evidence. Chapter 16 discusses in detail the proper recognition, documentation, and collection of physical evidence. The following discussion provides a general guideline for only the photographic documentation of evidence of interest. All evidence must first be documented in the place where it was found. These photographs show the condition of the evidence and its relationship with other items of interest. Evidence pictures generally follow the three-shot sequence described in the scene documentation section of this chapter. (See Figure 17–5.) One additional image is usually necessary when specific items are documented—the fourth picture in this series is the specific item of interest with a scale. These additional images with a scale may be taken at the scene or under controlled circumstances, such as a laboratory, office, examination room, or studio. The use of a copy stand may be helpful for this detailed documentation at a later time, especially if an alternate light source is used. These additional photographs are critical because they are also used for comparison and analysis by other forensic examiners.

If evidence is to be processed, enhanced, or altered in any way, images should be taken at each step to document the process. Most processing methodologies alter, destroy, or change the evidence from its original condition. Capturing images at each step will preserve the item or pattern so that any following alternations will not interfere with the value that may have preceded the next examination. Once you destroy the patterns or remove the evidence it can never be put back to its original condition.

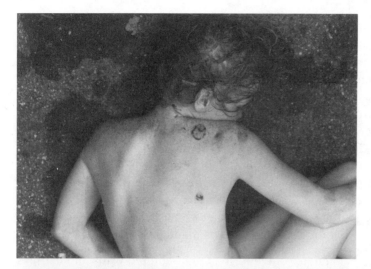

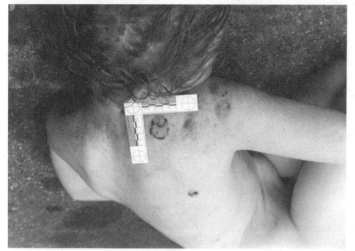

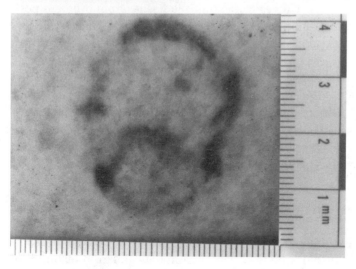

Figure 17–5
Documentation at a homicide scene by a death investigator using the three-step photographic process. The top picture depicts an overall view of the decedent as she was found at the scene; the middle photograph is a closer view of her upper torso showing an area of injury; the last picture is a close-up view of the bite mark on the decedent's shoulder. (Note a scale has been placed in the area for size reference.)

Flash Usage at the Scene

A supplementary flash unit is used to provide illumination when no or limited ambient light is present. This allows the photographer to control the light, giving the camera a standard to calibrate to. Today electronic flash units can produce enough light to illuminate an outside street crime scene up to 100 feet away from the camera position. By using the program modes and through-the-lens (TTL) metering, a flash unit will provide sufficient light to properly expose the image to be created. Tests should be done with the equipment being used so the photographer will know what the capabilities and limitations of the particular system are. These tests are referred to as Guide Number tests, and depend on the flash, subject matter, and film being used. A detailed explanation of these tests can be found in your owner's manual.

The photographer can take advantage of light-colored walls and ceilings to provide soft, even illumination when documenting an area. This procedure is called the "bounce flash" technique. When the flash is aimed at these surfaces the flash will reflect off ("bounce back"), giving an indirect lighting effect. Using a bounce effect will eliminate intensity differences in the lighting and "fall off" that can produce sharp and distracting shadows. This type of lighting is useful when trying to show the orientation of several objects at various distances from the camera lens. The bounce flash technique also may provide additional details and eliminate misleading shadows.

When dealing with scenes at night or in wide, poorly lit spaces, the forensic photographer can compensate for these light problems using a process called "painting with light." Painting with light requires coordination with other people at a scene and is therefore not suitable for documentation of an area if the forensic nurse is the only trained person documenting the scene. This technique involves using multiple flashes from different positions. To ensure the film frame does not move, the photographer mounts the camera on a tripod or other stable base. With the shutter of the camera set at "T" (time exposure), so the lens iris remains open during the entire process, the photographer places a black card over the lens except when the flash is used. A second person sets off the flash at various locations around the periphery of the area of interest. Painting with light is a way to expose the film such that the entire area is evenly illuminated, revealing the detail necessary for proper documentation. The forensic nurse should clearly identify those exposures in which this technique is used.

DIGITAL PHOTOGRAPHY IN FORENSIC NURSING

The use of digital imaging or digital photography may be considered as an alternative to instant film (Polaroid) technology. Polaroid instant film produces a finished photograph in about 90 seconds. This is of benefit because the photographer can quickly determine whether the photograph has critical focus and proper exposure, and if it depicts the necessary information about the subject. Some of the principal benefits of digital capture are:

- The photographer is independent of other photographic processing labs, and images can be processed and printed by a computer.
- The photographer can reasonably (but not critically) proof the image directly on the camera screen. In other words, the anxiety of whether the images "came out" can be relieved by proofing it on the spot before altering or releasing the subject. Because the victim may be covered with dressings obscuring the injury or other important details, photographing the area in question beforehand may be important.
- Viewing and critically evaluating the image on a monitor is the preferred method, because the image delivered to the camera's built-in display is quite small and of low resolution or quality.
- A digital file is capable of being exactly reproduced any number of times. The twentieth copy is of the same quality as the original.

It is these characteristics of digital photography that have made it the method of choice for quick documentation and storage of multiple images. The choice of camera and the type of storage medium that camera uses are critical considerations for the forensic nurse. As shown in Figure 17–6, digital cameras can range from expensive, professional-style to affordable consumer models. The forensic nurse can view the subject on a screen as soon as the photograph is taken. Thus, the photographer can decide immediately if it is necessary to rephotograph the subject. If additional photographs are necessary, this can be done with minimal change in the environment or discomfort to the subject. When choosing a camera or other digital capture device, image quality is of great importance. Image quality is usually stated in megapixels. Image sizes typically used in e-mail attachments and for Internet display (72 dpi) are unsuitable for evidentiary documentation and/or analysis. A camera used for documentation should be toward the higher end of the scale in image quality. The final output will be only as good as the captured images. Storage media, the type of media to which the images are written in the camera, vary with different manufacturers. At the present time the common media are compact flash cards, microdrives, and compact discs.

Digital cameras also come with enhancements. For example, there should be a white balance capability as well as the ability to set your capture device to the light source (fluorescent, incandescent, daylight, electronic flash, etc.). Most digital systems also provide some close-up photographic capability. The extent to which the photographer can

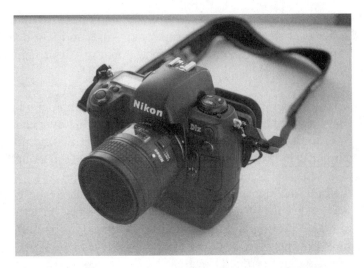

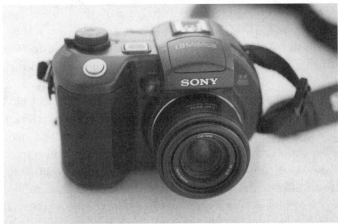

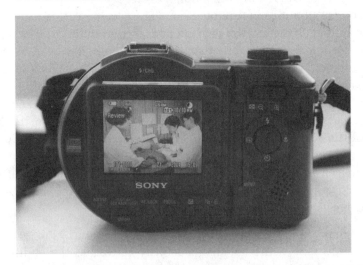

Figure 17–6 A professional-style digital camera is shown in the top photograph. A front view and the viewing screen of a consumer-style digital camera are shown in the lower figures.

zoom in on the subject to capture close details is of particular importance when imaging contusions, lacerations, damage to clothing, and similar alterations. After photographs are taken, the forensic nurse must consider additional, practical parameters:

- How will the images be output? Will they be printed, transmitted via a network, or burned to a CD?
- Which software will you use for organization, display, access, and archiving of your images? Will it be the software included with the camera or something more specialized such as iPhoto, Adobe Album, or ImageAXS Pro?

The cost of a professional or advanced amateur digital camera system is well in excess of $1,000. Although a serviceable consumer-oriented capture device may be purchased for less, not all cameras are suitable for proper evidentiary documentation. Most cameras produced today are geared toward typical amateur snapshot usage such as birthday parties, graduations, sports events, and vacation scenes. At the very least, any digital camera used by the forensic nurse should be capable of producing quality close-up photographs.

The obsolescence factor is a large consideration with digital equipment. Image processing requires powerful hardware in order to work efficiently. Operating systems and software require frequent updates and upgrades to keep in sync. Because many images taken by the forensic nurse may need to be accessed years from the date of capture, he or she must make every attempt to use a system that will allow this access. Thus, it is a real concern whether the software that created the files will soon be obsolete and whether the storage media will still be widely used, or at least readable, when the photographs are required. Also, forensic nurse's working environment may be unsafe for some digital image capture devices. Electromagnetic radiation, such as microwaves, can adversely affect or "erase" images on digital storage media, while LCD displays on any camera can be damaged when brought in proximity to MRI devices.

Digital image capture is well suited for low volume output; that is, for images that will be stored and displayed or viewed electronically on a monitor or printed in very small quantities. Although you may save some money on film and processing, outputting (printing) digital images is actually more expensive than regular photography and is more time consuming. When images are printed on paper, quality paper and inks must be used to produce quality photographs that show the detail required in court. In addition, characteristics of images printed on a desktop printer are typically poor because they tend to shift color. Color may play a key issue in a true and accurate representation of evidence that is of concern to the forensic nurse. Printer images also fade rapidly, especially when displayed. The so-called "archival" inks and papers currently available require further exploration. The cost of storage media for archiving digital images is also a concern. Additional media must be purchased and redundancy is often urged by experts in digital imaging. For example, multiple external hard drives and multiple duplicate CDs stored in separate locations are suggested to preserve some case materials. Clearly, photographs produced for criminal, civil, and death investigations must be handled and preserved to address legal admissibility and authenticity issues. The forensic nurse must be prepared to respond to questions concerning the potential for alteration or loss of digital images.

PHOTOGRAPHY IN THE COURTROOM

Photographs are usually offered by the forensic nurse as demonstrative evidence (i.e., to show the existence of fact as depicted in the photograph). Although a more detailed discussion of evidence admissibility can be found in Chapter 16, this section addresses several issues specifically related to the use of photographs in the courtroom. The first area of concern relates to the training and experience of the photographer; the second set of issues concerns the photograph itself.

In most circumstances the forensic nurse has had some training in proper photographic documentation techniques. Some forensic nurses may enroll in courses on advanced scene techniques and procedures in specific environments, such as in the emergency room. However, few forensic nurses have extensive training and experience in photography that includes technical issues using various cameras, film, and lighting techniques. However, the fact that photography is not the primary function of the forensic nurse is not necessarily a problem. As a trained forensic observer, the forensic nurse must be able to state conclusively that the photograph accurately depicts the object or location recorded on film. If the photographs are used as part of the documentation record, information related to what was photographed and any special lighting or other techniques must be noted. The forensic nurse must know the effects of these procedures and the equipment used on the image in the photograph. To understand those effects a basic knowledge of the camera, film, and other basic components is critical. Although additional knowledge may be desirable, the skill and experience of the photographer with the particular type of evidence being documented is the key to confidence in the photographs used by the forensic nurse. Thus, it is important that the photographer take many test shots under various conditions using the available equipment prior to use in an actual case. This experience will provide the forensic nurse with the background necessary to take photographs confidently. Some attorneys may attempt to draw the forensic nurse into a discussion of the fine points of photographic theory and camera operation. A witness should not hesitate to say "I don't know" when asked a technical question concerning the photographic process. In most cases such knowledge will have little relevance to the accuracy and reliability of the photograph. If the forensic nurse follows the guidelines for thorough and appropriate photographic documentation, most images will be useful for future study or admission during testimony.

As stated previously, the primary purpose for photographic documentation by the forensic nurse is to provide a clear and accurate record of what was seen at the time of the incident. As such, a person (the photographer or someone else present) testifies in court to the accuracy of the depiction. It is this testimony—the authentication of the image—that is most significant. The photograph is used to convey to the trier of fact the appearance of the scene, evidence, or injury. In essence, the witness testifies to the condition observed, using the photograph as a means to demonstrate those observations. Although some differences between photographs and other demonstrative evidence have been noted by the courts, the witness is usually required to provide an explanation of the circumstances surrounding the production of an image. The opposing attorney will make every attempt, when appropriate, to point out discrepancies or variations between the witness's oral description or other witnesses' observations and the photographic depiction. Similarly, problems with the photographic technique may result in purported misrepresentations that can keep a photograph from the jury's inspection. Ultimately, the court will make every effort to see that a complete and accurate representation is shown in an image. For example, if only a close-up photograph of an injury is shown, the jury may misinterpret the size and extent of an injury. By allowing the three or four photographs taken in the step-wise approach to documentation, the court ensures an accurate record for the jury to consider. Similarly, the court may limit the number of photographs admitted when a scene or injury is particularly gruesome. By limiting the exposure of the jury to such potentially shocking depictions, the court limits the potentially unfair bias that may be created in some of the jury as a result of the natural, human response to such evidence. If the forensic nurse is familiar with documentation guidelines and the abilities and limitations of available equipment, he or she can readily satisfy the basic requirements for use of photographs in court.

SUMMARY

The practice of forensic nursing involves numerous areas of specialization. Key to good practice in all of these areas is proper and complete documentation. Whenever documentation of physical characteristics, a pattern, or other physical evidence is required, some form of photography should always be used to supplement and enhance other forms of documentation. As discussed in this chapter, the forensic nurse has several options when choosing what photographic equipment to use in his or her practice. Whatever equipment and techniques are employed, the forensic practitioner should be facile enough with these to produce quality images that will satisfy any legal and scientific requirements for the use of the photographs.

The forensic nurse may be asked to photograph evidence in adverse conditions or with little time for preparation. By following a standard procedure such as suggested in this chapter, the forensic nurse can document thoroughly without wasting valuable time or adding to the client's stress. Practice with the various pieces of equipment under different circumstances outside an actual case experience is important to ensure the forensic nurse will be able to obtain good images under the adverse circumstances that often exist in case situations.

Photographs are also invaluable in refreshing the forensic nurse's recollection when preparing for testimony, even if the pictures themselves will not be entered into evidence. Alternately, good photographic documentation provides a solid basis for discussing findings with attorneys, other experts, and the trier of fact. Many issues that may arise in forensic cases are not known at the time of the initial examination and documentation. Photographs may often be the only source of objective information that can answer those subsequent questions. When the forensic nurse produces accurate photographs, the justice system always benefits.

QUESTIONS FOR DISCUSSION

1. Describe the test for a photograph to be entered into a court of law as a full exhibit.
2. What are the basic components of a well-equipped photography bag, and why is each item important for forensic documentation?
3. Forensic photography presents unique challenges for the forensic nurse. Identify some of those situations and develop strategies for meeting the photographic challenges encountered in each environment.
4. What factors might determine the type of photographic documentation used in a forensic setting? Which factors would be most important to consider when documenting injuries? When making a photographic record during a death investigation?

SUGGESTED READINGS

Blaker, A.A. (1989). *Handbook of scientific photography* (2nd ed.). Stoneham, MA: Butterworth.

Davies, A. & Fennessy, P. (1998). *Digital imaging for photographers* (3rd ed.). Woburn, MA: Focal Press.

Davis, P. (1995). *Photography* (7th ed.). Stoneham, MA: Butterworth.

Hedgecoe, J. (1982). *The photographer's handbook* (2nd ed.). New York: Random House.

McDonald, J.A. (1992a). *Close-up & macro photography* (2nd ed.). Arlington Heights, IL: PhotoText Books.

McDonald, J.A. (1992b). *The police photographer's guide.* Arlington Heights, IL: PhotoText Books.

Miller, L.S. (1998). *Police photography.* Cincinnati, OH: Anderson.

Redsicker, D.R. (1991). *The practical methodology of forensic photography.* New York: Elsevier Science.

Russ, J.C. (2001). *Forensic uses of digital imaging.* Boca Raton, FL: CRC Press.

Scott, C.C. (1969). *Photographic evidence* (Vols. 1–3). St. Paul, MN: West.

Sexual Assault Intervention and the Forensic Examination

Patricia LaMonica
Elaine M. Pagliaro

Sexual assault is one of the most frequently committed crimes in the United States and has the highest annual victims' costs, estimated at $127 billion per year. Although sexual assault most frequently occurs with females, males may also be sexually assaulted. The role of the sexual assault forensic examiner is multifaceted and encompasses a wide array of client needs following a sexual assault, such as: Providing medical and/or nursing care to the client while performing forensic procedures that include objective documentation, which may be utilized in a legal setting at a future date. By providing expert care and information to the client throughout the exam, the forensic examiner allows opportunities for the client to make informed decisions about his or her care, and thus begin the healing process.

CHAPTER FOCUS

Definitions and laws
Effects of sexual assault on victims
Special circumstances and concerns
Sexual assault forensic evidence collection
Drug-facilitated sexual assault
Medical/legal examination of sexual assault victims

KEY TERMS_____

colposcope
drug-facilitated sexual assault
forensic evidence
known comparison specimens
prophylaxis
rape
rape trauma syndrome
SACS
sexual assault
sexual assault response team
TEARS

INTRODUCTION

Sexual assault is one of the most frequently committed crimes in the United States and has the highest annual victims' costs, estimated at $127 billion per year (U.S. Department of Justice [DOJ], 1994). It has been estimated that as many as one in every three women and one in every five men is at risk of being sexually assaulted at some point during their lifetime (Federal Bureau of Investigation [FBI], 2004). That abuse is often perpetrated by close family members, friends, or adults in positions of authority. Various studies have shown that approximately 60%–80% of assailants are known to their victims. Riggs, Houry, Long, Markovchick, and Feldhaus (2000) studied the cases of 1,076 sexual assault victims and found that 61% of the victims knew their assailants. Statistics also indicate that *date rape* (assault by a known social acquaintance) occurs to approximately one out of every six college women. One of the most startling aspects of sex crimes is how many are unreported. According to recent Justice Department statistics, only 39% of rapes and sexual assaults were reported to law enforcement officials (U.S. DOJ, 2002). When sexually abused children in grades 5 through 12 were questioned, 48% of the boys and 29% of the girls did not tell about their abuse, not even to a friend or sibling (Commonwealth Fund Survey of the Health of Adolescent Girls, 1998). Common reasons given by victims for not reporting these crimes include guilt, self-blame, the belief that the abuse is a private or personal matter, and that they fear reprisal from the assailant.

Sexual assault is a violent crime most frequently perpetrated against women (Aiken, 1993). That violence is not committed for sexual gratification, but rather is usually a sexual expression of aggression. Often the focus of a sexual assault involves power and control for the assailant (Burgess & Holmstrom, 1974). Further discussion of the relationship between violence and sexual assault may be found in Chapter 9. The effects of sexual violence on victims and their families or significant others can be devastating. All are impacted in some way—psychologically or physically—and these effects can last a lifetime.

THE SEXUAL ASSAULT FORENSIC EXAMINER

The role of the sexual assault forensic examiner (SAFE) is multifaceted and encompasses a wide array of patient needs after a sexual assault. Often the examiner meets multiple needs of the patient simultaneously, providing medical and/or nursing care to the patient while performing forensic procedures along with objective documentation that may be utilized in a legal setting at a future date. Patients may seek assistance by entering the system with the chief complaint of rape or sexual assault or, at times, the sexual assault examiner may discover that the patient has been sexually assaulted through assessment findings, when the patient has entered the system for an entirely different reason. Clients may also enter the healthcare system as a result of victim conduct or through referrals from other sources, such as ruling out child abuse that may include sexual assault. Thus, it is essential that assessments of those clients be holistic in nature, such that the client is able to disclose when a sexual assault has occurred.

The role of the sexual assault forensic examiner as described by the International Association of Forensic Nurses (IAFN) addresses the comprehensive needs of the patient (IAFN, 1996). The practice includes assessment, evaluation, diagnosis, and implementation of comprehensive care designed to restore and promote the bio/psycho/social health of the client, which is the primary focus of the examiner. As part of this process, the forensic examination may consist of the following:

1. Obtaining the history of the assault
2. Providing crisis intervention
3. Obtaining the history of the patient's pertinent health issues
4. Performing a physical exam and assessment with a focus on inspection and evaluation of the forensic evidence of the body
5. Collecting forensic evidence
6. Treating and/or referring the client for subsequent medical treatment
7. Documenting all findings objectively
8. Interacting with clients in an objective and neutral manner that promotes informed decisions related to the available treatment options and the collection of forensic evidence

The forensic examiner is uniquely qualified to fulfill these requirements for a comprehensive examination.

DEFINITIONS

An understanding of the legal definitions of rape and sexual assault and of the physical and psychological effects of sexual assault on the client are essential if the sexual assault forensic examiner is going to meet the immediate and long-term complex needs of the client. Both the definition and legal implications of rape or sexual assault vary from state to state. Historically the term *rape* has been used primarily to connote the sexual assault of a female by a male (other than her husband), usually involving vaginal penetration by the assailant's penis. Rape is more currently considered forced sexual intercourse that includes both psychological coercion and physical force. Forced sexual intercourse may involve vaginal, anal, or oral penetration by a body part such as a penis or finger, or by a foreign object such as a bottle. More recently the term *sexual assault* has been used interchangeably with the term *rape*, and refers to both male and female victims of any age. Sexual assault is often defined as any type of sexual activity or act performed without a person's consent. *Consent* is considered a cooperative act of free will and can be granted only when a person is able to provide consent. In most circumstances, an adult of a statutorily specified age who is of sound mind may provide consent. By law, depending on the state the assault occurred in, people may not be considered capable of providing consent due to their age (minors), cognitive impairment (such as being under the influence of a drug or alcohol), or disability (such as being comatose). Sexual assault includes a wide range of victimizations, distinct from rape or attempted rape. These crimes include completed or attempted attacks generally involving unwanted sexual contact between the victim and offender. Sexual assaults may or may not involve force and include such acts as grabbing or fondling. Additionally, there are common informal subclassifications of rape or sexual assault that may include the following:

- *Acquaintance rape:* Unwanted sexual contact or activity performed by someone known by the victim (accounting for 75%–85% of sexual assaults)
- *Date rape:* Unwanted sexual contact or activity performed by someone with whom the victim is in a dating relationship
- *Drug-facilitated rape:* The use of drugs, both legal and illegal, by a potential rapist who sedates the victim prior to unwanted sexual contact or activity
- *Incest:* Sexual contact or activity performed by someone who is related to the victim

- *Statutory rape:* Sexual contact or activity performed with a minor (age determined by law) by someone who is older by a specific number of years (age determined by law)
- *Spousal or partner rape:* Unwanted sexual contact or activity with one's spouse or partner

Each sexual assault classification is defined by statute and differs slightly from state to state. For example, the definition of statutory rape may vary in the age of the victim or number of years' difference between the perpetrator and the victim.

EFFECTS ON VICTIMS OF SEXUAL ASSAULT

The effects of sexual assault can be devastating to its victims and victims' families in a multitude of ways, and its consequences may produce both physical and emotional sequelae. Those close to the victim of sexual assault can also experience feelings of rage, helplessness, and vulnerability, and may also benefit from intervention. Not all victims will present with physical injury or obvious signs of trauma. It is essential for the forensic examiner to be aware of the potential psychological effects of sexual assault, which can be far-reaching but may not be immediately evident. Individual emotional styles of clients lead to different reactions to the stress of sexual assault. Other factors affecting responses of the client include age, coping skills, culture, gender, and support systems (Ledray, 1990).

In 1974, Burgess and Holmstrom studied the emotional effects of sexual assault on victims. The cluster of emotions or emotional responses that are specific to the extreme stress surrounding sexual assault was designated rape trauma syndrome (RTS) by these authors. This response is very similar to post-traumatic stress disorder (PTSD), which is experienced by victims who are exposed to other types of extreme stressors, such as war. RTS can be divided into two phases: the acute phase and the reorganizational phase (Burgess & Holmstrom, 1974). The acute phase may occur immediately or within a short period of time following the assault. During the acute phase the victim experiences a period of disorganization. The victim's observable reaction may vary from no apparent response to being completely out of control. The specific response depends on the emotional style of the client and other influences. Although the victim is dealing with the immediate trauma of the sexual assault, he or she may also experience a variety of somatic symptoms, such as gastrointestinal problems, genitourinary problems, difficulty sleeping, or hypervigilance. According to Burgess and Holmstrom, victims also experience a wide gamut of feelings. The range of responses can include fear, guilt, humiliation, embarrassment, and self-blame. Fear of physical violence including death was the primary feeling described.

The second stage of RTS includes a period of reorganization. It is during this period that the victim attempts to gain mastery of the event. These attempts may include changing address, changing telephone numbers, leaving school or a job, or changing/ending relationships. It is important to note that some victims of sexual assault, for a variety of reasons, may be at high risk for depression, suicide, or inappropriate/dangerous behaviors during this time. The process of coping with the assault may begin at various times for each individual.

Understanding the potential effects of sexual assault on clients should enhance the forensic examiner's ability to communicate with them. This understanding can be beneficial to both the client and his or her intimate circle. Because of his or her unique training and experience, the forensic examiner can provide the client and others with educational and anticipatory guidance. Interactions that the examiner has with the client may positively impact the recovery phase of the client and others because it enables those individuals to regain hope for the future and a return to the previous level of functioning or better. Not all clients will agree to further intervention in an attempt to regain control.

Special Circumstances and Concerns

Sexual assault is a crime that affects all socioeconomic, cultural, ethnic, and religious groups. These differences may affect the manner in which the client responds to the assault and to the subsequent forensic and medical examinations. When the sexual assault forensic examiner is aware of the effect these parameters may have on the client and his or her perception of the process, modifications in language or actions should be made to make the client more comfortable with the forensic examiner and the examination process. Several circumstances that should involve special consideration include the age of the client (children, the elderly, and adolescents), any client disability, the client's gender, and the sexual orientation of the client.

Age is a critical consideration when dealing with a client who has been sexually assaulted. The client's age may affect his or her ability to describe the incident, relate symptoms, and understand the examination process as it proceeds. In addition, age will likely impact the client's response to the assault as well as the legal implications of that attack. Elderly clients often experience extreme humiliation, shock, and disbelief similar to that of other victims of sexual assault. In addition, the elderly may be acutely aware of their vulnerability and mortality as a result of the assault (Commission on the Standardization of the Collection of Evidence in Sexual Assault Investigations, 1998). Elderly victims of sexual assault may also experience more extreme physical injuries because they generally are physically more fragile or may be suffering from age-related conditions. Some studies support that post-menopausal women who have been sexually assaulted sustain more genital trauma than younger victims (Ramin et al., 1992). The recovery process for the elderly can be lengthier than for other victims due to their lack of resilience. Additionally, they may experience feelings of loss of independence and self-reliance or experience overwhelming shame and guilt (Girardin, Faugno, Senski, Slaughter, & Whelan, 1997). Recovery is dependent on nurturing and sensitive, appropriate interventions by significant others with counseling geared toward the needs of the older client. The older client also may require more frequent medical follow-up. Most states currently have mandatory reporting for the abuse of the elderly, including sexual assault.

The special needs of children who are victims of sexual assault are well documented. Although it is difficult to obtain true figures of the rate of child sexual assault, most authorities agree that there is widespread underreporting. Additionally, research shows that exposure as a child to sexual behaviors may be linked to early onset of sexual activity and increased sexual vulnerability in adolescence, including an increased risk for sexual revictimization (Fergusson, Horwood, & Lynskey, 1997). A study by Fergusson and colleagues demonstrated a higher rate of teenage pregnancy, early onset of sexual activity, unprotected intercourse, and sexually transmitted diseases in women who reported childhood sexual assault as compared to women who were not assaulted as children.

Many children are abused in various ways over long periods of time. As a result, the collection of forensic evidence may not be possible at the time of the exam, especially in cases where the child is under 12 years of age. Most jurisdictions have detailed guidelines for the pediatric physical examination, and the forensic examiner should always proceed according to those guidelines. In general, however, additional support personnel including parent or guardian, child advocates, or other professionals should assist the SAFE, when appropriate, to obtain the child's medical history (New Hampshire Sexual Assault Protocol Revision Committee, 1998; Adams, Harper, Knudson & Revilla, 1994; State of CT Supplemental Guidelines, 1998). Because statistics have shown that the offender is often a family member or close acquaintance whom the child trusts, the examiner should interview the child away from any potential offender. Children require special interview techniques to obtain clear, objective history, so the interview should be performed by a specially trained interviewer whenever possible. Additionally, specialized equipment may be needed for the physical examination.

As with all other clients, the sexual assault forensic examiner should take the time necessary to explain procedures to the child victim and to reassure the child as much as possible during the examination. It may be helpful to the examiner to utilize a developmental staging tool such as the Tanner Scale, which stages out female and male reproductive development to assist with further medical treatment and care.

Female adolescents are especially at risk for vaginal injury and for acquiring a sexually transmitted disease (STD) because they may be physiologically more susceptible, depending upon their developmental stage.

Special concerns also exist regarding clients with physical, mental, or communicative disabilities. These people may have limited cognition or difficulties that impair their perceptual abilities. These difficulties may cause clients to be frightened, unsure of exactly what occurred during the assault, or unable to understand that they have been a victim of a crime (Commission, 1998; American College of Emergency Physicians, 1999). As with the pediatric population, assaults within this population may go undetected for a long period of time because the offender is often a family member or a caretaker (Haddix-Hill, 1997). If speech or other communication appears to be difficult, the SAFE should make every opportunity to obtain the proper assistance in the form of an interpreter or electronic communication device. Most protocols recommend that victims with disabilities and their circle of support be given the highest priority. Extra time must be taken with the disabled client to communicate effectively during the examination process and to understand the questions or concerns of the client. Ideally, the interviewer has received specialized training regarding interviewing techniques in order to obtain a clear and objective history of the assault. The examiner may need to assist the patient in assuming the necessary positions for complete forensic collection and medical examination. Reporting of sexual abuse of disabled persons is mandated in every state.

Gays and lesbians comprise another population who require special considerations. Like other victims of sexual assault, there is often a resistance to report the sexual assault due to a fear of judgment by the police but also due to potential rejection from the gay community. Contrary to common public opinion, both gays and lesbians are more frequently assaulted by heterosexual males. The exam process is similar to that for heterosexual victims; however, the forensic examiner should be sensitive to their special needs, and counseling is best done by someone from the gay community whenever possible.

Many experts believe that sexual assaults of males are among the least reported of any group (Bureau of Justice Statistics, 2003). Other men commit most of the sexual assaults of boys, male adolescents, and adult men. It is not uncommon for the male victim to have multiple assailants and to have a high degree of nongenital trauma. In fact, males may often seek medical attention for physical injuries and initially may only disclose the physical assault. An awareness of this fact allows the forensic examiner to investigate further whether the male was sexually assaulted.

Male victims demonstrate the same responses to sexual assault as discussed previously. The male victim will have additional concerns about his inability to protect himself and his maleness, and may feel less masculine (Girardin et al., 1997). The extent to which male victims attempt to control their environment after a sexual assault may cause them to be less communicative during the medical examination and the collection of forensic evidence. Men may be less willing to discuss in detail the types of abuse they have suffered, which makes it more difficult to obtain appropriate forensic samples and to provide the necessary health care. The male victim may be embarrassed or concerned that the examiner or the police will question his masculinity. Sensitivity to these concerns on the part of the forensic examiner can often help to obtain an objective and clear history and may lead to obtaining appropriate forensic evidence.

THE FORENSIC EXAMINATION

It is critical that the forensic examiner maintain an objective and neutral approach during the examination and subsequent interaction with the client. Initial contact should occur in an environment that is both private and comfortable for the client. Adequate time for explanations of care and forensic procedures is critical; clients should not be rushed through the exam. The client should understand all that is about to occur and be given the opportunity to refuse those procedures with which he or she does not feel comfortable. Knowing that exams can be refused meets some of the client's need to assume some control of the situation after the assault and also provides education to allow the client to make informed decisions about care (Hampton, 1995).

Initial Considerations

Prior to starting the examination, the sexual assault forensic examiner should bring the client into a private location and establish a rapport with the client utilizing a neutral and objective approach. Whenever possible, clients should be interviewed alone at some point to avoid inadvertently being questioned in the presence of the offender, as in the case of a child. Also, prior to starting the exam, the assistance of the local sexual assault crisis service (SACS) should be offered. Their services are invaluable to both the client and the examiner. For the client, the SACS counselor can become a long-term connection to counseling and legal advocacy. SACS often serves as a lifeline for any needed future assistance. Generally, their services are free of charge and available 24 hours a day, 7 days a week. The SACS counselor assists the forensic examiner by providing support to the client during the physical examination and the evidence collection process. This allows the examiner to focus on the actual exam, evidence collection, and documentation. Should the client choose not to have a SACS counselor present at the time of examination, local SACS information should be provided to the client at discharge so that the client has the option of calling them at a later date. In addition, if the client wishes to have another person present during the examination, those wishes should be respected. It may take some time to establish rapport with the client and to provide the desired people for support during the process. However, the forensic examiner will be able to conduct a more thorough examination and to provide better care for the client if the necessary time is spent prior to initiating the actual examination process.

The SAFE should begin by explaining what she is planning to do and allow the client to control the speed of the exam and participate by selecting the order of the exam, whenever possible. The client always maintains the right to refuse any part or parts of the exam, and this should be explained to the patient before any action is taken and prior to each step in the process, thus allowing the client to make informed decisions. The examination must be done in a nonhurried way and allow opportunity for explanations and education by the SAFE. In addition, the client must have ample opportunity to ask questions throughout the examination. The client should also be told that he or she may stop the exam at any time.

The examiner should obtain a detailed history of the assault from the client, documenting on the medical record or other examination documentation form (see Figure 18–1). The SAFE should quote the client's own words as much as possible. This history should include all events surrounding the assault, where the sexual assault occurred, and when it occurred. A critical factor in sexual assault prosecution is often consistency between the assessment findings and the history of the sexual assault as related by the patient. Thus, no detail provided by the client should be omitted from the history, no matter how insignificant it may initially appear. The examiner should also obtain a health history from the client that includes current medical problems and a listing of medications that the client is taking, including when the client last took the medications. During the initial stages of the exam, the SAFE should determine if the client wishes to report the assault to the police, if he or

STATE OF CONNECTICUT
SEXUAL ASSAULT MEDICAL REPORT
(Additional writing space provided in Section 9, If needed.)   CGS19a-112a

HEALTH CARE FACILITY: _____

1. CHIEF COMPLAINT: _____

A. Date and Time of Arrival _____
    Month Day Year Time

B. Date and Time of Assault_____
    Month Day Year Time

2. MEDICAL HISTORY AS RELATED BY PATIENT:

A. History of Assault: _____
_____
_____
_____
_____
_____
_____
_____
_____
_____
_____
_____
_____

B. Nature of Sexual Assault:

	Contact By					Penetration By					Ejaculation		
	Penis	Hand	Oral	Other	Unsure	Penis	Hand	Oral	Other	Unsure	Yes	No	Unsure
Mouth:	☐	☐	☐	☐	☐	☐	☐	☐	☐	☐	☐	☐	☐
Breasts:	☐	☐	☐	☐	☐	☐	☐	☐	☐	☐	☐	☐	☐
Vagina:	☐	☐	☐	☐	☐	☐	☐	☐	☐	☐	☐	☐	☐
Penis:	☐	☐	☐	☐	☐	☐	☐	☐	☐	☐	☐	☐	☐
Anus/Rectum:	☐	☐	☐	☐	☐	☐	☐	☐	☐	☐	☐	☐	☐
Other:	☐	☐	☐	☐	☐	☐	☐	☐	☐	☐	☐	☐	☐

(specify): _____
C. Between the assault and present has the patient: ☐ douched

☐ wiped/washed off   ☐ rinsed mouth   ☐ defecated
☐ bathed/showered   ☐ brushed teeth   ☐ vomited
☐ changed clothes   ☐ ate or drank   ☐ urinated

(specify): _____

D. Nature of Physical Assault (specify, e.g., struck, bit, choked,etc.):
_____
_____
_____
_____
_____

PATIENT STAMP (If handwritten, record name, unit number and birth date.)

E. Did assailant: Use lubricant?   ☐ Yes ☐ No ☐ Unsure
                  Use condom?   ☐ Yes ☐ No ☐ Unsure
                  Insert foreign object(s)? ☐ Yes ☐ No ☐ Unsure

(specify): _____

	Yes	No	Unsure
F. Was the patient menstruating at the time of assault?	☐	☐	☐
If yes, is tampon present?	☐	☐	☐
G. Any additional physical injuries?	☐	☐	☐

If yes, describe: _____
_____
_____

If yes, any bleeding? ☐ ☐ ☐
H. Any injuries to assailant resulting in bleeding? ☐ ☐ ☐
If yes, describe: _____
_____
_____

3. PAST MEDICAL HISTORY:
A. Any sexual intercourse in the last 72 hours? ☐ ☐ ☐
If yes, type: ☐ Vaginal ☐ Anal ☐ Oral ☐ Other
If yes, date:_____ time:_____
Was condom used? ☐ ☐ ☐
B. Is contraception used? ☐ ☐ ☐
If yes, type:_____
C. Last menstrual period: _____
Is the patient pregnant? ☐ ☐ ☐
If yes, duration of pregnancy:_____

D. Additional medical history: _____
_____
_____
_____
_____
_____

Sections 1, 2 & 3 completed by _____

Figure 18–1   Victim interview and initial examination documentation sheet.

she has not already done so. The examiner should be familiar with the mandatory reporting requirements independent of the client's consent. If the SAFE is required by statute to report the sexual assault to law enforcement, this fact and the reasons for the report should be explained to the client. These laws vary from state to state. However, one law that appears to be consistent throughout the United States requires that sexual assaults of a minor be reported to the police. Reporting may also be mandated with other populations, such as mentally handicapped persons, elders, and assaults that include the use of a firearm.

Although some clients access the system immediately following a sexual assault, many victims of sexual assault initially experience a sense of disbelief or shock, which delays access to any form of assistance. Often the victim will not go directly to a hospital or police department, but may shower or bathe, or tell a friend or family member of the assault. The timing of an official report is critical because it will determine if a sexual assault evidence kit should be used. In general, forensic evidence collection is most useful within 72 hours of the sexual assault. After 72 hours most of the physical evidence useful to confirm the crime or identify the assailant has been lost, especially if the client has showered or bathed.

Adult patients may refuse forensic evidence collection with a sex crimes kit for a variety of reasons. These reasons include fear of retaliation by the perpetrator, embarrassment, and cultural influences, as mentioned previously. Depending upon the state in which the assault occurred, a sexual assault evidence kit may be used only if the assault is reported to law enforcement. Other states, however, allow for the collection and storage of the evidence for the statute of limitations, allowing the client to revisit the decision not to make an official complaint. Those states provide an option of allowing a patient to have forensic evidence collected using a sex crimes kit that can be entered anonymously for a period of time; the client can then take more time to make a decision concerning the filing of an official complaint. In these delayed reporting situations, the evidence will be given a specific code and then transported to the police or laboratory to maintain the appropriate chain of custody. This holding procedure benefits those patients who are ambivalent about the legal aspects of the assault. The forensic examiner should help the client make informed decisions about reporting the crime by providing information about the use of the evidence and related matters. Clients should also be informed of the potential loss of some types of forensic evidence due to delays in collection. It is important to keep in mind, however, that even if a forensic evidence collection kit is not used, the medical record of the client may provide evidence of the assault through the accurate documentation of the assessment findings.

Collection of Forensic Specimens

Before beginning the physical assessment, all equipment that the examiner needs for the examination should be available in the room. The ideal situation is to collect forensic evidence simultaneously with the medical specimens during the physical assessment. Usually, the examiner should perform any procedures for medical management of the patient after forensic and medical specimens are collected. All forensic evidence collected should remain in full view of the examiner and never be left unattended, to maintain an intact chain of evidence.

If the patient chooses to have forensic evidence collected, a sex crimes kit may be used. Kits vary from state to state depending on what types of analyses are recommended by the forensic laboratory of that jurisdiction. Figure 18–2 shows a typical sexual assault evidence collection kit. Most kits are designed to provide the examiner with the materials to collect and preserve samples in an appropriate manner. These kits also allow for flexibility in specimen collection, based on the client's wishes

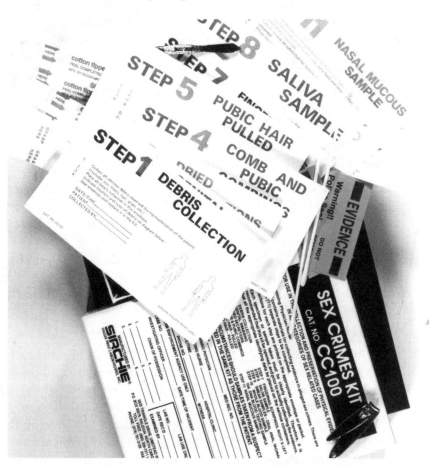

Figure 18–2 Typical sexual assault evidence collection kit and contents.

and the history of the sexual assault. The examiner should assure that the kit is fully sealed and has not been opened prior to being used. Before opening the examination materials, the SAFE should put on latex or nitrile gloves. The examiner should remain gloved during the examination, changing into new gloves as necessary to avoid contamination of the forensic specimens. Some examiners use a Woods Lamp to perform a cursory inspection of the client's body. Body fluids such as semen appear fluorescent in that light and may provide the examiner with an additional site for forensic specimen collection.

The following paragraphs outline a suggested sequence for the examination of the client and the collection of forensic evidence using a standardized sex crimes kit. Many variations in these procedures exist, although some attempts have been made to formulate national guidelines for the collection of sexual assault evidence. Often the examination is performed from the least invasive to most invasive procedure, or from external to internal examinations. Forensic evidence collected during this examination includes materials used as standards for comparison, samples used to prove that a sexual assault occurred, and specimens that may be linked to the perpetrator(s) of the crime. Those items that may be included in the forensic evidence collection include the following: blood from the client; fingernail scrapings/cuttings; hair from the client's head; oral swabs and smears; dried secretions found on parts of the body other than the genital area; pubic hair combings; pubic hair of the client; genital swabbing; vaginal swabs and smears; anal swabs and smear; and any other physical evidence that may be evident, such as a condom, tampon, or debris on the patient.

Fingernail scrapings and cuttings may provide trace materials or tissue/blood samples of the perpetrator. If the forensic laboratory conducts hair analyses, hair from both the head and pubic area are used in comparison to other hairs collected as evidence, such as in the pubic combings. Oral, anal, and vaginal swabs and smears are collected to identify seminal fluid or spermatozoa; if semen is found, DNA analysis may be conducted on those samples. Similarly, dried secretions collected from other parts of the victim's body, such as from bite marks, may be used to identify the perpetrator.

The forensic examiner may be able to obtain only an incomplete history of the sexual assault as the client may not recall portions of the assault or may be too embarrassed to provide details of all aspects of the assault. For example, older women often may be too embarrassed to relate that the assault included oral penetration. Therefore, it is important that the sexual assault forensic examiner perform a thorough physical assessment to identify any injuries and collect all significant forensic specimens, even if not indicated by the history at the time of the initial examination.

Steps in Evidence Collection

The following steps for sample collection are presented in a common sequence, based on the recommendations of several states. The exact order in which samples will be collected from the client will depend on the type of evidence, the guidelines of the locality in which the examination takes place, the physical and emotional condition of the client, and any particular requirements based on the assault history. Any procedures used by the sexual assault forensic examiner should be flexible enough to satisfy the legal requirements for evidence admissibility and the forensic requirements for evidentiary analysis while addressing the concerns and health needs of the client during the examination.

I. *Clothing*

The first step in the examination is usually the collection of clothing. Before the client undresses, the examiner should determine if the client is still wearing the clothing that he or she had on during the sexual assault. If the client has not changed clothing, these items should certainly become part of the evidence collected with the client's consent. In addition, even if the client has changed clothing since the assault, the forensic examiner may choose to collect the underpants if there was a vaginal or anal assault or if the victim did not bathe prior to changing clothes.

Before the client undresses, the examiner should place a paper sheet from the sex crimes kit on the floor. The client should stand on this paper while he or she removes each item of clothing. Standing on the paper will catch any debris, such as fibers or vegetation, that may fall off the clothing during the disrobing process. As each item of clothing is removed it is placed in a separate paper bag. Each bag is sealed and clearly marked with the contents, the patient's name, the date and time of collection, and the examiner's name. In general, the examiner should *not* remove any substances from the clothing prior to packaging. The location of material or the pattern of deposits may be significant forensic information that can be used during analysis or during the trial. Rather, when necessary, the forensic examiner should assist the client while he or she is taking off clothing to prevent loss of these types of physical evidence. Only if there is danger of evidence being lost or destroyed when the client disrobes should the examiner remove and package appropriately any loose materials. (Refer to Appendix 2 for evidence packaging guidelines.) If the foreign material is removed from an item of clothing, the examiner should note in detail the location and amount of that sample.

When collecting clothing from a male victim, the forensic examiner should take every precaution to prevent contamination of any body fluids with those that may have originated from the client. For example, the underwear of a male victim may contain semen from the client that should be kept away from areas that may represent seminal deposits of the assailant; paper between the folds of the clothing may help to prevent this cross-contamination.

After all of the clothing is removed, the paper on which the client is standing should be carefully folded, so evidence is not lost or contaminated, and properly packaged.

Clothing should be packaged in folded paper or paper bags. Paper bags are preferable to plastic bags or containers because plastic promotes mold and bacterial growth that can cause deterioration of the evidence. Any wet items of clothing should be air dried whenever possible prior to packaging. If items are soaked with blood or body fluids and they cannot be air dried, those items may be placed temporarily in a plastic bag; however, if this occurs the examiner should turn over the evidence as soon as possible to law enforcement for further drying or transport to the forensic laboratory. If a wet item has been placed in plastic, the SAFE should draw attention to this fact by placing prominent stickers or notations on the outer packaging. A "liquid biohazard" or "wet" designation alerts the police or the laboratory that special handling of this evidence is required.

2. Known Specimens for DNA Comparison

Collection of known blood specimens is often the next step in the examination process. Collection of blood at this time provides the opportunity to process specimens and to obtain results that are required for medical treatment before the end of the examination. Blood specimens needed for forensic DNA analysis should also be collected at this time. DNA testing protocols recommend the use of a purple cap (EDTA) tube to collect blood. Client-identifying information should be placed on the blood tube, along with the name of the person collecting the sample, the date, and the time. Because only a small amount of sample is required for DNA analysis utilizing current standard procedures, some states collect buccal swab samples as standards for DNA analysis instead of blood samples. If buccal swabs are used, the known DNA standard from the client must be collected so that there is no possibility of contamination by other swabs or fluids from the kit or persons at the time of collection. Buccal swabs for DNA standards should be collected after all other evidence has been collected from the oral cavity, and the victim should rinse thoroughly with distilled water prior to sampling the buccal epithelial cells.

3. Debris and Foreign Material

Examination of the client often reveals the presence of blood, semen, or saliva on the body in various locations. These body fluids are the most common secretions deposited by the assailant, although urine and feces may also be encountered. When these foreign materials are observed, the sexual assault examiner should collect each foreign sample using a sterile swab. The swab should be moistened with a minimum of sterile water for collection and allowed to air dry before packaging. In addition to body fluid deposits, debris and other materials may be noted that can be associated with the scene of an assault or with the perpetrator of the crime. This debris may include vegetative material, fibers, soil, hairs, or other types of trace material. For example, in one case, after a woman was sexually assaulted in a vehicle, fine metal shavings were collected by the SAFE from her hair. When a suspect was identified both his car and his garage work area contained metal shavings determined to be of the same composition and appearance. Use of an ultraviolet (Woods) lamp or other alternate light source to examine the patient may aid in locating very small samples of body fluid, fibers, and other trace materials that should be collected.

Bite mark evidence is one of the more common situations in which foreign body fluids, usually saliva, may be found. Bite marks are seen on clients who are the victims of sexual assault and other violent crimes. When bite mark evidence is recognized, it is important that the evidence in this area be processed prior to cleaning the wound. After appropriate photographic and written documentation of the bite mark, the saliva should be collected. It is important to use a minimal amount of sterile water on the swab when collecting from this area. The bite mark should be gently swabbed, rotating the swab and applying light pressure during collection. Use of too much force when swabbing bite marks may result in a sample that contains too little foreign material in relation to the amount of client cells, often leading to an inconclusive DNA profiling result.

4. *Fingernail Scrapings and Clippings*

Fingernails may be important specimens, especially if they contain biological material such as tissue or trace evidence from the assailant or crime scene. Factors that will determine whether fingernail scrapings should be taken include the amount of time since the assault, whether the client has bathed or washed his or her hands since the assault, and the history of the incident. Some protocols advise taking scrapings and clippings even if the client has no specific memory of scratching the perpetrator. The forensic examiner should obtain the client's permission before clipping fingernails.

5. *Known Hairs from the Client*

If the forensic laboratory conducts microscopic hair analysis, known head and pubic hairs should be collected from the client at the time of the examination. This step is usually carried out after pubic combings are collected from the client. The pubic combings will be examined at the laboratory to determine if any hair evidence was transferred from the assailant during the incident. The recommended method of hair collection differs among jurisdictions. These various methods reflect some of the different philosophies among sexual assault response teams, sexual assault counselors, and laboratories. Some procedures recommend that no hairs be collected at the time of the examination; those protocols often state that known hairs can be collected at a later date if foreign hairs are identified in the other evidence. Scientifically this is the least desirable situation because of the physical and microscopic differences that can occur in the hairs, even over a short period of time. It is important to collect contemporaneous hair samples for analysis because of the effect that time, diet, stress, physiological or physical conditions, and other factors can have on the morphological characteristics of hairs.

After conducting hair comparisons scientists are only able to determine whether a hair is "similar" and could have originated from an individual, "dissimilar" to hairs from an individual, or "inconclusive." Microscopic hair comparisons do not serve as a positive means of individualization. Because of the limitations of this type of analysis, some experts recommend that only combed hairs be obtained as standards and that pulled hairs be collected at a later date, only when necessary. Those forensic nurse examiners believe that the potential for pain that pulling hairs may cause the patient outweighs the limited evidentiary value of pulled hair specimens. However, opponents of obtaining only combed hairs point out that there is no way to associate definitively the source of those hairs in a combing—a comb will collect telogen (about to be shed) hairs from the client as well as any loose hairs transferred from the assailant during the incident. A mixture of hairs may be present in the combing that can present difficulty during legal proceedings. Clearly, there is a need to associate or exclude questioned hairs in a forensic sample, especially because mitochondrial DNA analysis of hairs can now be conducted (and is usually done after microscopic examination includes a person as a potential source of the hair).

One compromise, which allows the collection of an identifiable standard while preventing any further trauma to the client, is to cut known hairs at the skin line. This method provides the entire length of the hair for microscopic examination, but employs a painless collection process. Another approach is to have the patient pull his or her own head or pubic hairs. This method often reduces the client's embarrassment and the trauma of collection. Hairs should be cut or pulled as standards from various areas of a particular location to obtain a random sample of hairs that represent the various types of hair in the region. For example, hairs should be collected from the top, back, front, and sides of the client's head. The total number of hairs recommended varies, but ranges from 20 to 100 total hairs. The sexual assault forensic examiner should follow the specific recommendations of the state protocols or the healthcare facility or state when collecting hair samples.

6. Swabs and Smears

It is important to take swabs from each body orifice to collect evidence of penetration in the sexual assault. When collecting samples, the sexual assault forensic examiner should take every precaution to prevent contamination of the swabs with other samples or secretions. It is usually recommended that swabs and smears from the mouth, vagina/penis, and anus be collected, even if the client does not relate during the examination that such contact took place. However, as stated previously, if the client insists that he or she does not want a sample collected, that refusal should be honored. Swabbing of the mouth, vagina, and/or anus and the smears made from those swabs will be checked for the presence of spermatozoa or seminal fluid. If identified, DNA analysis can be conducted in an effort to individualize the source of that semen. If no semen is identified, condom lubricants may be detectable on the swabs. Penile swabbing of the male victim may reveal the presence of saliva on the penis that could indicate oral-genital contact. In some cases, such as the statutory sexual assault of a boy, the penile swabbing may be checked for the presence of vaginal epithelial cells and a female DNA profile.

Sterile swabs should be moistened with a minimum of sterile distilled water before swabbing the area being examined. Since swabs may be tested for the presence of condom lubricants and trace material, the forensic examiner should wear only nonlubricated, powder-free gloves during the swab collection process. Subsequently, the swabs are used to make a smear on a glass slide that will be examined for spermatozoa at the laboratory. The swabs and smears should be air dried before packaging.

The following swabs should be collected:

- Oral swabs should be collected using at least two swabs. Particular care should be taken to swab those areas in the mouth where material, including semen, may become lodged, such as between the gums and lips and in the pockets around teeth.
- Vaginal swabs should be collected without diluting the secretions or aspirating the area. Collection of vaginal swabs should take place after external genital swabbings and pubic combings are collected.
- Penile swabs should be collected using light pressure. All outer areas of the penis and scrotum should be swabbed.
- Anal/rectal swabs may be moistened with a small about of sterile water to reduce the discomfort to the client during swabbing. Whenever possible, avoid heavy deposits of fecal matter on the swab or smear.

7. Pubic Hair Combings

Contact between two people will result in the exchange of various materials, depending on the extent and type of contact. During a sexual assault, contact may result in the transfer of hairs, fibers, and other trace materials from the assailant, as well as materials from the crime scene. Combing the pubic area provides for the collection of these trace materials for identification and comparison at the laboratory. The sexual assault examiner should comb the area using a clean comb after placing a specimen envelope or paper under the buttocks. This location for the collection envelope or paper will prevent the loss of trace materials during the combing process. If any clumps of material are noted adhered to the hairs or if there are apparent deposits of semen or other liquid, the SAFE should ask the patient if the hairs in this area can be cut for collection. If the client does not agree to have the hairs cut, the forensic examiner should swab the deposits prior to combing the area.

8. Genital Swabbing

The exterior genital area should be sampled using a slightly moistened swab. When swabbing any visible secretions in this area, ensure that all the swab surfaces are exposed to the sample by turning the swab during collection. If the client is female, the vulva and inner thighs should be swabbed, even if no secretions are visible. If the client is male, the SAFE should use one swab to collect samples from the glans and shaft of the penis, a second swab for the base of the penis and the testicles, and a third swab for the thighs.

9. Additional Evidence, as Noted

At times there may be additional materials that should be collected that may provide valuable information about the perpetrator or provide evidence of a crime. When such evidence is encountered, such as a condom or tampon, that evidence should be collected, appropriately packaged, and included in the sexual assault evidence kit.

DRUG-FACILITATED SEXUAL ASSAULT

During the past decade, information concerning drug-facilitated sexual assault (DFSA) has become readily available to the public. Many popular magazines, television shows, and news programs have provided good background on the problem and various ways that potential victims of DFSA can protect themselves. In spite of this awareness, the problem persists, especially among young adult females, and many clients express the fear that they have been the victims of DFSA. Drugs are frequently mixed with alcohol or other beverages to incapacitate the victim. Once the victim recovers from the initial effects of the drug, it may be difficult for her or him to recall the event or any details concerning the assailant. According to Welner (2001), the *modus operandi* of perpetrators who employ drugs to incapacitate or otherwise affect a chosen victim has four components: means, setting, opportunity, and a plan to avoid arrest and prosecution. As this list implies, there is no one drug, one type of perpetrator, or one situation in which DFSA occurs. Various types of drugs are used, depending on the social setting, access to different drugs by the perpetrator, and the relationship between the victim and the assailant (more opportunities to use a drug will arise when there is a pre-existing relationship). Although no one particular group appears to be at risk, studies indicate that there may be an increased incidence of drug-facilitated sexual assaults among college and university students during the past few years (Fisher, Cullen, & Turner, 2000).

A study by ElSohly in 1999 showed the presence of various types of drugs in the urines of more than 2,000 victims who believed they had been drugged prior to a sexual assault. More than 20 different chemical substances were identified in those urine samples, but the most prevalent drug detected was alcohol (ethanol); approximately 40% of the samples tested were positive for this compound. Other common drugs identified in those urine specimens were marijuana, 18%; cocaine, 8%; gamma hydroxybutyrate (GHB), 3%; and flunitrazepam (rohypnol) 0.3%. Remarkably, tests in more than one-third of the urine samples (37%) failed to reveal the presence of *any* drug. However, it should be noted that many of the drugs used in DFSA are quickly metabolized and remain detectable for relatively short periods of time in the blood and urine. If the client delays reporting a DFSA, evidence of the drug may be irretrievably lost.

The identification of alcohol as the most common drug in these urine samples should not be a surprising fact. Alcohol is a legal substance that is readily available and acceptable in most social environments. Alcohol is common at many social gatherings and at parties on campuses around the country. In fact, much of the social contact of university students revolves around alcohol or takes place where alcohol is served. The symptoms of intoxication are well known and include a reduction in inhibitions, decreased motor coordination, reduced ability to think logically, and increased response time. This is the perfect drug for an assailant who can induce his victim to consume a sufficient amount of alcohol to achieve the desired effects.

Symptoms of the use of rohypnol and GHB are similar to each other and may last several days. They include drowsiness, lightheadedness, dizziness, fatigue, decreased blood pressure, and memory loss. It should be noted that GBL (gamma butrylactone), the chemical precursor to GHB, is available in many legal, commercial products. (GBL is not approved for human consumption.) (LeBeau, 1999).

Collection of Evidence in Drug-Facilitated Sexual Assault Investigations

In general, the sexual assault forensic examiner should not collect samples for forensic toxicology screening unless the client exhibits symptoms or a history that indicates DFSA or if it is medically indicated. The collection of DFSA evidence should be considered if:

- the patient or companion states that the client was or may have been drugged,
- or the client suspects drug involvement because there is no recollection of the event,
- or in the opinion of the examiner, the client's medical condition appears to warrant screening for optimal care (i.e., he or she exhibits symptoms consistent with the presence of a drug),
- and the amount of time since the alleged incident does not exceed the recommended time for collection. In general, if ingestion was within 48–72 hours, the collection of toxicology samples is indicated.

Even if these criteria are met, the SAFE should collect a blood or urine sample for forensic toxicology testing only with informed consent from the client. Informed consent requires that the forensic examiner discuss the following information with the client:

- the effects of time since the incident on the ability to detect and identify any drugs that may have been used;
- the inability to predict the success of the toxicology analysis;
- the fact that toxicology testing is not limited to well known "date rape" drugs, but will detect the presence of many other drugs, including legal and controlled substances that the client may have voluntarily ingested;
- the refusal to undergo testing, when it is indicated, may have a negative impact on the criminal investigation.

Before any evidentiary samples for toxicology testing are collected it is important to thoroughly advise the client of these factors. It is usually a good idea to involve a sexual assault crisis counselor during these discussions. Because of the potential implications and impact of toxicology testing for forensic purposes, most protocols require the client to sign a separate consent form prior to the collection of toxicology samples. Figure 18–3 shows a typical consent form for toxicology evidence collection.

**CONSENT FOR
TOXICOLOGY SCREEN**
CGS19a-112a

PATIENT STAMP (If handwritten, record name, unit number and birth date.)

To Examining Clinician:

Please review information in this form with patient, allowing ample time to discuss any questions the patient may have. **It is important that the patient understand all segments of this form prior to signing it.** If patient chooses to consent to toxicology screen:

    (1) Have patient sign and date the form in the space(s) indicated

    (2) Provide your signature and date in the space(s) indicated

    (3) Place and maintain this form in patient's medical record

---

To Patient:

Please read and review all information in this form with the clinician prior to signing it. Please discuss any questions you may have to ensure that you understand all of the information presented. If you choose to consent to toxicology screen, provide your signature and date in the space(s) indicated.

I consent to and authorize the collection of urine and/or blood samples for the purpose of detecting the presence of drugs or other substances that may have caused sedation and/or amnesia in the context of a sexual assault.

I understand that any samples must be obtained within 72 hours of ingestion.

I understand that the toxicology screen may detect any substances, medications or drugs (both legal and illegal) that may be in my system from the weeks prior to the sexual assault.

I understand that the results of the toxicology screen may be very important for the possible arrest and prosecution of the offender.

I have discussed toxicology screen with the clinician and have had an opportunity to ask questions and discuss concerns.

_____   _____
Signature of Patient   Date/Time

_____   _____
Signature of Clinician   Date/Time

Figure 18–3   Specialized consent form for collection of drug-facilitated sexual assault evidence samples.

Collection Procedures

The specific requirements in each state or county may vary, as outlined in the guidelines for toxicology collection established by the healthcare facility in conjunction with the local forensic toxicology laboratory and law enforcement organizations. Guidelines commonly recommend the collection of both urine and blood samples if ingestion occurred within 24 to 48 hours. If ingestion occurred between 48 and 72 hours, only urine should be collected. Collection of samples for toxicology after 72 hours is not recommended in most circumstances (LeBeau, 1999).

Blood samples should be collected in gray-top vacuum tubes using sterile procedures. Gray-top tubes contain sodium fluoride, a preservative, and potassium oxalate, an anticoagulant. Approximately 10–20 milliliters of blood should be collected. Failure to use a blood tube with the correct preservative may lead to false negative results upon testing. It should be noted that the blood tubes used for DNA testing that are present in the standard sexual assault evidence collection kits contain EDTA and are unsuitable for toxicological analysis. Thus, if there is no standard DFSA kit at the healthcare facility, the sexual assault examiner should obtain the proper tubes from hospital stock.

Urine is collected in a sterile urine collection vessel. Approximately 30–50 milliliters of mid-stream urine is recommended for toxicology testing. The urine vessel should be placed in a plastic bag that is sealed in a tamper-evident manner.

After the blood and the urine samples are collected, each should be labeled with the client's name and control number, along with the initials of the person collecting the sample, and date and time of collection.

Toxicology samples should be appropriately labeled as biohazardous materials and forwarded immediately to the appropriate laboratory for testing. Most healthcare facilities do not have the appropriate equipment or procedures in place for testing of some drugs commonly seen in DFSA investigations. More importantly, the necessary "chain of custody" must be maintained for the results of the testing to be admitted during a trial; hospitals and other healthcare facilities usually are not equipped to meet the legal requirements for chain of custody and admissibility of toxicology evidence.

PERPETRATOR EVIDENCE COLLECTION

At times, it is necessary to collect specimens from alleged perpetrators accused of sexual assault. Some states provide a "suspect evidence collection kit" that is similar to the sex crimes kit used for victims. The evidence often includes the collection of blood, hairs, fingernail scrapings, or other samples for comparison and standards for DNA analysis. Depending on how soon after the assault the perpetrator is apprehended, additional specimens may be collected, such as clothing or swabs, which can be used to search for materials transferred from the victim at the time of the assault. Suspect evidence is collected in a manner similar to that of evidence collected from victims. Documentation should be concise and clear. Because of the rights of the accused, suspect evidence collection takes place only after appropriate consent from the suspect or a search warrant is obtained by law enforcement officers. Proper protocols for the collection and preservation of evidence and proper chain of evidence are vital with this evidence. At times, the attorney representing the accused may also request assistance when biological samples are required for defense purposes. The forensic examiner should follow the same type of collection and documentation protocols required when assisting police with evidence collection.

THE PHYSICAL EXAMINATION

Clients entering the healthcare system should be initially examined and treated for life-threatening injuries. It is not uncommon for clients to appear uninjured or to present with minor injuries, such as abrasions or bruises. The physical examination and collection of specimens for medical treatment ideally should be performed at the same time as the forensic examination and collection of forensic evidence.

The forensic examiner will begin the physical examination with a general body survey of the patient. If no critical injury or condition requires immediate attention, the physical examination then proceeds from the least invasive assessment, such as listening to the patient's breath sounds, to more invasive procedures, such as the pelvic exam, while maintaining the privacy and dignity of the client. As previously stated, the use of a Woods lamp to perform a cursory general inspection of the body may be performed at this time. As the forensic examiner completes each step of the exam, she should clearly, objectively, and thoroughly document all findings. Specific, detailed forms for physical examination documentation are often provided in the sex crimes kit, although this type of form should be used whether utilizing a sex crimes kit or not. These forms provide specific cues to the examiner in addition to diagrams of both the anterior and posterior body and both male and female genitalia to aid in documenting the client's condition and any injuries or other findings noted during the examination. When injuries are identified, complete documentation should include the locations, dimensions, and descriptions of those findings.

The examiner looks for all abnormal findings, and may categorize most injuries according to the acronym *TEARS:* tears, ecchymosis, abrasions, redness, and swelling (Slaughter & Brown, 1992). Following this sequence to make observations and notations during the physical examination simplifies and standardizes documentation of injuries. It is critical that the examiner use a point of reference adjacent to the site of the injury to provide the appropriate perspective of size. This reference may be any appropriate scale, such as a tape marked with millimeters or centimeters on it. When making notations during the physical examination, the examiner should state clearly and objectively what was found and should avoid any attribution to the cause of an injury unless readily deduced from the actual observation of the injury. The SAFE should also use consistent terminology in any descriptions throughout the examination process. Careful examination of the oral cavity should be performed, especially if it is reported as a site of assault. Forensic and medical specimens may be obtained at this time.

Patterns of injuries may be determined through examination and description of injuries, such as a circular ecchymotic area, which could indicate a finger imprint, or a bite mark pattern. These patterns are important to note because they may provide consistency with the client's history. Photographs of injuries are helpful as they provide a visual document of the injuries. Forensic cameras are available that have magnifying features so that nongenital injuries may be more easily visualized. It is advisable to obtain the client's written consent to use photographs as part of the documentation prior to doing so. Photographs generally remain with the client's medical record, and the number of photographs taken as well as what areas of the body are being photographed should be clearly documented in the record. Each photograph should also be individually identified, along with the client's name, date, time, and name of the examiner. No photograph should ever be discarded, even if not well developed. A system should be developed to maintain the integrity of the photograph, including appropriate storage. If photographs are handed over to law enforcement, a chain of evidence should be maintained. A more detailed discussion of this documentation process may be found in Chapter 17 of this text.

After all areas of the body have been examined, the forensic examiner should then conduct the pelvic and rectal examinations. Only water should be used to lubricate the speculum initially if one is used, so that forensic specimens may be obtained. Following the collection of forensic specimens, a lubricant may be used to conduct the rest of the exam. If available, a colposcope may be used for the pelvic exam. The client should be informed of the use of the colposcope as it is a large piece of equipment and may be intimidating to the client. Studies have shown that using the colposcope improves the detection of genital trauma in sexual assault cases, as opposed to a gross visual exam, because it allows magnification of the sites (Slaughter, 1991). A study by Slaughter and Brown (1992) reported that genital trauma or injury visualized with a colposcope was as high as 87%, as opposed to detecting 10% to 30% with unaided visual examination. If a colposcope is used, it should be noted in the documentation along with the degree of magnification. A stain, such as Toluidine Blue, can be applied to stain the mucosa, which may enhance the visibility of any injuries (Lenahan, Ernst & Johnson, 1998). Some colposcopes are equipped to take photographs or videos of genital injuries. If this feature is used, the client should provide written consent. Chain of evidence should be maintained with colposcope photographs, as with other evidence.

A standardized and accepted method of describing the location of injuries in the female genital area is to mentally superimpose the face of a clock over the genital area, with 12 o'clock at the mons pubis, and 6 o'clock at the perineum (Girardin et al., 1997). Any injuries visualized may then be described on the medical record by using the acronym *TEARS* along with measurements and location within the context of the clock (e.g., a 2 cm tear at 6 o'clock at the posterior fourchette). Multiple studies have shown the most common location of genital injury in the female client is the posterior fourchette. Slaughter (1997) determined that the most common sites of injury by penile penetration of the vagina included the posterior fourchette, labia minora, hymen, and fossa navicularis. Once injuries have been identified, forensic and medical specimens may then be obtained.

The rectal area should also be inspected at this time, along with appropriate specimen collection. Depending upon assessment findings, it may be necessary for the examiner to use an analscope for better visualization. Superimposing the face of the clock over the anal area can also be helpful in the description of the location of any identified injuries, again using the acronym *TEARS*.

Once the examiner has completed the physical assessment and has obtained appropriate specimens to medically treat the patient and forensic evidence for the sex crimes kit, the topics of prophylaxis of both pregnancy and STDs should be discussed. Adults should be allowed to make informed decisions surrounding these issues. The examiner should be aware of any drug allergies or other health issues that the client may have at this time. The examiner should also be sensitive to the person's religious and other beliefs and provide factual information to the client. In fact, the religious orientation of the organization in which the client is being treated at times may be a factor in providing pregnancy prophylaxis. (The examiner should have addressed any potential conflicts in this area and developed acceptable protocols prior to providing care to any client.) Generally, pregnancy prophylaxis may be provided when the sexual assault occurred within 72 hours of the exam and the patient has tested negative for pregnancy. Testing can be done with serum or urine. There are a variety of prophylactic medications available, and more recent medications have very few side effects.

Untreated, STDs cause major health problems with far-reaching consequences, with treatment expenses as high as $8.4 billion annually (Reid, 1999). STDs may include gonorrhea (GC), chlamydia, syphilis, human papillomavirus, herpes, trichomoniasis, and bacterial vaginosis. The most frequently transmitted include GC, chlamydia, trichomoniasis, and bacterial vaginosis (Centers for Disease Control and Prevention, n.d.). Factors affecting the transmission of STDs include the type and nature of the assault, the extent of the injuries, number of assaults, multiple perpetrators, susceptibility of the client, and known STD status of the perpetrator(s). This information should be assessed and discussed with the client to determine prophylaxis and follow-up care. Baseline specimens for STDs may be taken during the exam; however, depending upon the timing of the assault, this testing may only provide information related to the client's condition prior to the assault. This fact should be discussed with the adult client.

STD testing is often carried out with children because assaults are generally repetitive and occur over a period of time; however, the type and nature of the assault(s) are taken into consideration, along with the child's presentation.

The decision to obtain specimens for STDs should be made prior to the exam so that the appropriate specimens may be collected at the same time as the forensic evidence collection. For many clients, it is advisable to provide STD prophylaxis at this time because many clients will not continue with follow-up appointments. Ideally, clients should be retested again in 2 weeks regardless of findings to assure that test results remain or become negative for sexually transmitted diseases. Also, testing for syphilis should be repeated 12 weeks after the assault. Many protocols provide for prophylaxis of GC, chlamydia, trichomoniasis, and bacterial vaginosis following CDC guidelines.

Hepatitis B may also be transmitted from a sexual assault. Transmission depends on the nature and type of assault, extent of injuries, and the known hepatitis B infection state of the perpetrator. The clinician should determine whether the client has previously received the hepatitis B vaccination series. Often, administration of the hepatitis B vaccine provides sufficient prophylaxis; however, depending upon the nature of the assault or the infection state of the perpetrator, it may be advisable to administer hepatitis immunoglobulin (HBIG) vaccine. Clients should be referred for follow-up doses as needed.

One of the greatest fears of many clients is the contracting of human immunodeficiency virus (HIV) from a sexual assault. Some studies have indicated that there is generally a low risk of transmission from a single encounter (Giardino, Datner, & Asher, 2003). Like other STDs, however, transmission is dependent upon the type and frequency of the assault (oral, vaginal, or anal), the type of injuries sustained along with exposure to blood and secretions, the presence of other STDs, and if known, the serological and clinical status of the perpetrator (Gostin et al., 1994). Prophylaxis is based upon this risk assessment, and all information should be discussed with the client to provide reassurance and allow for consideration of risks and benefits of prophylactic treatment. It is often considered more appropriate to have a lengthier discussion surrounding baseline testing and/or HIV prophylaxis at a follow-up exam, allowing for more time to weigh the risks and benefits of treatment. Clients, however, should make informed decisions as to how to proceed. In some situations, the forensic examiner may consult with the infectious disease specialist in order to provide the client with specific data related to the nature of the assault and enhance decision making related to testing and prophylaxis. Additional testing may be required at 3 and 6 months postassault.

Following the examination, the patient may be provided a shower and change of clothing, along with something to eat and drink. Specific referrals should be made for medical follow-up, along with individualized needs such as counseling. It is critical that the client be provided with simple discharge instructions that include telephone numbers of identified resources such as the forensic examiner or the investigating officer. Additionally, the client should have an information sheet that describes exactly what was provided to the client at the time of the exam, and what to do next. The examiner should assist the client with discharge to a safe environment, and supportive family or friends to transport the client there. At times the SACS counselor can assist with these arrangements.

Many states also have an Office of Victim Services that can provide financial assistance for those clients who are victims of a crime and cannot afford ongoing medical or other related expenses. Generally, the only obligation of the client is to file a police report. The SACS counselor can assist the client with completing the forms to apply for reimbursement.

Care of the sexually assaulted client is both comprehensive and lengthy. Based upon the setting that the examiner will be working in, it is advisable to develop protocols in caring for clients that allow specific direction and guidance to simplify the care and direct the examiner as needed. Also, it is helpful to have other specialists available for consultation, such as the communicable disease specialist, to address more complex needs of the client.

SEXUAL ASSAULT RESPONSE TEAMS

Many communities have started sexual assault response teams (SART) that provide a multidisciplinary approach to the client. One of the original SART models was developed in California and involved a coordinated response to the needs of the client from the time the client reported the assault, through any services necessary to assist the victim, to the prosecution of the crime. Generally, team members include the SAFE, emergency department medical personnel, law enforcement, prosecutor, and counselor(s). A SART may also include other types of professionals who are available as needed, based upon the location and needs of the community or individual client. In some locations, the actual team arrives and works together with the client to provide comprehensive care. Other models involve the team meeting at regular intervals to establish a better understanding of each other's roles, to utilize each other as resources and experts, and to share data to enhance the care provided to all clients.

SUMMARY

The forensic examiner provides a highly skilled level of care from the onset of the client seeking care. They provide physical, emotional, forensic, and legal care that continues to benefit the client long after the client has left the examiner.

QUESTIONS FOR DISCUSSION

1. What is sexual assault?
2. Who is at risk for sexual assault?
3. What are the consequences of sexual assault?
4. What is the role of the sexual assault forensic examiner?
5. What does the forensic exam involve?

REFERENCES

Adams, J., Harper, K., Knudson, S., & Revilla, J. (1994). Examination findings in legally confirmed child sexual abuse: It's normal to be normal. *Pediatrics, 94*(3), 310–317.

Aiken, M. M. (1993). False allegation. *Journal of Psychosocial Nursing, 31*(11), 15–20.

American College of Emergency Physicians. (1999). Evaluation and management of the sexually assaulted or sexually abused patient. Washington, DC: US

Dept. of Health and Human Services, Health Resources and Services Administration, Maternal and Child Health Bureau, Contract No. 98-0347(P).

Burgess, A. W. & Holmstrom, L. L. (1974). Rape trauma syndrome. *American Journal of Psychiatry, 131*(9), 981–986.

Centers for Disease Control and Prevention. (n.d.). 2002 Sexually Transmitted Disease Treatment Guidelines. *Morbidity & Mortality Wkly, Report.* 51 (RR06), 1–80.

Commission on the Standardization of the Collection of Evidence in Sexual Assault Investigations. (1998). *State of Connecticut Technical Guidelines for Health Care Response to Victims of Sexual Assault.* State of Connecticut.

ElSohly, S. J. S. (1999). Prevalence of drugs used in cases of alleged sexual assault. *Journal of Analytical Toxicology, 23,* 141–146.

Federal Bureau of Investigation. (2004). *Uniform crime reports, 2002.* Retrieved June 3, 2004, from www.fbi.gov.

Fergusson, D., Horwood, J., & Lynskey, M. (1997). Childhood sexual abuse, adolescent sexual behaviors and sexual revictimization. *Child Abuse and Neglect, 21*(8)790–803.

Fisher, B., Cullen, F. T., & Turner M. G. (2000). *Research report: Sexual victimization of college women.* Washington, DC: National Institute of Justice.

Giardino, A., Datner, E., & Asher, J. (2003). *Sexual assault victimization across the life span.* St. Louis, MO: G.W. Medical, 331–332.

Girardin, B., Faugno, D., Senski, P., Slaughter, L., & Whelan, M. (2002). Developing a Sexual Assault response team. Frankfurt, KY: KY Association of Sexual Assault Programs.

Gostin, L., Lazzanini, Z., Alexander, D., Brandt, A., Mayer, K., & Silverman, D. (1994). HIV testing, counseling, and prophylaxis after sexual assault. *Journal of American Medical Association, 271*(18), 1436–1444.

Haddix-Hill, K. (1997). The violence of rape. *Critical Care Nursing Clinics of North America, 9*(2), 167–174.

Hampton, H. (1995). Care of the woman who has been raped. *New England Journal of Medicine, 332*(4), 234–237.

International Association of Forensic Nurses. (1996). *Sexual assault nurse examiner standards of practice.* Silverspring, MD: Author.

Juvenile Justice Volume V1, Number I, October 1999; *The Commonwealth Fund Survey of the Health of Adolescent Girls: Highlights and Methodology.* Annual Report, 1998. Grand Rapids, MI: Nokomis Foundation. Available at: http://www.ncijrs.org/html/ojjdp/journal1099/nat8.html. Accessed on July 13, 2005.

LeBeau, M. (1999). Toxicological investigations of drug-facilitated sexual assaults. *Forensic Science Communications, 1*(1). Retrieved from http://www.fbi.gov/hg/lab/fsc/backissu/april1999/lebeau. htm. Accessed June 3, 2004.

Ledray, L. (1990). Counseling rape victims: The nursing challenge. *Perspectives in Psychiatric Care, 26*(2), 21–27.

Lenahan, L., Ernst, M., & Johnson, B. (1998). Colposcopy in evaluation of the adult sexual assault victim. *American Journal of Emergency Medicine, 16*(2), 183–184.

New Hampshire Sexual Assault Protocol Revision Committee. (1998). *Sexual assault: A hospital protocol for forensic and medical examination* (2nd ed.). Concord, NH: New Hampshire Office of the Attorney General.

Ramin, S. M., Satin, A.J., Stone, I.C., Jr., Wendel, G.D., Jr. (1992). Sexual assault in postmenopausal women. *Obstetrics and Gynecology, 80*(5), 860–864.

Reid, J. (1999). Sexually transmitted disease in the U.S. *ADVANCE for Nurse Practitioners, 7*(8), 45–50.

Riggs, N., Houry, D., Long, G., Markovchick, V., & Feldhaus, K. (2000). Analysis of 1,076 cases of sexual assault. *Annals of Emergency Medicine, 35*(4), 358–362.

Slaughter, L. (1991). Cervical findings in rape victims. *American Journal of Obstetrics and Gynecology, 164,* 528–529.

Slaughter, L. (1997). Patterns of genital injury in female sexual assault victims. *American Journal of Obstetrics and Gynecology, 176*(3), 609–616.

Slaughter, L. & Brown, C. (1992). Colposcopy to establish physical findings in rape victims. *American Journal of Obstetrics and Gynecology, 166*(1), 83–86.

State of Connecticut Supplemental Guideline. (1998). *Child sexual abuse examination.* Hartford, CT: St. Francis Hospital and Medical Center.

U.S. Department of Justice, Bureau of Justice Statistics. (1994). The cost of crime to victims. *Crime Data Brief.*

U.S. Department of Justice, Office of Justice Programs, Bureau of Justice Statistics. (1985). The crime of rape. *BJS Bulletin.*

U.S. Department of Justice, Office of Justice Programs, Bureau of Justice Statistics. (2003). *Criminal Victimization 2002 NCJ 199994.*

Welner, M. (2001). The perpetrators and their modus operandi. In LeBeau, M., and Mozayani, A. (Ed.) *Drug facilitated sexual assault* (p. 41). San Diego: Academic Press.

The Use of Biological Evidence and DNA Databanks to Aid Criminal Investigations

Carll Ladd
Henry C. Lee

The development of DNA analytical methods and their application to forensic analysis have changed the face of forensic science. DNA technology has revolutionized areas such as genetic counseling, paternity testing, and criminal investigations. One of the most significant advances in criminalistics is the creation of statewide and national DNA databases that contain DNA profiles of convicted offenders. When DNA is obtained from evidence in "no suspect" cases the resulting profiles can be compared to the data on file in the offender database. Thousands of cases that would have previously remained unsolved have been adjudicated due to the implementation of the DNA databanks.

CHAPTER FOCUS

Sources of biological evidence
Modes of evidence transfer
Collection and preservation of biological evidence
History of biological evidence examination
Individualization of biological evidence by DNA analysis
Felon DNA databanks
Challenges to DNA admissibility
Summary

KEY TERMS

allele
base
CODIS
deoxyribonucleic acid
DNA database
frequency
mitochondrial DNA
nucleotide
polymerase chain reaction
profile

INTRODUCTION

Beginning in the 1960s, crime rates in the United States rose dramatically. As a result, the public grew increasingly concerned about the impact of crime on our society. Even before the attacks of September 11, 2001, Americans routinely identified "improving public safety" as a key national priority (Lee & Ladd, 1997). Crime rates, though decreasing significantly in the last decade, remain unacceptably high, especially in the area of interpersonal violence. The amount of violent crime is staggering. Nationwide, more than 1 million aggravated assaults and sexual assaults are reported to the police each year. U.S. Justice Department victimization surveys put the number even higher (U.S. Department of Justice, 2002).

During this period of heightened concern about public safety, physical evidence has become increasingly important in criminal investigations. Courts often view eyewitness accounts as unreliable or biased. Numerous studies have shown this distrust is well founded. Physical evidence, however, such as deoxyribonucleic acid (DNA) may independently and objectively link a suspect or victim to a crime or develop important investigative leads. Physical evidence may also prove invaluable for exonerating the innocent.

The natural consequence of the greater emphasis on physical evidence is increased legal scrutiny. Evidence integrity begins with the first investigator at the crime scene or with the collection of physical evidence in the emergency room. Celebrated court cases such as the Nicole Brown (Simpson) and JonBenet Ramsey homicides highlight standard challenges to the use of physical evidence in criminal investigations and suggest that scrutiny of evidence collection, preservation, and handling will continue unabated. An entire case may be jeopardized if evidence is mishandled during the initial stages of the investigation. Indeed, evidence that is not properly recognized, documented, collected, and preserved may ultimately be of no probative value. Physical evidence is generally classified as biological, chemical, or pattern evidence (imprints, impressions, etc.). This chapter reviews the use of biological evidence, including the recognition, collection, preservation, identification, and individualization of that evidence in criminal investigations. This chapter will also examine some of the legal challenges to the collection and use of DNA evidence.

SOURCES OF BIOLOGICAL EVIDENCE

Biological evidence has been associated with numerous crimes, but is typically seen with violent crimes such as homicide, assault, sexual assault, child abuse, and hit and run accidents. Although any substance of biological origin may be useful for analysis, common sources of biological evidence submitted to forensic laboratories include:

- Blood and bloodstains
- Body fluid stains
- Tissues and organs
- Objects contacted by persons
- Nonhuman sources

Table 19–1 lists various sources of biological evidence that are used in forensic investigations. The identification of the type or source of biological material may be as significant as any subsequent testing for genetic markers. The sources of biological evidence listed can be used to link one individual to another, to a piece of physical evidence, or to a crime scene. In addition, the evidence may substantiate or disprove an alibi, or assist with crime scene reconstruction.

Table 19–1   Sources of Biological Evidence

Source	Types of Materials
Body fluids	Blood, semen, saliva, urine, tears, bile, perspiration, vaginal fluid
Soft tissue	Skin, organs, hairs, fingernails
Structural tissue	Teeth, bones
Other human sources	Fecal matter, vomit
Objects contacted by persons	Lipstick, toothbrush, hairbrush, razor, cigarette butts, drinking glasses/bottles, articles of clothing
Nonhuman sources	Animal, vegetative, microbial

BIOLOGICAL EVIDENCE TRANSFER

Although the identification of the type of evidence is the first vital step in analysis of biological samples, the method of deposit of that sample may be of equal or even greater importance in case analysis and interpretation. In general, biological evidence can be transferred by direct deposit or by secondary transfer.

Blood, semen, body tissue, bone, hair, urine, saliva, and other body fluids can be transferred to an individual's body or clothing, to an object, or to a crime scene by direct deposit from the source of that sample. Once liquid biological materials are deposited, they adhere to the material on that surface, the substratum. Those deposits become stains. The exact characteristics of those stains depend on the nature of the substratum, movement before the liquid dries, and other factors. Space does not allow for an extensive discussion of the factors that will affect the general appearance of a body fluid stain. However, the forensic nurse must be aware of those characteristics of stain patterns that may be important for future analysis, and he or she should consider those characteristics when collecting and preserving biological materials.

Nonfluid evidence, such as tissue, bone, or hair, can also be transferred by direct contact with the primary source of that biological material. Because these types of biological materials often sit on top of the target surface, subsequent actions may dislodge nonliquid samples. Liquid biological material may also be associated with these nonliquid samples, such as blood on tissue or bone, resulting in a deposit with characteristics of both types of materials.

Blood, semen, tissue, hair, saliva, or urine may also be transferred to a victim, suspect, witness, object, or location through an intermediary. This process is referred to as *secondary transfer.* With secondary transfer, there is no direct contact between the original source (the donor of the biological evidence) and the final target surface. Rather, some type of contact between the first stained substratum or individual and another surface or person results in a second transfer of the biological sample. For example, seminal fluid on a rape victim's clothing may rub against a car seat, leaving some semen in the vehicle. If a second individual sits in the same location, an additional transfer of the semen may occur. Another example of secondary transfer is when a person picks up a victim's hair from the suspect's vehicle onto his jacket. The hair has now been transferred from the victim to the car and then from the car to a piece of clothing. The transfer intermediary can be a person, an object, or a scene. The secondary transfer of physical evidence may, but does not necessarily, establish a link between an individual and a specific crime.

It should be noted that the stain or pattern of deposit that results from evidence transfer may be as important as or more important than the individualization of the material itself. For example, whether semen found on a carpet is an ejaculated direct deposit or a smear-type transfer may be important in supporting the victim's description of a sexual assault.

COLLECTION AND PRESERVATION OF BIOLOGICAL EVIDENCE

The ability to successfully analyze biological evidence recovered from a crime scene, person, or object depends greatly on the types of specimens collected and how they are preserved. Thus, the technique used to collect and document such evidence, the quantity and type of evidence that should be collected, the way the evidence should be handled and packaged, and how the evidence should be preserved are some of the critical issues in an investigation. Unless the evidence is properly recognized, documented, collected, packaged, and preserved, it will not meet the legal or scientific requirements for admissibility into a court of law. If the evidence is not properly documented prior to collection, its origin can be questioned. If it is improperly collected or packaged, cross-contamination may occur. Finally, if the evidence is not properly preserved, sample degradation may result. Therefore, it is extremely important to follow established procedures and use standardized techniques to collect and preserve biological evidence. An overview of sample documentation, collection, and packaging procedures for the forensic nurse may be found in Chapter 16 of this book. Many other publications discuss the collection and analysis of biological evidence in detail. (Lee, Pagliaro, Zercie & Maxwell, 1995; Lee, Ladd, Scherzinger & Barke, 1998).

Collection of Sexual Assault Evidence

The collection of evidence using a sexual assault kit warrants special consideration. Unlike most other crimes where typically the police collect the evidence, victims of sexual assault, domestic violence, and child abuse are examined by medical professionals in hospitals, clinics, or other centers. If no SANE/SAFE program exists at the facility, critical biological evidence may be collected by medical personnel who historically have been less familiar with the forensic and legal issues pertaining to chain of custody and evidence collection. This may become an issue during DNA analysis or interpretation of DNA profiles obtained from the biological evidence. Most jurisdictions have developed standardized sexual assault evidence collection kits and procedures. Table 19–2 lists the types of evidence typically collected for subsequent forensic analysis.

Table 19–2   Evidence Collected for Forensic Examination in Cases of Personal Violence

Type of Evidence	Source	Use
Swabs and smears	Genital, vaginal, oral, anal	Identification of foreign DNA in mixture
Questioned hair, trace	Head & pubic combing	Identification of foreign hairs/trace
Fingernail scrapings/clippings	Victim or suspect	Identification of foreign DNA in mixture, hairs, and/or trace
Reference samples	Blood or buccal swab	Comparison to DNA from evidence
Reference samples	Victim/suspect head & pubic hair	Comparison to unknown hair materials
Other biological material	Varies, depending on type of case & evidence	Identification of foreign DNA & trace materials

For the successful resolution of any criminal investigation, it is essential that all medical personnel attending victims or suspects have the requisite knowledge and experience to recognize, collect, and preserve potential evidence for forensic analysis. In addition, communication and cooperation among hospital staff, police, and the forensic laboratory is extremely important.

Body fluid evidence is commonly associated with other crimes against people and plays a particularly important role in the successful prosecution of these crimes. (DeForest, Gaensslen, & Lee, 1983). Sources of biological material such as blood, hair, and saliva have been very important in the prosecution of child abuse, assault, homicide, and sexual assault cases. Several evidence collection issues that may have an impact on the analysis of biological samples and subsequent interpretation of the DNA profiles obtained are worth emphasizing.

- Always collect the victim's or suspect's clothing to minimize the loss of important trace evidence such as blood crusts, hairs, and fibers. In addition, preserve any pattern evidence.
- All items of evidence be must be packaged *separately*. The evidentiary value may be seriously compromised if several articles of clothing or other evidence are packaged together.
- Wet clothing should be air dried prior to packaging in paper in a manner that limits the possibility of contamination or degradation of the biological sample. Under no circumstances should the evidence be packaged in plastic or any airtight container; this type of packaging causes samples to retain moisture, thus promoting bacterial growth.

When following standardized procedures, care must be taken to avoid collection techniques that may raise subsequent analytical issues. For example, it is useful to place the swabs in a specially designed cardboard swab collection box to ensure complete drying and minimize contamination. To minimize the recovery of skin cells from the body, collect any blood/body fluid stains as gently as possible. This can be accomplished by *lightly* swabbing the stained area. If fingernail scrapings or clippings are collected, it is important to avoid applying excessive force in this process; doing so will minimize the chance of collecting the victim's blood or skin.

After the evidence is collected, a cool, dry environment is optimal for preserving biological samples for DNA analysis. Moisture and heat can promote bacterial growth, which may seriously degrade DNA in the sample.

Statutory sexual assaults, which have been vigorously prosecuted in recent years, may also involve evidence collection by the forensic nurse. Sexual assault kits are not routinely collected in statutory or juvenile sexual assault cases because those assaults may not be reported until weeks or months after the incident. However, because consent cannot be a defense in the statutory sexual assault case, if a pregnancy has occurred as a result of the rape, the product of conception is itself proof of the crime. In such cases, the samples collected are typically blood from the suspect, from the mother, and from the child or the abortus. In the event of an abortion, tissue samples should be placed in a specimen jar and submitted for forensic testing as soon as possible. It is vital that the specimen *not* be put in any preservative, such as formalin, which will seriously degrade DNA. If the pregnancy is terminated early in the first trimester, it may be necessary for a medical examiner or other trained professional to examine the sample to isolate tissue of fetal origin before collection or testing.

HISTORY OF BIOLOGICAL EVIDENCE EXAMINATION

Serological Testing

The identification of an individual by analyzing his or her biological material, such as blood, semen, hair, and bone, has been reported in forensic science literature since 1904 (Lee, 1982). Over the years, numerous red blood cell antigen systems, isoenzyme markers, red cell protein variants, serum protein markers (Gaensslen, 1983; Gaensslen & Lee, 1984), and human leukocyte antigens (HLA) have been characterized and applied to forensic work (Lee, Gaensslen, Pagliaro, Mills, & Zercie, 1991). Historically, variation was detected by either immunological reactions, such as with the ABO blood group system and secretor status; Rh typing;

HLA histocompatibility antigens; or the electrophoretic separation of isoenzymes and serum proteins such as phosphoglucomutase (PGM), adinosine diaminase (ADA), or group-specific component (GC) variants (Gaensslen, Desio, & Lee, 1986). Some of these, such as typing stains for ABO group antigens, were very useful methods with old samples; other markers were temperature and time sensitive and of limited forensic use. For decades these tests were the standard techniques applied to biological samples. Figure 19–1 is an overview of methods utilized in forensic biology for the identification and individualization of biological evidence.

DNA Testing

During the last 10–15 years, DNA typing procedures have become increasingly important in the fields of forensic science and forensic medicine. (Lee, 1994; Lee, Ladd, Bourke, Pagliaro & Tirnady, 1994). Several DNA typing methods have been widely implemented for forensic use. If the examiner adheres to applicable national guidelines and standards (DNA Advisory Board, 1998), DNA analysis is generally considered reliable. At this time, DNA evidence and testimony are accepted by most courts. DNA testing may assist greatly in the resolution of criminal and civil investigations.

Genetic variation can be detected by many DNA-typing techniques, including restriction fragment length polymorphism (RFLP) analysis, polymerase chain reaction (PCR), and DNA sequencing. Developments over the past decade, such as more sensitive and discriminating PCR typing methods, the felon DNA databank, and increased federal and state funding, have greatly enhanced DNA typing in forensic casework.

The first widely publicized forensic use of DNA technology was in 1985 in the United Kingdom. Dr. Alec Jeffries of the University of Leicester applied his newly developed DNA "fingerprinting" procedures during the investigation of a double rape-homicide case in England. DNA was first applied to casework in the United States in late 1986 in the case *Pennsylvania v. Pestinikas* (cited also as *Penn. v. Pestinikas*). The FBI began accepting DNA cases in 1989, and widespread use of DNA testing occurred in the 1990s. Today more than 130 laboratories in the United States, both public and private, perform forensic DNA analysis. Each year, over 40,000 DNA cases are processed by these facilities (Federal Bureau of Investigation, 2003).

The two major applications of DNA typing in forensic science are paternity testing and criminal investigation. The former application, because it deals with fresh blood samples, is relatively straightforward. However, the quality of DNA samples from criminal cases is generally unpredictable, so the latter application has been challenged more vigorously during trials and hearings (U.S. Congress, Office of Technology

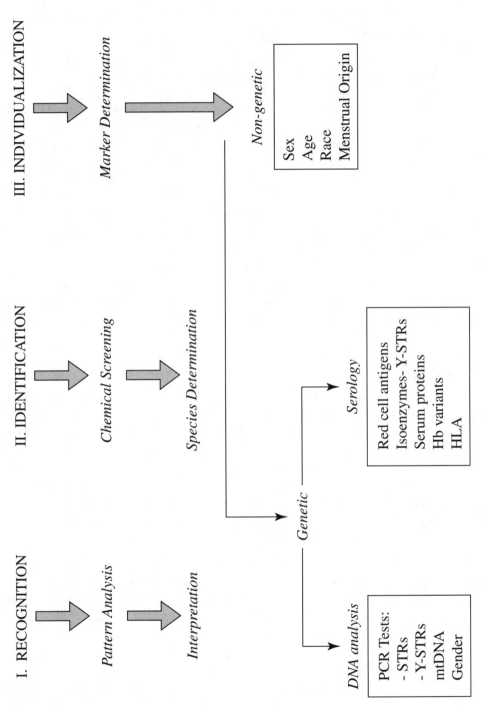

Figure 19–1   Methods used to analyze biological evidence.

Assessment, 1990). Several national and international committees have been formed to address the use of DNA in criminal cases, and extensive studies have been conducted in this area (Committee on DNA Technology in Forensic Science, 1992, 1996).

LABORATORY ANALYSIS OF BIOLOGICAL EVIDENCE

Prior to the widespread use of DNA testing in crime laboratories, forensic serology and immunology were employed to identify the source of the biological evidence, to determine if the sample was of human origin, and then to include (or exclude) an individual as a potential source of that sample. As more forensic laboratories developed DNA capabilities over the past decade, serological methods (especially ABO blood grouping and isoenzyme typing) have been significantly scaled back or eliminated. Today, serological analysis is generally limited to identifying the type of biological evidence collected. Nevertheless, sample identification is key in supporting the elements of crimes such as sexual assault and in interpreting the results obtained from subsequent testing. After the type of biological material is identified, the evidence is individualized; that is, linked to (or excluded from) a particular person by DNA typing.

Serological Methods for Identifying Body Fluids

The process of examining items for the presence of biological evidence begins with recognizing and identifying likely materials for further testing. Various screening tests exist that determine if a stain could be blood, saliva, semen, and so on. Evidence screening saves considerable time and money by eliminating those stains that are not consistent with the body fluid of interest. The acid phosphatase (AP) test, for example, is a well-known screening test for seminal fluid. Confirmatory tests conclusively demonstrate the presence of a particular body fluid. Lastly, the body fluid is individualized by DNA.

Reddish-brown stains that may be blood are also screened prior to DNA typing. Screening tests for blood are based on the reaction of the heme component of hemoglobin with chemicals such as o-tolidine, phenolphthalein (Kastle-Mayer reagent), luminol, and tetramethylbenzidine. These tests are extremely sensitive; however, reactions with enzymes or oxidizers may result in false positives. Thus, a positive reaction with any of these reagents indicates that the sample *could* be blood. Microcrystal tests such as that developed by Takayama confirm the presence of blood, but do not indicate the species of origin. A positive crystal test can be obtained from both human and animal blood. The presence of *human* blood can be determined using any immunological method that tests for human hemoglobin.

This one-step procedure is the preferred method in forensic laboratories today, because it consumes a smaller amount of sample and is extremely sensitive.

The most commonly analyzed body fluid in criminal cases is semen. As stated earlier, the common screening method for semen is the acid phosphatase test. Acid phosphatase is usually present in high levels in semen, but can also be found in other substances such as plant matter. In addition, lower levels of AP can be found in other biological samples (e.g., vaginal secretions, saliva, and fecal matter). The presence of semen must be confirmed by identifying spermatozoa microscopically or by detecting the human seminal protein p30, also called PSA. Recent developments in forensic science have greatly increased the sensitivity of some of these confirmatory tests.

Other enzyme and biochemistry tests may be conducted to identify biological substances such as saliva, urine, gastric fluid, and fecal matter. Microscopic examination may also be used for analysis of biological stains. For example, hairs are examined microscopically and compared to reference samples from the victim and suspect(s) and checked for the presence of hair root material.

INDIVIDUALIZATION OF BIOLOGICAL EVIDENCE BY DNA ANALYSIS

The forensic application of DNA typing methods constitutes a major advancement in the examination of biological evidence and the successful investigation of many crimes. DNA is important because it is remarkably sensitive, tremendously discriminating, and stable. DNA has become a key focus in the fields of forensic science, forensic medicine, anthropology, and paternity testing. Figure 19–2 shows an overview of the DNA analysis of a biological sample.

The Genetics of DNA

Deoxyribonucleic acid (DNA) is the genetic or hereditary material in living cells. DNA is a polymer with individual building blocks called nucleotides. Each nucleotide consists of a sugar (deoxyribose), a phosphate group, and a nitrogenous base. The four different nucleotides found in DNA are classified by the corresponding base in the structure— adenine (A), guanine (G), cytosine (C), and thymine (T). The functional DNA molecule contains two strands of DNA bound together by complementary base pairing (hydrogen bonding) to form a double helix. Adenine always pairs with thymine, and cytosine always pairs with guanine. DNA is primarily located in the nucleus of the cells, arranged into long threadlike structures called chromosomes. Humans have 23 pairs of chromosomes. One set is inherited maternally; the other is

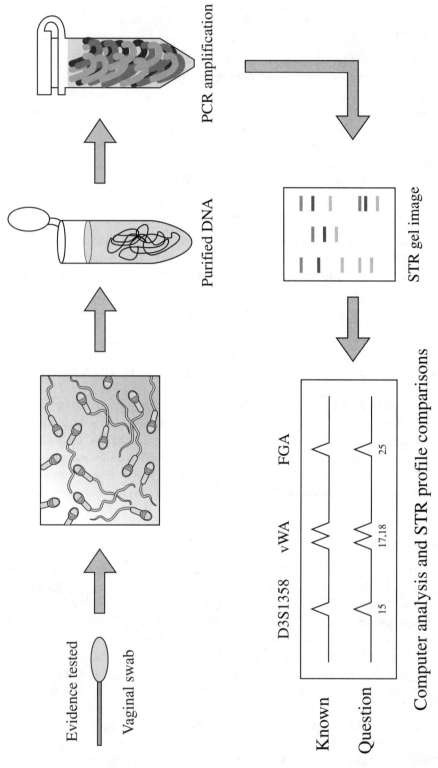

PCR amplification

Purified DNA

STR gel image

Evidence tested

Vaginal swab

Computer analysis and STR profile comparisons

D3S1358   vWA   FGA

Known

Question

15   17,18   25

Figure 19-2   Overview of the STR typing procedure.

derived paternally. The estimated 3–4 billion base pairs of DNA in the human genome encode approximately 30,000 genes on those chromosomes.

Scientists have estimated that more than 98% of the human genome is the same or very similar in most individuals (Lander, Linton, & Birren, 2001). However, considerable genetic variation exists in the DNA of noncoding regions (which are not genes); these areas are exploited by forensic DNA typing systems.

Sources of DNA

Evidence that is suitable for DNA typing, with the exception of mitochondrial DNA (mtDNA), is limited to biological samples containing nucleated cells. Table 19–1 earlier in the chapter lists sources of those biological samples suitable for conventional DNA analysis. Note that conventional DNA typing is possible only on hairs with roots. The hair shaft does not contain nuclei and can be typed only by mtDNA analysis methods. Other types of biological evidence, such as tears, perspiration, serum, and other body fluids without cells, are not amenable to standard DNA analysis. DNA has been isolated from materials such as gastric fluids and fecal stains; however, it is difficult to obtain sufficient DNA from these sources in case samples. It should also be noted that although DNA can often be recovered from the specimens mentioned in Table 19–1, in many cases the quality and/or quantity of the sample proves inadequate for DNA analysis.

Four factors affect the ability to obtain DNA typing results. The first issue is sample quantity. PCR-based DNA typing methods are very sensitive, but not infinitely so. The second factor is sample degradation. For example, prolonged exposure of even a large bloodstain to the environment or to bacterial contamination can degrade the DNA and render it unsuitable for further analysis. It is important to note, however, that degradation will not change DNA profile "A" into profile "B." The third consideration is sample purity. Although most DNA typing methods are robust, dirt, grease, some dyes in fabrics, and other materials can seriously inhibit the DNA typing process (Lee et al., 1998). The last issue is the ratio of DNA in mixtures of fluids from more than one person. DNA profiles can readily be detected with approximately equal amounts of material (e.g., 1:1 and 3:1 DNA mixtures). However, with mixture ratios such as 25:1 or 50:1, the quantity of the major DNA specimen (larger quantity) prevents the detection of the minor source (smaller quantity of DNA). This situation occurs with some vaginal swab samples where semen is detected. In such cases, the standard DNA tests detect only the victim's DNA.

Genetic Variation and Forensic DNA Typing

Two different classes of genetic variation are exploited by forensic DNA typing methods: sequence variation (single base changes) and length differences produced by variation in the number of tandem repeats. Important features of the two classes of genetic variation are illustrated in Figure 19–3.

DNA tests that detect length differences are currently the most common type of variation studied in forensic DNA analysis. Many well-characterized genetic regions (loci) contain sets of nucleotides (core elements) that are tandemly repeated. The number of these repeated units can vary from person to person. Certain base sequences called recognition sites flank these repeats. Specialized enzymes called restriction enzymes will cut the DNA at those recognition sites that

Sequence and Length Variation

(A)   Type 1 CGATCGGAATGGC
         Type 2 CGATCGG**T**ATGGC
         Type 3 CGAT**G**GGAATGGC

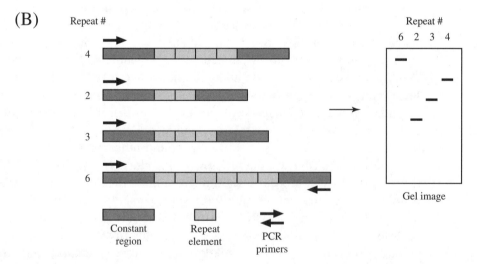

Figure 19–3 Types of genetic variation. (A) Sequence variation. DNA variations are highlighted. Only one strand of the DNA double helix is shown. (B) Length variation. PCR primers bind to the constant regions flanking the repeats.

flank the repeats. This restriction endonuclease digestion results in DNA fragments ranging in size from 500 to 22,000 base pairs long. The resulting fragments are separated by agarose gel electrophoresis. This process is termed restriction fragment length polymorphism (RFLP), and is the oldest DNA typing method for both criminal and paternity cases. The most commonly used DNA testing method today (a PCR method termed STRs, discussed in the following section) omits the restriction enzyme step. Instead, small synthetic pieces of DNA, known as primers, target the site of interest and bind to DNA flanking the repeats (see Figure 19–3B).

POLYMERASE CHAIN REACTION

The ability to amplify small segments of DNA by PCR constitutes one of the more significant developments in molecular biology. PCR has facilitated revolutionary advances in many scientific disciplines and has proven an invaluable tool in biological research as well as in the diagnosis of genetic disorders and infectious diseases.

PCR was invented in 1985 and was subsequently adapted to forensic science. The procedure amplifies (duplicates) small segments of DNA. This process is sometimes called "molecular photocopying." At the end of the amplification process, the target DNA molecule has been copied 1–10 million times.

As a forensic tool, PCR-based strategies have several advantages over RFLP analysis. First, PCR requires only trace quantities of DNA—typically, approximately 1 nanogram (ng) of human DNA is optimal for PCR, compared with 300–500 ng for RFLP typing. One ng is the amount of human DNA that typically can be obtained from a single hair root. Consequently, PCR permits DNA typing of evidence with minute samples, such as a cigarette butt containing epithelial cells. Second, PCR generates a large quantity of product in a very short period of time, considerably less time than required for typing by RFLP analysis. Third, degradation of the DNA sample is less of a concern when using PCR because it amplifies small segments of DNA. In contrast, RFLP typing requires samples with predominantly high molecular weight DNA. The DNA must be relatively "undegraded" because the DNA fragments analyzed by RFLP are much larger.

The first PCR tests in widespread forensic use were DQA1, Polymarker (PM), and D1S80. DQA1 and PM alleles display sequence variation that was detected by a colorometric assay. DQA1 and PM DNA profiles are determined by the pattern of blue dots that develops. D1S80 typing, also called amplified fragment length polymorphism (AMP-FLP) analysis, is a PCR-based DNA-typing strategy that detects length variation. D1S80 alleles contain different numbers of repeats similar to RFLP.

These three PCR systems are very sensitive; hence they permit the analysis of minute samples. However, they are much less discriminating than RFLP. Since the development of short tandem repeat procedures, the DQA1, PM, and D1S80 tests are seldom used in forensic casework.

Short Tandem Repeats

The standard DNA typing method employed by the forensic community today involves the analysis of short tandem repeats (STR). Conceptually, STR analysis can be thought of as a combination of PCR and RFLP. As with RFLP, the different STR types exhibit variation in the number of repeated core elements they contain and have tremendous discriminating power. In addition, like other PCR methods, STR typing is very sensitive. Furthermore, the use of different fluorescent dyes allows the analysis of multiple STRs in a single reaction with the aid of a laser and computer. This saves considerable time and limits sample consumption. For these reasons, STR analysis has replaced the first generation of PCR tests (Hott, Buon Cristiani, Wallin, Nguyen, Lazaruk & Walsh, 2002). Figure 19–4 shows typical results obtained when multiple loci are detected using a fluorescent dye and a laser detector.

Y-chromosome STR typing, which is in the early stages of implementation, constitutes an important new forensic method for processing sexual assault samples. For example, sexual assault cases routinely require the testing of intimate samples that are a mixture of male and female body fluids. In some cases, as described previously, only the female profile or a predominantly female profile can be detected using standard STR systems, even when spermatozoa or semen are identified by serological or microscopic methods. This is usually due to the large amount of female cellular material in the sample collected when compared to the number of male epithelial cells or spermatozoa. A Y-chromosome STR system significantly overcomes the problems associated with a large female-to-male DNA ratio that can lead to incomplete or no amplification of the male DNA. This ability to selectively target the male contributor(s) is a substantial tool for the DNA analyst in these cases. Indeed, in sexual assaults where the semen donor is aspermic (e.g., vasectomized males), Y-STR typing may be the best approach for detecting a foreign DNA profile (a profile that does not originate from the victim). In addition, Y-STR typing may assist in evaluating mixtures by providing information regarding the number of male contributors.

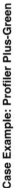

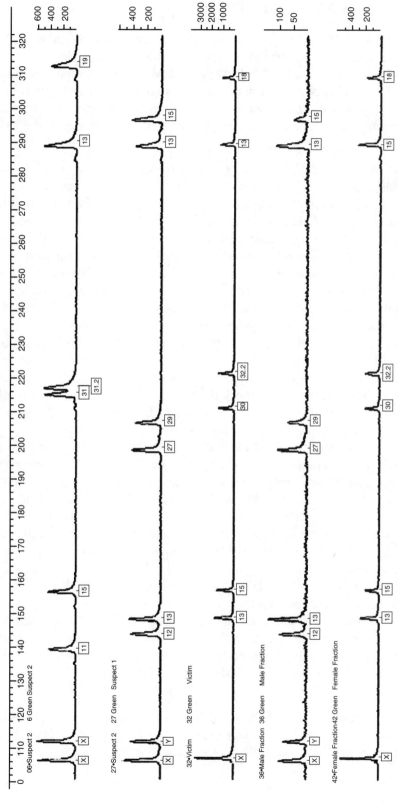

Figure 19–4 DNA typing results by STR analysis. Samples were amplified using the AmpF/STR Profiler Plus kit (Applied Biosystems). The results for the green loci (XY, D8S1178, D21S11, D18S51) are shown for a sexual assault case where a vaginal swab sample was submitted for STR analysis and comparison to known DNA profiles. A differential DNA extraction procedure was performed to separate the male and female DNA from a vaginal swab. Fluorescent DNA profiles were detected using the ABI Prism 377 DNA Sequencer (Applied Biosystems). Open boxes indicate the STR profile for each sample. The results are consistent with suspect 1 being the source of the DNA profile from the male fraction (vaginal swab, sperm DNA profile). The female fraction (vaginal swab, epithelial DNA profile) matches the victim.

FORENSIC DNA ANALYSIS CASE STUDIES

The value of DNA analysis in forensic casework is well known. The forensic nurse is well aware that a DNA profile generated from physical evidence can be used to identify a perpetrator or to exonerate the innocent. Thus, it is not necessary to discuss extensively the strength of this type of evidence. The two case studies that follow should suffice to demonstrate the impact DNA analysis has had on casework in the 21st century.

In the first case, DNA was the key evidence from a young woman who was sexually assaulted by a male unknown to her. This sexual assault was similar in several elements to two other rapes that had occurred in the neighborhood. The woman was able to give a description of her assailant to law enforcement, but could offer few other details about the incident. The police conducted a standard investigation and developed a suspect after consulting a number of their regular informants. The person who was the focus of the police investigation was a homeless male who roughly fit the description provided by the victim. After several hours of interrogation by detectives, the suspect confessed to all of the sexual assaults, although his version of the crime differed in some details from the actual assault. As part of their investigation, the police collected known blood and hair samples from the suspect for comparison to the biological materials in the sex assault evidence kits collected in all three cases. Laboratory scientists conducted DNA testing on vaginal swabs in the three cases. All three sperm-rich samples yielded identical DNA profiles—there was indeed a serial rapist in that city. The evidentiary profiles generated, however, did not match the person arrested for the crimes. Initially, detectives were sure that some error was made during the lab analysis because of the confession. The profiles generated in these cases were entered into the local and national DNA offender databases, but no match was found initially. Several months later, a sample collected from a convicted offender matched the profile generated in those three cases. The person identified by his DNA "hit" pled guilty to all three crimes. Certainly without DNA analysis an innocent person who confessed for some reason to crimes he did not commit would have gone to jail for many years. At the same time a dangerous sexual predator would have been released into the community. The DNA databank provided investigative information that would not have been possible only a few years earlier.

In another case, DNA did not identify a suspect when the search of the database against the evidentiary profile did not produce a match. That case involved the investigation of an almost 30-year-old homicide. A woman was stabbed to death in a parking garage. Based on the blood-stain patterns and other evidence at the scene it was apparent that the killer had been injured during the incident. When a suspect was finally identified 25 years after the crime through a search of the auto-mated fingerprint identification system database, the prosecutor wanted additional corroboration of this individual as the perpetrator of the murder. A few aged blood samples that had been stored in less than optimal conditions, some of which had been treated with numerous chemical reagents, were available for DNA testing. Although many other stains were originally recovered, years of serological testing reduced the number and size of material available for DNA profiling. However, DNA was extracted from some of the remaining stains and PCR analysis was conducted. STR profiles were generated from many of these samples. Although some of the bloodstains showed the presence of more than one DNA profile, the suspect was included as a possible donor to those stains. Significantly, a 13-locus match to the suspect was obtained from one of the bloodstains on a handkerchief found near the victim. The accused was convicted 29 years after the murder, and these DNA profiles were key evidence presented during the trial.

MITOCHONDRIAL DNA TYPING

Mitochondrial DNA (mtDNA) typing has also been adapted for forensic purposes. Mitochondria, organelles located in the cytoplasm of the cell, have their own DNA distinct from the DNA in the nucleus. The mito-chondrial genome contains 16,569 base pairs of circular DNA. Mitochondrial DNA is present in multiple copies per cell. In addition, mtDNA is maternally inherited. Typically mtDNA typing involves PCR amplification followed by direct sequencing of the DNA. Sequencing involves the determination of the exact sequence of bases composing the amplified portion of the DNA molecule.

Mitochondrial DNA testing is particularly useful with three types of biological evidence: old or degraded skeletal remains, human remains from mass disasters, and hair shafts that contain no intact cells and only mtDNA. An additional objective test provided by mtDNA analysis of hairs can be applied to hairs that could previously only be compared microscopically. Given its inheritance, an mtDNA profile can be compared to anyone with the same maternal lineage, and is not as discriminating as standard STR analysis. The procedure was first introduced in a U.S. criminal trial in the summer of 1996 (*Tennesee v. Ware*) (State of Tennessee v. Ware, 1999 WL 233592 [Tenn. Crim. App.]).

INTERPRETATION OF DNA RESULTS

The objective of forensic DNA analysis is to compare the evidentiary DNA profiles to the known profiles in a case, such as that of a victim or suspect. Whenever DNA results are generated in a case, one of three basic interpretations can be made:

1. *Inclusion:* DNA markers from known source "A" are present in the evidentiary or questioned sample. Therefore, person "A" could be the source of the DNA evidence.
2. *Exclusion:* DNA markers from known source "A" are not present in the evidentiary or questioned sample. Therefore, person "A" could not be the source of the DNA evidence.
3. *Inconclusive:* No conclusion can be made as to a possible source of the DNA evidence. Results, if any are obtained, cannot be interpreted.

Using these basic criteria, the DNA analyst can address an important but limited question: Could the individual tested be the source of the biological evidence? The more challenging question of guilt or innocence is the purview of the courts.

In the event of an inclusion or DNA match (interpretation 1), person A is the source of the sample, an identical twin of person A is the source of the sample, or another person who coincidentally has the same profile as person A is the source of the sample. Hence, the analyst must provide the court with a statistical assessment of the significance of the match—how common or rare the evidentiary profile is. This typically involves calculating the random match probability, which can be thought of as the expected frequency of individuals in the general population who could be the source of the evidence.

FELON DNA DATABANKS

One of the more significant developments in forensic science is the development and growth of felon DNA databanks. Given the high rate of recidivism associated with sexual assault, felon DNA databanks are particularly useful for solving these crimes; they also have been a valuable tool in the investigation of many other violent crimes. When the sexual assault victim or police are unable to identify a suspect, these types of sexual assaults are often referred to as "no-suspect" cases. Prior to establishing felon databases, forensic analysis of biological evidence was of little value because there was no known person other than the victim to compare with the evidence. With the creation of large felon databanks, however, it is possible to process a no-suspect case and compare the

DNA profile obtained from a sample of unknown origin to a "library" of felon DNA profiles. To date, databank technology has generated more than 10,500 "cold hits" nationwide, leading to numerous convictions (Federal Bureau of Investigation, 2005).

All 50 states have statutes that require biological samples to be taken from convicted felons, and over 4 million felon profiles have been collected. Indeed, a majority of states now collect DNA from all felony convictions, and some even mandate the collection of DNA from all arrestees. In 2002, all 50 states were linked to the national DNA databank system, CODIS (the Combined DNA Index System), which now contains approximately 3 million felon profiles and 100,000 forensic unknown profiles. This national CODIS databank allows states to compare no-suspect profiles that have not matched state or local databanks to the profiles from all 50 states in the national repository.

CHALLENGES TO DNA ADMISSIBILITY

The forensic use of DNA typing methods has played an important role in the successful resolution of many crimes. DNA is important because of its tremendous discriminating power and its stability. However, this very strength is also a prime reason that DNA tests have been challenged so vigorously in court.

Since their introduction into forensic science, DNA typing methods have been strenuously attacked in numerous protracted court battles. Initially, the general reliability of DNA typing procedures was questioned along with the statistical methods used to calculate DNA profile frequencies. In the last few years, legal challenges regarding the admissibility of DNA have shifted their focus away from the general reliability of the methods. Although most courts accept the basic methodology behind DNA analysis, some defense objections regarding DNA evidence continue to be effective. Indeed, successful challenges to the admissibility of DNA testing in court often attack the initial collection, preservation, and subsequent handling of the biological evidence. Thus, it is important for forensic nurses to be aware of the potential negative effects on DNA admissibility if physical evidence is mishandled or not documented correctly. A second type of challenge concedes that DNA typing methods are reliable *in theory*. Here, the defense argues that critical mistakes were made in testing that should invalidate the findings. With this strategy, typically the specific protocols and technical expertise of a particular laboratory or analyst are scrutinized.

With the sensitivity of PCR DNA typing systems, the issue of potential DNA contamination is often raised in court to challenge or minimize the significance of the DNA findings. Although contamination can occur, the greater impact may be on the prosecution. It is important to note that because multi-locus DNA profiles are rare, contamination will predominantly lead to a false exclusion or an artificial mixture rather than a false inclusion. Consequently, although contamination could complicate result interpretation, it would typically not include an innocent defendant.

SUMMARY

The importance of biological evidence has grown rapidly in the past two decades. Eyewitness accounts have often been viewed as unreliable or biased, and the courts have looked for more objective criteria to determine guilt or innocence. DNA analysis may *independently* and *objectively* link a suspect or victim to a scene or to each other. DNA's power as an exclusionary tool is equally noteworthy. Postconviction testing has been used to exonerate more than 130 wrongly imprisoned individuals, primarily those who were convicted based on eyewitness accounts and other less discriminating forensic procedures (Conners et al., 1996). The feasibility of postconviction relief has been greatly enhanced by the latest DNA typing methods, especially STR and mtDNA analysis. Those methods are particularly sensitive, and old evidence can now be re-examined. Clearly, DNA analysis has proven an extremely powerful tool for both prosecution and defense, and the technology continues to improve rapidly. Greater use of robotics and the development of plant and animal DNA analytical tools are well under way. The number of STR cases processed each year will continue to grow. In addition, mitochondrial and Y-STR DNA typing will be utilized on a much larger scale.

The efficacy of race or ethnic group–specific DNA markers that could provide important investigative leads in serial rapes, homicides, and other violent crimes is currently being debated. The problems associated with eyewitness accounts have been widely reported. The typing of race-specific DNA markers could point investigators in a more objective direction by providing typical, general physical information about the assailant (Wade, 2003). This information could result in considerable savings of time and resources.

Recently, the use of ethnic or race-specific DNA markers is reported to have been successful in the identification of a serial killer. By studying a set of DNA markers known as single nucleotide polymorphisms (SNPs), the laboratory at DNAPrint Genomics Inc. was able to measure the "biogeographical ancestry" of the individual allegedly responsible for five homicides in Louisiana (DNAPrint Genomics, 2003). This analysis provided investigators with information concerning the most likely characteristics of the perpetrator. It should be noted that some scientists, privacy advocates, civil libertarians, and other individuals have reservations regarding the potential for abuse of this technology.

Another area of debate has been the national database itself. The current trend is for states to expand their DNA databanks to include all felony convictions; some states are collecting samples from people upon felony arrests. Needless to say, this has sparked great debate about the rights of individuals not convicted of crimes, as well as the privacy rights of those whose samples are in the databanks. As greater resources are provided for processing no-suspect cases, the number of "cold" cases solved at both the state and national level will continue to rise. These developments will contribute significantly to solving sexual assaults, homicides, and other interpersonal violent crimes.

Although technological advancements in evidence processing are noteworthy, they are only one part of the solution. It is arguable that the biggest problems in forensic DNA analysis, as in forensic science generally, involve issues of judgment, ethics, and attitude, and not inadequate technology or funding. Job performance failures prominently aired in high profile cases such as those of O. J. Simpson and JonBenet Ramsey, and "exposés" of laboratory problems (such as with the FBI lab and the Oklahoma Crime Lab), may have significantly eroded public confidence (Lee & Ladd, 1997). Forensic nursing is not immune to these problems, as evidenced by appellate court decisions in several states. Further discussion of the problems that may arise when a forensic nurse acts as expert witness, for example, may be found in Chapter 22.

We can correct these problems, but in many ways we have not moved effectively to do so thus far. Accreditation and certification programs will not satisfy objections raised by defense attorneys, in part because present accrediting and certifying bodies are run primarily by the applicable division of the forensic community. Efforts to impose individual certification and facility accreditation are often seen by critics as little more than superficial exercises in self-policing. In addition, because the overwhelming majority of forensic practitioners already know their trade technically, the discipline may not be significantly improved by formal certification measures.

The greater challenge in the forensic community today is in finding ways to maintain independence and impartiality within an *intentionally* adversarial system. Effective solutions may require "cultural change" (Bromwich, 1997). Forensic practitioners must place greater emphasis on dispassionate and professional testimony. Forensic nurses must avoid the traps of emotion and advocacy. Furthermore, the current system built around the expert witness, discovery, and cross-examination can be very effective and deserves renewed appreciation. Lastly, thorough "quality control" programs are clearly the best vehicles for monitoring the technical skills and knowledge of forensic personnel.

The forensic nursing community needs to enhance its standing in the eyes of both the public and the courts if it is to make a greater contribution as an advocate for victims of sexual assault and other personal violence. Integrity and honesty are the cornerstones of public trust. We must submit to the discipline of the results. Avoid anything that could be seen as whitewashing when questions are raised. If science is served, justice will be well served.

QUESTIONS FOR DISCUSSION

1. What steps in forensic analysis are preferred before conducting DNA analysis? How do evidence documentation, collection, and preservation affect the DNA typing process?
2. What is polymerase chain reaction? In what ways did it revolutionize clinical and forensic testing?
3. How has the development of DNA profiling affected the ability to analyze evidence such as vaginal swabs in a sexual assault case?
4. What challenges may be brought against the collection of evidence from convicted felons for inclusion in a DNA database? Explain why some state that the issues change when samples are collected from persons arrested for certain crimes.
5. Data shows that ethnic origin may be indicated from certain DNA testing. Discuss whether you think this information should be developed for investigative purposes and stored in national databases.
6. How do DNA databanks contribute to the successful resolution of many crimes?
7. How can new developments such as Y-STR typing and mtDNA analysis assist in the investigation or prosecution of sexual assault cases?

REFERENCES

Bromwich, M. R. (1997). Justice Department investigation of FBI laboratory: Executive summary, Department of Justice Office of the Inspector General. *The Criminal Law Reporter, 61,* 2017–2039.

Committee on DNA Technology in Forensic Science, National Research Council. (1992). *DNA technology in forensic science.* Washington, DC: National Academy Press.

Committee on DNA Technology in Forensic Science, National Research Council. (1996). *The evaluation of forensic DNA evidence.* Washington, DC: National Academy Press.

Conners, E., Lundgeran, T., Miller, N., & McEwan, T. (1996). *Convicted by juries, exonerated by science: Case studies in the use of DNA evidence to establish innocence after trial.* National Institute of Research Report NCJ 161258. Washington, DC: United States Department of Justice.

DeForest, P. R., Gaensslen, R. E., & Lee, H. C. (1983). *Forensic science: An introduction to criminalistics.* New York: McGraw-Hill.

DNA Advisory Board. (1998). *Quality assurance standards for DNA testing laboratories.* Washington, DC: U.S. Department of Justice, Federal Bureau of Investigation.

DNAPrint Genomics, Inc, Press Release. June 5, 2003.

Federal Bureau of Investigation. (2005). *CODIS statistics.* Washington, DC: U.S. Department of Justice.

Gaensslen, R. E. (1983). *Sourcebook in forensic serology, immunology and biochemistry.* Washington, DC: U.S. Government Printing Office.

Gaensslen, R. E., Desio, P. J., & Lee, H. C. (1986). Genetic marker systems for the individualization of blood and body fluids in forensic serology. In G. Davies (Ed.), *Forensic science* (pp. 209–240). Washington, DC: American Chemical Society.

Gaensslen, R. E., & Lee, H. C. (1984). *Procedures and evaluation of antisera for the typing of antigens in bloodstains: Blood group antigens ABH, RH, MNSs, Kell, Duffy, Kidd, Serum Group Antigens GmlKm.* Washington, DC: National Institute of Justice, U.S. Government Printing Office.

Holt, C. L., Buoncristiani, M., Wallin, J. M., Nguyen, T., Lazaruk, K. D., & Walsh, P. S. (2002). TWGDAM Validation of AmpFlSTR PCR amplification kits for forensic DNA casework. *Journal of Forensic Sciences, 47,* 66–96.

Lander, E., Linton, L. M., & Birren, B. (2001). Initial sequencing and analysis of the human genome. *Nature, 409,* 860–921.

Lee, H. C. (1982). Identification and grouping of bloodstains. In R. Saferstein (Ed.), *Methods in forensic science.* (pp. 267–337). Englewood Cliffs, NJ: Prentice Hall.

Lee, H. C. (Ed.). (1994). *Crime scene investigation.* Taoyuan, Taiwan: Central Police University Press.

Lee, H. C., Gaensslen, R. E., Pagliaro, E. M., Mills, R. J., & Zercie, K. B. (1991). *Physical evidence in criminal investigation.* Westbrook, CT: Narcotic Enforcement Officers Association.

Lee, H. C. & Ladd, C. (1997). Criminal justice: An unraveling of trust? *The Public Perspective, 8,* 6–7.

Lee, H. C., Ladd, C., Bourke, M. T., Pagliaro, E. M., & Tirnady, F. (1994). DNA typing in forensic science. *American Journal of Forensic Medicine and Pathology, 15,* 269–282.

Lee, H. C., Ladd, C., Scherczinger, C. A., & Bourke, M. T. (1998). Forensic applications of DNA typing: Collection and preservation of DNA evidence. *American Journal of Forensic Medicine and Pathology, 19,* 10–18.

Lee, H. C., Pagliaro, E. M., Zercie, K. B., & Maxwell, V. (Eds.). (1995). *Physical evidence.* Enfield, CT: Magnani and McCormick.

Pennsylvania v. Pestinikas (1992), 617 A. 2d 1339 (Pa. Super.)

State of Tennessee v. Ware (1999), WL 233592 (Tenn. Crim. App.)

U.S. Congress, Office of Technology Assessment. (1990). *Genetic witness: Forensic uses of DNA tests.* OTA-BA-438. Washington, DC: U.S. Government Printing Office.

U.S. Department of Justice, Federal Bureau of Investigation. (2002). Uniform crime reports. Retrieved March 1, 2004 from http://www.fbi.gov/ucr/cius_00/contents.pdf.

Wade, N. (October 1, 2002). For sale: A DNA test to measure racial mix. *New York Times*, p. 4.

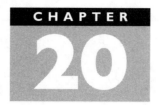

CHAPTER 20

Computer-Assisted and Internet Crime

Monique Mattei Ferraro
Rita M. Hammer

The computer has been in use since the last half of the twentieth century, and the Internet has been accessible to businesses and individuals for the last quarter of a century. Today there is widespread access to computers and the Web. The value of this tool in assessment and as a resource is obvious. However, certain populations, especially children and the elderly, are particularly vulnerable to exploitation and other computer-based crimes. Through research, experience, and opportunities to interact regularly with these victims, the forensic nurse can help identify victims of computer crimes and educate at-risk populations.

CHAPTER FOCUS

Computer-assisted and Internet crime defined
How computers and the Internet facilitate crimes
Focus on Internet crimes against children
Child pornography

KEY TERMS_____

actus reus
child pornography
computer
computer-assisted crime
denial of service
identity theft
Internet
Internet crime
mens rea
Ponzi scheme
pyramid scheme
spam
unauthorized access

INTRODUCTION

Crimes have two components. There is the act, called the *actus reus*. For the crime of larceny, for example, the *actus reus* is the act of taking something of value from another. But the act alone is insufficient to complete the crime. In order for a crime to be committed, there must also be a state of mind, called the *mens rea*. The state of mind is also sometimes called scienter. The state of mind is of great importance. Taking the larceny example, what if the individual has permission from the owner to take the thing of value? What if a person gets into an open car that has the keys in it and drives off, but he believes the car belongs to him? The car is the same color as his; it is the same make, model, and year; and the interior is the same. The act of driving off with another person's car is half of the crime of auto theft. The other half of the crime is the *mens rea*. There are varying gradations of *mens rea* that are determined by the level of intent and purposefulness on the part of the offender. A full discussion of the levels of intent necessary for a criminal offense is beyond the scope of this chapter. For the purposes of this chapter, it is sufficient for the reader to know that all crimes require that an offender must both commit the act and *intend* to commit the act in order for there to be a crime.

There are many ways to define the term *computer*. A computer could be defined as a personal computer, but there are so many devices that are so very similar to personal computers that limiting the scope of the term *computer* to *personal computer* would not do justice to the term. A broader, more functional definition of computer is: a programmable electronic device capable of accepting and processing data. That broader definition encompasses much more than personal computers, including such items as digital cameras, fax machines, mobile telephones, and personal digital assistants (PDAs). All of those items are electronic devices that accept and process data. Any of those machines may be used to commit, facilitate, or store evidence of a crime.

The *Internet* is a computer network, an association connecting computers so that they may communicate, share information, and share files. The Internet, an innovation that exposes its users to a wide variety of knowledge and opportunity, also exposes them to the potential of becoming a victim of computer-assisted crime. The expertise of the forensic nurse can be utilized in relation to such Internet crimes as healthcare fraud, including illegal prescriptions and solicitation of organs, illegal sexual encounters, and child pornography.

Computer-assisted crime is any crime in which a computer is used to commit the crime or to facilitate the crime. Computer-assisted crime also includes situations where the computer contains evidence of the crime. Similarly, *Internet crime* is a crime that uses the Internet to commit the crime, or to facilitate commission of the crime, or where Internet components contain evidence of the crime. The next section discusses the history of computer-assisted and Internet crimes and provides examples of the types of crimes most frequently committed.

HOW COMPUTERS AND THE INTERNET FACILITATE CRIMES

The basic computer crimes that we see today had their beginnings before the personal computer or the World Wide Web. When computers were first used, they were huge, expensive, and delicate. An interruption of service, misuse of the computer system, or destruction of data could cost staggering amounts of money. It may be hard to imagine, but the computing power that one can store in a space the size of a dime today would take up an entire room and require around-the-clock attention 35 or 40 years ago. Even during that time computer-associated crimes were being perpetrated.

The principal federal law governing traditional computer crimes can be found at 18 U.S.C. 1030 (2003). The federal law creates a class of protected computers, defined as any computer used by the U.S. government, by a financial institution, or in interstate commerce or communication, such as computers connected to the Internet. Most personal computers are used to access the Internet, so the federal law covers most computers. The federal law protects the computers from unauthorized access, theft or misuse of information stored by the computer, alteration or destruction of data or equipment, and physical harm or property damage as a consequence of the unauthorized access.

TYPES OF COMPUTER-ASSISTED CRIME

Unauthorized access to a computer system comes in a variety of flavors. Exceeding one's authority to access a computer or a system can be characterized as a "plain vanilla" type of computer crime. It isn't very exciting and it is fairly commonplace. In the world of violent crime, exceeding authority is similar to a crime of violence committed by a relative or friend. The attacker is known and the motivation most often stems from the relationship between the offender and the victim. Examples of exceeding authority include the help desk employee who is authorized to maintain the list of system users and their passwords in case an employee forgets. Bored one evening, the help desk employee uses the personnel officer's user identification number and password to access confidential files that include disciplinary histories, performance evaluations, and salary information on coworkers. Another example of exceeding authority would be an individual providing a friend with her Internet access account identification and password for a single use, and that "friend" using the account to send spam messages advertising pornography sites.

The other type of unauthorized access—a bit more exotic—is an outright intrusion. The intrusion type of unauthorized access is similar to violent crimes committed by strangers. The offender is often unknown to the victim and the motivation is less easily identified. The attack evokes more fear because of the stranger-to-stranger and seemingly unprovoked genesis of the activity. Examples of this type of unauthorized access are also easy to find. An individual sends an e-mail with an attachment that contains a virus. An unknown recipient opens the e-mail and the file attachment that contains the virus, which installs itself on the recipient's hard drive; subsequently, the virus reveals the person's user identification and password to the sender, who then accesses the e-mail recipient's account to send e-mail or to perpetrate identity theft.

This type of unauthorized access to a computer system is what many people refer to as "hacking" or "cracking."

Another type of computer crime is a denial of service, which can take many different forms. Attacks might affect one system, a network, a particular business, a website, or the entire Internet. Basically, anything that an individual does to interrupt or shut down a computer or network is a denial of service. Denial of service attacks range from the very simple to the extremely complex. A simple denial of service might be that someone accessed another party's Internet access account and sent a number of offensive e-mails. In response to the e-mails, several users reported the event to customer service, which shut the account down for violating the terms of service agreement. (Internet service providers usually have a terms of service agreement that forbids obscene or annoying behavior online.) A more sophisticated attack might target the internal network of a major utility, like the phone company or electric company. Hacking into the server and disrupting operations only briefly could affect service provision to all of the utility's users. The consequences of such a disruption or denial of service in the case of a utility can be life threatening. Imagine a hacking incident that causes phone service to be disrupted and at the same time there are users trying to call an ambulance or the fire department to report a fire, or a doctor is cut off while explaining a life-saving procedure to another doctor performing the procedure on the other end of the line.

Yet another vexing type of denial of service is the "distributed" denial of service attack, in which the attacker first breaks into other computer systems by sending out a virus or by other means. Software is installed on the victim systems that is later activated and used to launch the attack. The attacker sends a command to the compromised computers instructing them to begin the attack against a target. The exact method of attack varies, but often the attacker aims to overwhelm a service or website by sending too many messages or requests for it to handle. When a computer receives too many requests or is overloaded, it takes a time out, shutting down when it exceeds its capacity for processing.

Computer-assisted fraud is a primary target of the federal computer crimes law. Since the advent of e-commerce and online auctions, fraud has reached unprecedented levels. During 2002, the Internet Fraud Complaint Center received over 75,000 complaints—a 300% increase over the previous year (Internet Fraud Complaint Center, 2003). Almost half of the complaints related to online auction fraud. Most complainants lost less than $1,000.

Applying the same tactics used for thousands of years to part people from their money, fraudsters use the Internet to access millions of potential victims. The more people a fraud offender can access, the more likely that someone will participate in the scheme. The Internet has been used to further *pyramid schemes, Ponzi schemes,* sale of defective merchandise, and outright larceny. Figure 20–1 outlines the distinction between Ponzi schemes and pyramid schemes often in operation on the Internet.

By far the most prevalent of Internet frauds emanates from online auctions. Law enforcement receives hundreds of reports a day complaining that the merchandise paid for never came or that it doesn't work or that a seller sent merchandise and did not receive payment. A variation that has recently come into vogue is the use of counterfeit or forged checks to purchase merchandise. Usually the purchaser resides outside of the United States and sends the seller a bogus check for goods. By the time

The *Ponzi scheme* is named after its creator, Charles Ponzi. In the early 1920s Ponzi promised investors that he could provide a 50% return on their money in 45 days. The promise of such a large return brought him over $15 million. He was able to pay out the first investors with money from investors coming into the scheme later. The later investors were encouraged to invest because they saw that investors received the guaranteed return. Eventually, the money ran out and the Ponzi scheme failed. The smart fraudster takes the money and runs before the jig is up.

A *pyramid scheme* relies on contributors to recruit new contributors. Usually, the scheme centers around the sale of merchandise and is referred to as "multilevel marketing." It is called a pyramid scheme because there is someone at the top, then a few people under the top person, then more people under the second level, and so on, resembling a pyramid when sketched out. A new contributor or recruit gives money to the person who recruits them for training or for a "franchise" or membership as an investor. The new recruit makes money by recruiting new contributors or recruits. The people at the top make a proportion of whatever the people below them bring in. When the crop of new recruits runs out, the money stops and the scheme is over.

Figure 20–1 Ponzi schemes versus pyramid schemes

the check bounces, the goods are outside of the country, making it difficult to locate the "buyer." The amount of loss may vary, from $10 for a lipstick to thousands of dollars for an original painting or signed celebrity memorabilia.

A number of factors make Internet commerce a particularly rich avenue for fraudsters to be successful. First, almost all transactions occur across jurisdictional boundaries. It is time consuming and complex to trace Internet offenders, and the bulk of municipal and state resources are devoted to crimes against people (i.e., violent crimes), rather than property crimes like fraud. Second, the amount of loss is usually small. In order to justify either extradition (hauling a person into court in one jurisdiction when they reside in another state or country) or federal involvement, the amount of loss must warrant it. Usually, the amount of loss in an Internet fraud is under a few hundred dollars. Many times, the perpetrator resides outside of the United States, making the investigation and prosecution unlikely. Finally, Internet fraud victims contribute mightily to their victimization. Of course, it goes without saying that no one asks to be victimized and certainly no one is responsible for their victimization. However, there are commonsense precautions people can take to prevent being the victim of fraud on the Internet that most victims do not take.

A popular scam that is remarkably successful is the so-called "Nigerian Fraud Scheme." There are many different versions of the e-mail, but usually a "high-ranking" official or a doctor or lawyer from an impoverished or war-torn country sends out an appeal for someone to be kind enough to hold onto his or her money for a short period. In return for holding onto the individual's money, she or he will provide a fee— $10,000 or more—just for the seemingly simple act of allowing him or her to park some money in your account for a few days. Many people who receive these e-mails report them to law enforcement. Of course, there isn't much law enforcement can do with only the e-mail. Based on existing statutes, few jurisdictions would consider the e-mail an attempt to defraud. And often the sender of the e-mail is in another country, making it difficult or impossible to fully investigate the event. Of course, such e-mails are easily dealt with by simply pressing the Delete button. Surprisingly, some people do provide their bank account information and end up victims of theft, either directly from the person's bank account or through identity theft, which will be discussed shortly. A description of the Nigerian "4-1-9" scheme as highlighted by investigators is provided in Figure 20–2.

Many people approach the Internet with a reduced sense of suspicion. The same people who would never provide a social security number to a stranger over the phone enter it freely onto Internet forms. People send postal orders for goods purchased online. Many people send cash overseas freely, along with birthdates, addresses, and phone numbers. These factors are well known to Internet fraudsters who, like all criminals, seek to exploit the weakness in their justice system to conduct their illegal transactions with virtual impunity.

Identity theft is frequently perpetrated either entirely online or is greatly facilitated by the Internet. Identity theft occurs when an individual poses as another person in order to gain goods, services, or some other benefit. Without question, identity theft has quickly become the bane of our twenty-first-century existence. The victim of identity theft may suffer the consequences of the crime for many years, requiring constant vigilance to correct credit and criminal history information. Many victims do not learn they have been a victim of identity theft until most of the damage has occurred—when they apply for a loan or a credit card only to learn that dozens of accounts falsely taken in their name by the offender have been maxed out. By that time, the offender is often long gone and has assumed another person's identity. A series of recent commercials have done much to provide a comical warning to the public of the serious effects of identity theft.

Identity information is everywhere for thieves to plunder. Some thieves harvest identity information through their workplace. Anyone with access to credit card information can compile it and use it to co-opt the true owner's identity. For instance, retail cashiers and wait staff deal directly with credit card information. Also, people who have

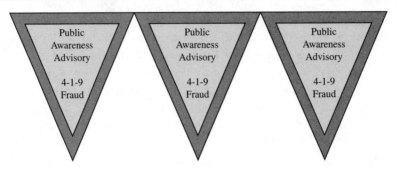

Nigerian Advance Fee Fraud "OPERATION 4-1-9"

The perpetrators of Advance Fee Fraud are often very creative and innovative. This fraud is called "4-1-9" fraud after the section of the Nigerian penal code that addresses fraud schemes. Nigerian nationals, purporting to be officials of their government or banking institutions, will fax or mail letters to individuals and businesses in the United States and other countries. The correspondence will inform the recipient that a reputable foreign company or individual is needed for the deposit of an overpayment on a procurement contract. The letter will claim that the Nigerian government overpaid anywhere from $10 to $60 million on these contracts. There is the perception that no one would enter such an obviously suspicious relationship; however, many victims have been enticed into believing they can share in such windfall profits.

Individuals are asked to provide funds to cover various fees and for personal identifiers such as Social Security numbers, bank account numbers, and other similar data. Once this information is received, the victims find that they have lost large sums of money. It is hard to pinpoint how much has been lost in these scams since many victims do not report their losses to authorities due to fear or embarrassment.

In response to this growing epidemic, the U.S. Secret Service established "Operation 4-1-9" to target Nigerian Advance Fee Fraud on an international basis. Indications are that losses attributed to Advance Fee Fraud are in the hundreds of millions of dollars annually.

Agents on temporary assignment to the American Embassy in Lagos, Nigeria, in conjunction with the Regional Security Office, supplied information in the form of investigative leads to the Federal Investigation and Intelligence Bureau (FIIB) of the Nigerian National Police. This project was designed to provide Nigerian law enforcement officials with investigative leads to enable them to enforce their own jurisdictional violations.

On July 2, 1996, officials of the FIIB, accompanied by Secret Service agents in an observer/advisor role, executed search warrants on 16 locations in Lagos that resulted in the arrests of 43 Nigerian nationals. Evidence seized included telephones and facsimile machines, government and Central Bank of Nigeria letterheads, international business directories, scam letters, and addressed envelopes and files containing correspondence from victims throughout the world.

Source: United States Secret Service (n.d.).

Figure 20–2 Nigerian advance fee fraud scheme.

access to their employer's database of customer information can harvest potential victims. Think about where your personal identifying information is stored. Usually information is in an insurance company database, your employer's human resources databases, everywhere you shop, and each place you have a credit account. Personal identifying information can also be obtained by "dumpster diving." Yes, people really do go through other people's garbage in search of personal identifying information. Discarded mail, such as preapproved credit card applications, bank statements, and credit card receipts, are rich sources of data that an identity thief can use to establish himself as the true owner.

Armed with another person's personal information, an identity thief can go online. The Internet greatly facilitates identity theft through the anonymous nature of electronic commerce. Before e-commerce, most transactions were face-to-face. If a white 21-year-old male presented a cashier with a platinum credit card bearing the name "Mrs. Antonio Hernandez," the cashier would likely have checked to make sure the card was not missing or stolen. Another e-commerce development is that one need not possess an actual credit card. Simply providing identifying numbers, like a social security number rather than a social security card or a credit card number rather than the actual card, is the rule rather than the exception online. When transactions are face-to-face, the card is usually required.

Shopping on the Internet, the identity thief can make a high number of purchases in amounts too little to merit immediate attention either by the vendor or the credit card company. Purchasing a little bit at one website and a little at another website, the identity thief hovers under the radar. Once detected by either the credit card company or the true identity owner, the identity thief has moved on. Sometimes, identity thieves are discovered before the goods are delivered and a controlled delivery of the goods is arranged. Often, though, victims and law enforcement remain frustrated.

In addition to fraud, a host of crimes can be facilitated by the Internet. The Internet provides greater access to victims and a resultant higher volume of completed crimes. Just as fraud schemes have enjoyed great success on the Internet, so has trafficking in narcotics. It does not require much searching to discover that one can obtain prescription drugs without the required prescription, as well as illicit narcotics, through the Internet. Using a credit card, check routing number, or cash, one may purchase any sort of drug. *Spam* (unsolicited commercial e-mail) fills Internet users' mailboxes advertising Viagra, Valium, and all sorts of prescription drugs. Some vendors offer an online service through which a doctor writes a prescription, but many others simply provide the drugs upon request and payment. Narcotics also can be obtained online. Through local chat rooms, newsgroups, and e-mail, buyers order what they want, and the transaction is completed either in person or by mail. Although there are legitimate vendors, clients need to be under the care of a professional for treating a medical condition, especially if they have self-diagnosed. Evaluation relative to the ordering of a medication to treat a specific illness requires a thorough medical history, a physical examination, instructions as to adverse affects, and provision for follow-up of the condition and the response to therapy. Thus obtaining medication is only a part of effective management of a condition. An individual can request the name of the prescribing physician and then check on his or her credentials through the state licensing board. The same can be done for the pharmacist involved. Any difficulty encountered in this process should send up red flags for the consumer.

The Internet is also used to facilitate prostitution. Hookers have flocked to the Internet with websites and webcams that provide live sex acts. Internet users can log onto a website and, for a fee, dictate the sex action. Individuals may also arrange to use the services of the hooker. Often, a sex transaction is something that takes place after a series of e-mails or online chat to ensure that the client is not a law enforcement officer or dangerous.

Gambling is another popular criminal activity facilitated by the Internet. Although laws against gambling may have lost their influence in the wake of legalized gambling in certain cities and states, many jurisdictions prohibit gambling. Although federal law prohibits online gambling, many websites located overseas make huge sums from online gambling. Even though it is illegal, there is no evidence that the law dissuades either the providers of gambling sites or online gamblers.

COMPUTERS AND CRIMES AGAINST PERSONS

So far, the discussion has been concentrated on traditional nonviolent computer crimes. However, the Internet also facilitates the crimes of murder, rape, robbery, assault, and child pornography. The remainder of this chapter discusses these crimes against persons in detail.

There are myriad ways to meet people on the Internet. There are dating services of all types. Some are specific to heterosexuals, others specialize in homosexual couplings, and others connect people with peculiar interests or fetishes. There are also countless chat rooms catering to every interest under the sun. Conversation in chat rooms often revolves around romance and sex. Online profiles—data entered by the Internet subscriber about him- or herself—can be accessed to find out about the people in the chat room. If a particular chat participant or profile sparks interest, individuals often instant message each other requesting further information.

People often meet people from the online world in the real world. Because of the anonymous nature of the Internet, it is impossible to guarantee that when one meets another in the real world that the person will be who they claim to be. Therefore, Web surfers should use a variety of methods to attempt to ensure their safety by confirming the identity of the person they intend to meet. They might request a picture, meet in a public place, talk on the phone first, and conduct a reverse directory check to confirm that the subscriber to the phone number is the same as the name the person provides. They might check the sex offender registry. All of these things can help to make a meeting with a stranger from the Internet more safe; however, it is important for Web surfers to be aware that none of these measures, alone or in combination, can guarantee that the meeting or potential ensuing relationship will be safe.

Focus on Internet Crimes Against Children

Younger people are particularly vulnerable to manipulation and are more likely to take risks by meeting people they communicate with via the Internet. A study by the University of New Hampshire of children between the ages of 10 and 17 found that 20%, or one in five, of the children using the Internet had been solicited for sex in the past year (Finkelhor, Mitchell, & Wolak, 2001). Over time, the probability that a child will be exposed to explicit sexual content or solicited for sex by a sex offender increases geometrically. The probability of solicitation is 20% in 1 year, but over a 2-year period the probability rises to 40%, and so on (Ferraro & Casey, 2004).

Researchers used the same sample to look more closely at why some preteens and teens developed romantic relationships through the Internet while others did not. (Wolak, Mitchell, & Finkelhor, 2003). Wolak et al. found that preteens and teens of both sexes who are troubled, or feel alienated from their parents, are more likely than preteens and teens who do not share those characteristics to form close online relationships. The researchers suspect that more troubled teens may be more likely to seek out support and nurturing relationships through the Internet, while better adjusted teens find satisfying relationships in the offline world. Table 20–1 provides some additional statistics related to sexual solicitation of minors on the Internet.

Table 20–1 Statistics Related to Unsolicited Exposure of Youth to Sexual Images on the Internet

Based on interviews with a nationally representative sample of 1,501 youth ages 10 to 17 who use the Internet regularly

- Approximately one in five received a sexual solicitation or approach over the Internet in the last year.
- One in 33 received an aggressive sexual solicitation—a solicitor who asked to meet them somewhere; called them on the telephone; or sent them regular mail, money, or gifts.
- One in four had an unwanted exposure to pictures of naked people or people having sex in the last year.
- One in 17 was threatened or harassed.
- Approximately one-quarter of young people who reported these incidents were distressed by them.

Source: Finkelhor et al., 2000.

ILLEGAL SEXUAL ENCOUNTERS

According to research conducted by the Crimes Against Children Research Center at the University of New Hampshire, an alarming number of children are victims of online sexual solicitations (Finkelhor, Mitchell, and Wolak, 2001). According to a survey conducted by this group, almost 1 in 5 young Internet users received an unwanted sexual solicitation within the past year. The majority of the youth were between the ages of 14 and 17 years. (Finkelhor, Mitchell, and Wolak). While not all of the youth who were exposed to unwanted sexual material were found to be distressed by the experience, many were reporting such things as intrusive thoughts and physical discomfort. Nearly half of the solicitations were not disclosed to anyone, possibly out of guilt or embarrassment. This lack of disclosure to parents and even to friends poses a problem in terms of providing counseling for the victim and regulating the illegal activity. Post-exposure trauma is an area that should be further researched by forensic nurses. Another issue raised by the survey was a lack of awareness of resources designed to deal with Internet offenses. It was found that parents and youth were not well informed as to where and how to report these solicitations.

While forming close relationships is typical adolescent behavior, the experience of forming these relationships online is a recent and potentially dangerous practice. The normal attraction of adolescents to risk taking combined with technologic proficiency in computers act in concert to create a very vulnerable population. All adolescents are at risk for involvement in this Internet activity, but some may be more inclined to carry on a virtual relationship to an actual one, occasionally with tragic consequences. Studies have shown that some adolescents are more at risk than others. Adolescents who are experiencing difficult relationships with their parents, those who have experienced prior victimization or depression, or are troubled in one way or another, may be more vulnerable to online exploitation (Wolak, Mitchell, and Finkelhor, 2003). The forensic nurse can act to promote the safety of children using the Internet through educational venues. Education for parents:

- Locate the children's computer in a common area where there is maximum family activity.
- Provide software that filters and monitors undesirable sites.
- Advise children to never provide personal information in an Internet chat room.
- Advise children to never send photographs of themselves over the Internet.
- Advise children to never arrange a meeting with someone they encountered on the Internet.
- Have children report any innocent looking Internet link that takes the child to an inappropriate site.
- Limit the amount of time the child can spend in chat rooms or surfing that does not have an educational purpose.
- Familiarize yourself and the children with resources and mechanisms for reporting undesirable unintended transport to objectionable sites.
- Do not overreact to a child's Internet activities, if inappropriate, as it may cause him to become less open about future activities.
- Encourage children to discuss their Internet experiences openly and freely.

Education for school personnel and health care professionals:

- Be alert for behavioral changes in children that may signal an inappropriate Internet relationship, such as avoiding classmates, acting aloof, and signs of depression.
- When counseling children and adolescents be sure to include an assessment of their Internet use along with other measures of social relationships.
- Collaborate with community members interested in the issue of Internet safety for children.
- Become actively involved in the process that seeks to address Internet safety for children through policy and legislation.
- Develop a system for evaluating Internet sites, chat rooms, and filtering software and make recommendations to school personnel.
- Conduct research aimed at understanding the impact of unwanted exposure to sexual material among children of varying ages (younger children report more distress after such exposure than older children)

- Involve children in the process of promoting safety and awareness of their responsibility for Internet standards.
- Facilitating the awareness of youth of sources of help for Internet offenses and ways to more easily report such offenses.

It is important to remember, however, that minors are not the only victims of Internet-facilitated rape. Because adults increasingly use the Internet to meet prospective partners, rapists increasingly use the Internet to find potential victims.

> Once an offender has selected a target, he/she can monitor potential or existing victims on several levels, ranging from participating in a discussion forum and becoming familiar with the other participants, to searching the Internet for related information about an individual, to accessing a potential victim's personal computer to gain additional information. Furthermore, by giving offenders access to victims over an extended period of time (rather than just a brief encounter) the Internet enables offenders to gain control of their victims or gain their victims' trust, and possibly arrange a meeting in the physical world. (Casey, McGrath, & Ferraro, 2004)

Child pornography is the scourge of the Internet. Child pornography is the graphic depiction of a minor engaged in sexual activity or in an explicit sexual pose. Child pornography is distinguished from erotica and adult pornography because the actions depicted in the images are criminal by their very nature. In the case of sex acts, the action is either statutory rape, forcible rape, or at the least a crime akin to impairing the morals of a minor or risking the injury of a minor. When the conduct depicted is a lascivious exhibition of the genitals, the act may not be a sexual assault or statutory rape, but in many jurisdictions, the soliciting of the suggestive pose by the photographer or adult is impairing the morals of a minor or risking injury to a minor. Minors are set apart from adults because they, by law and by developmental capacity, lack the ability to consent to certain conduct and obligations. For example, minors may not enter into contracts, enter into marriage, or consent to sexual activity. In the same vein, minors may not consent to a picture being taken of criminal activity in which they are also a victim. By the same force of argument, minors whose pictures have been taken while being victimized cannot consent to allowing those pictures to be distributed.

Before the Internet, due to heavy federal and state penalties for manufacturing and distributing child pornography, it was difficult to find sources of such materials. Transactions were all conducted either hand-to-hand, as in the case of a bookstore or other purveyor, or through the mail. It was easy for police to keep the lid on bookstore trafficking of child pornography because they knew where the stores were and who worked there. All police had to do was show up and walk around the store. They could see anything in plain view that was offered for sale, and if there was evidence that the store sold child pornography, a search warrant and arrest ensued shortly thereafter. The United States Postal Service postal inspectors have a keen eye for contraband, and especially child pornography. Postal inspectors often conducted undercover stings and controlled deliveries of suspicious materials. Between the actions of local police and the postal inspectors, the physical exchange of child pornography had been slowed substantially in the United States prior to technological advances that made digital images and their rapid exchange over the Internet possible.

Digital imagery revolutionized the child pornography trade. Before digital imagery was possible, child pornography was limited to photography, film, and video. Photography and film require at least some equipment and specialized knowledge to develop the film. To mass distribute photographs, one must employ a printer; to distribute film or videotapes in large quantities, a professional processor would be needed. Getting the product to the consumer posed other logistical difficulties. Issues of advertising and the physical distribution of the material were complicated by corporeal existence of the contraband. Thus, the expense of producing child pornography made it prohibitively expensive to most people to purchase. "Calculated in today's dollars, allowing for inflation, the child pornography magazine that sold for $25.00 in the 1970s in Chicago would go for about $108.00 and the $50.00 film would sell for $215.00 today" (Ferraro & Casey, 2004). Unfortunately, the ability to create, to store, and to traffic in child pornography in digital format has eliminated most of the traditional law enforcement and logistical barriers to mass producing and distributing that material.

Using a digital camera, one can sexually abuse a minor in the privacy of one's own home and record it as digital video or still images and instantly broadcast it to an unlimited number of recipients via the Internet. The one-time cost of the camera can be less than $50 for a small Webcam. The cost of distributing the image is next to nothing. A personal computer can be purchased for less than $500. A used computer costs much less than that. An Internet connection is as little as $10 a month, and through various offers can even be less.

Detection and Proof of Child Pornography

Detecting the distribution of child pornography is much more difficult for law enforcement when the images are in digital form. There are a myriad of issues beyond the reach of this chapter. Numerous articles and other publications can be found that provide a detailed analysis of this topic. (For a comprehensive overview, read Ferraro and Casey, 2004.) Briefly summarized, some of the issues include detection, jurisdiction, and proof.

Detecting the manufacture and distribution of child pornography in digital form is quite difficult. Because most trafficking is conducted via the Internet, the only reasonable way to detect the movement of child pornography through the network would be to monitor traffic. For many reasons, monitoring of Internet traffic by agents responsible for enforcing child pornography prohibitions is not possible. First, only agents charged with international intelligence responsibility, like the Central Intelligence Agency and the National Security Agency, are granted authority by Congress to monitor international Internet traffic. Second, monitoring Internet traffic within the borders of the United States would be prohibitively expensive and labor intensive. Third, the American people would never consent to close monitoring of their personal and private communications to detect a criminal activity such as trafficking in child pornography. For example, federal authorities have run into fairly strong opposition from civil rights proponents over new surveillance powers enacted since the September 11, 2001, tragedy, and those powers have been advocated for the limited purpose of monitoring, preventing, and interdicting in terrorist actions. Expanding surveillance authority to apply to child pornography, where there is no imminent threat of harm or a threat to a large number of potential victims, would be doomed to failure.

So, how does child pornography come to the attention of law enforcement, if law enforcement cannot monitor Internet activity proactively? Private citizens usually report the more obnoxious child pornographers— those who send spam e-mails advertising websites containing graphic images—websites stumbled upon inadvertently while searching for something else. Computer repair shops and employers also report child pornography trafficking and possession. Internet service providers also report child pornography trafficking when it comes to their attention. Since 2000, Congress has mandated that ISPs report child pornography to the National Center for Missing and Exploited Children (NCMEC) (42 United States Code § 13032 [2004]).

In response to citizen and Internet service provider complaints, the National Center for Missing and Exploited Children created a "CyberTipline" to accept reports of online child pornography. Since 1998, the CyberTipline has received over 117,000 reports of child pornography, online solicitation of minors, and other computer-assisted sexual exploitation of children (The Frontline, 2003). Several case studies of successful outcomes from CyperTipline reports are presented in Figure 20–3.

July 16, 2003

On October 8, 2002, NCMEC received a CyberTipline report indicating that a suspect was posting child pornography to an Internet Service Provider (ISP) Group. Once Exploited Child Unit (ECU) analysts confirmed that the suspect had posted graphic images of child pornography, they searched his online profile, which indicated an interest in the states of Pennsylvania and New York. ECU analysts forwarded the report to the Delaware County (PA) Internet Crimes Against Children task force and, within hours of receiving the report, the officers began an undercover operation. On July 10, 2003, the United States Postal Inspection Service and Elkland, Pennsylvania law enforcement executed a federal search warrant on the 53-year-old suspect's home in Elkland. The suspect's computer system, numerous floppy diskettes, and compact discs were seized as evidence. The suspect's case will be prosecuted by the U.S. Attorney's office in Harrisburg, PA.

June 26, 2003

On March 18, 2003, NCMEC received two CyberTipline reports from a registered Internet Service Provider (ISP) containing images of child pornography that allegedly had been distributed by a subscriber of that ISP. Exploited Child Unit (ECU) analysts conducted thorough Internet searches on the suspect's e-mail address and zip code, determined the suspect was in Orinda, California, and alerted FBI analysts at NCMEC. FBI analysts sent out a subpoena to the ISP requesting subscriber information for the suspect and the information was referred to the Orinda Police Department for an investigation. A warrant was executed and over 36,000 images were found on the suspect's hard drive. So far, 39 of the images have been confirmed as child pornography. The 17-year-old suspect was arrested and is currently being held in juvenile hall on suspicion of felony possession of child pornography for distribution and trading for his own personal use.

June 12, 2003

On April 8, 2003, NCMEC received a CyberTipline report revealing the online identity of a man allegedly attempting to lure a 12-year-old child to meet him for sexual purposes. When NCMEC's Exploited Child Unit staff conducted thorough Internet searches, they quickly found a photograph of the suspect and learned that he lived in Tennessee. The information was immediately forwarded to the Knoxville Police Department. A Knoxville police officer took on an undercover identity of a child under the age of 13 and began online correspondence with the suspect, which led to specific plans to meet so the suspect could engage with sexual activity with the child. The suspect arrived at a Knoxville hotel and was taken into custody. He was charged with the attempted rape of a child.

May 9, 2003

On January 30, 2003, NCMEC received a CyberTipline report detailing the possible sexual molestation of a 3-year-old girl by a man who, at the time, was living with the girl's father. The child disclosed this information to a relative, detailing the sexual acts the suspect had forced the child to perform with him. The caller was only able to provide NCMEC with a name and partial address of the suspect. Exploited Child Unit Analysts ran a public records database search on the suspect's information, confirmed a possible location for him in Clarkston, Washington, and forwarded the report to the Asotin County (WA) Sheriff's Office. Investigators were able to locate and interview the child, at which point she provided detailed information and drew pictures documenting the molestation by the suspect. Law enforcement then arrested the suspect at his home on February 5, 2003, and charged him with Rape of a Child in the First Degree.

Source: National Center for Missing and Exploited Children (2003).

Figure 20–3   Case studies: CyberTipline success stories.

Another way child pornography trafficking comes to police attention is during the course of investigation or forensic examination related to another crime. For instance, it is quite common for an individual attempting to entice a minor into sexual activity to send the prospective victim pictures containing child pornography as part of the "grooming" process. Child pornography may also be found on a suspect's computer during the course of a forensic examination relating to sexual assault, homicide, and, surprisingly, even counterfeiting or fraud.

The largest scale child pornography investigations were initiated when a website or payment service for child pornography websites was seized by law enforcement. A recent example is "Operation Avalanche," which resulted in hundreds of arrests and prosecutions of purchasers of child pornography website privileges. Figure 20–4 shows some of the coverage of the successful government sting.

Despite the many ways that child pornography trafficking comes to the attention of law enforcement, it is quite difficult for law enforcement to detect much of the trafficking that takes place. Compounding the limitations relative to detection are jurisdictional issues that make child pornography investigations difficult. There are usually multiple levels of jurisdiction involved in child pornography trafficking. State laws prohibit distribution of child pornography, as does the federal law. At the state level, state, county, and municipal police are all charged with enforcing the criminal laws. Which unit of law enforcement takes the child pornography case is often only dictated by which agency receives the complaint, rather than any designated official authority. At the federal level there are also multiple jurisdictional overlaps. Customs has jurisdiction over goods that travel in and out of the United States, the Postal Service has some jurisdiction, as do the Secret Service and the Federal Bureau of Investigation.

Shared jurisdiction over child pornography trafficking has inspired many federal, state, and local law enforcement agencies to join forces as task forces. The task force approach offers smaller organizations the opportunity to learn from and share the resources of larger agencies that have more experience investigating and prosecuting computer-assisted child exploitation. Task forces also help to relieve the workload of larger organizations by training local officers to investigate their own cases. Without the benefit of training and experience, the local officers would have to refer the cases to the state or federal authorities.

The Internet Crimes Against Children Task Forces, funded by the United States Department of Justice, Office of Juvenile Justice and Delinquency Prevention, were established to bring the various agencies together to combat online child exploitation. The FBI's Innocent Images National Initiative is another program established to counter the flood of child pornography distributed via the Internet. Figure 20–5 shows the information provided at the federal website describing the Innocent Images program. The task forces have the distinction of unprecedented information and resource sharing among diverse levels of law enforcement. However, despite their success in building cooperation, even their united forces have had limited impact on the distribution of child pornography over the Internet. Frustrating law enforcement efforts even further, the task of proving that an image is child pornography is one of the most onerous tasks a prosecutor can face.

In 1996, Congress amended the child exploitation sections of the federal penal code to anticipate that "virtual" images—that is, digital images rendered by computer technology—would be used to depict sexually explicit images of minors. The new provisions also prohibited the depiction of individuals who "appear to be" minors in sexually explicit acts. These two provisions became lightning rods for free speech advocates and legitimate, adult pornographers. A group called the Free Speech Coalition sued Attorney General John Ashcroft, claiming that these elements of the law were overbroad and vague. The United States Supreme Court held in *Ashcroft v. Free Speech Coalition* that prosecutors must prove that there is an actual minor depicted in the picture and that minor must actually be sexually abused. The Court reiterated its holding in *New York v. Ferber* when it stated that the distinguishing feature that allows child pornography to be treated differently than constitutionally protected speech is that it is a visual preservation of a criminal act against a minor. There were many other features of the *Ashcroft v. Free Speech Coalition* case that are of importance, and the case is far more complex than the explanation here. Although this discussion of *Ashcroft* is a grossly simplified summary, it provides sufficient highlights of some issues relative to prosecuting a child pornography case following the *Ashcroft* decision.

Some prosecutors have interpreted *Ashcroft* to require that the state must prove beyond a reasonable doubt that the person portrayed in an image is not an adult or a computer-rendered image and that there is actual, prohibited sexual activity taking place. Thus, in order to try a child pornography case, investigators and forensic examiners often are required to prove that the person depicted in the picture actually exists and was the person depicted in the pictures. To facilitate these identifications, the National Center for Missing and Exploited Children (NCMEC) maintains a database of "identified" child pornography images. Investigators send images to NCMEC requesting a search of the database, and NCMEC confirms whether any of the images are of "known" victims. The NCMEC database has solved a small part of the problem of proving that a person depicted in an image is a minor being

The U.S. Postal Inspection Service Teams with Internet Crimes Against Children Task Forces in Operation Avalanche

Attorney General John Ashcroft and then-Chief Postal Inspector Kenneth Weaver announced in August 2001 the successful conclusion of a two-year investigation that dismantled the largest commercial child pornography enterprise ever uncovered. Following the "take down" of Landslide Productions, Inc., a multimillion-dollar child pornography business, 30 federally funded ICAC task forces throughout the United States partnered with U.S. Postal Inspectors to launch Operation Avalanche. This proactive, undercover investigation resulted in an unprecedented sentence of life in prison for Landslide's owner, the execution of over 160 state and federal search warrants across the country, the arrest to date of more than 120 offenders for trafficking child pornography via the U.S. Mail and the Internet, the identification of child molesters, and the rescue of child victims.

The Internet Crimes Against Children (ICAC) Task Force Program was created in 1998 by Congressional mandate. Administered and funded through the Department of Justice's Office of Juvenile Justice and Delinquency Prevention (OJJDP), ICAC provides grants to state and local law enforcement agencies, which use them to build regional task forces that address and combat Internet-related crimes against children.

Operation Avalanche began in 1999, when Postal Inspectors discovered that a Ft. Worth, Texas, company, Landslide Productions, Inc., operated and owned by Thomas and Janice Reedy, was selling child pornography websites. Customers from around the world paid monthly subscription fees via a post office box address or the Internet to access the hundreds of websites, which contained extremely graphic child pornography material. Ft. Worth Postal Inspector Robert C. Adams and Dallas ICAC Task Force Detective Steven A. Nelson teamed together to initiate what would become a child exploitation case of unprecedented magnitude.

During the investigation, while Landslide Productions was still in business, the National Center for Missing and Exploited Children's CyberTipline received more than 270 complaints from people around the world related to the Landslide case. All credible complaints were forwarded to investigators.

Postal Inspector Bob Adams obtained federal search warrants for the business and personal residence of the Reedys. The warrants were executed by a task force of 45 officers and agents. They served seizure warrants on Landslide's bank accounts and two unencumbered Mercedes Benz vehicles valued at more than $150,000—and purchased with the Reedy's ill-gotten gains. Landslide was a highly successful financial enterprise, at one point taking in over $1.4 million in a single month.

Figure 20–4 Operation Avalanche: A successful sting operation.

After reviewing volumes of seized evidence and subpoenaed financial records, the Reedys were indicted in federal district court on 89 counts of conspiracy to distribute child pornography and possession of child pornography. Following a one-week jury trial, the Reedys and their company were convicted on all counts as charged. Thomas Reedy was given an unprecedented sentence of life in prison, and his wife Janice received a 14-year prison sentence.

Putting Landslide Productions out of business and the Reedys behind bars struck a major blow to the global child pornography industry, but the investigation did not end there. Using intelligence gained from Landslide's customer database, Postal Inspectors joined with 30 federally funded ICAC task forces across the country and, with legal guidance from the Department of Justice's Child Exploitation and Obscenity Section, designed and implemented a nationally coordinated, undercover operation.

Working out of the Dallas ICAC Task Force office, Postal Inspectors and other investigators initiated undercover contacts with the most egregious suspects. As cases were developed, the suspects were passed off to other Postal Inspectors and ICAC task forces throughout the United States for further investigation. Investigators obtained and served search warrants, seized huge volumes of child pornography images and materials, identified child molesters, and rescued victimized children from further sexual abuse. To date, over 160 search warrants have been served and more than 120 child sex offenders and pornographers have been arrested.

In one instance, Postal Inspectors and ICAC Task Force investigators searching the home of a 36-year-old computer consultant in North Carolina found videotapes he had produced depicting the sexual abuse of a number of young girls, one of whom was only four years old. The offender recorded the activities with a pinhole camera he had hidden in a bedroom smoke detector and which was connected to a VCR and a computer. On August 7, 2001, the man was sentenced to 17 and 1/2 years in federal prison on various charges of sexual exploitation.

The Internet has not only cut across global boundaries, it has cut across jurisdictional lines. Few cases that originate on the Internet remain in the same jurisdiction—nearly all cross state lines and involve multiple jurisdictions at federal and state levels, with extensive interagency collaborations. Operation Avalanche exemplifies law enforcement teamwork at its best. Over 60 foreign countries and their citizens have benefited from this cooperation, which has identified thousands of suspected child pornographers and molesters around the globe and continues to track down and halt these criminals.

Source: United States Postal Service (n.d.).

Internet Crimes Against Children Task Force Program

In 1998, the Missing Children's Program of OJJDP initiated its Internet Crimes Against Children (ICAC) task force program, a national effort to combat the threat of offenders who use the Internet to sexually exploit children. Through this program, state and local law enforcement agencies can acquire the skills, equipment, and personnel resources to respond effectively to ICAC offenses. The program encourages law enforcement agencies to develop specialized multijurisdictional, multiagency responses to prevent, interdict, investigate, and prosecute Internet crimes against children. As of mid-2000, 30 ICAC task forces were participating in the ICAC task force program. Each task force is composed of federal, state, and local law enforcement personnel; federal and local prosecution officials; local educators; and service providers such as mental health professionals. These task forces serve as valuable regional resources for assistance to parents, educators, prosecutors, law enforcement personnel, and others who work on child victimization issues. You can obtain more information on this and other law enforcement programs from the OJJDP website at ojjdp.ncjrs.org/programs/programs.html

Source: U.S. Department of Justice. Office of Justice Programs home page. Retrieved October 25, 2004 from www.ojp.usdoj.gov.

HISTORY OF INNOCENT IMAGES

While investigating the disappearance of a juvenile in May 1993, FBI Agents and Prince George's County, Maryland, police detectives identified two suspects who had sexually exploited numerous juveniles over a 25-year period. Investigation into the activities of the suspects determined that the adults were routinely utilizing online computers to transmit child pornography. Further investigation and discussions with experts, both within the FBI and in the private sector, revealed that the utilization of computer telecommunications was rapidly becoming one of the most prevalent techniques by which some sex offenders shared pornographic images of minors and identified and recruited children into sexually illicit relationships. Based on information developed during this investigation, the Innocent Images National Initiative was started in 1995 to address the illicit activities conducted by users of commercial and private online services and the Internet.

During the early stages of Innocent Images, a substantial amount of time was exhausted on commercial online service providers that provide numerous easily accessible "chat rooms" in which teenagers and pre-teens can meet and converse with each other. By using chat rooms, children can chat for hours with unknown individuals, often without the knowledge or approval of their parents. Investigation revealed that computer sex offenders used chat rooms to contact children. Chat rooms offer the advantage of immediate communication around the world and provide the pedophile with an anonymous means of identifying and recruiting children into sexually illicit relationships.

Figure 20–5 Federal task force programs.

TODAY'S INNOCENT IMAGES

Today, the FBI's IINI focuses on:

- individuals who indicate a willingness to travel interstate for the purpose of engaging in sexual activity with a minor; and
- major producers and/or distributors of child pornography.

In addition, the IINI works to identify child victims and obtain appropriate services/assistance for them.

Online child pornography/child sexual exploitation is the most significant cybercrime problem confronting the FBI that involves crimes against children. Throughout the FBI, there was a 1,997% increase in the number of IINI cases opened between fiscal years 1996 and 2002, from 113 to 2,370. It is anticipated that the number of cases opened and the resources utilized to address the crime problem will continue to rise during the next several years.

The FBI has taken the necessary steps to ensure that the Innocent Images National Initiative remains viable and productive through the use of new technology and sophisticated investigative techniques, coordination of the national investigative strategy, and a national liaison initiative with a significant number of commercial and independent online service providers. Innocent Images has been highly successful. It has proven to be a logical, efficient, and effective method to identify and investigate individuals who are using the Internet for the purpose of sexually exploiting children.

Source: Federal Bureau of Investigation (n.d.).

sexually abused. But, the database cannot deal with pictures of new victims that enter the stream of trade every day.

A full two-thirds of offenders who were con~icted of sex crimes against minors were found to be in possession of child pornography, the majority of which depicted children between the ages of 6 and 12. Many successful cases of prosecution have come about as a result of individuals reporting instances of the crime to the CyberTipline (http://www.cybertipline.com).

Forensic nurses need to be aware of the methods by which they can facilitate the reporting of such crimes. The forensic nurse can be an advocate for the protection of children through assessment, counseling, and parent and community education.

HEALTH CARE FRAUD

Individuals diagnosed with chronic illness, particularly progressive or life-threatening conditions, frequently seek information and products to treat their conditions on the Internet. Almost 100 million adults in the

United States use the Internet as a resource for health information for themselves, family members, or friends (Bren, 2001). The populations most at risk for healthcare fraud are adolescents and the elderly. Adolescents regularly seek remedies for or advice about health-related issues such as weight, acne, depression, eating disorders, plastic surgery, and exercise. One might think that the elderly, a large segment of the population with chronic illness, might not be computer literate, and therefore not risk falling prey to such fraud. However, this is increasingly not the case, as even those elders who do not own their own computers often become proficient in their use through Internet classes offered at senior centers, libraries, and assisted living facilities.

Healthcare fraud is defined by the Food and Drug Administration (FDA) as the "promotion, advertisement, distribution, or sale of articles, intended for human or animal use, that are represented as being effective to diagnose, prevent, cure, treat, or mitigate disease (or other conditions), or provide a beneficial effect on health, but which have not been scientifically proven safe or effective for such purposes" (Stehlin, 1995, p. 3). It is estimated that healthcare fraud costs Americans an estimated $30 billion dollars per year. More ominous is the fact that these practices, in some cases, may cost individuals their lives.

There are many websites that advertise products of little or no therapeutic value. In some instances the claims for the products are simply without proven merit. In other instances, the clients order and pay for products and then do not receive them. Clients may also illegally obtain prescription medications on the Internet, some approved but many not yet approved by the FDA. Counterfeit drugs have also found their way onto the Internet.

In vitro diagnostic (IVD) tests are marketed freely and if used as the sole predictor of health or disease can be potentially disastrous for vulnerable populations. Using these products, individuals may self diagnose and self treat themselves inappropriately and dangerously. Examples of tests available from the Internet include tests for HIV, hepatitis, drugs of abuse, and cholesterol, among others. Physicians routinely use such tests but only in conjunction with other standard medical practice such as physical examination, medical history, evaluation of other presenting symptomatology, additional more sophisticated IVD testing and so forth (CDRH, 2001). Such self diagnosis could rely on a test that yields either false positive or false negative results. Tests that yield quantitative data may be misinterpreted by the individual and could compromise their health if not followed up by a visit to a certified professional healthcare provider. Thus the advertising of products for use at home without further medical oversight is misleading at best and possibly quite dangerous for the clients using them. In addition, while some IVD tests are effective, many are of poor quality and some are clearly illegal; that is they are being marketed without approval by the FDA. Others may be approved for professional use but are marketed for unapproved uses. (CDRH). Potential users must be educated about the fact that all such products should first be researched and approved by the FDA.

It is estimated that 1 in 3 clients avail themselves of some form of alternative therapy, the majority of whom do not disclose the information to their healthcare provider. Some of these therapies are fraudulent and others, while not illegal, are purported to have beneficial effects that are clearly without scientific validation. The availability of these products on the Internet can have potentially dangerous consequences as the (illegally obtained) medications or ineffective treatments may interact adversely with those already legitimately prescribed for the client, or in other cases substitute for proven conventional medical treatments that could help. Some examples of recently prosecuted cases include a claim that St. John's wort was a safe treatment for clients with HIV or AIDS when there exists a potentially dangerous interaction with protease inhibitors used to treat the disease and the marketing of a device that claimed it could kill the agents of diseases such as cancer and Alzheimer's disease by delivering a mild electric current (Bren, 2001). While one cannot blame clients who are experiencing major illness for which there is little hope and who wish to try anything that might prolong their lives or at least relieve their suffering, the problem is that some may be foregoing proven medical therapies that could help. Although many alternative therapies are helpful or at the least, not harmful, the forensic nurse can act as an advocate to ensure that clients do not rely on products that are clearly fraudulently advertised and will not improve their state of health. Forensic nurses must be aware of these potentially dangerous websites, monitor them where feasible, and actively engage in policymaking to curtail this type of healthcare fraud. Workshops and/or educational seminars held for the elderly in senior settings or for adolescents (in educational settings) should also strive to aim their program toward educating these vulnerable populations as to the dangers involved in engaging in activities related to personal health on the Internet. Observing and assessing clients through a forensic lens may alert the nurse to situations in which the clients may be being victimized and/or are compromising their health. Educating clients should include the following points:

- Always consult your healthcare provider when using any products obtained through the Internet.
- Avoid products that claim to treat a wide array of illnesses.
- Be suspicious of products that claim to be "all natural," as this implies a level of safety that may not be justified.

- Avoid products that can only be obtained through one supplier.
- Obtain full information regarding the firm's name, address, and phone number.
- Do not rely on the results of any one IVD test without medical validation.
- Be wary of any product described in grandiose terms such as guaranteed cure.

ORGAN TRANSPLANTATION

A report by the secretariat of the World Health Organization (2003) acknowledges that while payment for human organs and tissue is illegal in most countries, there are many reports from various countries that living donors, particularly of kidneys, have received direct payment for their donation and may indeed have been exploited in the process (WHO, 2003). While it is a violation of federal law in the United States to receive or provide remuneration in exchange for a body part, Internet solicitation of organs for transplantation exists and may in some cases involve a financial transaction. One such Internet site, http://www.matchingdonors.com, claims to have over 1700 willing donors. The first transplant of an organ from a donor solicited from this site was performed in October 2004. However, in another instance, a potential recipient describes receiving several offers from a similar website (http://www.organgiving.org), from potential donors who expected payment of some sort which she could not afford, not all of which would be considered legal (Healy, 2004).

In cases of living donation of organs from strangers, referred to as altruistic donors, the forensic nurse should be attuned to the possible vulnerability of the donor. In some instances the donor may be considered to be the victim, since in many cases they are young, in need of money, and inadequately informed as to the long-term health consequences of their action, which in some cases are quite serious. To surrender a healthy kidney, for example, as a young adult may, if illness ensues in later life, places the donor himself in need of a transplanted organ. Careful psychological screening methods must be employed prior to allowing a young, healthy adult to donate a body part to a virtual stranger, one met on the Internet. An index of suspicion must be employed when caring for clients in areas where organ transplantation is involved, particularly in cases where the donor may not be fully informed of the risks and consequences. When caring preoperatively for a transplant donor, forensic nurses in clinical settings may be in a position to ensure that the consent form signed by the donor is truly "informed consent" as required by law. Forensic nurses in the community must be knowledgeable when providing services to families and community groups about the possible implications of deviating from the prevailing medical system of organ procurement.

The shortage of available organs for transplant, and issues of fairness of distribution of such organs through the United Network for Organ Sharing (UNOS), has fueled dialog about the need to formulate another method of encouraging and allocating organ donations. There is increasing discussion about the idea of providing some type of reward system for those individuals and families who might consider donating organs for transplant. The ethical issues associated with such a program continue to pose a significant challenge to the idea. It remains to be seen how widespread the use of the Internet by clients in need of an organ transplant will become.

SUMMARY

The dawn of the computer and Internet age has brought with it great benefits as well as great challenges. As with any technological breakthrough, computer technology has outpaced our ability to prepare for the unexpected, sometimes negative, consequences. Law enforcement, forensic science, and the law are in a chaotic state in the early years of the 21st century because all disciplines are trying to identify the consequences, formulate a response, and institute methods of dealing with computer-related crime. While this process of trying to make sense of things takes place, the Internet is similar to the "wild, wild West," the 19th century's "www." Lawlessness rules, and it is unclear whether or when the dust will settle. Amid this turmoil the forensic nurse can provide assistance by being an educator, an advocate for the victims of child pornography, and an activist for appropriate, effective legislation.

QUESTIONS FOR DISCUSSION

1. What computers do nurses use that might contain digital evidence?
2. How can nurses help to determine if a computer or the Internet was part of the crime?
3. What are the two components of a crime?
4. What is the difference between a pyramid scheme and a Ponzi scheme?
5. After reading this chapter, how would you change your Internet activities?
6. What will you recommend to others about using the Internet safely?
7. What is child pornography, and how might it play a part in child sexual assault or child exploitation?

REFERENCES

Ashcroft v. Free Speech Coalition, 122 S. Ct. 1389; 152 L. Ed. 2d 403; 2002 U.S. LEXIS 2789 (2002).

Bren, L. (2001). Agencies team up in war against Internet health fraud. *FDA Consumer Magazine,* 1–4. Retrieved November 17, 2004 from www.fda.gov/fdac/features/2001/501_war.html.

Casey, E., Ferraro, M. & McGrath, M. (2004). Sex offenders on the Internet. *In Digital evidence and computer crime: Forensic Science, Computers, and the Internet* (2nd ed.). Boston, MA: Academic Press.

Center for Devices and Radiologic Health. (2001). Buying diagnostic tests from the Internet: Buyer beware! *CDRH Consumer Information,* 1–3. Retrieved November 18, 2004 from www.fda.gov/cdrh/consumer/buyerbeware.html.

Federal Bureau of Investigation. (n.d.). *Crimes against children.* Retrieved October 25, 2004 from http://www.fbi.gov/hq/cid/cac/crimesmain.htm.

Ferraro, M. M. & Casey, E. (2004). *Investigating child exploitation and pornography: The Internet, law and forensic science.* Boston: Academic Press.

Finkelhor, D., Mitchell, K. J., & Wolak, J. (2001). Highlights of the youth Internet safety survey. *OJJDP Fact Sheet.* (4). Washington, DC: U.S. Department of Justice, 1–2.

The FrontLine. (2003). Newsletter of the National Center for Missing and Exploited Children. (Spring 2003, vol. XXXXIX).

Healy, M. (2004). Organ donation incentives revisited. *South Bend Tribune,* November 10, 2004. Retrieved November 28, 2004 from https://www.southbendtribune.com/stories/2004/11/10/living.20041110-sbt-MICH-D3-Organ_donation_incen.sto.

Internet Fraud Complaint Center. (2003). *Welcome to IFCC.* Retrieved October 24, 2004 from www.ifccfbi.gov.

Mitchell, K. J., Finkelhor, D., & Wolak, J. (2001). Risk factors for and impact of online sexual solicitation of youth. *Journal of the American Medical Association, 285*(3), 3011–3014.

National Center for Missing and Exploited Children. (n.d.). Home page. Retrieved October 25, 2004 from www.missingkids.com.

New York v. Ferber, 458 U.S. 747; 102 S. Ct. 3348; 73 L. Ed. 2d 1113 (1982).

Stehlin, I. (1995). An FDA guide to choosing medical treatments. *FDA Consumer.* Retrieved November 18, 2004 from www.fda.gov/oashi/aids.fdaguide.html.

United States Postal Service (n.d.). *Home page.* Retrieved July 7, 2005 from www.usps.com.

United States Secret Service. (n.d.). *Home page.* Retrieved October 25, 2004 from www.secretservice.gov.

Wolak, J., Mitchell, K. J., & Finkelhor, D. (2003). *Internet crimes against minors: The response of law enforcement.* Alexandria, VA: National Center for Missing and Exploited Children, 1–14.

World Health Organization. (2003). Human organ and tissue transplantation: report by the Secretariat. Retrieved April 26, 2005 from http://www.who.int/gb/.

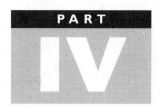

SPECIALIZED FORENSIC NURSING ROLES

Correctional Nursing

Anita G. Hufft

In a 1979 film from the American Medical Association, *Out of Sight—Out of Mind*, Dr. Alvin J. Thompson remarked, "Professionalism in medicine depends on our ability to provide quality care to the least of us" (Anno, 1991). If the care and treatment provided to the incarcerated is a reflection of the degree of professionalism attained in a healthcare field, it seems logical that advanced practice nurses working as correctional specialists provide leadership in the care of those in our jails and prisons, instituting best practices, supervision, and role modeling in secure settings.

CHAPTER FOCUS

Advanced practice correctional nursing
Growth of correctional institutions as healthcare settings
Factors affecting health care in corrections
Major healthcare challenges
Prisoner populations: culture of corrections
The prison subculture
Special prison populations
Advanced practice nursing in correctional settings
Professional correctional nursing development

KEY TERMS

adjudication
deterrence
evidence-based practice
federal prisons
incapacitation
jails
lock-up
malingering
manipulation
maximum security
minimum security
rehabilitation
restitution
restoration
state prisons
subculture

INTRODUCTION

It has been said that to understand society, one only needs to look within its prison walls where one can see people affected by racism, poverty, and illiteracy. During 2003 the U.S. prison population increased to 2,166,260, a 2.6% increase, which is the largest since 1999 (*Corrections Today,* 2003). Observations of prison settings reveal the fact that a majority of prisoners are people of color and underrepresented minorities, and those from economically impoverished communities. As a result, prisons comprise a microcosm of marginalized and oppressed populations normalized within a unique structural and cultural institution. The poor healthcare status observed in prisoners is not surprising given that poverty and race status are known factors affecting incidence and prevalence of communicable diseases and mental health problems. Within prison walls are individuals who have often lacked access to health care and who often have received poor healthcare services prior to incarceration. Consequently, prison offenders present unique challenges to the nursing and healthcare staff charged with their care.

On January 27, 2003, United Press International released a news brief from its chief White House correspondent regarding a report on inmate medical care in the United States. This report revealed the results of a National Institute of Justice study, which found that many prisons and jails in the United States did not meet the established guidelines for the delivery of healthcare services, resulting, upon release from incarceration, in the eventual introduction into the community of many offenders with serious health problems such as HIV/AIDS, tuberculosis, hepatitis, and mental disorders (Potter & Tewksbury, 2005). Ironically, correctional facilities are mandated to provide health care at a level that exceeds the experience of many Americans, and therefore often provide the best, and sometimes the only, health care many offenders have ever received (Hofacre, 2003). Correctional health care, and the nursing care within it, represents part of the overall healthcare delivery system for the most vulnerable of society. Because corrections directly impacts the overall delivery of health care to a very high-risk population, correctional nursing is in a position to help improve the health of offenders and, in turn, to positively impact the general public health.

ADVANCED PRACTICE CORRECTIONAL NURSING

This chapter is not intended as a comprehensive reference on correctional nursing. The purpose of this chapter is to review the role of advanced practice nursing in correctional settings and propose strategies for the identification and implementation of advanced practice correctional nursing as a specialty of forensic nursing. Advanced practice correctional nursing involves the direct care of incarcerated persons in traditional as well as expanded roles within secure settings of jails and state or federal prisons. Advanced practice correctional nurses are nurse practitioners or clinical nurse specialists prepared at the graduate level. They use in-depth knowledge of healthcare policy, organizational behavior of secure settings, ethical and legal issues in correctional health care, role development in correctional nursing, diversity and cultural competency in corrections, and health promotion and disease prevention among correctional populations. Advanced practice correctional nurses implement highly autonomous and collaborative nursing roles primarily aimed at conducting comprehensive health assessments, diagnosing and treating complex responses to actual or potential health problems of individuals and groups within offender populations, and formulating clinical decisions to manage acute and chronic illness and promote wellness in prison and jail settings. The range and depth of competencies and knowledge of advanced practice correctional nurses result in a broader repertoire of effective strategies to meet the needs of inmate patients and correctional healthcare systems, and they are therefore suited to manage more complex, more uncertain, and resource-limited situations that characterize correctional settings (American Association of Colleges of Nursing, 2002; American Association of Critical Care Nurses, 2003).

GROWTH OF CORRECTIONAL INSTITUTIONS AS HEALTHCARE SETTINGS

Although incarceration rates in the United States have leveled off since the dramatic increases in the 1980s and 1990s, the number of adults and juveniles in correctional facilities has seen unprecedented growth. At the end of the twentieth century, the United States put more people behind bars than at any other time; over 2 million people were housed in prisons or jails (Jamison, 2002). Unlike decades past, when rates of incarceration rose and fell with wars, depressions, and economic booms and busts, as well as with the rise and fall of crime rates, the current growth in incarceration has continued to increase. In 2002, 6.7 million people were on probation, in jail or prison, or on parole. More than 3% of all U.S. adult residents, or 1 in every 32 adults, is under the supervision of the criminal justice system. Between 1995 and 2002, the incarcerated population grew an average of 3.6% annually, with the largest growth occurring in federal prison (5.8%) and local jails (5.4%) (U.S. Department of Justice, 2003).

In the United States, the rights of offenders are based on interpretations of the Eighth Amendment to the United States Constitution, which prohibits "cruel and unusual punishment." Both federal and state laws, along with professional standards of correctional health care, serve as guidelines for the administration of safe and ethical health care to offenders. The basic assumption upon which professional and ethical standards of care are developed in correctional settings, and for which advanced practice nurses are responsible for providing oversight, is that incarceration does not, by itself, deprive individuals of rights, although these rights must be administered within the scope of legitimate needs of penal authorities to preserve security, control, and rehabilitation (American Psychiatric Association, 2000; American Nurses Association [ANA] 1998; Kay, 1991; National Commission on Correctional Health Care, 2002a). All correctional facilities are designated as providers of health care, either directly or indirectly through the establishment of contractual arrangements.

The introduction of professional nursing to prisons and jails has become common only within the last 20–30 years; it is therefore important for advanced practice correctional nurses to understand the evolution of jails and prisons as settings for societal sanctions available to the courts to deal with those who commit criminal offenses. The first prisons were created in the Middle Ages by the Christian Church to house those who offended canon law. Debtors' prisons followed in the 1400s for the purpose of housing those who violated civil laws (Schmalleger, 1999). The prison or jail, as we know it, emerged out of the 16th century with the building of the prototype house of correction, the London Bridewell. Prior to Bridewell, prisons were used as detention settings for those awaiting punishments such as the ducking stool, the pillory, whipping, branding, or the stocks (Howard League, 2003). Evidence suggests that the prisons of this period were badly maintained and often controlled by negligent prison wardens. Many people died of diseases such as typhus. Houses of correction evolved out of the "Poor Law," and were intended to instill habits of industry through prison labor. Most of those held in detention were nonviolent offenders convicted of petty theft, being vagrants, or being disorderly local poor. During the 18th century large numbers of British prisoners were transported to Australia and America for the purpose of imprisonment and hard labor. The first correctional institution in the United States, the Walnut Street Jail, opened in Philadelphia in 1790 and, unlike previous institutions, was established purely for the purpose of punishment (Wrobleski & Hess, 1997). Also referred to as the Philadelphia Penitentiary, the Walnut Street Jail housed offenders in solitary confinement so that they could "wrestle with the evils they harbored," study the bible, and be reformed (Schmalleger).

The rehabilitation era of the "Pennsylvania style" prison gave way to the "mass prison era" of the 1800s in an attempt to lower costs and increase access to group workhouses (Schmalleger, 1999). Between 1876 and 1890 Alexander Maconochie and Sir Walter Crofton's efforts in Australia and Ireland to change prison conditions and focus influenced Gaylord Hubbell, warden of Sing Sing prison in New York, to create a "reformatory" based upon concepts of earned early release if the inmate reformed himself. Men and women of vision met at the first National Prison Association conference in 1870 to propose the ideal prison system, emphasizing rehabilitation of first-time offenders. The eventual failure of this system has been attributed to cultural orientation of prison staff that overemphasized confinement and institutional security rather than reformation. It is important to remember that the conflict between custody and reform remains with us today, and is highlighted in the recurring role conflict between custody and caring experienced by correctional nurses (Maeve, 1997; Peternelj-Taylor & Hufft, 1997; Peternelj-Taylor & Johnson, 1995).

Three basic facilities make up the correctional institutions found in the United States today: jails, state prisons, and federal prisons. Jails are locally operated correctional facilities that confine persons before or after adjudication. Offenders sentenced to jail usually have a sentence of 1 year or less, although this can vary from state to state. Jails also incarcerate persons in a variety of other categories, such as persons being held pending arraignment, trial, conviction, or sentencing; those who have been returned to custody following violation of the terms of their release on probation or parole; and persons being transferred to the custody of other criminal justice or correctional authorities. Lock-ups, commonly located in city halls or police stations, differ from jails in that they are temporary holding facilities authorized to hold individuals for a maximum of 48 hours. Either a state or the federal government operates prisons, and they confine only those individuals who have been sentenced to 1 year or more of incarceration. Generally, persons sentenced to prison have been convicted of a felony offense (National Institute of Corrections, 2003).

Organization and delivery of nursing and health services is in part determined by the physical and procedural limitations of the correctional facilities in which they are offered. Offenders in prisons and jails are classified by security levels designated to match physical and procedural restrictions with the prisoner's risk to the population in terms of violence or escape. Maximum-security facilities house the most dangerous of offenders and tend to locate cells and other inmate living facilities in the center of the institution and place a variety of barriers between the living area and the institution's outer perimeter. Medium-security prisons generally afford more freedom of movement and activity, and are under less intense supervision than maximum-security facilities, particularly in relation to associations between offenders, movement in the prison yards, and use of facilities such as exercise rooms, libraries, showers, and bathrooms. Headcount is an important security measure and is usually taken several times throughout the day. All activities, including health care, must conform to security routines in correctional facilities. The lower a facility's security level, generally the more comfortable the environment. There is generally more room for movement, more windows, more programming, and more opportunities for social interactions. These environmental concerns are important factors affecting psychosocial and biophysical health, and an in-depth knowledge of facilities and the rationale for those facilities is a critical component to assessment and planning for advanced practice correctional nurses.

The federal prison system was implemented in 1895 with the conversion of Leavenworth Prison from military confinement to civilians convicted of violating federal law. The Federal Bureau of Prisons was established in 1930 to adequately oversee the 11 federal prison facilities existing at that time and to provide a professional framework for the development of prison standards. At present there are 100 institutions, 6 regional offices, a central headquarters, 3 staff training centers, and 28 community corrections offices. In addition, the Bureau of Prisons provides health care for most offenders within the correctional institutions. For those that need hospital care, there are 7 inpatient medical referral centers with about 2,000 inpatient and chronic care beds (U.S. Department of Justice, 2001).

Current trends in prisons and jails affecting nursing and health care include expanding populations of offenders and those ordered for evaluation prior to trial or sentencing, shortages of nursing staff, limitations in financial and physical resources, role ambiguity and role conflict as a consequence of caring and security goals, and the necessity of adapting to the values and transactions inherent in prison culture. A recent survey conducted by the National Institute of Corrections cited widespread deficiencies in medical staff in prisons or other units housing offenders with medical needs, particularly in women's care units and for mentally ill offenders (National Institute of Corrections, 2002). Advanced practice nurses with backgrounds in women's health care and psychiatric nursing are particularly needed in correctional settings.

FACTORS AFFECTING HEALTH CARE IN CORRECTIONS

Both physical setup and procedural restrictions serve as mechanisms to preserve security and promote control in correctional settings. Restrictions in movement, interactions with staff and other offenders, and physical barriers introduced to prevent escape are common in correctional environments. Locked doors, high fences, and barred windows are part of the physical reality of prisons and jails. Rigid schedules for daily activities, required attendance at scheduled meals and work details, along with mandatory silence at "lights out" are a few of the temporal limitations of life in a correctional setting. Understanding the relationship between the physical and logistical demands of a correctional setting, and the procedures used to implement health care, is essential for developing optimal systems of care.

Before seeing a healthcare provider, offenders must usually complete a written request, indicating the nature of the health problem for which care is sought. Depending on the institution, the request for health services may be evaluated by individuals with little or no medical training, and in some instances, correctional officers, whose knowledge and assessment of the conditions warranting routine or emergency care may be limited or biased by security concerns. When healthcare triage decisions are unduly influenced by security concerns, delay or denial of healthcare requests can occur. In some settings, the disorganization or limitation of services delaying routine sick call requests results in unnecessary declarations of emergency by offenders.

Like the emergency room used for routine health care, the misuse of emergency declarations overtaxes healthcare systems in corrections and may result in sanctions or higher levels of eligibility before an offender can be seen. Advanced practice nurses in correctional settings are responsible for the review of policies and procedures related to access to health care. Recommendations for procedures that facilitate the availability of healthcare services to inmates, along with the development of documentation systems verifying appropriate screening, referral, and delivery of healthcare services by qualified healthcare staff, require negotiation with security staff and health authorities. Advanced practice nurses must be aware of threats to security and a variety of options for the delivery of healthcare services so that recommendations can be adapted to the specific needs of the institution.

Growing numbers of correctional institutions require inmates to pay a minimal, but unaffordable to some, co-pay for care. Long waiting periods, sometimes in very uncomfortable conditions outside, without cover, serve as another deterrent to those seeking care. Often inmates are restricted to sick call-out at only one time each day. Sick call may be as early as 6:00 A.M., with the request needing to be posted the day before. Any healthcare concern that is not an emergency that occurs after that time would need to be postponed until the next day. When attending clinics or sick call, inmates miss meals, work assignments, or special programming. In some instances, missed days of work add days to the sentence, a disincentive to those seeking medical care. Many times inmates will postpone medical care until an emergency exists, making their conditions more severe and more difficult to manage.

Inmates on medication face difficulties related to accessing their medications, maintaining privacy in terms of what medications they are taking, and timing of medications. Any activity related to security, such as headcounts or lockdowns, interrupt any other activity taking place in the institution and may contribute to missed medication and medications dispensed without regard for food and beverage ingestion. When unable to take their medications with prescribed food or on an empty stomach, inmates may experience side effects, drug resistance, or exacerbation of a medical condition.

Perhaps the greatest barrier to inmates in accessing and using health care in correctional settings is the culture of the institution itself. Prison culture does not tolerate weakness, and those with medical problems can be viewed as outcasts and deviants by inmates and by correctional staff. Suspected of manipulation, inmates seeking health services, particularly those who complain of pain, are often marginalized and disrespected. Responding to the need for acceptance among their peers and out of a need for self-preservation, offenders may elect not to access healthcare services and become "no shows" in clinics. *Noncompliance* is a common term used in corrections, because many offenders view medication refusal as a way of asserting their independence in a setting in which they have very little control. Understanding the organizational behavior exhibited within corrections, among both staff and offenders, is a critical element to the organization of healthcare services. The advanced practice nurse is in a position to not only influence policy directly, but also, through the education and development of correctional staff, increase the manpower available to deal with special needs populations such as the mentally disordered and chronically ill (Tahir, 2003).

The prison healthcare setting is, by its very nature, an environment unconducive to clinical productivity. Low productivity among healthcare staff results in under-used healthcare resources and denial of access to facilities by inmates. Overcoming issues such as organization of efficient nursing staff to support medical and nursing interventions, management of laboratory reporting processes, and low administrative support of healthcare functions is a priority in all correctional settings (Anno & Dubler, 2002; Bachmeier, 2003; Paris, 2003). Advanced practice nurses must be able to implement productivity measures in order to develop staffing formulas appropriate for the setting. Warden's meetings, inmate transportation, inmate count or attendance, and reducing paperwork associated with documenting services are all points of activity for the management of effective and efficient correctional healthcare services.

MAJOR HEALTHCARE CHALLENGES

Although offenders represent the larger communities from which they come, individuals in prison and jail settings reflect major categories of acute and chronic illnesses at greater rates than the public. Major responsibilities of the advanced practice nurse in corrections include knowledge of policy, institutional culture and organizational behavior, and standards of correctional nursing care to establish nursing systems for implementation of the nursing process and attainment of institutional health benchmarks.

Screening and Assessment

Critical to the successful management of health care in correctional settings is the development of effective screening procedures and accompanying policies and protocols to deliver appropriate healthcare interventions. An example of an opportunity for critical assessment of screening tools is the use of instrumentation to assess drug use among offenders. Current legislation requiring mandatory sentencing for drug-related crimes has resulted in significant numbers of offenders with substance abuse histories. Presented with growing numbers of drug-involved offenders and limited resources, it is essential for advanced practice correctional nurses to provide oversight and guidance to the development of protocols for nursing involvement in drug screening and treatment facilitation. Instrumentation for nursing assessments of substance abuse in correctional settings are implemented to help mental health staff identify candidates for levels of treatment designed for maximum impact and avoid spending time and money on intensive treatment of low-risk offenders. Any mandatory and routine assessments or screenings done by nursing staff should be subject to review by nurses, who are accountable for ensuring that the cost, length of time to administer, scope, and application of drug and alcohol treatment options are appropriate for the instruments being used (Peters et al., 2000; Wells, 2003).

Identification of Nursing Priorities

Identifying major nursing diagnoses for those offenders presenting for nursing care is helpful in the development of plans of care for groups of offenders. Major infectious diseases such as HIV/AIDS, tuberculosis, and hepatitis B and C occur at significant rates in correctional settings.

PRISONER POPULATIONS: CULTURE OF CORRECTIONS

The goal of culturally competent care for clients in correctional settings is to encourage appropriate exchanges and collaborations among offenders, healthcare providers, and correctional staff. These collaborations should foster equitable health outcomes and result in the identification and provision of services that are responsive to issues of race, culture, gender, sexual orientation, and social and economic status. Being competent in cross-cultural functioning means learning new patterns of behavior and effectively applying them in appropriate settings.

The American Nurses Association has asserted that culturally competent nursing care goes beyond cultural sensitivity and awareness of different cultures to specific knowledge and skills that can help the nurse change situations of oppression and avoid stereotypical assumptions (ANA, 1998). Based on the anthropological concept that all human communities develop through learned and shared information about what is acceptable and expected behavior, nursing has evolved as a scientific practice discipline rooted in our own cultural values of caring, compassion, and technical competencies. The prison or correctional setting represents a challenge to nursing as offenders represent a multitude of cultures within a unique culture of the prison itself. Culture is a distinctly human capacity for adapting to circumstances and transmitting this coping skill and knowledge to future generations. The prison culture has its own attributes, forming a sense of identity, a set of expected behaviors, and distinct goals for those who are incarcerated and for those who care for them. Prison becomes a setting in which persons from various cultures and criminal backgrounds come together in a contrived culture derived from values and dictates of the criminal justice system and the participants in the operations of the institution.

Prisons mirror those characteristics of any culture through expression of values and norms, beliefs and attitudes, relationships, communication and language, sense of self and space, appearance and dress, work habits and practices, and food and eating habits. Correctional nurses who are aware of the cultural backgrounds and characteristics of offenders are in a position to adapt healthcare practices to meet client needs and avoid imposing their own attitudes and approaches on others.

Historically, prisons have served five major purposes in American Society, retribution, deterrence, incapacitation, rehabilitation, and restoration (Schmalleger, 1999; Wrobleski & Hess, 1997). Retribution represents punishment for the sake of punishment—also referred to as revenge. Retribution focuses on the crime itself rather than on the offender's needs or the needs of the community. Deterrence relies on incarceration as a means to prevent future criminal actions and is more proactive and functional than retribution. Incapacitation refers to making it impossible for offenders to commit other crimes and has the goal of segregating offenders from the rest of society to protect them. Rehabilitation has the goal of correcting deviant behavior. In and out of favor in the criminal justice system and dependent upon funding, rehabilitation is the focus on medical and mental health treatmnet for many offenders whose offense is related to their pathology. Due to critical levels of funding and questions about the effectiveness of rehabilitation in light of high rates of recidivism among offenders, the prevailing approach of the criminal justice system in relation to corrections currently focuses on punishment or retribution. An evolving paradigm of justice, called restorative justice, focuses on problem solving and repair of social injuries incurred through criminal behavior (Wrobleski & Hess, 1997). Restorative justice acknowledges the relationship between the offender and the victim, the rights of the victim and the need for society to be repaired through the offender making retribution for injuries perpetrated in criminal offenses. This approach recognizes the ability of the stigma of offense to be removed through repentance and forgiveness and, while implemented in probation sentencing, does not represent the current model of prison culture.

The prison culture values order and obedience, power over the weak or disenfranchised, and strict adherence to policies and procedures. Many prisons are characterized by a culture of fear (Ramsbotham, 1999), and underscored by actions by offenders and staff suggesting racism and sexism. Normative behavior often includes widespread use of drugs and physical and mental abuse among offenders. Prison culture is heavily oriented toward security, with offenders being kept powerless and forced to rely on correctional officers for the delivery of services, particularly health care (Blair, 2002).

Prisons are overcrowded and occupied by individuals convicted of violent crimes (49%), property crimes (20%), and drug crimes (21%), the latter being the most rapidly increasing category (U.S. Department of Justice, 2001). The prison population in general is characterized by low levels of formal education, socially disadvantaged backgrounds, and a lack of significant vocational skills. Most adult offenders have served considerable time in juvenile correctional facilities and evidence acculturation to the prison.

Correctional nurses must be aware of the culture shock most offenders experience upon first entering a correctional setting. Culture shock is a psychological disorientation related to inaccurate interpretation of role expectations or cues from another culture (ACA, 2003). In addition to being cast into interactions with persons of diverse and often unknown cultural backgrounds, the prison itself presents an environment requiring adaptation. Offenders must adhere to sets of policies dictating every movement and event from when they eat and sleep to what they wear, when they can speak, and what work they will do each day. They are cut off from family and social support systems and subjected to lack of privacy, changes in stimulation and recreation, and limited access to physical and emotional stress management options. Offenders in prison must learn vocabulary and postures in order to fit in. They must quickly identify the power structures among the other offenders and among the staff in order to avoid becoming a victim of abuse or ridicule. Offenders with physical problems, developmental problems, or mental disorders are particularly vulnerable to segregation and victimization. All offenders share common deprivations of liberty, goods and services, heterosexual relationships, autonomy, and personal security. These are the common stressors that link the offenders in prison.

One approach to the study of prison culture is based on the work of Erving Goffman (1961b). He described total institutions as places where the same people work, play, eat, sleep, and recreate together on a daily basis. Such places include prison concentration camps, mental institutions, and seminaries. Total institutions are small societies cut off from the larger society either forcibly or willingly. They evolve their own distinctive values and styles of life.

THE PRISON SUBCULTURE

Two realities exist in prisons. One is the official structure of rules and procedures dictated by the state department of corrections or the federal government. The other is the more informal but more powerful inmate culture—the prison subculture.

Offenders have to learn all the rules and regulations set by the corrections administration, but they must also learn very quickly the unwritten rules dictated by the prison subculture incorporating inmate concerns, values, roles, and even language (Schmalleger, 1999). The inmate learns an unwritten code that dictates five common elements:

1. Do not interfere with the interests of other offenders. Never rat on a con.
2. Do not lose your head; play it cool and do your own time.
3. Do not exploit offenders. Do not steal. Do not break your word, be right.
4. Do not whine. Be a man.
5. Do not be a sucker. Do not trust the guards or the staff.

Prison subculture is constantly changing and probably represents the greater culture of criminals existing outside of prisons. Structural dimensions of prison subculture often determine how prison culture is described. These include the degree to which the staff and the offenders are alienated, the three general categories of offense types among the offenders, how work gangs and cell houses are organized, racial groups, the power of inmate leaders, the degree of sexual abnormality presented by an inmate, and personality differences existing among individuals (Schmalleger, 1999).

SPECIAL PRISON POPULATIONS

Since the 1960s a growing concern for the rights of ethnic minorities, women, the physically and mentally challenged, and many other groups has extended to the issue of unfair and inequitable treatment by the criminal justice system. A special population is identified as any group of individuals who present patterns that distinguish them from other individuals and whose patterns of behavior or physical characteristics affect their health or experience of health and health care. Within the prison culture there are specific groups needing nursing assessment and intervention. Major groups identified as special prison populations upon which one can focus culturally competent nursing intervention strategies include women, homosexuals, juveniles, gang members, ethnic and racial minorities, the elderly, and those with chronic illnesses.

Women

Although women represent only 10% of the country's correctional population, they are the fastest growing group in jails nationwide (Harrison & Beck, 2005). On average, female offenders are 2.5 years older than their male counterparts, are less likely to be convicted of a violent offense, and are more often than not victims of sexual or physical abuse, involved in drug use or drug trade, and have children (Greenfeld &

Snell, 1999). Women live in prison within complex social systems based on close emotional relationships with other offenders. Women find prison life harder than men, crave affection, and are more vulnerable to homosexual relationships (Heidensohn, 1995).

Women are especially vulnerable to the stress of separation from family and children. Women's correctional facilities often suffer from a lack of resources as compared to men's, due to a lack of funding equity. Fewer women in prison results in numbers too low to justify many programs. In addition, women in prison are subject to sexual misconduct in the form of sexual contact between women offenders and staff, name calling, and inappropriate leering. The great imbalance of power between health or correctional staff and offenders makes the notion of consent impossible and the resulting vulnerability serves as a constant source of stress (Coolman, 2003).

Incarcerated women use healthcare services at a significantly higher rate than men due to the greater complexity of a woman's reproductive system, a high rate of sexually transmitted disease, and pregnancies. Women entering correctional settings report problems with alcohol abuse, headaches, fatigue, drug abuse, and sexually transmitted diseases (National Commission on Correctional Health Care, 2001; National Institute of Corrections, 2002).

Women in prison present unique healthcare challenges due to poor self-care, high levels of drug use and histories of abuse, high-risk pregnancy, and dysfunctional family histories. Diets high in fat and carbohydrates often lack nutrients considered essential in the prevention of heart disease and hypertension, loss of bone mass, and anemia.

Although women tend to resist prison subculture and are more likely to have more trusting relationships with staff, they are often viewed by the correctional staff as complainers and whiners. Their physical and emotional complaints are often viewed as malingering or manipulation. Women are typically underserved in correctional settings due to under-programming, fragmentation of services, inconsistent treatment philosophies (especially in areas of mental health and co-morbidity), and lack of gender-specific treatment alternatives (Dolan et al., 2003).

Women tend to organize themselves into "prison families," creating artificial relationships that mirror the outside world. These relationships produce three primary responses and distinct personality types; square, cool, and life (Pollock, 1998; van Wormer, 2001). The squares identify predominantly with conventional norms and values and have had little previous experience with the criminal justice system. Cools represent those women who isolate themselves and are career offenders. Lifers are full participants in the prison culture, usually taking leadership roles.

Lifers represent those women who have no meaningful relationships or identity outside prison and find prison culture their only source of self-concept and status. A new category of female offender, the "crack kid," exhibits a lack of respect for traditional prison values, for their elders, or even for their own peers. They are frequently involved in fights and their lack of even simple domestic skills estranges them from others.

Homosexuals

Homosexual activity in prisons is universally condemned and prohibited by formal prison policy and, at the same time, encouraged and promoted by the environmental and social structures supporting prison subculture. There are two major male types of homosexual activities in prison. One type of homosexual activity involves predatory behavior of heterosexual males reacting to the constraints of prison life that prohibit heterosexual liaisons. The other involves those men who participated in a homosexual lifestyle outside of prison. Homosexual activity among females is less aggressive than males and involves the need for attention and affection (Potter & Tewksbury, 2005).

Newly admitted offenders may be sought out by older offenders looking for a sexual union. They will ingratiate themselves by offering cigarettes, money, drugs, and other favors and then demand sexual favors in return. The inmate code calls for the payment of debt and the inmate is therefore obliged to perform sexual favors or be subject to inmate "justice."

Rape among male offenders has been reported as high as 28% (Lockwood, 1978). Although most sexual aggressors do not consider themselves homosexuals and sexual release is not the primary motivation for sexual attack, many aggressors continue to participate in gang rape activity in order to avoid becoming a victim of rape. Twelve percent of all hate crimes in prison are perpetrated against males believed by their victimizers to be homosexuals (Schmalleger, 1999), and this aggression often continues into the correctional setting against homosexual offenders.

Juveniles

As juvenile drug use, gun use, and gang involvement increase, the presence of juveniles in correctional settings has increased by more than 300% over the past decade. Mirroring the adult population, most juvenile offenders are male, and the female population is growing at an unprecedented rate (U.S. Department of Justice, 2002).

Taken as a broad category of the correctional population, juveniles are characterized as "rejecting middle class values of social duty and personal restraint" (Schmalleger, 1999, p. 578). Increasing experience with problems of drug and alcohol abuse, violence, gang membership, separation from family and home, and sexual and physical abuse affect the growth and development of the juveniles seen in the criminal justice system. The rates of self-destructive behavior such as self-mutilation and attempted and completed suicide are on the rise among juveniles in the correctional population at higher rates than in the general population (American Academy of Pediatrics, 2001).

Ethnic and racial diversity among juveniles is a complicating factor influencing diagnosis and implementation of responsive and appropriate healthcare strategies, particularly in mental health (Canino & Spurlock, 2000). Inability to focus on the subtleties of cultural variance in symptoms of illness can delay onset of treatment or selection of appropriate treatment. This has been a factor in the persistent lack of resources and adequate health care for youths in detention and correctional facilities.

Routine childhood and adolescent developmental issues must be integrated into any plan of care for juveniles in corrections. A complete assessment includes immunization updates, the need for crisis intervention and suicide prevention, and risk factors such as domestic violence, drug use, and assaultive behavior. In addition, specific policies related to parental notification and consent for treatment must be instituted. Unlike adult populations, the impact of healthcare services may be greater among juveniles. If juvenile offenders receive intensive intervention while incarcerated, during their transition to the community, and while they are under community supervision, they will benefit from improved family and peer relations, education, job skills, substance abuse levels, mental health, and recidivism levels (Bradley & Kalfs, 2003).

Gang Members

Prisons began to have noticeable increases in gang activity when states enacted tougher laws for gang-related crimes in the 1980s. Documented as an inner city phenomenon in the United States since the 1920s, gangs have experienced a growth in numbers and power inside prisons. Many individuals who had previously never associated with gangs become gang members during incarceration (Egley, 2005; Egley & Arjunan, 2002; Schmalleger, 1999; Thornberry, Huizinga, & Loeber, 2004). Correctional facilities bring members of gangs together in a setting without natural boundaries, creating tensions over "turf" and opportunities for competition for space, power, and membership. Male gang members tend to adopt a defensive world view evidenced by a feeling of vulnerability and suspicion, a general mistrust of others, the need to maintain social distance, a proclivity toward violence as a problem solving mechanism, and an attraction to others who are defensive. Gang members tend to come from dysfunctional families and are less likely than nongang members to complete high school. They are known as predators, taking advantage of and exploiting other juveniles and adults. Extreme risk takers, gang members are frequently involved in accidents as well as altercations, making them frequent visitors to the infirmary (Esbensen, 2000; Howell, 2000; Howell & Lynch, 2000; Wright & Wright, 1995).

Gangs can be extremely well organized, many holding regular meetings with a rigid set of rules and even requiring regular payment of dues. Violence is often used as a right of passage, and up to 40% of gang members report rape of females and other violent crimes, especially on rival gang members (Schmalleger, 1999). Most gangs are ethnically diverse (70%), but few allow female membership or female leadership roles. Exclusively female gangs are increasing in number, particularly among the Hispanic population. The one thing that most gang members have in common is a tendency to violence and delinquency before joining a gang (Esbensen, 2000). However, most gang members claim that, if given a second chance, they would not have joined a gang. The correctional environment, however, with its emphasis on sustaining tightly controlled reference groups, does not promote the success of programs designed to discourage gang affiliation.

Ethnic and Racial Minorities

The recognition of hate crimes—offenses in which aggression is based on actual or perceived race, color, religion, national origin, ethnicity, gender, or sexual orientation—emphasizes the segregated and heterogeneous nature of American society. White supremacist and separatist groups adhering to an "identity theology" further marginalize and segregate ethnic and racial groups (Marable, 2000; Schmalleger, 1999). Racial and ethnic minorities such as African Americans, Native Americans, and Hispanics are overrepresented in U.S. prisons and jails. Factors contributing to this minority overrepresentation in our correctional systems include biases and deficiencies in our justice system, socioeconomic conditions, educational systems, and trends in family structures and instability (Devine, Coolbaugh, & Jenkins, 1998). Although African American males are so visible in our prisons, they are more likely to be a victim of violent crime than any other segment of our population. In contrast, the correctional staff and healthcare professionals caring for correctional populations are predominantly white.

African Americans account for over 50% of the correctional population and Hispanics represent 15% of those incarcerated, far exceeding their numbers across the nation. In predominantly Hispanic or African American communities, these statistics are even higher (Harrison &

Beck, 2005). Correctional communities solidify segregation of racial and ethnic minorities, increasing opportunities for friction and suspicion based on racial and ethnic identity and differences.

Growing numbers of non-English-speaking offenders from ethnically isolated Asian or Middle Eastern communities present special needs. Restricted financing for prisons and jails and difficulty recruiting a diverse workforce in corrections limits the ability to provide multilingual services.

The Elderly

The elderly (those 55 years of age and older) represent a growing population in correctional settings. Growing numbers of elderly in prisons are the result of 1) increasing crime among those over 50; 2) the gradual aging of society from which the offenders come; 3) a trend toward longer sentences, especially for violent offenders with previous offenses; and 4) the gradual accumulation of older habitual offenders in prison. Similar to overrepresentation in other prison age groups, elderly offenders serving life sentences or long sentences tend to be African American (Neeley, Addison, & Craig-Moreland, 1997; Harrison & Beck, 2005).

Common characteristics among elderly offenders include physical impairments and chronic illnesses, a lack of sustained contact with family or regular visitation, and a lack of interest in rehabilitation programs. Elderly offenders may have chronic, pervasive stress levels that are subsumed under a stoic or tough outward appearance and behavior, particularly if they have been institutionalized for a long period of time. Dealing with the threat or experience of violence present in correctional settings can be especially difficult for this population (Parrish, 2003; Smyer, Gragert, & LaMere, 1997; Yates & Gillespie, 2000).

The Chronically Ill

The growth of HIV and AIDS among prison offenders is a serious health-care problem facing the United States. Positive HIV seroprevalence rates vary from region to region, from 2.1% to 7.6% of all men and between 2.5% and 14.7% of women (Day, 2004; Seiter & Kadela, 2003). HIV appears to be spreading in prison through homosexual activity, intravenous drug use, and the sharing of tainted tattoo and hypodermic needles. Most offenders report high-risk behaviors before entering prison, especially intravenous drug use. Most reports indicate that HIV transmission within prisons is minimal (Macalino, 2004). Often offenders who are HIV positive do not have their confidentiality protected. Knowledge of their status results in avoidance by staff and offenders, and denial of certain jobs, home furloughs, and visitation.

Other special populations can include those with terminal illnesses, those living on death row, and political offenders, who, by nature of their unique circumstances and backgrounds, each provide distinct cultural characteristics and considerations. They are often grouped together, segregated by the nature of their offenses, and therefore bonded by collective notions of victimization or unjust treatment. Many offenders with chronic illnesses will eventually be reintegrated into society after incarceration. The period of incarceration provides an opportunity for effective treatment and illness management.

The moral and social philosophies associated with the definition of crime and the associated appropriate and proportionate justice response are integral to the understanding of individual and collective healthcare response to patient needs among offenders (National Commission on Correctional Health Care, 2002c).

CULTURALLY COMPETENT NURSING IN CORRECTIONAL SETTINGS

Nurses working in corrections must adapt to the culture and mandates of the setting. Healthcare priorities are subsumed into the larger mandate for confinement and punishment, and resources for rehabilitation are often diverted to structures and staff focusing on security. Nursing efforts must be highly focused and clearly substantiated through accurate and reliable assessments of patient needs that incorporate advanced health assessment skills. The use of master assessments of physical, psychosocial, and cultural indicators is essential for efficient and effective care. The preservation of ethnic identity and personal self-concept is a right that must be sustained within the confines and restrictions of correctional environments that demand close inspection of and impose restrictions on verbal and nonverbal communication. Acceptance of authority, particularly from female correctional officers or healthcare staff; ways in which stigma or shame are dealt with; and the struggle to maintain individual identity, particularly in the area of healthcare choice, need to be included in any health promotion plan of care (DuPont & Halasz, 1998).

Specific strategies for the implementation of culturally competent care include the assessment of the cultural groups present in the correctional facility and an inventory of practices, beliefs, and needs affecting health behavior that distinguish those groups. Advanced practice correctional nurses are expected to provide leadership in this endeavor and provide education to healthcare personnel. An understanding and respect for differences, although critical to cultural competency, is difficult to promote in an environment that emphasizes conformity. Advanced assessment skills are essential to quality health care for offenders in correctional settings and must be grounded in awareness of population characteristics, differentiating them from myths about inmates. Biases toward prisoners greatly impact the care they receive while in correctional settings and revolve around several myths. Many people believe that all prisoners are dangerous and need constant surveillance and restraints, despite the fact that most prisoners have not committed violent crimes. Additionally, a myth exists that all offenders are drug seekers, noncompliant with medications, not interested in health, malingerers, and manipulative. Although it is true that some inmates exhibit these characteristics, it is not the case with all, and designation of such should be on the basis of assessment and evidence, not myth. It is essential that advanced practice correctional nurses understand these labels and reserve them for appropriate circumstances, based on evidence collected in health history and assessment.

Drug seeking behavior is a common phenomenon in correctional settings. Requests for narcotics or psychotropic medications are accompanied by common complaints of back pain, headache, extremity pain, and dental pain. Without a thorough history and assessment, the nurse will not be able to confirm the frequency of those requests and physical complaints not supported by physical assessment findings. The challenge to the advanced practice correctional nurse will be to accurately assess the need for medication and appropriately avoid rewarding drug seeking behavior, while avoiding using the label "drug seeking" without sufficient cause. Many inmates will present physical or psychological symptoms in an effort to avoid work details or other undesirable assignments, to escape exploitation by other inmates, to defy or control the "system" and its authority figures, or to self-manage undiagnosed psychological disorders or substance abuse withdrawal.

Manipulation is a way of life and a primary means of goal-oriented behavior and satisfaction for those with whom many advanced practice correctional nurses work. A behavior common in personality disordered individuals in secure settings, manipulation has primary aims of securing privileges to which individuals are not eligible, escaping boredom, establishing or maintaining a sense of power, and sustaining inappropriate boundaries for self-image and self-esteem. Mastering techniques for recognizing manipulation and dealing positively with this behavior is essential in forensic nursing. It is important for the nurse not to take manipulation personally, because one of the most powerful outcomes of manipulation is to make someone in authority angry, self-conscious, or fearful.

Although manipulation cannot be totally eradicated among the incarcerated, it can be managed. Systematic, thorough assessment based on fact and observation, along with consistency in the application of policies and procedures, is crucial to limiting the impact of manipulation among inmates. The use of a matter-of-fact, nonjudgmental approach to interactions with inmates strengthens interventions aimed at understanding what the inmate hopes to achieve and how he or she understands his or her acts of manipulation. Underlying effective nursing responses to manipulation is the ability to communicate the absence of power, the need, or the interest in assisting the inmate to achieve the goals of manipulation.

Malingering is the fabrication or exaggeration of psychiatric symptoms occurring in association with a clearly identifiable secondary gain (American Psychiatric Association, 1994). Malingering is characterized by significant exaggeration or faking of psychiatric symptoms for a conscious gain or purpose; the malingerer is fully conscious of the intended purpose of personal gain or advantage. Malingering is prevalent in correctional populations, estimated to occur in 8–37% of individuals referred for pretrial evaluations and up to 46% of inmates claiming psychological impairment (Norris & May, 1998). Motivation to malinger is similar to that of manipulation and includes benefits such as avoidance of responsibility or punishment, better living quarters, medications, declaration of incompetence to stand trial or the insanity defense, or obtaining medical benefits after release from prison. Screening measures specific for malingering are being used with some success in correctional settings and are more successful in identifying malingerers than a structured clinical interview, distinguishing most malingerers in correctional settings as less educated and younger than nonmalingerers (Hall, 2000; Hall & Pritchard, 1996; Norris & May; Reid, 2000). This finding may imply that malingering is an adaptation tool for those less capable of sophisticated decision making and those who are more impulsive. Often malingerers begin malingering before they are incarcerated, subsequently obtaining a psychiatric diagnosis that is assumed to be a preexisting condition upon admission to the correctional facility. Familiarity with current specialized screening and assessment tools is an essential skill of advanced practice correctional nurses in order to determine the correlation between inmate patterns of behavior and complaints of psychiatric illness.

Factitious disorders are similar to malingering in that the offender presents physical or psychological symptoms in order to assume the sick role and associated benefits. Unlike the malingerer, who is conscious and aware of the intended benefit to be derived from their feigned illness, the person experiencing a factitious disorder is not aware of the drive underlying the intent to mislead (American Psychiatric Association, 1994). Although the act of malingering can sometimes be adaptive, as in the case of hostages, the absence of external incentives for the presenting symptoms in factitious disorders always signifies psychopathology. It is important to understand that, in the correctional setting, the object or goal, whether conscious or not, often is placement in the healthcare unit and the adoption of the sick role as a means to receive caring that is not present in other correctional settings. Although there is no known cause for factitious disorder, some theories suggest a history of abuse or neglect as a child, or a history of frequent illnesses that required hospitalization, may be factors in the development of the disorder. Advanced practice correctional nurses have the responsibility to ensure that health history forms and data collection include nursing assessment of history of abuse in order to affirm or add to the findings of other healthcare providers. Significant numbers of female offenders express their disorder as Munchausen Syndrome by Proxy, an extreme form of the disorder manifested by the creation of symptoms in their children, particularly infants, in order to present to healthcare providers as a heroic and tragic parent figure. Held in particular disdain by other offenders and staff, these patients present challenges for the advanced practice correctional nurse in terms of effective management of staff and inmate behavior as well as establishment of therapeutic care (Eminson & Atkin, 2000; Maden, 1996).

Nurses must work with correctional staff and administration to identify appropriate opportunities for individualization of healthcare interventions and link these to an overall plan for health promotion for offenders and staff within the institution. Acknowledging the importance of staff health and concerns is an important first step to gaining the cooperation needed to implement individualized care for offenders. Opportunities to substantiate outcomes of nursing intervention with scientific or databased information can be a powerful tool in enlisting support. The nurse who links the provision of privacy during medication administration and teaching offenders about their treatments and medications with decreased problems of noncompliance and/or disruptive behavior during pill call will be very successful in getting the administration's attention. Nurses must recognize the importance of their roles as *continuous* change agents.

Over 80% of all offenders will return to the communities from which they came, having served their time. There has been steady growth in the offender populations with special needs such as the mentally ill, women, and the elderly. Responsibilities of the advanced practice correctional nurse include the discharge planning and case management of offenders, particularly those with chronic physical and mental health illnesses. Among successful approaches used to promote health in community-based offenders is the Girls Assets Program, a combination of therapy and mentoring used to decrease recidivism among at-risk youthful offenders (Eels, 2003; Evans, 2003). The nurse must build documentation of assets and resources for the offender within the correctional setting and in the community into which the offender will go upon release. Assets can be grouped into two categories: external and internal. External assets include positive resources such as social support systems, activities and goals for empowerment, setting boundaries, and assistance for time and resource management. Internal assets include those values and skills the offender has acquired in order to promote his or her health and to maintain medical compliance.

The experience offenders take with them, including the type and nature of health care provided to them, can be a determinant of whether or not they re-offend. Culturally competent nursing care in corrections is dependent on the incorporation of fundamental principles: inclusiveness, reflecting the diversity of the community served, valuing cultural differences, employment equity, service equity, and involving everyone in the setting.

The first obligation of the culturally competent correctional nurse is to become exposed to information about and opportunities to be involved with the cultures represented in the correctional setting. Accepting the value of differences is a personal decision necessary to cultural competency and precedes all other professional development. The culturally competent nurse recognizes the personal responsibility and accountability for continuous professional development through formal educational opportunities or informal lectures and events. The nurse must organize information about cultural groups for whom care is provided and document standards of care incorporating interventions that have meaning specific to individual cultural considerations. Hiring practices and the recruiting of new staff should be guided by a commitment to inform and educate potential staff regarding the cultural groups represented in the institution (American Correctional Association, 1993; DuPont & Halasz, 1998).

Language, customs, and practices should be maintained as much as possible, within the security restrictions of the setting. Healthcare staff must work with correctional staff to identify maladaptive or dysfunctional cultural behavioral patterns, such as tattooing or gang raping as an initiation to a gang, and target them for extinction through therapeutic as well as policy mechanisms.

Core symbols of culture need to be examined within each cultural group to verify how they are acted out in the correctional setting. Issues of collectivism, individuality, positivism, genuineness, assertiveness, orientation to time, and secrecy are common themes distinguishing cultural groups that are modified in correctional settings. Nonviolent posturing as a form of emotional expressiveness among African Americans must be distinguished from intent to act. Understanding that Hispanic male youths often act out aggressively rather than withdraw when they are depressed is essential to assessment of emotional and psychiatric state. Additionally, understanding that among Muslims, Islam is always the determining factor in decision-making processes and there is no distinction between secular and religious life, is critical to explaining why even small concessions to dietary or dress rituals demanded in correctional settings is intolerable and is a source for violent response (American Correctional Association, 1993).

Nurses must break down barriers to culturally competent care from within their own ranks, learning how to recognize and confront prejudice, stereotyping, and discrimination. We need to think about ways we apply "profiling" to groups of offenders or clients, whether it be assuming all victims of rape should be willing to report the assault, or assuming that nurses who work with drug addicts must themselves be in recovery. Nurses must identify sources of "friendly fire" in the form of biased language, grouping people as having a characteristic simply because of where they come from, mislabeling groups, addressing persons in a familiar way when is it not warranted, and using inappropriate titles and terms. Nurses must learn to apply principles of physical and psychosocial assessment in a culturally competent way, particularly in corrections where eye contact may be discouraged not only as part of cultural heritage, but also as learned behavior initiated by expectations of punitive correctional staff. Recognizing when behavior is consistent with the correctional culture and when it is a product of another cultural context is a difficult and ongoing process that correctional nurses must master. Even nursing goals for patient behavior may be inconsistent with expectations of the prison culture, such as promoting trust and openness during psychiatric encounters, when this behavior may actually be life-threatening in the correctional setting.

Finally, nurses must take an environmental inventory of the ecological factors affecting and predominating in the correctional setting. Nurses need to take the lead in asking the questions that raise awareness of and appreciation for the need for cultural competency.

PROFESSIONAL CORRECTIONAL NURSING DEVELOPMENT

The development of programs for discipline-specific training and continuing education for correctional nursing staff is a major responsibility for advanced practice correctional nurses. Topics for continuing professional development should be based on a needs assessment specifically identifying competencies and interests directly associated with nursing productivity, positive nursing intervention outcomes, nursing work satisfaction, and the expectations of those interfacing with nursing. Among topics common for development are physical and mental healthcare issues of offenders, especially special populations, and the role of the professional forensic nurse working in correctional facilities. Issues such as ethical/legal implications of practice in correctional settings, acute and chronic disease management, and special vulnerabilities in the areas of communicable diseases, suicide and self-destructive behavior prevention, and assaultive behavior management are high priorities in correctional settings. More training is needed in mental health issues related to offenders and the relationship of race and ethnicity to mental health assessments, which are important education areas. The mastery of boundaries of practice and relationships with correctional staff and the offender are recurrent dilemmas for correctional nurses. Primary learning needs are centered on the correctional culture and how nurses reconcile the demands of the correctional setting with their professional code (Hufft & Peternelj-Taylor, 2000). In addition, there is a need for strong leadership in correctional nursing, reflected in the feelings among nurses that they are undervalued and neglected in major decision making related to nursing services. Advancing the skill sets in areas of leadership, management, and administration are essential to advancing the correctional nursing role.

Expectations for professional performance emphasize evidence-based practice, and individual and departmental accountability in corrections. Major cultural changes for the nursing staff are outcomes of professional role modeling:

1. Policies and procedures are revised to conform to national standards, rather than focusing on specific institutional correctional preferences.
2. Nursing roles are defined in terms of the healthcare agency rather than correctional confinement or control goals.
3. Relationships with correctional officers are redefined from subservient to collaborative.
4. Institutional policies are not an excuse for lack of professional accountability.
5. Success is defined in terms of healthcare outcomes of offenders, rather than in terms of logistical expediency or security goals.

These changes are a necessary foundation for the transition to better health care for the offenders and part of the overall change in values that are the responsibility of advanced practice nurses in corrections. Although security and confinement will always be very important factors affecting the healthcare delivery system, the roles of correctional officers and nursing staff must be clarified, freeing nurses to care for and be responsive to the needs of the people in their care.

SUMMARY

Advanced practice correctional nurses must intervene sensitively, creatively, and responsibly on the basis of scientific and evidence-based knowledge, and must also extend their roles to include that of personal advocate for competent care for offenders in correctional facilities. Their roles include development and implementation of correctional healthcare policy, development of organizational culture to promote collaborative models of healthcare delivery, advancement of ethical and legal nursing practice, development of professional nursing roles within correctional facilities, and facilitation of diversity and culturally competent health promotion and disease prevention. Increasing inmate satisfaction and the effectiveness of health care received in correctional facilities may provide a basis for offenders trusting and participating in healthcare strategies and self-care health promotion during their incarceration and after their release.

Advanced practice correctional nurses are in a unique position to provide leadership in the efficient and effective implementation of nursing and healthcare standards in correctional settings. New standards for health services in prisons and jails were published by the National Commission on Correctional Health Care (NCCHC) in 2002, which distinguished between prisons and jail settings and emphasized educational material enabling facilities to assess their compliance with the standards using the same indicators used by NCCHC accreditation surveyors. Advanced practice correctional nurses are well prepared to serve as surveyors for the NCCHC.

Internal classification systems, those used to determine appropriate custody, housing, and programming within a facility, use policies and procedures for screening and evaluating prisoners who are management problems and those who have special needs. In particular, these criteria and procedures are used to assign offenders to administrative segregation, disciplinary segregation, and protective custody. Mental health and medical health care units must be part of the system. Advanced practice correctional nurses involved in the assessment of offenders for classification not only will provide expert administration of reliable and valid instruments, but also will advise and collaborate in decisions regarding options for using the results of such assessments in determining appropriate designation of offenders, ensuring involvement of the inmate in the process. The nurse should ensure that the inmate is informed and has a copy of the classification assessment. In addition, the nurse should ensure periodic review of any nursing assessments and be involved in the design and implementation of the classification process as it involves nursing and health assessments (Schneider, 2002).

Managing risk in a correctional healthcare setting is an especially important priority for advanced practice nurses due to the increased threats to security and the unique nature of the offenders, including the health risks they present. Significantly higher proportions of inmate populations, as compared to nonprison populations, are exposed to HIV and tuberculosis, experience substance abuse and physical trauma, and have mental disorders. Suicide rates in jails have been reported as high as 40% (Goss et al., 2002; Robertson, 2004). The advanced practice role includes surveillance, infection control, and risk management roles and the implementation of a systematic approach to problem identification and analysis of adverse events related to correctional health care (Valente, 2002). Suicide, exacerbations of psychiatric conditions, undetected or delayed diagnoses of medical conditions, and detection of active tuberculosis represent major foci of risk management programs in correctional settings. The advanced practice correctional nurse uses the public health model to construct nursing policies and procedures to document critical health events occurring in inmate and staff populations.

Advanced practice correctional nursing roles include that of mentor. Designed to improve the professional lives of correctional healthcare staff, mentoring focuses on the support, counsel, friendship, reinforcement, and constructive feedback necessary for successful professional practice. The Academy of Correctional Health Professionals has established a formal mentoring program and provides training at national meetings (National Commission on Correctional Health Care, 2002). Nurses in advanced practice are expected to possess skills in listening and demonstrating caring for coworkers. Bringing new generations of correctional nurses into professional and social maturity occurs best through close and nurturing relationships with experienced expert nurses who not only provide practical information related to the policies and procedures of secure settings, but also provide guidance and modeling of evidence-based approaches to analytical problem solving and culture building. Building trusting relationships with correctional officers and establishing meaningful boundaries with staff and offenders is essential to successful professional practice. A correctional nursing mentor focuses on his or her career and institutional goals while maintaining professional standards of practice and upholding ethical and intellectual principles supporting nursing.

Privacy provisions established by the Health Insurance Portability and Accountability Act of 1996 (HIPAA) represent a unique challenge for correctional healthcare settings (Orr & Hellerstein, 2002). Impacting primarily the operations and finances of healthcare providers and payers, HIPAA privacy requirements regarding general consent and the privacy practice notification specifically exclude offenders. Translating these protections into best practices reflecting appropriate policies for correctional healthcare settings requires analysis and input from advanced practice nurses.

Establishing a therapeutic relationship with any patient can be a challenge, particularly if that individual has a mental disorder or is otherwise suspicious or paranoid. When the patient is an inmate, challenges to the therapeutic alliance include suspiciousness associated with prison culture and inmate socialization, and conditions imposed on professional and personal boundaries related to security. Advanced practice nurses are prepared to present nursing models of care that incorporate strategies for adapting and caring for unique interpersonal relationships represented in the correctional population.

In extraordinary circumstances, patients are informed specifically not to engage in treatment, as in the case of sex offenders, because information revealed to counselors or nurses can be used to confine them in a post-release treatment facility. Since 1999, the U.S. Supreme Court has allowed sex offenders to be confined in treatment facilities after their release from prison, if it is determined they are at risk for re-offense. There is no current data on how many sex offenders in correctional facilities refuse treatment or reasons why those refusing treatment do so. Advanced practice nurses are positioned and educated to collaborate with other healthcare providers to deliver therapeutic programs for special populations such as sex offenders.

Correctional health care provides a means to advance the public health agenda by caring for those who are among society's most vulnerable. Advanced practice correctional nurses are positioned to create and manage a closed healthcare system in which they can identify and treat high risk patients, monitor their care, and support lifestyle changes. Advanced practice correctional nurses have the skills and knowledge needed to advance nursing care as the most powerful change agent in correctional settings (Vitucci, 2001). Ultimately, the health care of the community is positively impacted.

QUESTIONS FOR DISCUSSION

1. What does the dress code adopted in a correctional setting, for staff as well as offenders, say about us?
2. How do the furnishings and layout of the physical setting affect emotions, perceptions, stress, and functional ability to carry out daily routines?
3. What does the vocabulary we use in the correctional setting say about our attitudes, beliefs, and philosophy of nursing care? Does it matter whether we use the terms *inmate, patient, client, youth, felon,* and *perp*?
4. What does the history of the institution tell you about how we nurse those in our care? What roles have nurses taken? What part of the budget has been given to nursing? At what meetings or activities have nurses regularly been included? Where and when are nurses mentioned in official documents? How often and in what context do nurses interact with administration?

REFERENCES

American Academy of Pediatrics. (2001). Health care for children and adolescents in the juvenile correction care system policy statement (RE0021). *Pediatrics, 107*(4), 799–803.

American Association of Colleges of Nursing. (January 2002). *AACN white paper: Hallmarks if the professional practice environment.* Retrieved May 16, 2005, from http://www.aacn.nche.edu/Publications/positons/hallmarks.htm.

American Association of Colleges of Nursing. (2002). *The essentials of master's education for advanced practice nursing.* Washington, DC: Author.

American Association of Critical Care Nurses. (2003). *What is an advanced practice nurse?* Retrieved June 12, 2003, from http://www.aacn.org/AACN/Advanced.nsf.

American Correctional Association. (2003). *Understanding cultural diversity.* Lanham, MD: Author.

American Nurses Association. (1998). *Culturally competent assessment for family violence.* Washington, DC: Author.

American Nurses Association. (1998). *Legal aspects of standards and guidelines for clinical nursing practice.* Washington, DC: Author.

American Psychiatric Association. (1994). *Diagnostic and statistical manual of mental disorders* (4th ed.). Washington, DC: Author.

American Psychiatric Association. (2000). *Psychiatric services in jails and prisons* (2nd ed.). Washington, DC: Author.

Anno, B.J. (1991). *Prison health care: Guidelines for the management of an adequate delivery system.* Chicago: National Commission on Correctional Health Care.

Anno, J. & Dubler, N.N. (2002). Confidentiality in corrections: Examining the ethical issues. *CorrectCare, 16*(4), 12.

Bachmeier, K. (2003). Addressing quality health care in the correctional setting. *Corrections Today, 65*(6), 76–77.

Blair, P. (2002). Correctional nursing: What's wrong with this picture? *CorrectCare, 16*(4), 8.

Bowling, M.A. (2003). Root cause analysis: A systematic approach to managing risk. *CorrectCare, 17*(2), 1, 18.

Bradley, J. & Kalfs, E.M. (2003). Identification and management of chronic medical problems in juveniles. *Corrections Today, 65*(6), 86–89.

Canino, I.A. & Spurlock, J. (2000). *Culturally diverse children and adolescents: Assessment, diagnosis and treatment.* Amherst, MA: BOSC Books.

Centers for Disease Control (2003). Routine HIV testing of inmates in correctional facilities. Divisions of HIV/AIDS Prevention retrieved January 4, 2005, from http://www.cdc.gov/hiv/partners/Interim/routinetest.htm.

Coolman, A. (2003). Sexual misconduct in women's facilities: The current climate. *Corrections Today, 65*(6), 118–120.

Corrections Today (2003). U.S. prison population rises 2.6 percent. *Corrections Today, 65*(6), 13.

Day, R.F. (October 2004). HIV/AIDS in prison: Crisis of the confined. *Body Positive.* Retrieved June 30, 2005, from http://www.thebody.com/bp/oct04/prison.html.

Devine, P., Coolbaugh, K., & Jenkins, S. (December 1998). Disproportionate minority confinement: Lessons learned from five states. *Juvenile Justice Bulletin (NCJ 173420)*. Washington, DC: Office of Juvenile Justice and Delinquency Prevention, Office of Justice Programs, U.S. Department of Justice.

Dolan, L., Kolthoff, K., Schreck, M., Smilanich, P., & Todd, R. (2003). Gender-specific treatment for clients with co-occurring disorders. *Corrections Today, 65*(6), 100–107.

Dumond, R.W. (2000). Inmate sexual assault: The plague that persists. *The Prison Journal, 80*(4), 407–414.

DuPont, K. & Halasz, I.M. (1998). *Diversity: Communicating effectively: Professionalism in corrections.* Lanham, MD: American Correctional Association.

Eels, S. (2003). Providing therapeutic mentoring. *Corrections Today, 65*(6), 20–22.

Egley, A., Jr. (2005). *Highlights of the 2002–2003 national youth gang surveys. OJJDP Fact Sheet.* Washington, DC: U.S. Department of Justice.

Egley, A., Jr. & Arjunan, M. (2002). *Highlights of the 2000 national youth gang survey.* OJJDP Fact Sheet #04. Washington, DC: Office of Juvenile Justice and Delinquency Programs.

Eminson, D.M. & Atkin, B.L. (2000). The dangerousness of parents who have abnormal illness behavior. *Child Abuse Review, 9*(1), 68–73.

Esbensen, F. (2000). *Preventing adolescent gang involvement bulletin. Youth Gang Series.* Washington, DC: U.S. Department of Justice. Office of Justice Programs, Office of Juvenile Justice and Prevention Programs.

Evans, D.G. (2003). New AAPA president faces today's challenges. *Corrections Today, 65*(6), 24–27.

Feldman, M.D., Ford, C.V., & Reinhold, T. (1994). *Patient or pretender: Inside the strange world of factitious disorder.* New York: John Wiley.

Fletcher, B.R., Shaver, L.D., & Moon D.G. (Eds.). (1993). *Women prisoners: A forgotten population.* Westport, CT: Praeger.

Goffman, E. (1961). On the characteristics of total institutions. In D.R. Cressey (Ed.). *The Prison.* New York: Holt, Rinehart & Winston.

Goss, R.J., Peterson, K., Smith, L.W., Kalb, K., & Brodey, B.B. (2002). Characteristics of suicide attempts in a large urban jail system with an established suicide prevention program. *Psychiatric Services, 53*(5), 574–579.

Greenfield, L.A. & Snell, T.L. (1999). *Bureau of Justice Statistics: Women offenders.* Washington, DC: U.S. Department of Justice

Hall, H.V. (2000). *Detecting malingering and deception: Forensic distortion analysis* (2nd ed.). Los Angeles: CRC Press.

Hall, H.V. & Pritchard, D.A. (1996). *Detecting malingering and deception: Forensic distortion analysis (FDA).* Delray Beach, FL: St. Lucie Press.

Harrison, P. & Beck, A.J. (2003). *Bureau of Justice statistics, prisoners in 2002.* Washington, DC: US Department of Justice.

Harrison, P.M. & Beck, A.J. (2005). *Prison and jail inmates at midyear 2004.* Washington, DC: Bureau of Justice Statistics, Office of Justice Programs, U.S. Department of Justice.

Heidensohn, F. (1995). *Women and crime* (2nd ed.). New York: New York University Press.

Hofacre, R. (2003). The correctional health care debate. *Corrections Today, 65*(6), 8.

Howard League (2003). *A short history of prison.* London: The Howard League for Penal Reform Publications.

Howell, J.C. & Lynch, J.P. (2000). Youth gangs in schools. Young Gang Series Bulletin. Washington, DC: U.S. Department of Justice, Office of Justice Programs, Office of Juvenile Justice and Delinquency Prevention.

Howell, J.C. (2000). *Young gang programs and strategies.* Summary. Washington, DC: U.S. Department of Justice, Office of Justice Programs, Office of Juvenile Justice and Delinquency Prevention.

Hufft, A.G. (2004). Supporting psychosocial adaptation for the pregnant adolescent in corrections. *MCN, American Journal for Maternal/Child Nursing, 29*(2), 122–127.

Hufft, A.G. & Kite, M. (2003). Vulnerable populations and cultural perspectives for nursing care in correctional systems. *Journal of Multicultural Nursing & Health, 9*(1), 18–26.

Hufft, A. & Peternelj-Taylor, C. (2000). Forensic nursing. In J.T. Catalano (Ed.), *Contemporary Professional Nursing* (2nd ed.). Philadelphia: Davis.

Jamison, R. (2002). The punishing decade: Prison and jail estimates at the millennium. Retrieved from http://www.cjcj.org/pubs/punishing/punishing.html.

Kay, S. (1991). *The constitutional dimensions of an inmate's right to health care.* Chicago: National Commission on Correctional Health Care.

Lock, J. (2003). Preventing violent incidents in a maximum-security forensic psychiatric hospital. Retrieved July 10, 2003, from http://psychservices. pscyhiatryonline.org/cgi/content/full/50/11/1481.

Lockwood, D. (1978). *Sexual aggression among male prisoners.* Ann Arbor, MI: University Microfilms International.

Macalino, G.E., et al. (2004). Prevalence and incidence of HIV, hepatitis B virus, and hepatitis C virus infections among males in Rhode Island prisons. *American Journal Public Health, 94*(7), 1218–1223.

Maddow, R., Phil, D., & Bick, J. (2003). The management of end stage liver disease in the correctional setting. *HIV Education Project, 6*(12), 1–8.

Maden, T. (1996). *Women, prisons, and psychiatry: Mental disorder behind bars.* Oxford: Butterworth-Heinemann.

Maeve, M.K. (1997). Nursing practice with incarcerated women: Caring within mandated alienation. *Issues in Mental Health Nursing, 18*(5), 495–510.

Marable, M. (2000). Racism, prisons, and the future of Black America. Along the Color Line. Retrieved September 21, 2003, from www.manningmarable.net.

McClelland, G. M., Teplin, L.A., Abram, K.M., & Jacobs, N. (2002). HIV and AIDS risk behaviors among female jail detainees in Chicago: Implications for public health policy. *American Journal of Public Health, 92*(5), 818–825.

Minor, M. (2002). Understanding prison health care: Fostering competence and compassion in treating prisoners. Retrieved August 1, 2003, from http://movementbuiding.org/prisonhealth/index.html.

National Commission on Correctional Health Care (2001). *Women's health care in correctional settings position statement.* Chicago: NCCHC.

National Commission on Correctional Health Care. (2002a). *Standards for Health Services in Prisons.* Chicago: NCCHC.

National Commission on Correctional Health Care. (2002b). *Standards for Health Services in Jails.* Chicago: NCCHC.

National Commission on Correctional Health Care. (2002c). *The health status of soon-to-be-releates inmates: A report to congress.* Retrieved January 19, 2005, from http://www.ncchc.org/pubs_stbr.html.

National Commission on Correctional Health Care. (October 2002). Mentoring: A great way to give back to your profession. *CorrectCare,* 4.

National Institute of Corrections (2002). *Special issues in corrections: Women's prisons and special prison populations.* Retrieved on June 2, 2003, from www.nicic.org/pubs/2002/018602.pdf.

National Institute of Corrections (2003). Frequently asked questions. Retrieved July 15, 2003, from http://www.nicic.org.FAQ.aspx.

Neeley, C., Addison, L., & Craig-Moreland, D. (1997). Elderly offenders: the forgotten minority. *Corrections Today, 44,* 14–16.

Norris, M.P. & May, M.C. (1998). Screening for malingering in a correctional setting. *Law and Human Behavior, 22*(3), 315–323.

Orr, D. & Hellerstein, D. (2002). Controversy, confusion herald HIPAA. *CorrectCare, 16*(4), 1, 22.

Paris, J.E. (2003). Overcoming barriers to correctional physician productivity. *Corrections Today, 65*(6), 72–75.

Parrish, A. (2003). Reaching behind the bars. *Nursing Older People, 15*(3), 10–13.

Peternelj-Taylor, C.A. & Hufft, A.G. (1997). Forensic psychiatric nursing. In B.S. Johnson (Ed.), *Psychiatric-Mental Health Nursing: Adaptation and Growth* (4th ed.). (pp. 771–785). Philadelphia: Lippincott-Raven.

Peternelj-Taylor, C.A. & Johnson, R.L. (1995). Serving time: Psychiatric mental health nursing in corrections. *Journal of Psychosocial Nursing and Mental Health Services, 33*(8), 12–19.

Peters, R.H., Greenbaum, P.E., Greenbaum, M.I., Steinberg, Carter, C.R., Ortiz, M.M., Fry, B.C., & Valle, S.K. (2000). Effectiveness of screening instruments in detecting use disorders among prisoners. *Journal of Substance Abuse Treatment, 18*(4), 349–358.

Pollock, J.M. (1998). *Counseling women in prison.* Thousand Oaks, CA: Sage.

Potter, R.H. & Tewksbury, R. (2005). Sex and prisoners: Criminal justice contributions to a public health issue. *Journal of Correctional Health Care, 11*(2), 171–190.

Ramsbotham, D. (1999). Report on a full announced inspection of HMP Exeter. Retrieved January 14, 2005, from http://www.homeoffice.gov.uk/docs/exetcpe.html.

Reid, W.H. (2000). Malingering. *Law and Psychiatry, 6*(4), 226–229.

Robertson, J.E. (Summer 2004). Inmate suicide litigation redux. *Special Issue: Jail Suicide/Mental Health Update, 13*(1), 1–20.

Sable, M.R., Fieberg, J.R., Martin, S.L., & Kupper, L.L. (1999). Violence victimization experiences of pregnant prisoners. *American Journal of Orthopsychiatry, 69*(3), 392–397.

Schmalleger, F. (1999). *Criminal justice today: An introductory text for the twenty-first century* (5th ed.). Upper Saddle River, NJ: Prentice Hall.

Schneider, J.W. (2002). Managing inmate populations. *Correctional News, 8*(6), 20–21.

Seiter, R.P. & Kadela, K.R. (2003). Prisoner reentry: What works, what does not, and what is promising. *Crime and Delinquency, 49*(3), 1–7.

Smyer, T., Gragert, M.D., & LaMere, S. (1997). Stay safe! Stay Healthy! Surviving old age in prison. *Journal of Psychosocial Nursing & Mental Health Services, 35*(9), 10–17.

Tahir, L. (2003). Supervision of special needs inmates by custody staff. *Corrections Today, 65*(6), 110–111.

Thomas, R.L. (2003). Bioethics and corrections: An experiment in bioethics in the Florida Department of Corrections. *Corrections Today, 65*(6), 66–71.

Thornberry, T.P., Huizinga, D., & Loeber, R. (2004). The causes and correlates studies: Findings and policy implications. *Juvenile Justice, 9*(1), 3–19.

Toch, H. (1992). *Living in prison: The ecology of survival.* Washington, DC: American Psychological Association.

U.S. Department of Justice. (2001). *About the federal bureau of prisons.* Lompoc, CA: Federal Bureau of Prison Industries.

U.S. Department of Justice. (2001). Criminal offenders Statistics. Retrieved November 9, 2003, from http://www.ojp.usdoj.gov/bjs/crimoff.htm.

U.S. Department of Justice. (2002). *Bureau of Justice Statistics: Demographic trends in jail populations.* Retrieved September 21, 2003, from http://www.ojp.usdoj. gov/bjs/glance/tables/jailagtab.

U.S. Department of Justice. (2003). *Corrections statistics.* Retrieved September 20, 2003, from http://www.ojp.usdoj.gov/bjs/correct.htm.

U.S. Department of Justice. (2003). *Nation's prison and jail population 2002.* Retrieved May 16, 2005 from http://www.ojp.usdoj.gov/bjs/pub/press/ pjim02pr.htm.

Valente, S. (2002). Overcoming barriers to suicide risk management, *Journal of Psychosocial Nursing and Mental Health Services, 40*(7), 22–33.

van Wormer, K. (2001). *Counseling female offenders and victims: A strengths-restorative approach.* New York: Springer Publishing.

Vitucci, N. (2001) Innovation leads to DC jail transformation. *CorrectCare, 15*(1), 1, 12.

Wells, D. (2003). Drug-assessment instruments: Making wise choices. *Corrections Today, 65*(6), 28–30.

Wright, K.N. & Wright, K.E. (1995). *Family life, delinquency, and crime: A poli-cymaker's guide.* Washington, DC: Office of Juvenile Justice and Delinquency Prevention.

Wrobleski, H.M. & Hess, K.M. (1997). *Introduction to law enforcement and criminal justice* (5th ed.). Minneapolis, MN: West Publishing.

Yates, J. & Gillespie, W. (2000). The elderly and prison policy. *Journal of Aging and Social Policy, 11*(2–3), 167–175.

Expert Witness Testimony and a Domestic Violence Paradigm

Evan Stark
Elaine M. Pagliaro

The battered woman represents a segment of the population that is among the most vulnerable, from a psychological, physical, and in many instances financial perspective. In addition, the still lingering tradition of viewing intimate partner abuse as a tolerated social phenomenon compounds the burden of proof that such a victim must produce in order to receive proper protection and justice within the court system. Thus the provision of expert testimony becomes critical to the case. This chapter seeks to highlight the conduct and importance of expert testimony through compelling case studies of actual instances of woman battering. It also illuminates some of the negative fall-out that may result from the provision of such testimony.

CHAPTER FOCUS_____

Portions of this chapter were published previously as "Chapter 11: Preparing for Expert Testimony in Domestic Violence Cases" by Evan Stark, from *Handbook of Domestic Violence Intervention Strategies* edited by Albert R. Roberts, copyright 2002 by Oxford University Press, Inc. Used with the permission of Oxford University Press, Inc.

KEY TERMS

    battered woman syndrome (BWS)
    coercion
    criteria-based content analysis
    cultural integrity
    dangerousness assessment (DA) scale
    Daubert decision
    evidence admissibility
    expert witness
    Frye standard
    learned helplessness
    post-traumatic stress disorder
    risk assessment
    spousal assault risk assessment (SARA) tool
    Stockholm syndrome
    Wanrow instruction

INTRODUCTION

On a December evening, a distraught woman gave police in Torrington, Connecticut, a signed description of abuse by her husband, Anthony Borrelli. The statement read in part:

> . . . about 3 am. We went to bed and he began to accuse me of cheating on him. He started cutting up my clothes, underwear and things with his knife . . . cut up my license and social security card because they have my maiden name on them . . . he said he was going to tie me up and I said not to. He took a pillow and put it over my face. I couldn't breathe. I gasped for air. He let me go and took a rope and tied my hands and feet together behind my back. It hurt. He kept putting the knife on my mouth and chest while he sat on my chest and put his knees on my arms. He said he was going to kill me. He cut the top of my lip and the bottom of my lip . . . He kept saying he was going to kill me and my family, my two daughters and two sons. He got up, said it didn't matter if he went to jail—no matter how long he was in jail he would get out and kill us. He also put a lighter near my genital area . . . he had a lit cigarette which he threw on the bed. It landed next to me. I thought the bed sheets would catch on fire. He then said "I missed you," picked up the cigarette and put it on my chest . . . ." (*State v. Borrelli,* 1993, pp. 88–89)

Mr. Borrelli was charged with kidnapping, assault, criminal mischief, unlawful restraint, and threatening. At the jury trial, Mrs. Borrelli surprised the prosecution by testifying that her husband had not committed the acts she had alleged in her statement. Instead, she claimed, it was actually she who had tied up and physically abused the defendant. She also testified that she made up her initial story because she wanted to get her husband into drug treatment.

Apart from sparse physical evidence, a previous domestic violence arrest, and the "excited utterances" of Mrs. Borrelli, the police provided no independent support for the prosecutor's case. The state's attorney asked an expert specializing in domestic violence to explain to the jury what might motivate a woman in Mrs. Borrelli's situation to recant. In his testimony, the expert defined woman battering; provided general information about its incidence, demographic dimensions, and consequences; and reviewed common misconceptions about the dynamics in abusive relationships, including the myth that abuse wasn't really serious if a woman remained with the partner. He also described how the typical strategies batterers used to dominate their partners could create a hostage-like situation that caused their wives to deny, minimize, or blame themselves for abuse. The prosecutor described hypothetical situations based on the statement signed by Mrs. Borrelli and asked whether these were consistent with general knowledge in the field to link the expert testimony to Mr. Borrelli's crimes. The jury found Mr. Borrelli guilty.

On appeal, Mr. Borrelli argued that the trial court erred in admitting the expert testimony. Traditionally, the admission of expert testimony was governed by a three-part test: 1) the subject matter had to be "beyond the ken of the average laymen"; 2) the expert had to possess sufficient skill, knowledge, or experience in the field to aid the trier of fact in his search for truth; and 3) the state of the scientific knowledge involved had to be sufficiently developed to allow an expert opinion to be rendered (Strong, 1999). Borrelli's attorney insisted that neither the sociologist nor the domestic violence field, as a relatively new area of inquiry, met the "*Frye* test" for admissibility of scientific or clinical evidence (*Frye v. United States*, 1923). In a precedent-setting decision, Connecticut's highest court disagreed. Rejecting the stringent test suggested by *Frye*, it found that expert testimony was proper as long as the expert was qualified by his educational background, work experience, and/or research; the testimony focused on a subject not familiar to the average person; and it was helpful to the jury. That Connecticut ruling reinforced a Supreme Court decision made that same year in *Daubert* (*Daubert v. Merrell Dow*, 1993).

Expert testimony in criminal cases involving domestic violence is by no means uncontroversial. However, standards for expert testimony similar to those established in Connecticut make it possible for the forensic nurse and other experts to present testimony to help a judge or jury assess evidence or to correct misconceptions about various forensic specialty areas, such as woman battering and its effects. Standards for admissibility have been developed through Supreme Court and state court decisions. A discussion of those standards and how they must be satisfied to testify as an expert witness can be found in Chapter 7 of this book.

This chapter provides a broad overview of the role of the forensic nurse expert witness in criminal and civil cases. Drawing on case examples involving battering of women, the role of the expert witness, case preparation, and courtroom presentation will be addressed. In addition, some of the difficulties and dilemmas that confront the expert witness will be discussed.

ROLE OF THE EXPERT WITNESS

People who are familiar with the judicial system only through watching television or reading crime novels believe that the most important work conducted by an expert witness is in the courtroom. At that time the expert can provide the "smoking gun"—the information that the attorney can use to find the real criminal or to nail a conglomerate whose flouting of the law resulted in harm to an unsuspecting community. However, most of the work of a good expert is accomplished outside of the courtroom. Through a disciplined, scientific approach to his or her area of expertise and the case facts provided, an expert witness assists the legal team in many ways. For example, the forensic nurse consultant may provide important insight into improper procedures that led to injury of a patient in the emergency room. In addition, he or she may point out that all guidelines were properly adhered to, saving the attorney much time and energy in pursuing what would ultimately be an unsuccessful challenge in a medical malpractice case. In fact, the attorney will depend on the forensic nurse to act as a true professional, pointing out both strengths and weaknesses in a particular incident. The forensic nurse must have the knowledge necessary to support his or her viewpoint with theory and practical examples. She or he must also provide an overview of contrary opinions that may be offered in a case and the strength of those arguments. In addition, the forensic nurse must be aware of the limitations of his or her expertise. Although the expert may have sufficient knowledge to review a case, detailed scientific knowledge of other experts may be required to effectively assist the client or attorney.

How an expert witness proceeds from the first contact at the beginning of a case through testimony and any subsequent contacts about his or her involvement will ultimately determine his or her success. Table 22–1 provides a list of guidelines for the expert witness during this process. Although not exhaustive, these guidelines should provide a roadmap for the successful and ethical expert witness. The following discussion will expand on some of those points, although space does not permit a thorough treatment. Several very good references and many articles are on the market today to help the beginner become an effective and ethical witness. Expert testimony is illustrated in the second part of the chapter, which discusses the process of providing expert testimony in the area of domestic violence.

Table 22–1   Guidelines for the Expert Witness

* Discuss parameters of the case prior to case acceptance.
* Set fees and expectations in a written agreement.
* Establish limits of expertise early in case discussions.
* Review all available, pertinent case materials.
* Offer both strengths and weaknesses of the case during evaluation and discussion with client or attorney.
* Testify only after pretrial conference.
* Maintain a dispassionate, professional demeanor.
* Let the truth of your testimony speak for itself.
* Answer all appropriate questions without argument.
* Learn from each experience as an expert witness.
* Seek advice if ethical issues arise.

The Expert Witness

As stated previously, whether someone can testify in a court of law or at a legal proceeding as an expert witness is ultimately determined by the judge. Acting as gatekeeper, it is up to the judge to determine who is an "expert" and what the area of expertise is about which that person may testify. However, many experts never go to court, but provide information and services to attorneys, managers, and others responsible for handling investigations, trials, and hearings. This is a very common aspect of the expert witness experience, so it is important to consider how user groups determine who is a suitable expert for a case. It is equally important for experts to consider whether a case is suited for their particular skills and temperament.

Many expert witnesses, even when hired as full-time employees, list their general qualifications and areas of expertise in an expert witness registry or advertise in legal and bar association publications. This is an efficient and cost-effective method of reaching those people most likely to need the expert's services. Once an expert is well established in his or her field, advertising is often not necessary and the expert has more work than can be accepted. However, even the well-seasoned expert may find it necessary or desirable to expand potential clients. Because only a small amount of information, and perhaps a C.V., can be provided prior to involvement in a case, it is extremely important that the expert witness discuss his or her areas of expertise and limitations prior to accepting any case. One of the biggest mistakes some expert witnesses make is to go beyond their specializations. For example, one forensic odontologist was reported as testifying to tool marks made by a knife at the crime scene, even though he had no specific training in that area (Saviers, 2002). Unfortunately, this can happen even to people who frequently act as experts. This problem can be avoided from the beginning, however, if the expert has clearly delineated the knowledge, skills, and abilities he or she has to offer. Once the parameters have been established it is easier for the expert to maintain those boundaries. Many attorneys are not aware of the different backgrounds and training necessary for some specialties. Or they may misunderstand scientific and medical information. It is therefore up to the expert witness to explain any unique aspects of forensic nursing that are applicable in a case. For those who are employed full-time by a firm or institution, although sometimes difficult, it is still important for the expert to review the facts and to determine if it is appropriate to take on a case without assistance.

Initial Consultation

The initial consultation is a critical step for the expert witness. This initial discussion need not take a long time, but should provide the expert with sufficient information to gauge the situation and to decide if he or she is suited for the case. Because people seeking an expert often have little time and do not want to waste resources, they may provide little unsolicited information. Develop a series of questions to ask someone seeking your professional assistance. Questions such as, "How do you think I can help you?" or "What are the basic facts in dispute?" may quickly get to the heart of the matter. During an initial contact in a legal case, for example, an attorney should provide a short outline of the case, the specific expertise that is being sought, and a time estimate for the expert's work review/report and testimony, if necessary.

Often attorneys will ask colleagues for expert witness names, especially those experts who have been successful supporters and advocates for their "side." Some who require specialized expertise will go "expert shopping," seeking a witness who will support their view of a situation no matter what the facts may indicate. All experts should be wary of this possibility. You should make it clear during the initial contact that an unbiased, scientific approach to data evaluation and only appropriate testimony will be provided. For example, although the forensic nurse may be an advocate for victims of domestic violence, the attorney should not assume that this will slant her expert opinion.

If the expert cannot meet the expertise required or the time restraints presented in the initial inquiry, it is important to state that fact up front. If the time factor is critical to the case, then the expert may provide the names of people who may be more appropriate for the case needs. It is ethical behavior and proof of your professionalism to do so. Many experts get into trouble because they have case overloads and cannot complete work in a timely fashion. No matter how important an issue appears or intriguing a case may sound, if you cannot fulfill your professional obligations that information will soon become general knowledge.

If an expert is unsure about a case or may not have time for a particular case, it is usually a good idea to request further information for review and consideration prior to committing to the project. Usually the expert can be provided with materials with the understanding that those materials are confidential, even if he or she decides not to act as the expert after case evaluation.

After the basic outline of the problem has been provided, the expert should also make a clear statement about his or her fees, including any requirements if he or she needs to testify. It is difficult for some people to discuss fees, especially if they are accustomed to doing the same work for someone else at a salary or as government employees. Fees are necessary, and an expected part of dealing with an expert witness. All fees should be reasonable and customary. For example, if you normally charge $200/hour for your expert services, this would likely be considered reasonable to review case materials and consult with the attorney about your findings. However, if in a similar case involving a well-known celebrity you charged $800/hour for the same type of work, there may be some question about the ethics of your agreement. Inevitably a question concerning fees will be asked during the testimony of a private expert witness, but most jurors understand that seeking payment for one's special skills is reasonable and necessary. Usually, only when the fees appear to be unreasonable or to be influencing ("buying") the expert's testimony will the jury consider those funds a factor in the credibility of the expert witness. Once you have agreed to participate as an expert witness, the terms should be written in a letter of agreement from you, the other party, or both.

Case Review and Evaluation

The expert witness provides appropriate assistance in a case only when all relevant materials are provided from the client. Some clients will not always pass along all information in a case because they do not realize what is relevant or are in the habit of passing along only minimal information. Every expert witness should ask for all documents, interviews, photographs, depositions, and other significant material pertaining to the case or fact at issue. The expert should make a list of information not provided that might clarify points and should note all questions that arise during the case evaluation. Rules of evidence recognize that many opinions of experts rely on data other than that presented in court to reach their conclusions.

It is obviously common practice to interview a party when physical or psychological status is at issue in a case, such as with an insanity or syndrome defense. As discussed later in this chapter, several approaches exist for carrying out these interviews. No matter the approach, the effectiveness of an expert will depend on the thoroughness of his or her preparation for that interview. Appropriate documentation and notes must be maintained during this process. Some experts are afraid that notes may be subpoenaed in criminal cases. However, without such notes there may be little factual information that the expert can provide in a trial or hearing that takes place years after the evaluation. In addition, notes and other documentation provide material to refresh the recollection of the expert prior to testimony. If an expert has been objective, professional, and thorough in his or her evaluation, she or he should not be afraid to have an expert from the other side review that documentation. Often, when the forensic nurse acts as an expert the situation provides opportunities for interaction with the client or patient. Although this relationship may provide added insight for the expert and the opportunity to assist the client in many ways, the expert must be careful to maintain an unbiased approach to the case. Even if the witness is personally committed to the client, emotional separation is necessary in the courtroom to best serve the client's interests. Although some experts may find this professional separation difficult to maintain, the forensic nurse has training and experience that is especially useful in situations that require such professionalism.

After thorough evaluation and study of supporting materials, the expert witness will usually prepare a report of his or her findings. This report should answer the overall question and provide the necessary data to support his or her conclusions. This report will be the basis of the expert's subsequent testimony in most cases. Both parties in the case will be able to see those factors the expert considers significant and the logic applied when analyzing the case. Theories of outstanding experts in the field that substantiate conclusions are important to point out. In addition, when appropriate, the expert witness should point out opposing theories, especially if they may have an impact on the case if presented by opposing counsel's expert. This approach to case evaluation and report writing is an extension of the scientific objectivity that the expert must maintain throughout the case.

Expert Witness Testimony

Most cases in which an expert is involved never come to trial. The information that the expert provides in her written report may be used by the attorney to negotiate a settlement in a civil case or plea bargain before a criminal trial. As important and common as that process is, the expert should always be prepared to testify to her findings and support her conclusions on the witness stand. During oral testimony the expert has the opportunity to explain to the trier of fact opinions and interpretations of the data obtained. Prior to testifying, the expert witness should always have a pretrial conference with the attorney. Even if there have been several previous conversations concerning her report, no expert should get on the witness stand without such a meeting. The purpose of the pretrial is two-fold. First, the expert will have a final opportunity to review her or his position and highlight significant points with the attorney. The attorney should review with the expert the questions he or she will ask and make sure of the likely answer. Second, if any additional issues have arisen during the trial, the pretestimony meeting is the only way that the expert can be aware of any changes in strategy or possible unanticipated questions that opposing counsel may raise. There is nothing more frightening to the conscientious expert than an attorney who will spend little time with her before testimony; when the attorney says, "Don't worry, I know what I'm doing," the expert witness may be justified in beginning to worry!

Prior to being qualified as an expert witness by the judge, the expert will be asked a series of questions designed to outline his or her educational background, training, and experience. Questions about membership in professional organizations, publications, and faculty appointments will also be put forth. The expert should be careful not to inflate his or her qualifications in an effort to impress the court or the jury. Even small overstatements, such as claiming association with illustrious scientific leaders when having taken only a course from that expert, can be fatal to one's career. In a recent case, when the expert presented himself as having been on the faculty of a university, this statement was effectively challenged by the defense attorney who knew that the "expert" only worked under an on-site, grant-funded project. Once the facts came to light, the judge barred any further testimony and warned of possible perjury charges (*North Carolina v. Peterson,* 2003). In another instance, the state's expert in a murder trial testified that he had a master's degree; in fact, he had completed the coursework, but not his thesis and did not have a graduate-level degree.

Oral testimony is a somewhat unique situation. Although testimony provides an opportunity to educate the trier of fact to the issues and the expert's opinion, it is unlike a typical educational setting. Generally, direct testimony provides a setting in which the expert can present clearly, in his or her own way, significant data and opinions. Even on direct examination, however, the attorney controls the flow of the discussion and decides which questions will be asked in what order. With appropriate preparation and a pretrial meeting with the attorney, the expert should be able to lay out her opinion in a clear and concise manner with few interruptions.

The expert witness is usually asked to give her opinion according to reasonable scientific certainty. This terminology is sometimes difficult for the expert witness to deal with, because experts often deal with possibilities and likelihood and not certainty. When an attorney asks about "reasonable scientific certainty," this does not mean that there is no uncertainty associated with the opinion. As explained by Fields (1999), this term is usually thought of as a likelihood of more than 90%, "derived from the statistical data on the sources of measurement" and not taken as an absolute. However, it goes without saying that this certainty must be based on information gathered using practices acceptable to the relevant medical community.

Rightly or wrongly, the expert's demeanor during testimony plays a large part in his or her effectiveness. The expert does not have to maintain a solemn expression, but there are few opportunities in court to make jokes during testimony. This does not mean that the expert should be wooden or expressionless. On the contrary, the animated expert usually retains the attention of the jury. An expert's presentation style may go a long way in getting a jury to listen carefully to the expert's opinion. Usually it is more difficult for the expert who appears condescending or pompous to testify effectively. Unfortunately, the expert witness may not be aware of her or his pomposity. Using medical terminology without defining it to the jury may confuse them; explaining procedures and opinions in a condescending manner has reportedly caused juries to ignore a witness. An expert witness should seldom lose his or her temper, even when being pressured in a continuous attack by a ruthless attorney. In fact, that is usually the questioner's purpose. In such a situation, the expert actually wins high points with the jury for remaining cool under fire. Some experts who are even-tempered during direct examination have been known to become argumentative on cross. Behaving in this manner will give the impression that the witness is biased or has something to hide from the court. Remember that it is the attorney's job to represent his or her client vigorously. The witness should not take personally any attempts of the attorney to do so.

An expert witness should have an open, natural manner and look often into the eyes of the jury. This personal contact instills a feeling of trust and maintains the interest of the jury during testimony. Of course, the most important aspect of the expert's testimony is a strict adherence to an ethical code that requires scientific objectivity.

The expert testifies ostensibly because her opinion will support the side calling her to court. The expert will explain clearly any conclusions and support these with studies and facts from other experts, where appropriate. Being an advocate for a particular viewpoint does not remove the responsibility to acknowledge other possible interpretations of the same data. When asked about other theories that could be in opposition to the expert's testimony, the witness should be prepared to explain why his or her explanation or application is more reasonable under the specific case circumstances. A forensic nurse should be aware of any limitations of the tests performed or interpretations of data and the error rate associated with any statistical analyses. Similarly, the expert should be careful not to allow any previous role as an advocate to color testimony.

In *Hussen v. Commonwealth of Virginia* (1999), the sexual assault nurse examiner testified that in her opinion injuries noted during her medical examination of the victim were the result of rape. When pressed further, she stated that consensual sex was "out of the question" because injuries such as those observed did not occur when the sexual response was triggered. Although the Virginia supreme court upheld the SANE as an expert in the examination and medical evaluation of sexual assault, some of the defense community are still disturbed by her testimony. Few still argue that the judge erred when he recognized the years of experience in the emergency room and the training as a SANE that gave the forensic nurse an appropriate background as an expert. However, some defense attorneys believe that the SANE's refusal to consider any other modalities, even when the victim had not had intercourse previously, pointed to a biased and unscientific medical evaluation. Supporters of the forensic nurse argue that as an expert she gave her opinion based on direct observation of the injury and her expertise, and the SANE role as an advocate for the victim did not color her testimony. Similar controversies will no doubt occur in the future, especially in areas in which the forensic nurse combines her medical training and advocacy role.

Follow-up After Testimony

After an expert has testified, he or she should directly leave the court or hearing room in a professional manner. The effective expert will never stop to shake hands with the attorney or client, which can communicate a bias to the jury. When the trial is finished, the expert may want to contact the attorney and analyze the testimony or discuss the more effective testimonial techniques. In addition, the expert witness should seek feedback from both attorneys, if possible, to improve her testimony skills. Some experts refuse to seek the opinions of opposing counsel, especially after criminal trials. Since the opposing counsel did not invest much time or money in the other side's witness, comments from that attorney may prove most helpful, especially to the novice.

EXPERT WITNESS TESTIMONY IN BATTERING CASES

This section presents the stages of developing expert testimony in a domestic violence case. Identification and qualification of the expert witness, initial consultation, thorough case preparation, and likely areas of testimony are covered in detail. In addition, an overview of the theory applied and assessment tools used by the expert during case preparation are also discussed. Additional information related to partner violence can be found in Chapter 10.

Who Is an "Expert"?

As stated previously, before the expert can testify, the court must qualify that witness as able to provide the special knowledge being claimed. This process of information gathering is known as a *voir dire*. To qualify as an expert on battered women, the judge or attorneys would likely review the expert's education, professional preparation and affiliations, credentials or licenses, employment, experience with victims and/or offenders, research, publications in the area, honors or awards, and any special training (including conferences attended) that bears on domestic violence. Clinicians or advocates might be asked what proportion of their clientele are battered women. Qualification as an expert in the area of domestic violence will usually be expedited if the expert has been previously admitted to testify; however, this is not a prerequisite or a guarantee that the court will qualify the expert in the case at hand.

Initial Consultation

During an initial consult with an attorney, prosecutor, or client, sufficient information is gathered to determine what kinds of domestic violence expertise are relevant to the case, fees or related costs are described, the time frame is explored, and the access needed to relevant parties and documents is explained. Does the attorney want consultation, a preliminary assessment, a report, and/or generic or case-specific testimony, for instance? What are the strengths and limits of the expert's involvement compared with other potential witnesses with other skills? A common misconception in domestic violence cases is that only a licensed clinician can provide expert testimony because it involves a mental health assessment. In fact, woman battering is a condition of victimization, and a psychiatric diagnosis is usually not appropriate.

In civil cases involving battering, victims usually make the initial contact and pay the fee. Calls are often prompted by experience with attorneys who have been insensitive or whose understanding of domestic violence is limited. Although it is important to validate a woman's need for support, successful testimony depends heavily on a positive working relationship with the attorney. The expert should be prepared to educate attorneys about abuse; provide them with relevant reading or citations; and work as a partner in developing questions, scheduling and interrogating witnesses, preparing clients for trial, and making recommendations for disposition (e.g., custodial arrangements). Consultation is a legitimate role for an expert, even if neither a report nor testimony is required.

The Role of Evaluation

Unless directed to special issues, the purpose of a pretrial evaluation is to answer three questions: 1) Is the client a battered woman? 2) If so, what were the dynamics of abuse? 3) What are the consequences of abuse for the client and/or any children? If the battered woman is charged with violence or another alleged crime, an assessment may also consider, 4) how the history of battering affected her perceptions and behavior related to the event. Documents and interviews with friends, family members, or witnesses may help answer these questions. But the critical information is almost always provided by the client interview.

The assessment begins with a working definition that is experience- and research-based rather than limited to the discrete acts of physical assault or threats typically covered by domestic violence statutes. For example, experts rely on the coercive control model, where battering is defined as a malevolent course of coercive conduct wherein one social partner dominates another through the use of violence (abuse), coercion (isolation, intimidation, and emotional abuse), and control.

Following this definition, the assessment explores whether and to what extent the partner employed violence, coercion, and control; the interplay of these strategies over the course of the relationship; how the woman responded; how she was harmed; and how these experiences shaped her perceptions and behavior.

Choosing a Framework for Examining Harms

An appropriate forensic framework should be selected based on the facts in a case and the victim's presentation. Many cases of what Johnson (1996) calls "common couple violence" involve allegations of injurious physical assault only. Although emotional or psychological abuse can play a role in such cases, evaluation and testimony focus on the degree, frequency, and effects of violence on the safety of the woman and her children. Such an assessment may be relevant in a "duress" defense to a criminal charge (such as embezzlement, drug involvement, or signing a false tax return) or to custodial disputes where the court simply wants expert opinion about whether the client is or is not a "battered woman."

In this instance, evidence of psychological harm is kept to a minimum because it can impugn a woman's credibility or parenting capacity.

Psychological models of victimization are relevant when clients charged with a serious crime evidence adaptations to severe physical abuse that include symptoms of battered woman syndrome (BWS), post-traumatic stress disorder (PTSD), or a related complex that mitigates their criminal responsibility. Drawing on the vast trauma literature, the evaluator may administer formal psychological tests and/or clinically assess whether changes in feeling, perception, attitude, and behavior are the result of abuse. Here again, the clinical assessment should be sensitive to its potential misuse to impugn the credibility of the victim as a witness to her abuse. A complete investigation of objective constraints in a battering relationship will often explain why fears and perceptions seem "exaggerated."

Evidence of PTSD or BWS may be relevant for explaining a victim's behavior in a specific situation, but the absence of traumatic reaction in no way negates the reasonableness of a battered woman's fear. To the contrary, battered women frequently remain relatively intact psychologically despite multiple episodes of physical abuse, deprivation, isolation, and control. In cases where the principal presentation of battering is a state of subjugation (or "duress") rather than severe physical injury or psychiatric disease, the working definition of battering as coercive control is most appropriate. Here, the evaluator's attention is directed toward the existential condition of "entrapment" that compromises a woman's capacity to escape the battering, act independently, or protect herself or her children.

Documentation

Depending on whether the case is criminal or civil and whether it is relatively new or ongoing, prior to meeting the client, the evaluator reviews available records and evaluations from courts; corrections; criminal justice, medical, mental health, and behavioral health agencies; court-ordered evaluations of children; investigative reports of friends, witnesses, and family members; and records of related legal proceedings (depositions, trial transcripts, visitation orders, protection orders, judicial rulings, etc.). Although official documents rarely mention domestic violence explicitly, they may describe injuries, complaints, and other presentations suggestive of abuse (e.g., frequent "falls," "unwanted pregnancies," nonspecific complaints of pain, suicidality) as well as psychiatric and pseudo-psychiatric diagnoses frequently misapplied to abused women such as "hysterical" or hypochondriac. In one case, when a client supported her supposed "delusions" with a daily record of abuse stretching back 7 years, her court-ordered treater changed her diagnosis to "obsessive." Conventional documentation of domestic violence is the exception rather than the rule, however, even where a victim has sought help aggressively.

A written chronology of abusive events prepared by the client is an important source of documentation that can help prompt memories prior to the interview, date episodes in relation to key life events, and help prepare the evaluator for the assessment and testimony. A Palestinian woman who had paralyzed her husband with a club was dubbed "of limited intelligence" by her attorney, primarily because she spoke little English. But the 50-page record of abuse she provided in Arabic proved key to acquittal. A chronology also saves the client time and money. With the client's written consent, the expert garners collateral information from witnesses, family members or friends, and treaters.

Unconventional sources often provide the most important supporting information in domestic violence cases. A common misconception is that the severity of domestic violence can be measured by injuries that come to the attention of doctors or the police. In fact, the high-risk condition of entrapment typically results from the cumulative effects of minor, but frequent, abusive episodes, in combination with isolation, intimidation, and control. Sources used to document these events may include date books, log books, telephone messages, diaries, letters (including threatening letters from partners), tapes, photographs, and other records. Unconventional documents may also help the court understand the pattern and degree of abuse. For example, in the case of Donna B., the key to acquittal was a log book in which her husband had her record her daily activities (including any purchases, menus, thoughts of him, etc.). He would call her downstairs nightly to defend each entry, then beat her for not doing enough to advance their family.

The Interview

Depending on the framework adopted, the interview is structured to determine the fact of abuse as well as its dynamics, consequences, and significance. A preliminary discussion of the purpose of the interview and previous experience with battered women help reduce a client's anxiety about revealing painful and potentially embarrassing details to a stranger. Victims are urged to share as much detail as they can, even if they don't consider the acts queried abusive. However, clients should also be informed that, in contrast to other clinical interviews, the information provided may be available to opposing counsel, to other experts, or even to partners via counsel.

Accurate recall can often be a serious problem in domestic violence evaluations. Battered women often adapt to coercion and control by repressing, denying, minimizing, or normalizing the danger they face as well as by medicating the stress associated with abuse with substances that distort their memory. Conversely, victims may blame themselves for what happened or exaggerate their culpability, particularly if they feel guilty about their own violence. Donna B.'s husband sent her to Weight Watchers (which she liked because she got out of the house), then put her on a scale and beat her for not losing weight. Overeating is a common adaptation to abuse, but, Donna blamed her "stupidity" and "forgetfulness" for the assaults, a conclusion the prosecutor tried to exploit. Ironically, self-blame can be protective because it helps clients maintain a sense of "control in the context of no control." Although evaluation is not counseling, it is appropriate to help clients understand their partner's culpability and weigh appropriate expressions of their own responsibility against defensive postures that could increase their vulnerability at trial. For example, prosecutors often exploit the propensity for battered women to recall abusive episodes they initially denied. In fact, as Hermann (1992) suggests, the revision of a woman's story as memories surface is a sign of recovery from trauma and should be reframed as such for the court.

To maximize accurate reporting, some practitioners recommend an intensive, all-day interview that follows events in a chronological order, moving gradually from neutral questions about family background, early dating experiences, and the like to more emotion-laden episodes (Thyfault, Browne, & Walker, 1987). This approach has the added benefit of simulating courtroom testimony. Walker and her colleagues also suggest structuring questions about violence—and testimony—around four different battering incidents: the first occurrence of violence in the relationship, the worst episode, the typical episode, and the most recent or fatal incident. Each of these narratives is followed by matching sets of detailed questions about the specific circumstances (e.g., time, place, duration), acts (e.g., slap, hit, knife), and outcomes of the incident (e.g., injury, help seeking, retaliation) before moving to the next episode. Obtaining consistent details about incidents provides a picture of violence that allows comparisons over time that can identify escalation or other changes in behavioral patterns.

Other experts prefer repeated, shorter interviews spaced over several weeks and proceed from a semi-structured narrative in the first meeting to a more structured assessment schedule that probes the occurrence of specific events. Repeat, shorter interviews exploit the fact that recall improves dramatically over time, particularly if the abuse has culminated in an event involving extreme violence, and have the added advantage of allowing the interviewer to fill gaps and clarify ambiguities.

The initial interview (or phase of the interview) captures the woman's "story" as she understands it (i.e., in a rough chronological and narrative form). After reviewing the incident precipitating the evaluation, the interview takes a standard psychosocial history that includes any familial history of violence; sexual abuse or substance use; a history of earlier relationships, abusive or not; schooling; work history; and a history of major medical, mental health, or behavioral problems. The oft-claimed link between current victimization and violence in childhood is greatly exaggerated. Still, violence in the family of origin or in prior relationships contributes to a woman's understanding of the current relationship. An employment history can counter negative stereotypes of battered women or, conversely, illustrate how the abusive partner disrupted a woman's work life, caused her to lose a job (or workdays), or obstructed her career path. Information on prior pathology can also illuminate a woman's response pattern. However, the psychosocial history is also mined to provide baseline evidence of independence and resilience against which the effects of subsequent abusive experience can be weighed. Courts frequently want to know whether the victim's current state reflects abuse rather than long-standing personality problems.

The next phase of the interview focuses on the current relationship and, depending on the framework of harms adapted, seeks to establish the existence and interplay of abusive strategies, the consequences of battering, and how the woman responded. The narrative account is guided by frequent prompts to sharpen recall, direct attention to dimensions of experience not linked with abuse in the popular mind (such as isolation or control), and keep the focus. This is followed by questions targeting specific dimensions of violence, coercion, and control not covered in the narrative that research or case work suggest are common and/or are associated with an elevated risk of fatality or entrapment. Table 22–2 shows the information that an expert witness seeks concerning the history of violence in a battering case through the interview process.

Estimates of the number of abusive episodes can help neutralize the misconception that only injurious, life-threatening violence constitutes abuse, and dramatize the often "serial" nature of violence, where assaults occur once a week or more over many years. Donna B.'s husband first slapped her several days after they married, when she laughed on the phone while talking to her husband's uncle. A few nights later, she said she wasn't feeling well enough to make love and he tied her hands behind her back with a belt and "had his way." She recalled a dozen similar incidents during the first year. Early in the second year of their marriage, the couple moved away from his family into their own

Table 22–2   Information Sought by Experts Concerning Adult Trauma History

About partner's *violence*:

- The number, frequency, types, duration, and severity of assaults
- Injuries or chronic problems resulting from assault
- The typical assaultive incident
- The presence and/or use of weapons
- Sexual assault
- Assault during pregnancy
- Violence or other criminal conduct outside the relationship
- Violence in the presence of others, including children
- Violence while under the influence of alcohol or drugs
- Physical and/or sexual abuse of children

About *emotional abuse* and *intimidation*:

- Chronic putdowns of woman, friends, or family members.
- "Games" designed to make the woman feel "crazy" (called *Gaslight* games after the film by that name)
- Withdrawal from communication (e.g., the "silent treatment")
- Terrorizing or sadistic behaviors, particularly when the victim is sick or injured
- Paranoid, jealous, or homicidal fantasies
- Threats against the woman, family, friends, or pets, including threats to kill
- Monitoring or stalking
- Threats of suicide
- Use of children as "spies"

apartment and the husband implemented the nightly log ritual. From this point until she shot him 3 years later, the wife described beatings as occurring "nightly," "constantly," and "all the time." Using specific questions about the frequency of assaults during limited time periods bounded by watershed events, the expert estimated conservatively that there had been somewhere between 250 and 300 attacks in this relationship. The expert should be prepared to defend the estimate during cross-examination.

Evaluating a woman's access to helpers is an important piece of assessing control. Batterers frequently prevent women from seeking help, regulate their interaction with helpers, punish them for help seeking, or force them to terminate care while they are still at risk. In one case, a physician who was ashamed to have his colleagues see his wife "sick" sprayed her with RAID to cure her cancer. Then, 24 hours after surgery, he insisted she return home, where she contracted an infection and almost died.

Assessing Risk

Experts may be asked to assist in risk assessment at any phase of the judicial process, from pretrial assessment of offenders to correctional discharge and civil justice matters. Courts are increasingly turning to risk-assessment instruments to predict future violence by offenders in civil as well as criminal proceedings. Risk assessment is used to aid in custodial decision making and, more often, as part of a defense strategy, to demonstrate the level of risk a woman faced when she assaulted or killed an abusive partner.

A promising generic instrument available for predicting risk is the Spousal Assault Risk Assessment (SARA) (Kropp, Hart, Webster, & Eaves, 1998). The SARA is a set of guidelines composed of 20 items identified by the empirical literature and designed to enhance professional judgment about risk. Because the SARA is not a test (although it includes an analysis of psychological data), it can be used by the non-clinician. The procedure recommended resembles the evaluation discussed here in many respects, and includes interviews with the partner and the victim, standardized measures of physical and emotional abuse and drug and alcohol abuse, and a review of collateral records.

As part of a defense strategy in a criminal case, risk assessment can be designed to answer the following question: Based on the prior history of battering in this relationship, what was the risk that the battered woman would be killed at the time she used violence against her partner? Psychologist Angela Browne (1987) set the stage for this type of assessment when she reported that women who killed abusive partners could be distinguished from battered women who had not used violence by the level and frequency of physical and sexual violence to which they were subjected, the batterer's use of drugs and alcohol, the presence of weapons in the household, and the propensity of their partners to threaten or use violence against others, including their children.

Assessing Validity and Reasonable Scientific Certainty

Because the client interview is often the primary source of evidence that battering occurred, the court—as well as opposing counsel—naturally wants to know whether and why the expert finds the woman a credible source of information. In lieu of independent corroboration, the expert can only establish credibility with a reasonable scientific certainty based on the external and internal validity of her story. With respect to *external validity*, the paramount question for evaluation is whether the pattern of violence and control depicted is consistent with what is known about the dynamics in abusive situations, the personality and behavior of batterers, or the consequences of battering. In testimony, the evaluator may review basic knowledge about battering, then show why the material provided in the interview was consistent with this knowledge. Consistency between the narrative account and documents reporting specific episodes or witness accounts also helps to validate descriptions of other facets of abuse that are undocumented. But expert assessment never hinges on the occurrence of a single abusive episode. Even setting aside the defense mechanisms that lead victims to minimize or blame themselves for abuse, the complexity and duration of domestic violence often make it impossible to reconstruct the actual sequence or nature of events. Instead, the major focus of evidence gathering is on the pattern or course of abusive conduct, on routine or typical incidents, and on strategies used to coerce and control victims, as well as to hurt them physically. Clients may mislead even a skilled interviewer about particular episodes, but they are extremely unlikely to credibly simulate a lengthy course of conduct that resembles coercive control.

One way to assess *internal validity* is to use "criteria-based content analysis." This test, which was originally developed to assess truthfulness in cases of alleged sexual abuse, involves looking for repetition in word patterns and phrases (which indicates that a story is rehearsed), as well as repeating key questions. Additional factors that suggest internal validity include victims sharing responsibility for events, admitting their own acts of violence, and remembering extraneous details of traumatic events.

SUMMARY

Early work on women's self-defense stressed the positive role that expert testimony might play at trial in complementing the defendant's testimony and making her particular experience plausible to a jury. More recently, however, even sympathetic commentators have questioned whether its benefits in specific cases are worth the risk that expert testimony on battering and its effects will replace rather than support women's voices in the courtroom. To the extent that the court relies on an expert to provide a window on common experiences, the authority and credibility of women as witnesses to their own experience may be reduced, a possibility reflected in the popular conceit that battering occurs "behind closed doors" (i.e., without a credible witness). The ambiguous political status of expert testimony is further reinforced by the dominant psychological models of abuse used in defense cases.

Deciding how to best support a woman's voice in the legal setting is sometimes difficult, particularly when the state requests expert testimony to discount a victim's recantation or refusal to testify. Noninterference with a victim's choices is a basic tenet of the empowerment approach to women's self-defense work. Further, victims are assumed to be the best judge of their risks. Balanced against this individualized notion of empowerment is our civic obligation to protect vulnerable people from harm and uphold standards of community justice.

Another challenge faced by the expert witness is to help judge and jury "walk in the shoes" of a woman when the class or cultural underpinnings that frame her decision making are foreign, perhaps even alien, to your own. A week before Donna B. shot her husband she packed her clothes and son into her car and prepared to leave. Then, realizing how complete her isolation would be from the Albanian community (as well as her family) if she left her husband, she returned to the house.

To some, the hardest parts of expert testimony arise from the drama that attends a courtroom appearance, cross-examinations that seem mean-spirited, the need to simulate a level of certainty that is unfamiliar to researchers, or, conversely, to provide an objective appraisal that differs markedly from frank advocacy. If helping a client you believe is legally innocent avoid painful jail time is gratifying, it can be personally devastating when a client you have come to know and care about is convicted, goes to jail, or loses custody of her children. And there are few more frustrating experiences than sitting in the witness chair without being able to fully answer questions or tell the "story" as you know it because of the restraints of the courtroom.

The battered women in whose cases experts become involved have suffered extensive, sometimes shocking harms. In reporting these harms, the expert merely reflects their experience. But in asking the court to set aside the stereotypic imagery of victimhood and psychological dysfunction these experiences may evoke, the expert also does something more, asking judge and jury to suspend their pity and step inside the world battered women inhabit to discover what they are struggling to defend as well as to avoid or escape. Instead of wondering what sort of person would be drawn to this level of suffering, the expert must help the court envision the personhood needed to survive these incredible constraints. Through sheer will and raw courage, battered women propel themselves through a potentially paralyzing fear to find a hope that often has no objective confirmation in their immediate situation. If, despite the seeming totality of their oppression, battered women nonetheless regain a sense of control in the court context, this is because through reconstruction and authentication of their story, they are put in touch with a larger social context in which their right to safety and independence is affirmed through what Judy Hermann (1992) calls "an alliance of victim and witness."

QUESTIONS FOR DISCUSSION

1. Describe the desirable characteristics for an effective expert witness.
2. How are the credentials of an expert witness assessed?
3. Discuss the potential pitfalls that await the expert witness during trial testimony. What are some steps that can be taken to minimize or avoid them?
4. In what ways can a team of attorneys use an expert witness besides direct trial testimony?
5. Describe the important assessment indicators to be considered when interviewing a victim of violence.
6. Discuss some strategies for managing the potential conflict between the role of the nurse as advocate and the role of the expert witness in cases such as intimate partner abuse.

REFERENCES

Daubert v. Merrell Dow Pharmaceuticals, Inc., 509 U.S. 579 (1993).

Fields, R. (1999). The science of expert opinions. In M. Shiffman (Ed.), *Ethics in forensic science and medicine* (pp. 50–63). Springfield, IL: Charles C. Thomas.

Frye v. United States, 293 F. 1013 at 1014 (D.C. Cir. 1923).

Hermann, J. L. (1992). *Trauma and recovery.* New York: Basic Books.

Hussen v. Commonwealth, 414 S.E. 2d. 597, 243 Va. 262 (1999).

Johnson, M. (1996). Patriarchal terrorism and common couple violence: Two forms of violence against women. *Journal of Marriage and the Family, 57,* 283–294.

Kropp, P. R., Hart, S. D., Webster, C. W., & Eaves, D. (1998). *Spousal assault risk assessment: User's guide.* Toronto, Canada: Multi-health Systems.

Saviers, K. D. (2002). Ethics in forensic science: A review of the literature on expert testimony. *Journal of Forensic Identification, 52*(4), 449–462.

State v. Borrelli. (1993). Reported in *Connecticut Law Journal, 153,* 85–89.

State v. Peterson. (2003). [docket not yet decided, California]

Strong, V. W. (1999). *McCormack's book on evidence.* Eagon, MN: Westhorn.

Thyfault, R., Browne, A., & Walker, L. (1987). When battered women kill: Evaluation and expert testimony techniques. In D. J. Sonkin (Ed.), *Domestic violence on trial* (pp. 71–85). New York: Springer.

Disaster and Emergency Management

David Duff

Emergency preparedness is an essential concept to master for those who often serve as the interface between the legal field and the field of medicine. Those in forensic nursing play a unique role within this discipline because they are educated in medical response, in postmortem response, and in the potential medical-legal implications that a man-mediated disaster, such as arson, building collapse/structural failure, or a terrorist action, may have for patients.

CHAPTER FOCUS

What is a "disaster"?
The disaster cycle
Mitigation
Preparedness
Response
Recovery
Incident command
Basic types of disasters
Diagnostic criteria
Specialized response units
Hazard vulnerability analysis

KEY TERMS

awareness
disaster
disaster management
emergency operations
emergency operations center
hazard vulnerability
homeland security
incident command post
infrastructure
natural disaster
preparedness
recovery
technological disaster
terrorism
weapons of mass destruction

INTRODUCTION

The term *disaster management* conjures up the images of the terrorist attacks of September 11, 2001, and the subsequent response. This large-scale disaster served as a wake-up call, alerting the Western world that nontraditional warfare has become the preferred weapon for use by terrorists and/or religious zealots to advance their causes. The Western world, more specifically the United States, realized it was no longer immune to the actions of organizations based in many second- or third-world countries, as the members of these organizations are willing to attack the countries perceived as supporting their enemies. This nontraditional, limited warfare, also known as terrorism, is an ideal weapons platform for a less technologically advanced country or organization to confront a stronger opponent. One must query the purpose of the terrorist organization and their intended gains by performing such horrific actions against a civilian population. The goal is often as simple as wishing to disrupt the lives of the targeted country, using fear to alter how that country's inhabitants attend to their daily activities, or to force a change in how governmental policy is created or enacted. This disruption is most evident today in the United States, Great Britain, Australia, France, Germany, and other Western republics/ democracies. Such societies must now reconfigure their prevention and response apparatus to confront new threats. This has resulted in the construction of new government entities, with a tremendous channeling of fiscal and manpower resources toward the concept of strengthened homeland security. The creation of the Department of Homeland Security within the United States, with the concomitant commitment of resources, is intended to prevent or at least limit the impact of new disasters perpetrated by terrorist groups. As a study in the social sciences, this would generate endless perspectives to consider in the debate of what is terrorism vs. an act of war. However, as this chapter is designed to serve as a basic primer in disaster management, we will not delve further into the motivations of such actions. Rather, we will examine some of the steps that are taken to prepare for such actions and to reduce the impact of these activities.

Although terrorism preparedness and response is the overwhelming issue presented in media discourse, it is not the only concern of the emergency manager. Many disasters frequently impact the population. These disasters range from intense forest/brush fires (Australia, western U.S. states, and several of the European nations) to floods, hurricanes, blackouts, and earthquakes that may cause loss of life and property. The disaster/emergency manager must be prepared for a rapid response to both natural events and terrorist actions. The forensic nurse specialist may play an important role in responding to either type of crisis as well as assisting in the evaluation of the causative action/agent.

WHAT IS A DISASTER?

A disaster is an occurrence or event that exceeds the capabilities of the available resources of a business or governmental jurisdiction. The term *disaster management* not only includes the immediate response by a person, group, or agency to a traumatic event, but also encompasses a greater scope of management. Although a large, powerful storm may wreak havoc through a region, it may not be defined as a disaster if the local government meets the needs of the citizenry with the available resources. If the ability to respond to the event exceeds the available resources of the jurisdiction, then the event will be classified as a disaster. In the United States, the local government then seeks assistance from the next level of government. This process continues up the chain of governance until the disaster exceeds the capabilities of the state or group of states to adequately assist in the response. The governor of the affected state must request a declaration from the president of the United States for a situation to be deemed a federal disaster.

This leads to the next major tenet of disaster management, that all disasters are local events. Although the response may escalate to the federal level of government, the local agency retains primary management of the event. This allows the group most familiar with the incident to serve as the immediate command staff. As an event escalates in levels of response, other county, state, or federal agencies will then provide resources and support to the responding community. The only exception to this protocol would be in a suspected or confirmed terrorist event. In a terrorist event, the FBI is designated as the lead investigative agency per Presidential Decision Directive 39 (PDD39, 1995), the United States Policy on Counterterrorism. In an ongoing or suspected event, the FBI would also be the lead response agency and bring a vast array of resources to the incident.

THE DISASTER CYCLE: PHASES OF EMERGENCY MANAGEMENT

The disaster cycle, consisting of mitigation, preparation, response, and recovery, is a concept introduced by the Federal Emergency Management Agency (FEMA, 2003) to explain the essential interdependence of its components (see Figure 23–1). Those unfamiliar with the concept of the disaster cycle may think that "response" is the essential activity of emergency management organizations. Although this is the most visible phase of the disaster cycle, it is equally as important as the remaining components.

Mitigation

Mitigation is the cornerstone of emergency management. Often, when first introducing the phases of emergency management, they are described as "mitigation, mitigation, mitigation, and response," to

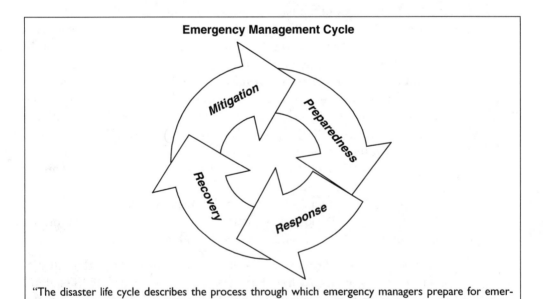

Emergency Management Cycle

"The disaster life cycle describes the process through which emergency managers prepare for emergencies and disasters, respond to them when they occur, help people and institutions recover from them, and mitigate their effects, reduce the risk of loss, and prevent disasters such as fires from occurring."

Source: *Principles of Emergency Management*, G-230, FEMA Emergency Management Institute.

Figure 23–1 The emergency management cycle.

emphasize the importance of the mitigation phase. Mitigation is the process of proactively reducing the potential impact that disasters may have on the community over the long term. Mitigation provides the emergency manager with the opportunity to save lives and reduce the future costs associated with responding to a disaster.

The forensic nurse and other members of the disaster response team should consider how the following activities could mitigate the impact a disaster may have on a community and its population:

- *Building codes:* Ensure that buildings conform to safety standards for earthquakes, fire safety, accessibility, exits, high wind safety, foundation depth, hazardous substance storage, flammables, emergency power requirements, and so on.
- *Zoning:* Keeps buildings out of flood plains, establishes buildings at sufficient distance to minimize impacting one another, keeps vital infrastructure components well protected and sufficiently spaced apart so that an incident at one location does not affect others, maintains industrial areas a safe distance from residential areas, provides adequate enforcement of zoning laws, and so on.
- *Equipment:* Provide programs for public safety agencies to acquire the needed equipment to operate effectively and help businesses to develop and maintain equipment safety programs; equipment maintenance programs; "a go-bag" for self, family, and family pets; and so on.
- *Training and public information:* Brief people on a building's escape plan, terrorism awareness, basic first aid, knowledge of select agents (a select agent is a biological agent or toxin that has the potential to pose a severe threat to the public's health and safety), family preparedness issues, computer system backups, and so on.
- Other mitigation activities common to natural disasters and terrorist events.

These mitigating factors should also be considered when determining what agencies or government acts (e.g., legislation) may be important in emergency management. The forensic nurse should be proactive in this area and is well situated to promote necessary changes in local and federal policies related to emergency or disaster management.

Preparedness

The second phase of emergency management is preparedness—the process of developing an emergency response plan for the family, the business, or the community. This process is necessary because it is impossible to mitigate 100% of the potential threats, whether natural or man-made. The development of this plan will include identifying specific functions, supplies, or resources required and redundant facilities to be used for a disaster. General considerations in the development of the emergency response/operations plan may include but are not limited to: public safety, fire suppression, public health/medical care, emergency communications, public information, utility management, search and rescue, public works, transportation, and mass care for the displaced. The terrorists on September 11, 2001, had two major goals— the first was to destroy the citizenry's confidence in the government to protect them, and the second was to cause a dramatic disruption to the economy. Since then, business continuity and redundant information technology infrastructure have become major preparedness goals.

Preparedness also includes the concept of awareness. In order for emergency planning to function, emergency managers must work with their constituents to educate them on the plans that have been developed. The constituent base must be made aware of and have a basic understanding of the plan, in addition to understanding its role in an event. Without this type of education and training for the people or agencies that will be relied upon in the event of a disaster, the plans that have been developed may prove difficult to enact. Therefore, it is essential that upon completion of thorough training, the plans should be drilled.

All preparations made for response to a potential event also require an evaluation to determine how each piece works independently and interrelates with the other components of the emergency response plan. This can be accomplished through the use of tabletop and live action drills. The drill will reveal weaknesses or potential conflicts within the plan, at a time when the plan's success or failure does not immediately impact the health, life, and safety of those people it was designed to assist. The weaknesses may then be evaluated and corrective measures taken to improve the plan.

Response

The third phase of the disaster cycle is response, the most closely scrutinized by the outside world. The primary function of this phase is to coordinate all activities to save the lives of the family, the workforce, or the citizenry. The response phase begins in very much the same way a nurse would begin care of a new patient. The disaster manager must make a brief, rapid assessment of the situation in order to determine what issue(s) should be addressed and how large of a portion of the available resources should be allocated. This approach remains true for any disaster, whether a natural event or a terrorist action; just as in nursing, there must be a continued reassessment to evaluate the effectiveness of actions taken and resources applied.

The emergency manager will be most concerned with protecting the lives of the citizenry and ensuring the safety and continued operations of the community's critical infrastructure. Traditionally, critical infrastructure represents the various utilities upon which the modern world depends for daily activities (electricity, clean water, natural gas, telephones, etc.). With the dramatic evolution of information technology, the concept of critical infrastructure has changed. Today, the unfettered flow of information and the security of that information are just as vital as the power generation stations. In fact, many of the traditional forms of critical infrastructure have come to rely on information technology, which makes them more susceptible to acts of aggression via the same technology. Presidential Decision Directive 63 (1998) defines critical infrastructure as "those physical and cyber-based systems essential to the minimum operations of the economy and government. They include, but are not limited to, telecommunications, energy, banking and finance, transportation, water systems and emergency services, both governmental and private."

While securing the critical infrastructure, the emergency/disaster manager must also consider the need to evacuate the citizenry and provide food, water, and shelter to those deprived of homes and services. In addition, medical care should be addressed, to accommodate both medications for pre-existing conditions and care for injuries resulting from an event. The medical care required for these people may often include crisis counseling on topics such as anxiety/stress management, posttraumatic stress, and managing grief and loss.

In a disaster, there is a natural inclination to help those in need. Although impromptu volunteerism may appear helpful initially, this abundance may create additional stresses for an overtaxed emergency/disaster manager. Many issues arise from an influx of spontaneous volunteers, such as:

- Accuracy of credentials
- Volunteer management issues
- Food
- Shelter
- The potential for injuries and legal actions on the part of the volunteers due to their actions
- A lack of dedication to complete the tasks at hand

Emphasizing these concerns is not meant to discourage volunteerism, but rather to encourage people to seek out volunteer organizations prior to a disaster. (Please contact your local emergency manager for more information on Volunteer Organizations Active in Disaster [VOADs] in your area.) By proceeding in this manner, volunteers may receive the appropriate identification and training to more effectively assist with a response. Not only would this benefit the volunteers, but also may help the VOADs and emergency managers pre-identify their resources as they develop their individual response plans.

Recovery

Recovery is the process of rebuilding the affected organization or community. The goal of the recovery process is the normalization of activities within the community, to return to life prior to the event. The recovery phase actually begins during the response phase as vital services are restored to the affected area. Recovery may be viewed in terms of both short- and long-term goals. The short-term goals may include the resumption of basic services and a normalization of many daily activities; the long-term goals may include a complete restoration of services, infrastructure, and economic activity for individuals and the business community within the affected area. The recovery process may take years to complete, depending on the extent of the damage. The psychosocial recovery of the individuals may also take many years. It is important to remember that traumatic events may require extended periods of counseling for some members of the community.

The recovery phase also heralds the beginning of retrospection. Following an emergency, an opportunity exists for the emergency/disaster manager to improve the level of preparedness within their jurisdiction. This is done through thoughtful analysis of the activities that occurred during the disaster and assessment of how future mitigation and preparedness projects may reduce the impact of similar events in the future. From this point the cycle repeats itself, causing the emergency manager to constantly seek refinement of operational planning and reduce the potential threats through mitigation activities.

DISASTER TYPES

Another basic concept to understand is how the Federal Emergency Management Agency (FEMA) defines a disaster. Currently, FEMA categorizes disasters into two types, natural and technological (FEMA, 2005). The term *natural disaster* includes events such as tidal waves, earthquakes, floods, forest fires ignited by lightning, blizzards, and heat waves. The term *technological disaster* refers to those disasters that are caused by man, including terrorist acts (chemical, biological, radiological, explosive, and incendiary), blackouts, computer system failures, failure of telecommunication systems, arson, computer viruses, and accidents that may involve hazardous material spills, oil spills, and shipping.

INCIDENT COMMAND

Given the large number of events that may be termed disasters, the forensic nurse specialist should have a basic knowledge of the incident management system used by most jurisdictions as well as many

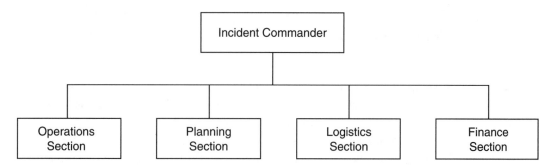

Figure 23–2   The incident command system.

private institutions to manage disaster response. The methodology used to manage most incidents/disasters is known as the incident command system (ICS). Incident command is a management structure used to coordinate both large and small events. ICS was originally developed by those involved in wildland fire management in the mid-1970s. It is designed to provide cost-effective management that may span multiple jurisdictions (National Wildfire Coordinating Group, 1994).

The following summaries were derived from the National Wildfire Coordinating Group's project to develop the National Interagency Incident Management System (NIIMS), which provided the groundwork for the incident command system. The incident command system is divided into five primary functions (Figure 23–2):

1. *Command/incident commander:* This position is responsible for the overall management of the response, setting the objectives and priorities that the team will attempt to accomplish.
2. *Operations section:* This section conducts the tactical operations to achieve the objectives set by the incident commander. The operations section chief develops tactical objectives, is responsible for organizational development, and directs assigned resources.
3. *Planning section:* This section is tasked with the development of the strategic objectives and the operations plan, as well as monitoring the long-term availability and deployment of resources.
4. *Logistics section:* This section provides and maintains the available resources and necessary supplies as well as supporting services to all staff (food, transportation, medical care, etc.).
5. *Finance and administration section:* This section monitors costs related to the incident, provides for accounting, establishes procurement contracts, monitors worker's compensation issues, provides time recording, and handles cost analysis.

The ICS is used by many different organizations to coordinate activities during a disaster or planned event. ICS provides many basic benefits, including:

- *Defined primary functions:* These functions provide a structural matrix upon which additional activities may be added and defined as the incident grows and evolves.
- *Chain of command:* ICS provides for an orderly ranking of management positions. A clearly defined hierarchical structure provides for a clear line of supervision and stability in the implementation of the emergency operations response guidelines.
- *Organizational flexibility:* Although a position is listed, there is no mandate that it must be filled. The functions required to accomplish the mission determine the necessity of positions.
- *Common terminology:* This common vocabulary is important when working with multiple agencies and jurisdictions. Common terminology is applied to organizational elements, position titles, resources, and facilities.
- *Span of control:* This is a critical ICS issue. Span of control describes how many people or units may safely and effectively serve under each position. This management concept includes up to seven people or units serving under each position, with five being the ideal number. When additional resources or units are required, the incident commander, using the organizational flexibility of ICS, may add an additional management position in order to maintain a safe operational response.
- *Planning by operational period:* The concept of developing a written incident action plan (IAP) for each operational period is novel to many responders. This plan is developed by the planning section in coordination with the operations section and supervised by the incident commander (IC).

The written action plan allows the logistics section chief greater precision in requesting additional staff, equipment, or materials needed for the upcoming operations instead of estimating the requirements. It allows the finance section chief to prepare funding requests, and it provides goals or targets to be achieved by the operations section. The written action plan provides a way to measure the effectiveness of response. The ability to review the strategy and outcomes against a standard of expectations allows the IC to address problematic areas in which success has been limited.

Incident Command Post vs. Emergency Operations Center

There is often confusion about the terms *incident command post (ICP)* and *emergency operations center (EOC)*. The incident command post is the location for on-scene management of an event, whereas an emergency operations center is the location where governmental entities and representatives of critical infrastructure meet to provide coordinated support to the responding agencies involved in disaster operations. The EOC may support several different command posts simultaneously during an event. In some cases the ICP and the EOC may be co-located in the same facility or room. In some instances the EOC may assume the functions of the ICP.

WEAPONS OF MASS DESTRUCTION

In the current sociopolitical milieu of terrorist threats and unstable nation-states, the threat of a weapon of mass destruction (WMD) being used appears to have increased. However, if we reflect on prior civilizations, we can see evidence that the threat of WMDs has actually existed since the time of the Assyrians and Athenians (6th century BC), who used toxins and biological agents to poison the water supplies of their enemies, or the Tartar army in 1346 AD, catapulting its own plague-riddled corpses over the walls of Kaffa (Decameron Web, n.d.). The main difference between the modern era and the ancient times is that science has allowed genocide on a larger scale through the purification of biological agents, the improved lethality of chemical agents, nuclear weapons that can destroy large cities, and radiological dispersal devices that seek to spread contamination throughout the blast area. In this section, we will discuss some of the various weapons as well as the impact that the term *weapon of mass destruction* has on society.

Presidential Decision Directive 39

In the event of the deliberate use of a WMD within the United States, the key governmental directive of concern to the forensic healthcare provider is Presidential Decision Directive 39 (PDD 39, 1995). PDD 39 clearly defines roles and responsibilities of federal agencies in the event of such an attack. The FBI is designated as the primary law enforcement agency responsible for preventing the attack and also for handling the postevent investigation. Although this appears to contradict the previous adage that all events are local, one must remember the potential scope that this investigation may entail. If a WMD is used, it would be considered an act of war if the action was sanctioned by a nation-state, or an act of aggression if committed by saboteurs/illegal combatants and/or terrorists. WMD use by terrorists may represent a cause with a multinational operational profile, like the group Al-Qaeda. A multinational profile impedes tracking and the identification of the terrorists; thus the FBI, in coordination with all of the available federal resources, becomes the ideal entity to deal with threat prevention and the capture of the fugitives postevent.

It is important for the forensic nurse specialist to understand the role that the FBI plays in responding to a potential act of terrorism involving a weapon of mass destruction. The forensic specialist may be required to assist in the collection or examination of evidence, such as bodies, clothing, visual imagery, and documented observations of survivors. If a weapon of mass destruction is used, there will be casualties of the attack and potentially many more people affected by the psychological impact of the attack. Early in the response to an event, these victims will require crisis and medical interventions. The response to such an event necessitates a combination of medical and legal knowledge, so the forensic nurse specialist appears the ideal candidate to assist the community, given the definition of forensic nursing provided by Lynch (1991). Lynch describes forensic nursing as the combined application of forensic science and clinical nursing in the scientific investigation and treatment of trauma, death, violence, and criminal activity.

This juxtaposition of medical care and forensic science seen in forensic nursing gains greater significance as institutions focus on initiating a proactive response to a WMD event. If people are believed to be "contaminated," one of the first responses is to remove all the clothing and douse water upon the person or patient presenting. This reaction is similar to the commonly observed response in the emergency department (ED), where the primary goal is to save the patient, without regard to the preservation of evidence. Lynch emphasizes that appropriate forensic nursing techniques are vital in the ED, as the nurse is frequently the first to see the patient, to handle patient property, and to handle lab specimens. The emergency nurse must recognize that any patient with potentially liability-related injuries, whether victim or victimizer, living or dead, is a clinical forensic patient (Lynch, 1995). This last phrase from Lynch highlights an important detail to consider when dealing with patients from a WMD incident—that some of the patients may have perpetrated the incident. Therefore, the application of appropriate forensic technique, even amidst the mayhem of the response, is critical. The development of this protocol should be a joint effort between forensic specialists, law enforcement, and healthcare institutions.

The most important aspect for a forensic nurse specialist to consider before being called to such an event is the early development of a positive working relationship with local and federal law enforcement agencies. One of the basic tenets within emergency management is that the first contact between responders or agencies should occur over coffee before an event, not during the event. The development of such a rapport is critical to all aspects of emergency management and will improve the interactions of the forensic nurse with those with whom he or she may be working.

PDD 39 also designates FEMA as the primary agency to oversee consequence management, which means FEMA will perform its normal functions of coordinating the resources available to the federal government in support of the actions of the state EOC.

Chemical Weapons

Chemical agents are classified by primary site of effect: blood agents (cyanide), nerve agents (tabun, sarin, VX), pulmonary/choking agents (phosgene or chlorine), blister agents (mustard types, lewisite), and incapacitating/riot agents (tear gas-type agents). In this section we will briefly review the pulmonary agents and the nerve agents.

The fact that many of the pulmonary agents are also common chemical precursors within modern industry means that there is a relatively abundant supply of these substances throughout the country. A terrorist who can effectively identify an opportune situation might decide to use one of these agents in an area that could affect thousands of people. The well-prepared emergency manager will understand the risks within the jurisdiction and develop a mitigation plan to reduce the continued threat that exists from this chemical type, whether it is an accidental release or an intended one aimed at creating terror, injuries, death, and financial impact.

Nerve agents were accidentally discovered in the mid-1930s by German scientists performing research to develop improved insecticides. The research into these agents, commonly known German Gas A (GA, a.k.a. tabun), German Gas B (GB, a.k.a. sarin), German Gas C (GD, a.k.a. soman), and German Gas F (GF, a.k.a. cyclosarin), was discontinued due to their extreme toxicity. Another nerve agent that is frequently mentioned is VX. VX, where the "V" stands for venomous, was originally developed in the 1950s in the United Kingdom. It is considered much more toxic than sarin and is considerably less volatile; therefore it may be more persistent in the environment.

Nerve agents are chemicals that act on the nervous system of victims, overstimulating the nerve receptors. Nerve agents bind acetylcholinesterase, preventing the enzymatic degradation of acetylcholine at the nerve receptors. The binding of the acetylcholinesterase leads to the overstimulation of muscles and glands. The acronym "SLUDGE" (salivation, lacrimation, urination, defecation, gastrointestinal distress, and emesis) may help people remember the effects of nerve agents on the human body. To counter these effects, atropine and pralidoxime chloride (2-PAM Cl) are provided to the victims via either intramuscular injection or intravenous access.

The threat of a chemical weapon to advance a political agenda may be significant for several reasons: the relative ease of acquiring the chemical intermediates required for the manufacture of the poison, the creation of immediate casualties and fear in the target population, the relative stability of the substance over a long period of time, and the use of modern devices to assist in the dispersal of the agent. However, there are also negative aspects for the terrorist to consider. A chemical attack is geographically limited in the extent to which it may effectively cause injuries to the intended target population. Another drawback is that a chemical exposure is unlikely to create additional patients from person-to-person contact. This lack of transmission is not only due to the agent's volatility, but also because responders have become aware of signs and symptoms of nerve agent intoxication and are more likely to take precautionary steps in dealing with these patients. The last drawback to consider is that it is possible for the terrorist to be overcome by the agent, becoming a casualty along with the targets. As was mentioned previously, this is an important consideration for the forensic nurse specialist—any patient with injuries related to a man-made disaster is a clinical forensic patient. The actions of the forensic nurse specialist may assist in the retention of vital evidence that may be used to further the investigation into the terrorist act and also within the courtroom if the perpetrators are apprehended.

Biological Weapons

One busy day, when you ask yourself the question "Why are all of these people in my emergency department?" you may be the first to recognize the signs of a potential biological attack. Unlike other forms of weapons of mass destruction, a biological agent released into the community may not announce itself for several days to several weeks because the agent requires time to incubate in the host. Many programs are in development across the United States attempting to create a practical disease surveillance platform. Until this is accomplished, it may be an alert member of the physician or nursing staff who will raise the alarm. To be prepared to deal with such a threat, the ability to grasp and enact the basic concepts of forensic epidemiology must be developed within the physician and nursing corps.

The Centers for Disease Control have designated several biological organisms or their toxins as potential weapons when used in a manner not conforming to legitimate research. These biological agents are divided into specific categories based upon those agents that are considered readily weaponized and those that have a strong potential to eventually be refined into weapons-grade material. The agents listed in the highest risk category (Category A diseases) by the Centers for Disease Control are:

- Anthrax (*Bacillus anthracis*)
- Smallpox (Variola virus)
- Plague (*Yersinia pestis*)
- Tularemia (*Francisella tularensis*)
- Botulism (botulinum toxin)
- Viral hemorrhagic fever

This section on bio-agents is intended only as a quick summary of the potential problems that such agents may create for the emergency/ disaster manager. It is not intended to provide the medical practitioner with care or treatment guidelines. Guidelines for the recognition, care, and treatment of patients that may have been exposed to these bio-agents can be obtained from the CDC website, www.bt.cdc.gov.

Although most known agents are not considered transmissible between humans, there are some notable exceptions. Smallpox (Variola virus), which was eradicated through a worldwide vaccination program, is considered to be highly contagious between humans (WHO, 2004). The last remaining known caches of the virus are held by the Russian and United States governments. There is considerable supposition that additional countries may have retained their virus stocks or may have stock that was surreptitiously obtained. Smallpox has proven itself as an efficient weapon, assisting the Europeans in their conquest of the indigenous people located in both of the American continents. The fear that it may be reintroduced has led to a dramatic policy change and the re-creation of a vaccine to limit its spread. Again, note that fear of man-mediated events drives security, political, and fiscal policy decisions of the government. The terrorist organizations have not needed to perform specific acts to cause several governments to respond by diverting funds and manpower; the terrorists have already instilled the belief and fear that they have the potential resources and desire to act in such a manner (Henderson et al., 1988).

For centuries, the plague (*Yersinia pestis*), otherwise known as Black Death, has remained a problem for man. The plague in fourteenth-century Europe is estimated to have led to the deaths of one-third of the population. Plague is still endemic in many regions of the world. This historical success makes the plague and smallpox such potentially lethal choices as weapons. Like smallpox, the plague has the potential for human-to-human transmission (*History of Bioterrorism,* 2004). Additional reasons why these agents may be considered potential weapons are:

- Stability for storage and transportation
- Known to produce stable aerosols
- Can be produced in large quantities
- High mortality
- Highly infectious
- Person-to-person spread—more limited in plague
- Most of the world has little or no immunity

When the concept of using biological agents as an offensive weapon was still a part of military doctrine, anthrax (*Bacillus anthracis*) was once considered an excellent choice for the field commander in a war situation. The benefits of using anthrax were its lethality, ease of production, stability during lengthy periods of storage, and the inability of the bacillus to re-aerosolize in a particle size small enough to enter the lower respiratory tract (thereby not infecting the troops who initiated the anthrax attack as they marched through the newly conquered territories). This theory was tested in the United States during the fall of 2001. A spate of letters containing anthrax spores led to several deaths across the eastern seaboard. The unusual feature of these attacks was that those infected were not necessarily the intended targets, but rather the victims of re-aerosolization of the bacillus caused by the use of automatic mail sorting machines. The bacillus was milled by the machines to a sufficiently small size to pass into the respiratory tract. Thus, the bacillus contaminated many different pieces of mail as it was mechanically sorted and sent to other parts of the country. The electrostatic charge of the anthrax bacillus was somehow neutralized so that it did not enlarge, because it did not attract other particles to it. The bacillus remained a small enough size to enter the respiratory tract (Rosenburg, 2002).

The bio-weapon is an antipersonnel weapon that provides an unusual set of challenges for the emergency manager, public health official, and healthcare professional, largely due to the current mobility of the population. An excellent example of how a disease can rapidly spread before it is recognized is the outbreak of Severe Acute Respiratory Syndrome (SARS) in the fall of 2002 to the summer of 2003. This disease spread from a rural Chinese province to many developed countries of the world in under a year. This inadvertent spread had a disastrous impact on many populations. An engineered bio-weapon containing a transmissible agent may have a far greater impact on the world.

The use of quarantine is a much debated topic in emergency management and public health circles. Quarantine was used with some mixed results during the initial SARS pandemic. Because of the varied results, albeit in very different cultural settings, the efficacy of both voluntary and involuntary quarantine measures is not fully understood. In addition to this question, there are still questions on how the implementation of mass quarantine would be accomplished within the United States, as this would depend on the potential scale of the disease outbreak. The political jurisdiction might be able to effectively limit the movements or isolate several individuals, but as the numbers of individuals affected by the epidemic increases, there may be increasing difficulty in implementing quarantine orders. This decrease in the ability to effectively implement quarantine orders may be linked to several issues, including lack of political will to order the implementation of quarantine, overworked public health employees, the need to cohort patients in specific healthcare facilities, media broadcasts fanning the anxiety of the populace, and civil resistance. The ability to quarantine may also be limited by the lack of empowering legislation or by potential backlash from individuals claiming that the quarantine order violates their civil rights.

Containment and quarantine are vital to the emergency manager and public health official. However, these programs raise many questions among forensic nurses and other healthcare professionals, politicians, and citizens. Among the issues that might be raised during a discussion of how to manage a biological disaster are:

- How does the local jurisdiction pursue the implementation of restrictions on the movement of its citizenry?
- Can a government force medical care upon its citizens?
- Can a government enforce quarantine orders on several citizens?
- What effects may be created or enhanced by the actions of the media?
- How can the emergency manager or public health official work effectively with the media and gain their trust and support?
- What happens to the above issues when the number of people presenting for care dramatically increases?
- What happens to the above issues when the number of confirmed or suspected cases escalates in a short period of time?

Another challenge presented by the bio-weapon is that it may be difficult to detect in the early stages of the disease outbreak. Several biological agents often present in a manner that is consistent with an outbreak of the influenza virus. The ability to recognize a bio-agent release is extremely time sensitive. Recognizing that the differential diagnosis for influenza includes some of these diseases is vital to the containment of the outbreak. Time is of the essence, not just for patient care, but also for evidence collection. In the time it takes to draw the distinction between a simple flu outbreak and the suspected use of a bio-weapon, damages may escalate from minimal fatalities to hundreds or thousands dead.

Radiological Dispersal Devices (RDD)

The radiological dispersal device (RDD), or "dirty bomb," is a threat for which the emergency manager must mitigate, prepare, and develop response plans. The RDD is a denial of territory device, as it is designed to contaminate the blast area with a radioactive substance, such as Cesium 137 or Cobalt 60. It is a true weapon of terror, as it plays on the fear that the uninformed populace has regarding anything radioactive. The aftermath of the RDD will require an extended recovery period, not only to remove or minimize the contamination, but also to encourage the citizenry to once again use the area after the remediation has been completed.

Psychosocial Issues of Terrorism and Weapons of Mass Destruction

Earlier in this chapter, the discussion of terrorism postulated that terrorists are attempting to make political changes or statements, to force policy changes within the targeted nation-state's foreign affairs, or to disrupt the economy and lifestyle of the targeted population. The essence of terrorism is to force expanded expenditures, to make life uncomfortable for the citizens of the targeted nation, and to force them to change how they live and thereby demand their government to change its policies. In the end, terrorism is more of a psychological weapon aimed at making socioeconomic and political changes than a weapon to destroy people.

Given that a terrorist group is interested in creating fear, the mere threat of using a weapon of mass destruction is often sufficient to achieve their goals. In their text, Maniscalco and Christen (2002) use the nomenclature of "weapon of mass effect" as a new way of viewing the potential use of WMD materials, as the terrorist seeks to disrupt society by creating fear and preventing normal operations. The threat of such weaponry may encourage a society to change its operations. Excellent examples of these adjustments can be seen with the CDC's efforts to restart the smallpox vaccination process, the creation of a new large governmental organization (Department of Homeland Security), and the reallocation of scarce monetary resources into counterterrorism activities. We have dramatically changed our priorities in the United States as a result of persistent threats.

As was mentioned previously, a disaster, whether natural or man-mediated, causes a disruption of societal norms. The physical damage may be great, but often the population's psychological response to a disaster may be much greater. The citizenry involved in a disaster or terrorist attack may respond in many ways. Each type of response will require different event and post-event recovery assistance. Psychosocial assistance is not meant to pathologize the response of the participants; on the contrary, the psychosocial response is meant to provide those affected with the tools required to cope with the immediate time period during and after the disaster. Psychosocial response recognizes that many people are by nature resilient to the effects associated with a traumatic event. This type of intervention is intended to enable disaster victims to retain at least minimal function. The psychosocial intervention is also meant to identify individuals who may require additional mental health assistance beyond the scope of the psychosocial assistance; these individuals would be immediately referred to psychiatric specialists for more intensive interventions.

The event may continue to significantly affect some individuals weeks, months, or years after the traumatic experience. These individuals may require extended medical care and mental health assistance. Post-traumatic stress disorder (PTSD) treatment is performed by licensed professionals over a lengthy period of time to assist with the coping of those involved in traumatic events. Figure 23–3 presents criteria for the assessment of post-traumatic stress disorder. A more thorough discussion of PTSD may be found in Chapter 14 of this book.

Diagnostic Criteria for 309.81 Post-traumatic Stress Disorder, DSM-IV

A. The person has been exposed to a traumatic event in which both of the following were present:
   (1) the person experienced, witnessed, or was confronted with an event or events that involved actual or threatened death or serious injury, or a threat to the physical integrity of self or others
   (2) the person's response involved intense fear, helplessness, or horror. **Note:** In children, this may be expressed instead by disorganized or agitated behavior

B. The traumatic event is persistently re-experienced in one (or more) of the following ways:
   (1) recurrent and intrusive distressing recollections of the event, including images, thoughts, or perceptions. **Note:** In young children, repetitive play may occur in which themes or aspects of the trauma are expressed.
   (2) recurrent distressing dreams of the event. **Note:** In children, there may be frightening dreams without recognizable content.
   (3) acting or feeling as if the traumatic event were recurring (includes a sense of reliving the experience, *illusions, hallucinations,* and dissociative *flashback* episodes, including those that occur on awakening or when *intoxicated*). **Note:** In young children, trauma-specific reenactment may occur.
   (4) intense psychological distress at exposure to internal or external cues that symbolize or resemble an aspect of the traumatic event
   (5) physiological reactivity on exposure to internal or external cues that symbolize or resemble an aspect of the traumatic event

C. Persistent avoidance of stimuli associated with the trauma and numbing of general responsiveness (not present before the trauma), as indicated by three (or more) of the following:
   (1) efforts to avoid thoughts, feelings, or conversations associated with the trauma
   (2) efforts to avoid activities, places, or people that arouse recollections of the trauma
   (3) inability to recall an important aspect of the trauma
   (4) markedly diminished interest or participation in significant activities
   (5) feeling of detachment or estrangement from others
   (6) restricted range of *affect* (e.g., unable to have loving feelings)
   (7) sense of a foreshortened future (e.g., does not expect to have a career, marriage, children, or a normal life span)

D. Persistent *symptoms* of increased arousal (not present before the trauma), as indicated by two (or more) of the following:
   (1) difficulty falling or staying asleep
   (2) *irritability* or outbursts of anger
   (3) difficulty concentrating
   (4) *hypervigilance*
   (5) exaggerated *startle response*

E. Duration of the disturbance (symptoms in Criteria B, C, and D) is more than 1 month.

F. The disturbance causes clinically significant distress or impairment in social, occupational, or other important areas of functioning.

Specify if:
Acute: if duration of symptoms is less than 3 months
Chronic: if duration of symptoms is 3 months or more

Specify if:
With Delayed Onset: if onset of symptoms is at least 6 months after the stressor

Source: Diagnostic and Statistical Manual of Mental Disorders, Fourth Edition, Text Revision. Copyright 2000 American Psychiatric Association.

Figure 23–3 Diagnostic criteria for post-traumatic stress disorder.

SPECIALIZED RESPONSE UNITS OF THE FEDERAL GOVERNMENT

The government of the United States has initiated many programs to assist the emergency manager and, therefore, the public, in the event of a natural or technical disaster. One such response unit created by the U.S. government is the Urban Search and Rescue (USAR) teams, which are specially trained and equipped units established by FEMA to perform search and rescue missions in collapsed or unsound structures. These units may also provide basic medical services to those trapped while awaiting extrication.

Emergency health services are a vital component of any response planning that an emergency manager must develop. Providing medical services under the stressful conditions of a disaster can be difficult for the existing medical facilities and staff. The U.S. Department of Health and Human Services developed the concept of the National Disaster Medical System (NDMS). One of the primary components of the NDMS is the disaster medical assistance team (DMAT), which is designed to provide self-contained medical services under austere conditions when the healthcare demands presented by the emergency exceed the available healthcare resources. DMATs are federal assets deployed to assist the local healthcare infrastructure to meet the needs of its citizens, either by establishing field hospitals or by serving as supplemental staffing for local hospitals. DMATs deploy with sufficient medical and personal supplies to operate for a minimum 3 days before requiring additional supplies. As part of the restructuring under the Homeland Security Act of 2002, the NDMS was moved from Health and Human Services to the new Department of Homeland Security.

A disaster does not just affect humans, but also man's best friends. To support animals in a disaster, NDMS has established veterinary medical assistance teams (VMATs). Like the DMATs, VMATs also respond rapidly to provide emergency medical care to animals affected by disasters. VMATs also may establish field hospitals or provide staff augmentation to existing veterinary facilities to assist them in meeting the needs of animal populations in the event of a disaster.

NDMS has another response group that plays an important role in a disaster with multiple fatalities, the disaster mortuary operational response team (DMORT). A DMORT consists of funeral directors, pathologists, forensic anthropologists, medical records specialists, fingerprint specialists, forensic odontologists, radiology technologists, mental health specialists, computer professionals, administrative support staff, and security and investigative personnel. The DMORT is responsible for the establishment of temporary morgue facilities; identification of remains; and preparation, processing, and assisting in final disposition of the remains.

HAZARD VULNERABILITY ANALYSIS

Disasters are by definition unforeseen events that are often accompanied by significant destruction and loss. However, as was previously discussed, the mitigation phase of the disaster cycle allows the emergency manager to minimize the amount of potential losses that may be incurred. To proceed with the mitigation phase in an organized fashion, the emergency manager performs a hazard vulnerability analysis (HVA). The HVA may be presented in several forms, including written analysis or a matrix format. The written analysis is normally the most complete form of threat analysis performed, but it may be difficult to decipher by those unfamiliar with the business or jurisdiction. The matrix format is a simple method that assigns a score to each potential disaster. The higher the score, the more likely the threat would cause damage or disruption in services. The matrix is the most common form used, at least within the healthcare community.

The first step that the emergency manager performs is to identify which hazards may confront the jurisdiction or business. This list of potential hazards is normally categorized as technological threats or natural threats.

Once the emergency manager develops the list of hazards, the next step is to evaluate the likelihood of the event occurring within the jurisdiction. Using the matrix format, the emergency manager assigns a number from zero (unlikely to occur) to three (highly likely to occur during the period covered by the HVA). In attempting to determine the probability of an event occurrence, it is important to consider historical occurrences, known threats, and any intelligence provided by the law enforcement community.

The emergency manager next evaluates the risk that the jurisdiction or business faces for each identified disaster. Risk is a category that evaluates the potential for harm or loss from each specified disaster. Risk may include posing an immediate threat to the life or health of the citizens/employees, the disruption of services (including information technology services), damage to critical infrastructure, the loss of goodwill or trust, financial impact, or legal impact on the business or governmental jurisdiction. Risk is scored on a scale of one (the lowest risk) to five (the highest level of risk to life and property).

The final component of the matrix is the evaluation of the jurisdiction's or business's level of preparedness to respond effectively to each specific hazard. This is often done using a scale of one to three. The lower the score assigned, the better the preparation of the jurisdiction or business in meeting the potential threat. In considering preparedness, the emergency manager should include such issues as insurance, availability of resources, readiness of response plans, and

Event	Probability				Risk					Preparedness			Total
	High	Med	Low	None	Life Threat	Health/ Safety	High Disruption	Moderate Disruption	Low Disruption	Poor	Fair	Good	
Score	3	2	1	0	5	4	3	2	1	3	2	1	
Terrorism— Chemical	3				5	4				3	2		45
Terrorism— Radiological Dispersal Device	3					4				3			36
Terrorism— Biological	3				5						2		30
MCI (HazMat)		2				4				3			24
Mass Casualty Incident (Trauma)		2			5						2		20
HVAC Failure	3					3					2		18
Fire, Internal	3				5							1	15
Terrorism— Nuclear			1		5					3			15
Structural Damage		2					3				2		12

Figure 23–4 A sample hospital hazard vulnerability analysis chart.

most importantly the training status of the responders and supervisors in the implementation of the plan. Having a plan is essential, but it is more important to know that the people who will implement it are not only familiar with the plan, but are comfortable with the role(s) in which they may function.

Computation is the final step in the development of this matrix HVA. For each event, multiply the probability, risk, and preparedness together to determine the vulnerability to that specific threat (Probability × Risk × Preparedness = Vulnerability). The results are then sorted in descending order. This provides an ordinal ranking of events. The higher the score, the greater exposure and vulnerability the institution has to that event. The purpose behind the HVA is to provide an ordered list of events for the emergency manager to address in the mitigation phase. By identifying the greatest vulnerabilities, the emergency manager may now address the most significant in the mitigation process. Figure 23–4 shows a sample hospital hazard vulnerability analysis chart.

PERSONAL/FAMILY PREPAREDNESS ISSUES

Disaster readiness is an issue not only for governments or businesses, but also for you and your family. If you are expected to respond to and provide assistance in a disaster, then the development of your own plan is imperative. Preparations that may be considered are:

- Arrangements for child care and pick-up from school. (The possibility exists that a disaster may occur that would preclude people from picking up their children. It is important to establish a system that would allow grandparents, aunts, uncles, or close family friends to pick the children up from child care or school. Many schools and day care centers require that alternates are preregistered with the office. This prudent step is to ensure that only those who actually belong with the children may pick them up.)
- Pet care
- Bottled water
- Medications
- Food that does not require refrigeration for the family as well as the pets
- Prearranged evacuation route and reunification location for family
- Entertainment that does not require power or batteries
- Flashlights with replacement bulbs
- Battery-operated radio
- Batteries
- Cash
- Prepaid calling card

Personal preparations include preparing a "go-bag" for each person that, at a minimum, contains:

- Clothing (socks, underwear, shirts, pants, and sweatshirts for 3–5 days)
- Shoes
- Personal care supplies (shaving kit, toothbrush, toothpaste, soap, shampoo, and other personal hygiene materials)
- Medications (30-day supply of prescriptions and photocopies of prescriptions)
- Cash
- Books, playing cards, or some other form of entertainment/diversion that does not require power or batteries

SUMMARY

The knowledge base of the forensic nurse specialist continues to expand, as does the variety of potential disasters. Basic concepts of emergency management have become one of many new tools for the forensic nurse. Though many may think of emergency management as the response and recovery from an act by a terrorist, it is actually based on developing a program to address the needs presented by all hazards. This "all hazards" approach to emergency management contends that the emergency management cycle needs to equally address the many potential threats presented by the modern world. Even though terrorism is the hot topic of emergency management, it is essentially just a disaster that is mediated by man to increase either the probability for an event to occur or the degree of impact of the event upon the community. Because of the use of an "all hazards" approach to planning, the prepared emergency manager should have, at a minimum, a basic response model for each event. A chemical terror attack is similar to a chemical release from a factory or transport vehicle, whereas a biological attack is an epidemic that was intentionally released on the target population.

Emergency management emphasizes mitigation as the best way to reduce the impact that disasters may have on a jurisdiction. By increasing training and readiness as well as improvements to the physical environment protected by the emergency manager, the potential impact that an event may have on the region is lessened. As responders, it is important that forensic nurses, as well as their families, be prepared to respond to an event. Personal and family preparedness will allow for a quicker response time as well as less time devoted to concern over the well-being of one's family. Having made adequate preparations, the responder should have fewer worries concerning the safety of their family and therefore be better able to concentrate on their performance.

The evolving field of emergency management depends on many different governmental agencies, businesses, nongovernmental organizations (Red Cross, United Way, etc.), and individuals prepared to enact their response plans in the event of a calamity. Regardless of the disaster, the trained forensic nurse has the potential to play an essential role in all phases of the emergency management cycle. It will be up to the forensic nurse specialist to engage in the process no matter where they are employed or living.

QUESTIONS FOR DISCUSSION

1. What are the steps in the disaster cycle?
2. What are some strategies for an organization to be prepared for and deal effectively with a disaster?
3. What governmental response units are available to respond to a disaster? What is the role of each unit and how do these interact with each other and with local management teams?
4. What difficulties are inherent in dealing with terrorist-type disasters?

REFERENCES

Decameron Web. (n.d.) *The coming of the plague to Italy.* Retrieved September 20, 2004, from http://www.brown.edu/Departments/Italian_Studies/dweb/plague/origins/spread.shtml.

Federal Emergency Management Agency; Emergency Management Institute. (July 2005). *The ICS/EOC interface.* Emmitsburg, MD: The Department of Homeland Security.

Federal Emergency Management Agency; Emergency Management Institute. (August 2003). *Principles of emergency management.* Emmitsburg, MD: The Department of Homeland Security.

Henderson, D. A., Fenner, F., Jezek, Z., Arita, I., Ladnyi, I. D. (1988). *Smallpox and its eradication: The history of smallpox and its spread around the world.* Retrieved September 20, 2004, from http://whqlibdoc.who.int/smallpox/9241561106_chp5.pdf.

History of bioterrorism: A chronological history of bioterrorism and biowarfare throughout the ages. Retrieved September 20, 2004, from http://www.bioterry.com/HistoryBioTerr.html.

Lynch, V. A. (1991). Forensic nursing in the emergency department: A new role for the 1990s. *Critical Care Nursing Quarterly, 4*(3), 69–86.

Lynch, V. A. (1995). Clinical forensic nursing: A new perspective in the management of crime victims from trauma to trial. *Critical Care Nursing Clinics of North America, 1*(3), 489–507.

Maniscalco, P. M. & Christen, H. T. (2002). *Understanding terrorism and managing the consequences.* Upper Saddle River, NJ: Prentice Hall.

National Wildfire Coordinating Group. (1994). Incident command system national training curriculum: History of ICS. Retrieved September 20, 2004, from www.nwcg.gov/pms/forms/compan/history.pdf.

Presidential Decision Directive 39, U.S. Policy on Counterterrorism. (June 21, 1995). Retrieved June 2004 from http://www.fas.org/irp/offdocs/pdd39.htm.

Presidential Decision Directive 63, Critical Infrastructure Protection. (May 22, 1998). Retrieved June 2004 from http://www.fas.org/irp/offdocs/pdd/pdd-63.htm.

Rosenburg, B. H. (2002). *Analysis of the anthrax attacks: Analysis of the source of the anthrax attacks.* Federation of American Scientists. Retrieved September 20, 2004, from www.911review.org/wget/www.fas.org/bwc/news/anthraxreport.htm.

World Health Organization. (October 2004). Fact sheet on smallpox. Retrieved June 17, 2004, from http://www.who.int/mediacentre/factsheets/smallpox/en/index.html.

Zkea Archives. (n.d.) *Category: Historical background, Native Americans, smallpox, history, demographics.* Retrieved September 20, 2004, from http://www.zkea.com/archives/archive06010.html.

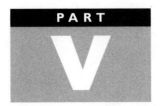

PART

V

CONCEPTS FOR
THE 21ST CENTURY

24

Media Management and Public Relations

Anne Klein

The forensic nurse interfaces with many individuals within the broad scope of forensic practice. The various roles of the forensic nurse may sometimes lead to interactions with the public in nontraditional ways. Because the forensic nurse may be involved in high profile cases or serve as an advocate or spokesperson, knowledge of how the media function and the best way to work with the media to achieve success for both parties is critical. In today's era of "all news, all the time," well-honed communication skills can often help bridge the gaps among the healthcare system, the justice system, and the public. As a forensic nursing professional, you must know how and when to work with the news media. You need to know what your role is in many professional situations. You need to know what you can say without compromising the case you are working on or jeopardizing the security, safety, or health of the people with whom you are working, while protecting your own credibility.

CHAPTER FOCUS

Understanding the media
Monitoring the media
Developing a strategy to work with the media
Developing a proactive plan to manage a crisis
Drills and media training
Understanding media terminology

KEY TERMS_____

broadcast media
follow-up questions
for background only
Internet media services
key message
not for attribution
off the record
on the record
outreach
preapprovals
print media
spokesperson
talking point

INTRODUCTION

As a forensic nurse, you might be called upon someday to be an official spokesperson to the news media. You may think that it is unlikely, but in today's era of "all news, all the time," chances are that sooner or later you will be contacted or confronted by at least one reporter seeking factual information, or just wanting your comments when something major occurs or as an advocate for a particular cause or group. Competition requires that reporters go to anybody they can find to give them responses to whatever questions they may have.

It won't matter what the occurrence. It might be a natural disaster or a case involving violence against a child or elderly person. It might be a case of sexual abuse. It might involve a crime scene investigation or an autopsy. Because forensic nurses help bridge the gap between the healthcare system and the justice system, the range of possible instances where reporters might seek you out for information or opinion, even when you are not an official spokesperson, is enormous. This is why it is so important that, as a forensic nursing professional, you know how and when to work with the news media. You need to know what your role is in any of these situations. You need to know what you can say without compromising the case you are working on or jeopardizing the security, safety, or health of the person you are working with. At the same time, you need to protect your own credibility.

This chapter will provide an overview of the news media and some basic coping skills when working with reporters and other news professionals. In this chapter you will learn:

- about different types of news media and how their roles and needs differ.
- the differences between proactive and reactive media relations.

- what you can and cannot say to the media—and when and how to say it.
- how to develop "key messages" and how to stay focused on them.
- how to prepare responses well in advance of actually being asked questions.
- how to answer questions you don't really want to answer, without having to say, "No comment."
- how to balance the media's need to know with HIPAA's privacy standards.

In all these and other matters you will learn how to work with the media so that both their needs and yours are satisfied without violating your professional code of ethics.

UNDERSTANDING THE MEDIA

All news media generally want the same information:

Who (Who was involved?)
What (What happened?)
When (When did it happen?)
Where (Where did it happen?)
Why (Why did it happen?)
How (How did it happen?)

But all media are not necessarily looking for identical answers. That is because each medium operates differently, with different time and space constraints, and with different audience needs. Consequently, what you say must be tailored to the needs of each specific medium.

Traditionally, news media have fallen into two broad categories—print and broadcast/cable. In recent years the Internet, which combines print and broadcast/cable with immediacy and instant availability, has been growing as a major source of news information.

Print Media

Print media include newspapers, magazines, and national news (also known as wire) services such as The Associated Press (AP), Dow Jones, and Reuters. Print media reporters often have more time than their broadcast brethren in which to research and write their stories. This often gives them the time and the ability to do in-depth research. It also enables them to look for more relevant material and different angles from what the broadcast media will have reported because of their earlier and more-or-less instant deadlines.

This difference can be especially beneficial when you need to explain complex material. Because print reporters generally have the time to delve into details, it gives you the opportunity to cover material that may have been ignored or played down by broadcast media in their rush to be first with the news. There is also a very good chance that more of what you have to say will be quoted in print. In turn, this enables you to be able to give perspective to your story for people who may have only gotten a quick summary from the broadcast coverage.

However, this opportunity can also pose a danger if you are not careful. Because so much more of what you say can and, most likely, will be reported, you need to be careful not to ramble on and on. The more you keep talking, the more there is a danger you may say something you shouldn't. If this *faux pas* appears in print, the likely result will be embarrassment for you and your organization.

There is also the danger that the reporter may go off in a wrong direction. If the reporter does not completely understand the subject, he or she can do a lot of harm. Therefore, when working with print media, use the opportunity to tell your story in depth, but make certain the reporter is properly focused and understands what you are saying at all times. Consider the interview an opportunity to educate the reporter. If the reporter is confused when he or she begins to write the story, the result can be a professional disaster.

Broadcast/Cable Media

In contrast to print media, broadcast media—that is, radio and television—and cable TV news channels are not usually interested in extended, in-depth reports. In most instances, stories prepared by broadcast reporters run anywhere from about 30 seconds to a couple of minutes. If you are lucky and have given the reporter a good, concise interview, you may have a chance to be quoted in your own voice as part of that news report. The problem is that you will usually have perhaps only 15 to 20 seconds in which to state your case. This means that the message you want to convey to the public has to be well organized and framed clearly in one or more concise "sound bites." If your answers are too lengthy, only a portion of one of your responses will be used to highlight a particular point that the reporter wants to make during the broadcast. Unfortunately, because the reporter is choosing the portion of the interview to air, unless you have chosen your words carefully, the report may not have the impact you intended.

There are significant differences among the various broadcast media. Because radio conveys sound only, you want to try to frame your comments for the listening audience in a way that will help them form mental pictures. A word of caution: In most instances radio reporters generally try to get their information and sound bites as quickly as possible, then depart. Don't be misled by that. Radio can still be an important news medium for your organization as long as you remember to speak your message clearly and concisely. When you do that you can be reasonably certain that what you have to say will be reported fairly and accurately on radio.

Television reporters, on the other hand, want more than just your voice. They are equally concerned about getting pictures to show along with their reports, so you may want to give thought beforehand to any picture possibilities to go along with your comments. It is not unusual for TV reporters to use the spokesperson's voice (but not his or her face) while relevant pictures are being shown. That is referred to in TV parlance as a "voice-over." Unlike radio where you have to be concerned with just your brief sound bite, when dealing with TV it is important to try to frame what you say to go along with particular images you may have in mind. The use of demonstrative "props" while speaking or requesting the interview be filmed in a setting that conveys part of your message are two examples of framing your message.

Another problem often encountered when dealing with TV is its use of live pictures as events are unfolding. Frequently, the anchorperson back in the studio who is trying to describe the pictures that are going out over the air has only scant information about what is happening, so he or she will keep repeating what has been previously said. This can be advantageous to you if you can get your quote on the air early. If studio news anchors keep repeating your perspective of the incident, it can help assure that your version of the story is getting out to the public.

Not all television news is the same. Local TV news broadcasts focus on events differently from network television newscasts, and both differ considerably from cable TV's 24-hour news channels. Local TV news programs generally focus on the local angle. They are concerned with the story's impact on their own viewing area, especially if someone from the local area is involved. Network TV news, on the other hand, focuses on stories that have broad national importance. If you are lucky (or unlucky) enough to be involved in a story covered by the networks, you may find that the entire event is capsulized in a single sentence or two during scheduled news broadcasts. On the other hand, cable TV news (where many channels compete in providing nonstop coverage) may devote hours to coverage of even relatively unimportant events. That magnifies the impact of the event and makes what the spokesperson has to say all the more important.

When TV, or occasionally radio, devotes extended time to a news story, reporters often have to fill a lot of air time with relatively few facts to report. That often leads to on-the-air speculation. In such situations, it becomes especially important that you not join in the speculation or allow yourself to be goaded into voicing your own speculative thoughts.

We have all seen forensic professionals asked to speculate about the types of evidence or other factors influencing high profile cases. Too often they provide on-the-spot commentary that later comes back to haunt them. Remember, when you are addressing the news media officially or unofficially, professionalism demands that you speak only from a strictly informational and factual perspective; otherwise, you risk your personal and professional credibility.

The Internet

The Internet is quickly becoming an important third major news medium. It has the unique ability to combine print, sound, photos, and moving images and present them on demand, thereby combining the best features of newspapers, radio, and TV, along with the major news services. Recent studies have shown that an ever-increasing number of people are turning to the Internet as their first source of information about breaking news.

Today nearly every major news outlet, from national to local newspapers and magazines and from national broadcasters to local broadcasters, has a website where people can turn for the latest news. Working with reporters for Internet news feeds is not any different from working with regular print or broadcast reporters; they are usually the same people, and that means we can expect their news reports will be professional, fair, balanced, and accurate.

Unfortunately, not all information on the Internet meets professional journalistic standards. Chat rooms, rogue websites, and "bloggers" who maintain online journals and diaries answer to no professional authority and often dispense disinformation, rumor, and innuendo. Monitoring such sites is extremely difficult, if not downright impossible. Therefore, it becomes even more important to maintain good relations with the professional mainstream media to ensure that your story is being properly told.

MONITORING THE MEDIA

This ability for news to be instantly disseminated—even incorrectly—by dozens of media makes it paramount that the various media be monitored for accuracy. The sooner an inaccuracy can be corrected, the less likely serious damage may occur. This is especially important during breaking news stories. If necessary, be sure that your organization appoints one or more individuals to monitor assigned media to see whether your story is being accurately reported. If it is not, immediately contact the appropriate news outlet and urge the editor to make a timely correction. Unfortunately, depending on the type of medium, that correction may not have the same impact as the original news story.

Working with the news media is like working with fire: It can give your image a warm favorable glow or it can burn you badly. Your experience will depend upon how well you perform your task of spokesperson when you are called upon to fill this role.

Develop a Proactive Plan for Working with the Media

Can you imagine any doctor or hospital undertaking a heart transplant operation without any advance preparation or planning? Of course not. Not if they want to maximize success and minimize risk. The same is true when it comes to working with the media. The more prepared you are, the greater the chance of achieving your goals.

The best way to work with the media is proactively. The more you work with the media before a serious situation arises, the more effective you will be working with the media when high profile incidents do occur.

Media Outreach

To start, build a list of reporters, editors, and broadcast news producers and directors at all of the local media outlets that might cover your organization, healthcare issues, and the justice system. Call them to introduce yourself and, in the process, explain to them how forensic nursing is the bridge between the healthcare system and the justice system. Then meet in person and get to know them (see Figure 24–1). The idea is to let them get acquainted with you before the need ever arises for them to have to seek you out.

Getting better acquainted means learning what kinds of stories interest them. It means learning what their deadlines are and honoring those deadlines. It means being open and friendly and willing to help the reporter or editor as much as you can. It means being prompt in returning phone calls or emails, and offering them help on stories on which they are working that may not even be related to your organization. It means holding seminars on purely technical subjects for no purpose other than to provide background information even when you are not looking for publicity or a credit line. It means introducing reporters who cover crime, healthcare, or legal issues to your key executives and other individuals in your organization who can provide information when needed. It means developing credibility in their eyes long before you may ever need it in reaction to a crisis situation.

You are a forensic nurse, a professional with a specific area of expertise. Reporters seek experts as they write their stories. If you are called by a reporter, remember these guidelines and you will have a good experience:

1. **Treat reporters as professionals** and recognize they have a job to do.
2. **Confine your responses to your area of expertise.**
3. **Know in advance what you want to say, and stick to it.** Write it down and keep your notes with key message points handy.
4. **When you are a spokesperson, ask to be briefed by the public relations staff prior to a media interview,** especially if the reporter has provided questions in advance. Anticipate other questions the reporter may ask.
5. **Take time to formulate your answers before responding,** especially for more difficult questions. If you need more time to prepare your answer, ask the reporter to repeat the question. Don't digress. Stick to the main facts.
6. **Never lie to a reporter. Be as honest, open, and helpful as you can** when answering a reporter's questions. Remember, a reporter's job is not to serve as an advocate or foe of a particular organization or individual. Reporters want a good story. You can put your best foot forward and help them by following this "open honesty" rule.
7. **Cooperate with a reporter** because he or she will get the story whether you help or not. If you don't give reporters the facts, they will find someone who will, including people who don't know the answers but will talk anyway. If you don't cooperate, you can't complain if the story that gets published or broadcast is based on hearsay and conjecture.
8. **Convey medical and technical information in lay terms** whenever possible. Be patient if reporters seem to have difficulty understanding the information you are conveying. Try using a second approach to explaining the material. If you can, give reasonable analogies that the public can relate to. You want the reporter to get the information right.
9. **Repeat information or review what could be considered confusing details.** This is particularly important during a crisis situation, when information must be accurate to avoid confusion of the facts.
10. **Provide plenty of background information** about your organization and your job. Use any background information you have available, especially about forensic nursing and your role as a responder.
11. **Do not answer a question if you don't have the facts and do not give out any unconfirmed facts.** Say, "I don't know, but I will get that information for you." Then, get back to the reporter as soon as possible.
12. **Stop talking after you have answered a reporter's question.** Don't ramble on. This is when many comments are made that were not meant to be made. Reporters will sometimes use "awkward" silences to their advantage. If there is a long pause after you have given an answer, ask "Do you have another question?"
13. **Always ask what a reporter's deadline is and honor it** when you must get back to him or her with information. If you cannot honor it, say so.
14. **Keep your word.** If you promise to arrange an interview or to get more information for an answer, be certain you follow through, even if it is only to let the reporter know you are still "working on it."
15. **Never play favorites when it comes to providing newsworthy information.** If you do offer a reporter an exclusive feature or background story, then it should remain exclusive until both you and the reporter agree it is not.
16. **Do not *ever* respond to a question with "No comment."** It is *never* an acceptable answer. If you cannot comment, explain why. (See Figure 24–6 on page 731.)

Figure 24–1 Guidelines for working with the news media.

17. ***Never talk "off the record."*** An excellent rule to remember is, "Never say anything you do not want to see in print or hear on the air." Assume the microphone is on whenever a reporter is present. Unless you have a long-established relationship with a reporter, "off the record" entails considerable risk.
18. **Never ask to see a story or news report before it is printed or aired.** Reporters and editors do not look kindly on this practice. They regard it as an intrusion on the tradition of a free press and an attempt on your part to censor their coverage.
19. **Be alert to inaccuracies in a printed or aired story.** If there are major inaccuracies in a printed or aired story, call the reporter, explain the error, and ask him or her to correct the file or database. Do not demand a retraction or correction unless absolutely necessary. You do not want to prolong the story.
20. **Do not offer the reporter gifts.** Good intentions can be misconstrued.
21. **Build relationships.** Get to know reporters you might be working with and what types of stories they like to work on. If you have a story idea for them or information to help them do their jobs better, call them.
22. **Provide telephone numbers** where you can be reached in an emergency.
23. **Avoid an initial overreaction during a crisis.** You are a professional. Try to remain calm and speak to the reporter in a conversational tone. When you get angry, you lose control of the situation and lessen the chances for ensuring that your information is reported properly and correctly. Do your best to be helpful. Don't guarantee how quickly you can provide answers.
24. **Notify the media before they contact you** if having the media first learn about a situation from someone else would damage you or your organization's image or credibility.

The Reality of Forensic Nursing

Forensic nursing is a relatively new specialty. The term was only introduced into the United States in 1991, and it was not recognized as a specialty by the American Nurses Association until 1995. So most people, including news people and many in the healthcare industry, have not yet heard of it.

One of the very first proactive conversations you should have is to educate the news media about forensic nursing—what it is, why it is a cutting-edge profession, and what you, as a forensic nurse, do. When television shows or movies focus on forensics for solving crimes, many may assume this to be your principal role. This is where being credible is essential. You will want to point out the differences between entertainment and real life, then take this excellent opportunity to explain the various specialties (in particular your specialty) within forensic nursing practices.

Build Goodwill

Build on your media contacts in positive ways. For example, with the assistance of public relations professionals in your organization, you might develop a series of news releases or feature articles introducing reporters to forensic nursing and covering the differences between fictional drama and reality. You could provide information on ways the public can protect itself should an environmental hazard occur. Or you might discuss the implications of school bullying and other antisocial behavior. Or, as still another example, you might identify risk factors and cues for violence in healthcare and workplace settings. These are only a few of the many informational news stories you could offer the news media that would not only help explain what it is you do, but also build a working relationship and establish credibility with the news people who cover your field.

The more goodwill you develop with the members of the news media during this proactive phase of your media relations, the more residual goodwill you will have when a crisis or disaster strikes and you are forced to go into reactive mode. Remember that the reporters who will most likely cover your organization when trouble strikes will be the same ones you will have been working with proactively. If you have already established your credibility with them and earned their trust, they will be far more likely to be receptive to what you have to say. And they will likely be more cooperative.

PLAN FOR A CRISIS

You can prepare for working with the media during a crisis. That process entails having your responses prepared even before disasters strike. It is not as difficult as you might think. In fact, it is nearly impossible to handle a crisis effectively from a communications point of view unless you have planned ahead. Reactive communications without planning can result in missteps and cause even more serious consequences. A guide to use during times of crisis is shown in Figure 24–2.

In the Chinese language, the expression for crisis is made up of two characters, one meaning danger and the other meaning opportunity. Every crisis situation actually can be an opportunity to polish and enhance your or your organization's image, provided you have carefully planned in advance what to do and how to respond. Here, then, is how to convert potential adversity into good fortune.

Identify Potential Scenarios

Start by identifying every potential situation or scenario you might have to face that could require interfacing with the media. Ask yourself such questions as: Where are the greatest risks in our organization? What specifically might happen? How likely is it? How severe could the impact be? What groups would be affected? What is our organization's

A crisis should not come as a surprise. As a forensic nurse, your work always has the potential to come to the attention of the news media. You should plan ahead for what you might do or say if the media calls during a crisis situation. Here is a checklist of action steps to help you prepare.

1. **Begin by making a list of potential crisis scenarios you could face.** Working with your department colleagues, develop statements (called key messages) that are appropriate and safe to say about each scenario.
2. **For each potential crisis scenario, know in advance who has the authority to speak for the organization.**
3. **If you are a designated spokesperson, be sure that key staff members know your role, your area of expertise, and when and how to contact you.**
4. **Prearrange needed clearances of your key messages for each potential scenario.** Identify the person who will need to provide clearance for comments on unanticipated events.
5. **Anticipate the questions the media might ask as a follow-up.** Know when to say, "I'm sorry, I just cannot say anything more because . . ." (See Figure 24–6 on page 731.)
6. **Establish a relationship with your organization's legal department and agree on your role before a crisis develops.**
7. **If you have a public relations or public affairs department in your organization, establish a working relationship with the staff members.** They will be a big help in working with the media.
8. **Be sure everyone in your organization knows your organization's definition of what constitutes a crisis.** This is especially true of receptionists, telephone operators, security guards, and administrative staff.
9. **Prepare general background information on forensic nursing and your role in a crisis situation that you can have ready for distribution to reporters.**
10. **Keep your prepared key messages and talking points up to date and instantly available.**
11. **Participate in tests of your organization's crisis and media preparedness, and ask for media training.**
12. **Work with reporters as much as you can in noncrisis situations.** You will build credibility with them and confidence in yourself.

If you plan for potential crises, you will feel confident in your role as a spokesperson.

Figure 24–2   A crisis communications checklist.

position if this type of incident occurs? What is our organization's philosophy on how to respond to this situation? What is my role?

Some potential situations and scenarios that readily come to mind include:

- Child, elder, and spousal abuse
- Sexual assault
- Environmental hazards
- Internet crime
- Pornography, especially if it involves children
- Bullying in schools
- Issues of competence

- Treatment of prisoners in custody
- Treatment of crime victims
- Criminally induced trauma
- Maladaptive social behavior
- Assessment of inmates in a psychiatric facility
- Preservation of evidence
- Investigations of death and violence

You may encounter other situations in your work. They, too, should be considered, because if you don't know how you will respond to that very first reporter's call, it is almost a foregone conclusion that the first story written or broadcast will be negative or, at best, simply incorrect. Unless you handle the call properly, your credibility or your competence—or both—will be questioned.

Identify Spokespersons

Once you have identified the potential crisis scenarios you might face, then determine who within your organization or sphere of work will be the official spokesperson. Will it be someone from the public relations or public affairs department? Someone from legal? Someone from management? You?

Where and when do you fit into the picture? Regardless of your assigned or unassigned role, it is still a safe bet that sooner or later you will be approached by someone from the news media, so it is best to be prepared. This is especially true if you have taken the time to develop a relationship with the media in your area. You will be their "go to" person, whether or not you are the official spokesperson or even directly involved in the crisis situation.

Develop Key Messages

Once all the potential situations and scenarios have been identified, the next step is to determine how you or other designated spokespersons will respond to the media should any of these incidents occur. That means developing key messages and talking points for each potential incident. You cannot respond adequately to a crisis unless you have prepared in advance. There are too many other things to think about and do when the crisis occurs.

Key messages are simply short, concise statements (sound bites) that help you explain the main points you want to make. Talking points are additional statements that expand, explain, or support your key messages. In working with the media, your key messages will help them understand who you are, what you do, and how well you do it; for example: "I am a forensic nurse. This is what I do. . . . These are the steps or protocols involved in a situation such as this. . . ." Your talking points then become the facts you use to describe how you do your job.

It is essential that you give your key message up front before discussing or addressing other issues. In a fast-paced environment, you never know when you will be interrupted. Unless you are focused on your messages, it is easy to be led off the topic to other subjects by reporters. When that happens, you never get to talk about what *you* want to talk about. In more extreme cases, you may need to consider how to respond to a hostile reporter; points to consider in this situation are outlined in Figure 24–3.

Your key messages should be the three or four most important sound bites that you want the reporter to use. They should not be rambling sentences. A good guideline to remember is that you should be able to complete a response in the time it takes for a short elevator ride to the third or fourth floor.

Somewhere in the course of your relationship with the news media, you can expect to be confronted by a hostile reporter. How you manage that situation will not only affect how that reporter handles your story, but it could also have an influence on other reporters' reactions. That's why the first rule for dealing with a hostile reporter is to remain calm and cool.

Don't let a hostile reporter get you rattled or angry. You will make a very poor impression on a reader or listener. Instead, be calm, friendly, and pleasant, no matter what the reporter says, and no matter how many different ways he or she tries to get to you.

Here are eight other suggestions for diffusing a hostile situation.

1. Bridge to another subject by saying, "That's an interesting point, but you'll be more interested in . . ." and say it.
2. Restate the hostile question in a positive way. You can say, "If by that you mean . . ." and ask a more positive question that you can then answer.
3. Disagree with the premise if it is incorrect. Never let incorrect assertions remain unchallenged. A simple "that is not correct" will do. Then give the correct information before you go on to answer the question.
4. Refuse to comment on alleged facts you don't know to be true or on out-of-context statements. Explain that you can't answer until you have all the facts or have heard the full statement in context.
5. Never respond to a hypothetical question. Just say that you don't respond to hypothetical questions because they involve speculation, and it is not your job to speculate.
6. Don't let reporters shame you into responding to hostile questions by making personal attacks against you. Learn to resist the urge. Restate the key message points you want to make.
7. Don't let yourself get trapped into a "yes" or "no" answer, if that is an inadequate response. Keep repeating your key message points.
8. Never use offensive language even if quoting someone else. If you say it, regardless of the context, it can become your quote.

Figure 24–3   How to respond to a hostile reporter.

Prepare for Follow-up Questions

After you have determined your key messages, you are not yet finished. Reporters always ask follow-up questions. Anticipate media questions in advance. Remember that reporters always want the answers to questions that start with the words who, what, where, when, why, and how. Here are a baker's dozen questions you can almost always expect to be asked:

- What happened?
- Who was involved?
- Where did it happen?
- When did it happen?
- Why did it happen?
- How did it happen?
- Who was hurt?
- How badly?
- What are you going to do about it?
- Who else is working on this?
- When will you know the answers?
- How are you going about it?
- Why will it take so long?

Knowing what questions to expect makes preparing answers in advance that much easier. But unless you have carefully thought about the many crisis scenarios you could face, you won't know what to say to the media. You will hesitate or perhaps say the wrong thing and make matters worse. Your responses, especially to the question "What are you going to do about it," should be a reflection of your organization's ethics and feelings about how it operates. Most important, your responses should reflect your professionalism and competence in doing your work. (See Figure 24–4.)

---

1. Be mentally prepared. Know your role. Know what you can and cannot say. Always have your key messages about the role of a forensic nurse in your mind. Stick to them.
2. Never let a reporter badger you into answering simply yes or no when a fuller explanation is required. You do not have to respond only in the way the reporter wants you to respond.
3. Never answer "what if" hypothetical questions. They serve no purpose except to lead to more hypotheticals and endless discussion.
4. Do not comment on any purported statements by others unless you personally have seen or heard them and have had time to formulate an opinion and give a response.
5. Answer only questions about which you have information. Refer the reporters to others who may have the answers or offer to get the answers.

Figure 24–4 How to respond when you are ambushed by a reporter.

Obtain Preapprovals—A Must

You should have a preapproved list of the kinds of information you can provide to the media without having to clear every word through the legal department while the crisis is actually under way. This would include telling the media what happened, when it occurred, and what you are doing to remedy it. In addition, the restrictions placed on the forensic nurse by HIPAA and similar regulations may have a significant impact on the type of information that may be shared with the media, as shown in Figure 24–5.

The best way to obtain preapprovals is to simply introduce yourself to staff members in the legal and public relations departments so they can get to know you and you can get to know them. That will make it easier to learn what they expect or require in working with the media and, in turn, help guide your own responses to the media.

Know Your Job

In many instances, your best response to reporters' questions, regardless of the incident, may simply be to describe for them what protocols you follow in the performance of your duties in response to a specific incident. It might be a statement that begins, "I am a forensic nurse. In a situation such as this, involving (fill in the incident: child abuse, sexual assault, autopsy assistance, etc.), these are the protocols I normally follow." Or, "This is what I normally do in such situations," or "This is what I am going to be doing," and then begin to describe for the reporter or reporters how you perform your duties in this matter. The advantage of this type of response is that it grounds your answer in fact, not speculation, and you don't need to worry about having given an answer that may violate professional ethics. This is an especially effective way to respond to questions from the media when an ongoing criminal investigation prevents any discussion of the particulars of the specific case, evidence, or your involvement. Answering in this fashion also educates the reporter about your professional role and relieves you of having to say "No comment." (See Figure 24–6.)

The most important thing to remember when you are working with the media is that you can control what you say. You have the ability to give out as much or as little information as you choose. Never forget that!

Review Your Plans

Review your crisis scenario plans periodically. Try to determine whether you need to update the anticipated situations or your planned responses. Refresh your key messages and talking points, depending on the situation. Hone them to the point they make good 20- to 30-second sound bites for broadcast and then practice, practice, practice saying them.

The generally accepted rule for working with news media is to tell as much as possible as quickly as possible, and as honestly and forthrightly as possible.

However, where medical facilities and patients are involved, this guideline may be difficult to follow. Most healthcare organizations have in-house restrictions to safeguard the privacy and confidentiality of patients in their care. The Health Insurance Portability and Accountability Act of 1996 (HIPAA) also puts restrictions on what healthcare institutions and organizations can and cannot reveal to the news media. (Note: In the event state law is more restrictive than the HIPAA privacy regulations, the state law applies.)

Unfortunately, some medical organizations and medical professionals use HIPAA guidelines as an excuse not to talk to the news media or provide any information whatsoever. This approach can only exacerbate a difficult situation, and it may even tarnish an organization's image. Remember, reporters will keep contacting people until they find an alternate source who is willing to give them the information they are seeking.

It is interesting to note that police, other law enforcement agencies, and firefighters are not considered covered entities under HIPAA. HIPAA restrictions do not extend, for example, to police incident reports, fire incident reports, court records, autopsy reports, or records of agencies that do not provide either health care or insurance for health care. Also not restricted are records that an individual has authorized to be disclosed. In addition, family members, witnesses, Good Samaritans, or anyone else not affiliated with a healthcare provider can provide information without running afoul of HIPAA.

You may find that reporters today know as much or more about HIPAA's guidelines than medical organization spokespersons. Various professional journalism organizations have had attorneys review the HIPAA guidelines for the benefit of reporters so that they know their journalistic rights. One journalism group even goes so far as to suggest to its members that they challenge blanket refusals to disclose information based on HIPAA by asking, "Where in the law does it say you are prohibited from releasing that particular information?"

So rather than taking a negative stance in dealing with the news media, consider looking for some common ground that balances their need to know with the need for confidentiality and protection of privacy. Here are some common-sense guidelines for what kind of information you could divulge that most professionals would agree can work, especially in a crisis situation.

• Description of the general nature of the incident (i.e., what happened).
• Corrective measures being taken at present (e.g., fire department has situation under control, a triage center has been set up, everyone has been safely evacuated, etc.). This is an opportune time for the forensic nurse to explain his or her role as a professional.
• Description of the emergency response at the scene, including police, firefighters, physicians, and forensic nurses.
• Presence or absence of injuries (but not the names of individuals involved unless you have received permission). If it is absolutely necessary to give more detail, provide an anonymous, nonspecific description (a 64-year-old male, for example), but nothing that would directly identify or strongly hint at the victim's identity. If the family members insist on keeping the victim's name confidential, you must abide by their wishes.
• Names of hospitals being used in case of injuries.

Kathleen Kirby, legal counsel for the Radio-Television News Directors Association & Foundation, goes so far as to note that whether an institution can confirm a patient's death depends on where the body is. "If the patient is still within the facility, then it is arguable that death is a condition that may be disclosed as part of the directory information. If the deceased patient has been removed from the hospital, then the hospital must obtain a signed authorization from the patient's personal representative to release information about the patient's death," she writes.

Other directory information (except for the patient's religion) may also be released to the media if the media or public asks for the patient by name and only *after* the patient has been given the opportunity and consented to the release of directory information. This includes the patient's location in the hospital as well as the patient's general condition.

If a patient has agreed not to restrict his or her information, the American Hospital Association recommends the following terms:
Undetermined: Patient awaiting physician and assessment.
Good: Vital signs are stable and within normal limits. Patient is conscious and comfortable. Indicators are excellent.
Fair: Vital signs are stable and within normal limits. Patient is conscious but may be uncomfortable. Indicators are favorable.
Serious: Vital signs may be unstable and not within normal limits. Patient is acutely ill. Indicators are questionable.
Critical: Vital signs are unstable and not within normal limits. Patient may be unconscious. Indicators are unfavorable.
Treated and released: Patient received treatment but was not admitted.

A more detailed statement regarding a patient's condition and injuries or illness can be released only with written authorization from the patient. If the media ask for additional information, you should politely but firmly explain that you cannot provide the information because the patient has requested privacy.

Note: When the media ask you for information, start by asking yourself a very basic question: Is the information you are about to divulge going to affect people and have an impact on their lives or decisions, or is this information just going to satisfy idle curiosity? If you answer the latter, then do not respond to the media, and explain why you are taking this position.

Figure 24–5 HIPAA vs. the media's need to know.

The best way to receive fair and balanced news coverage is to be open with the media. But sometimes you may find yourself being asked questions you really don't want to answer.

Saying "no comment" automatically implies guilt or that you are hiding something. And the more often you repeat "no comment," the more certain you can be that the reporters will seek out and find someone else who *will* say something—and very likely not favorable to your situation.

Here are some ways to fend off questions you don't want to answer without saying "no comment."

1. If you don't know the answer to the question, just say so. It's far better to state on the record that you don't know, because at least you are being truthful and reporters will respect that.
2. If you don't know the answer, but think you can find someone who does, say so. Tell the reporter you will try to find out and get back to him or her. But don't just say it; *do it* as well!
3. If you don't yet have enough facts to give a meaningful response, say so. Then use your key messages to get across the information you want the media to know.
4. If the information you would have to provide is proprietary, point that out and explain why you cannot respond without divulging this information.
5. If there are relevant HIPAA restrictions or institutional privacy guidelines that may prevent releasing information, cite them.
6. If the reporter is basing his or her question on a faulty premise, explain why the premise is incorrect.
7. If you don't like the subject of the question asked, bridge to an entirely different thought instead. Watch political debates or Sunday morning talk shows and observe how politicians often don't answer the question asked, but instead respond with something else they prefer to talk about.
8. If the reporter's statement is true, but you have more information that provides a fuller perspective, say something like "Let me tell you more about . . ." and paint the bigger picture.
9. If you don't know personally that the information the reporter is giving you as part of his or her question is true, just say you haven't been told that yet and therefore are not in a position to answer the question at this time.
10. If the question involves conjecture or speculation, note that it is not your job to speculate.
11. If you are asked a hypothetical "what if" question, respond that a hypothetical answer to a hypothetical question would serve no purpose and might even raise unnecessary concern on the part of the public.
12. Use your key messages and talking points as an answer.

Figure 24–6 A dozen ways to avoid saying "no comment."

Follow up from time to time with the public relations department to determine whether there have been or should be any changes in who will speak for the organization to the news media. Similarly make certain you have a designated backup spokesperson and that he or she has been brought up-to-date on the various scenarios and the prepared responses.

Review your prepared responses with the legal department and make sure you understand all of the legal ramifications involved. Because attorneys are, by professional training, sometimes overly cautious, work with them to strike a balance between the privacy guidelines in HIPAA and the media's need to know.

Prepare in advance any needed background information about forensic nursing and your role. Work with both PR and legal departments to determine when written statements should be issued to the media, and get them cleared and approved beforehand.

Make certain that your organization has a continuous media monitoring system set up and that each individual charged with following coverage knows which media he or she is responsible for monitoring. Monitoring ongoing news coverage in the midst of a breaking story is especially critical. Errors or misinformation need to be caught and corrected as quickly as possible before they are more widely disseminated. Mistakes are much harder to correct after first impressions have been formed.

Finally, and most important of all, when a crisis occurs and the need to go into reactive mode arises, stay calm. Take your time to assess the situation carefully, then begin to implement your plan. Remember that you have control over what you say, when you say it, and how you say it. If you have carefully planned, regularly updated your plan, and periodically practiced implementation of your plan, you will have your media communications under control.

DRILLS AND MEDIA TRAINING

There's an old vaudeville joke that goes something like this: A tourist in New York stops a person on the street and asks, "How do you get to Carnegie Hall?" The person answers: "Practice."

Corny as that joke is, it contains a serious grain of truth. Nothing is ever successfully accomplished without lots of practice. The same is true with regard to media relations and managing the media. Skills are perfected through repeated training exercises.

If your organization holds disaster or crisis training drills, be sure media response is included. Drills can give you an opportunity to practice your skills as a spokesperson and measure the effectiveness of your media relations plan under more realistic circumstances. Coworkers are usually assigned to play the role of reporters during such a drill, and the questions they ask are usually pretty tough because they know a great deal more about you and your organization than any reporter does. Sometimes organizations invite a few members of the media to participate in the drill. Both reporters and organization staff benefit from the training exercise, but a more important and lasting benefit is the opportunity to enhance the bond between your organization and the news media.

If your organization conducts periodic media training exercises for executives and managers, insist on being included in this training.

Not enough can be said about the importance and benefits of a good media training program. You will learn when and how to issue formal statements. You will learn how to condense and capsulize your key messages and talking points into effective sound bites. You will learn how to face a crowd of questioning reporters coolly and calmly. You will learn how to control the questioners and how to maintain your composure in a hostile environment. You will learn how to take your time to consider your answers to questions before responding. You will learn how to maintain your credibility and objectivity. You will learn the do's and don'ts for working with the media. You will learn the meanings of media terminology. In short, you will learn and become skilled in your role as a spokesperson working with the news media.

Practice, Practice, Practice!

Dancers who worked with the award-winning choreographer-director Bob Fosse like to tell how he would make them rehearse dance numbers, sometimes hundreds of times, before the opening of a show. And they were grateful, because when they finally stepped on stage in front of an audience, they did not have to consciously remember their dance steps. Their feet and their bodies just moved automatically, exactly as they were supposed to. Their bodies were so conditioned that they couldn't make a mistake if they tried. The moral of the story is, of course, that it is not enough simply to train how to do something. It requires practice to perfect one's skills.

The same is true with media relations. It is not enough to know how to work with the media or to plan your key messages and talking points beforehand. Without practice, there is no assurance that when the time comes to perform for real, you will be able to execute your plan flawlessly. Only with repeated practice can you be relatively certain of meeting your goal.

Start by reviewing the potential scenarios and situations you have identified as requiring responses. Review the key messages and talking points you have developed and written down for each of these. Edit these messages as often as needed to reduce them to meaningful 20- to 30-second sound bites, then periodically rehearse saying them while facing someone with a television camera or with a microphone stuck in your face.

In other words, try to get the feel of "performing" in an actual working environment so that you become comfortable in such a setting. Like Bob Fosse's dancers, you want to be able to say and do all the right things before your news media audience without ever thinking about your steps. And that can only come from constant, repeated practice.

UNDERSTANDING MEDIA TERMINOLOGY

Members of the news media operate under an unwritten code of ethics that spells out what they may and may not print or air based on agreements they make with news makers. But, if you expect reporters to adhere to these agreements, it is important that both you and the reporter have the same understanding about what you have agreed to. This is why it is critical that you learn the meaning of some basic media terms. Otherwise you may think that what you are telling a reporter in an attempt to be helpful will not be printed or used on the air and then be shocked or horrified when it becomes public.

On the Record

This means exactly what it sounds like. Everything you say can be used or reported at the reporter's discretion. If you say it, its use is fair game. You can't take back anything you said—even if you didn't mean to say it.

Off the Record

This is the opposite of on the record. It means that anything you say "off the record" may not be reported. But it is not that simple. There are protocols to be followed; otherwise, despite what you think, you may still be on the record, not off.

First of all, if you want something to be off the record, you must say so in advance, not after you have spoken it. Once the cat is out of the bag, you cannot change your mind and declare the previous remarks to be off the record. It just doesn't work that way.

The reason for telling reporters that what you are about to say is off the record is to give any of them a chance to say, no, they do not wish to go along with an off-the-record presentation. Sometimes reporters don't want to accept off-the-record information because they want to be free to report it. Agreeing to accept off-the-record information in effect commits the reporter to secrecy (until you put it on the record) and blocks him or her from reporting that information. Even then, if the reporter should learn the off-the-record information from another source without violating your off-the-record agreement (and can confirm this), he or she will still be free to report it.

In other words, just saying something is off the record is no guarantee it will not be reported. But you can minimize the risk by asking reporters to agree in advance before you tell them what they can't report.

Not for Attribution

This is pretty much what it seems. It means reporters can use the information you gave them, but they cannot identify you as the source. As with off the record, not-for-attribution remarks must be prefaced in advance and agreed to by those present. The purpose of not-for-attribution remarks is to help reporters round out their stories with more facts or details than they otherwise could if it would appear the information came from you. When, for instance, you read a news story that attributes the source as "a high government official," it sometimes may even be the president or vice president of the United States. But by speaking not for attribution, they can say things or reveal information they otherwise could not say formally on the record.

For Background Only

This is also sometimes known as "for deep background only." Either way the meaning is the same. As with not for attribution, the information given out is intended to put developments into perspective or context for reporters so they can write a more accurate and meaningful story for their audiences. For example, background information may explain how or why something came about, or it may make reference to similar situations or incidents, or developments that reporters would not otherwise know about that would better help explain their stories.

The important point to remember in talking with the news media is that you can control what you say so that you and your organization gain the maximum benefit. Knowing how and when to go on or off the record, on background, or not for attribution maximizes that control. But still that control is not absolute. It is the reporter, not you, who ultimately controls what gets reported. That's why the *best* policy is simply to forget about off the record, not for attribution, and background. You will never get burned if you follow this simple advice: Never say *anything* that you wouldn't want to see on the front page of the newspaper or on the evening TV news.

SUMMARY

In this chapter you have learned the importance of developing good media relations and how to comport yourself with reporters when and if you are ever called upon to serve as a spokesperson for your organization. You have learned:

- what comprises the news media, how they differ in their presentations of the news, and how their news-gathering needs differ as well.
- the importance of proactive media relations not only to educate reporters and editors about forensic nursing and the role it plays in

society, but also to prepare for the day you may have to meet reporters in reaction to a crisis, disaster, or other major event.

- how to anticipate potential scenarios and situations that would be covered by the media, and how to develop and prepare key messages and talking points in response.
- the importance of planning responses and obtaining needed clearances in advance.
- do's and don'ts for dealing with the news media, including differences between on the record, off the record, for background only, and not for attribution comments.
- the importance of striking a balance between HIPAA's privacy guidelines and the media's need to know, as well as guidelines for what you can and cannot say to the media.

And finally, you learned the importance of having a training program to practice how to work effectively with the media and the reasons to consistently practice media communications skills before the time ever comes to put them to use.

In essence, what you've learned about working with the news media is, to borrow the motto of the Boy Scouts, "Be prepared!"

QUESTIONS FOR DISCUSSION

1. Identify the common public media with which the forensic nurse often interacts. In what ways do these media differ? What different skills might be required with each?
2. In what ways can the forensic nurse work with the media to develop goodwill and to highlight areas of forensic interest for both parties?
3. A critical incident has occurred in a local healthcare facility that may involve intentional harm to patients caused by one of the staff. What special concerns might arise when addressing such a case with the media?
4. Discuss some strategies the forensic nurse can use to develop and to practice skills that will be helpful when working with representatives from the various media.

Leadership in Forensic Nursing

Ellen Russell Beatty
Maryann Glendon
Mary Jane M. Williams

This chapter explores the role of leadership in forensic nursing in relation to current leadership theory, and illustrates the application of leadership concepts to complex situations within the practice of forensic nursing, especially in the area of policy development. Concepts related to policy are defined, and examples of successful leadership strategies to influence policy changes related to forensic nursing practice are outlined. A rich array of examples from the authors' expertise and experiences serve as a resource and inspiration for the reader.

CHAPTER FOCUS

KEY TERMS

core competencies
forensic nursing
forensics
health policy
leadership
policy
policy strategies
professional organizations
public policy
transformational leadership

INTRODUCTION

Forensic nursing is a growing area of specialization within graduate nursing education and the profession. As the specialty develops and defines a unique area of practice for the public sector, an examination of the relationship between leadership and policy formation becomes essential. Forensic nurses must be prepared to take leadership roles in policy development at the local, state, regional, and national levels. This chapter examines leadership as defined in the current leadership literature with an emphasis on knowledge and skills necessary for future practice as workforce settings and environmental factors change. Core and correlated competencies that are essential for future leaders in forensic nursing are also discussed within the context of the political arena. To develop this necessary body of nursing knowledge for the creation of a forensic policy agenda, policy development and analysis as well as political strategies are presented. Policy formation, implementation, evaluation, and political influence as they apply to the state and federal levels are examined.

Isabel Maitland Stewart's quote that called on the profession to be courageous during crisis is as applicable today as it was in the early 1950s:

> It is evident that leadership in nursing . . . is of supreme importance at this time. Nursing has faced many critical situations in its long history, but probably none more critical than the situation it is now in, and none in which the possibilities, both of serious loss and of substantial advance, are greater. What the outcome will be depends in large measure on the kind of leadership the nursing profession can give in planning for the future and in solving stubborn and perplexing problems . . . if past experience is any criterion, little constructive action will be taken without intelligent and courageous leadership. (Stewart, 1953; as cited in *The Role of the Clinical Nurse Leader 2003,* p 11)

As a new era of leadership in nursing emerges, we still struggle with Stewart's challenge. The questions need to be asked again: Is nursing as a profession ready to assume a leadership role in the healthcare arena? Will there be qualified nurses to move into leadership roles in order to advance the profession?

THE HEALTHCARE WORKFORCE

Nurses, at 2.6 million nationally, are the largest group of healthcare providers in the nation; yet it has been argued that they have had the least political impact on the healthcare industry. That brings us to a major issue related to nursing in the 21st century: What is the current status of nursing in the United States? Some 2.2 million nurses are employed in the nursing profession, with approximately 60% of all registered nurses working in hospitals. It is reported that the healthcare industry job sector will increase by 2.7 million positions before 2005. A large part of this growth will be generated by the need to provide care for a growing population of elderly clients.

Coincidentally, nursing will suffer the most severe shortage in its history during this same time period. Some states have reported a decreased license renewal over the past decade but this latest shortage will not be remedied by using traditional strategies (e.g., overtime, flex-time, and bonuses) because the shortfall is also due to increased demand. It is predicted that by the year 2010, the demand for registered nurses will exceed the supply (Buerhaus, Staiger, & Auerbach, 2000).

Long-term changes in the registered nurse workforce over the next 6–15 years will be dominated by aging registered nurses leaving the field, accelerating the reduction in the supply. Registered nurses had a mean age of 43.3 years in March 2000, up from 42.3 in 1996. The registered nurse population under the age of 30 dropped from 25.1% of the licensure pool in 1980 to 9.1% in 2000 (U.S. Department of Health and Human Services, 2000). In the year 2003, 50% of the national nursing workforce was over the age of 45, presenting nursing leadership with a significant problem requiring attention. Buerhaus states that "the aging of nurses coupled with the decrease in enrollments of prospective students will create a major nursing shortage." It will also result in a significant loss of clinical and theoretical expertise (Buerhaus, 2001).

The total United States nurse population is growing at the slowest rate in 20 years. A July 2002 Health Resources and Services Administration (HRSA) report determined that the nursing shortage would deepen, because more nurses were returning to the profession than were entering it. Although 30 states experienced nursing shortages in 2000, HRSA indicates that the crisis will intensify, with 44 states plus the District of

Columbia expected to have RN shortages by the year 2020 (HRSA). The latest projections from the U.S. Bureau of Labor Statistics notes that "more than one million new and replacement nurses will be needed by 2012" (U.S. Department of Health & Human Services, 2000).

Buerhaus and colleagues published a report that stated "the U.S. will experience a 20% shortage in the number of nurses needed in our nation's health care system by the year 2020. This translates into a shortage of more than 400,000 registered nurses nationwide" (Buerhaus, 2000, p. 2948). The rapidly changing demographics in society and in nursing will mandate a new leadership and management style to address these issues.

WORK ENVIRONMENT

Changing practice environments have implications for the nursing profession. There is a growing demand for registered nurses in all settings including health maintenance organizations, home care agencies, managed care companies, primary care centers, nursing homes, community clinics, and outpatient facilities. There is also a concurrent growing need for nurses in critical care, intensive care, labor and delivery, and emergency and operating rooms within acute care settings. Despite efforts at consolidation, the demand for nursing is increasing as the prospective supply diminishes.

The role of the forensic nurse is essential in dealing with violence as a major national and world public health issue (World Health Organization, n.d.). "Forensic nursing is gaining momentum nationally and internationally" (Burgess, Berger, & Boersma, 2004, p. 59); thus, nursing leadership must be proactive in the healthcare delivery arena and in educational settings. The charge is to create effective educational and experiential preparation as well as proper utilization and certification of the forensic nurse to address the growing global issues of injury and violence prevention and treatment.

MANAGEMENT VERSUS LEADERSHIP

Nursing education has traditionally focused on preparing nurses to be managers of care versus leaders. Nurses have been educated to manage environments, patients, staff, and resources. However, with the changes in the industry, the growing shortage of nurses, and the baby boomer nurse retirements, the profession has been forced to re-examine the role of the nurse in health care, refocusing on nursing leadership as a core component of nursing education. This leadership preparation focuses on preparing practitioners to lead as well as manage, while participating in the decision-making process at the organizational policy and administrative level.

We know that leadership in the 21st century will be interdependent; nursing leaders will be experts in establishing relationships. Change is always about relationships. What are the relationships between the players in the system and surrounding the system? What are the connections for interdependence? What is the new paradigm? We are entering a new era in leadership and management and creating a new paradigm that will focus on partnerships, where risk is expected and shared. Our society is based on economic principles and is driven by the "bottom line." Healthcare reform will continue to change dynamically. Nursing must move forward with the social values on which the profession is based: caring, prevention, self-reliance, and health advocacy.

Leadership

Leadership has been defined extensively in the literature. Leadership "refers to the use of personal traits and personal power to constructively and ethically influence patients, families, and others toward an end point vision or goal" (Yoder-Wise, 2003, p. 2). Leadership is "liberating people to do what is required of them in the most effective and humane way" (DePree, 1989, p. 1). "Leadership is the capacity to create a compelling vision and translate it into action and sustain it" (Bennis & Nanus, 1985). "Enlightened leadership is the ability to elicit a vision from people and to inspire and empower these people to do what it takes to bring the vision to reality" (Oakley & Krug, 1994). A leader is someone who has the capacity to create a compelling vision that takes people to a new place and to translate that vision into action. "Leaders draw other people by enrolling them in their vision" (Bennis & Goldsmith, 1997, p. 4). Tappen (2001) identified the following components as essential for effective leadership: "knowledge, self-awareness, communication, energy, goals, and action" (p. 54). What are the common strands that run through all these definitions? They present the reader with the core competencies a future leader must bring to the practice setting. A leader is a visionary, someone who is capable of motivating others and who utilizes a participatory style of management. The new leader for the next millennium will emulate a positive attitude and be sincerely interested in his or her role and the effect it has on the practice arena. The new leader will be caring, humanistic, and intuitive.

Leadership Competencies

After considerable review of the literature, the authors believe that the leader in forensic nursing will come to the practice setting ready to transform and motivate others. In order to accomplish this vision, the leader must utilize the following competencies: communication skills, the ability to articulate in the written and spoken word, and comfort with silence. The forensic leader must have strong interpersonal skills and be capable of motivating others. Forensic practice mandates that the nurse be able to communicate therapeutically in the most difficult situations. The forensic nurse must be a risk taker, comfortable with change and creative in developing solutions. The forensic nurse leader must have expert knowledge in his or her area of specialization. It is essential to their work that forensic nurse leaders possess excellent conflict management and negotiation skills with the ability to understand and facilitate collaborative relationships. The forensic nurse leader must partner with related specialties to accomplish joint professional and political agendas. The development of leadership competencies is ongoing, learning is never static, and the development of leadership skills is a lifelong process. The leader in forensic nursing fosters the specialty by adhering to the standards of practice, as defined by the profession (see Figure 25–1). The expert forensic nurse works in collaboration with the healthcare, criminal justice, and mental healthcare systems. The rapid evolution of this nursing specialty attests to effective leadership and political competence.

Support of core competencies for leadership in nursing comes from the Robert Wood Johnson Foundation Executive Nurse Fellows Program (2002). Five core competencies are noted in this program as essential for successful leadership in the healthcare system: self-knowledge, interpersonal and communication effectiveness, risk taking and creativity, inspiring and leading change, and strategic vision. The program considers all five competencies to be interrelated to enhance an individual's leadership potential.

The American Association of Colleges of Nursing (AACN), which represents baccalaureate and graduate schools of nursing in collaboration with a variety of healthcare organizations, has proposed the new role of clinical nurse leader (CNL) to address needed changes in the healthcare system. O'Neil & Morjikian (2003) believe that the role and skills of the nurse as a provider of care will need to be reassessed as technology and patient care needs change. The forensic nurse specialist is a clinical leader and should possess knowledge of all of the core competencies.

The AACN proposed clinical nurse leader exhibits a proactive approach to the issues related to the labor shortage and work environments. The clinical nurse leader is envisioned as "a leader in the health care delivery system across all settings in which health care is delivered, not just acute care settings" (AACN, 2003). The clinical nurse leader provides and manages care at the point of service to individuals, clinical populations, and communities. This concept supports the role of the forensic nurse in the public health arena. The clinical nurse leader is responsible for clinical management of comprehensive client care, for both individuals and clinical populations, along the continuum of care and in multiple settings. The CNL must possess core competencies related to delegation, supervision, evaluation, and advocacy. This model recognizes advocacy for individuals, families, and communities who do not have the skills for self-advocacy for a variety of reasons. AACN conceptualizes the CNL as a member and a leader of the healthcare team, an educator, and a member of the profession. Several components are essential to the development of the CNL: a liberal education, professional values, core competencies, core knowledge, and role development.

Transformational Leadership

The literature begs the question: What is the leadership style that compliments the nursing workforce, the environment, and the clients the nurse leads? It seems that the answer to this question is transformational leadership. Transformational leadership is intelligent, courageous leadership. It is a process by which leaders and followers raise one another to higher levels of motivation and morality (Burns, 1978, p. 20). The transformational leader motivates individuals to perform beyond their own level of expectation. Transformational leadership is about change, innovation, and empowerment of others (Barker, 1990). Barker believes that in order to be transformational, the leader must create new visions, thereby giving new meaning to nursing.

The literature reveals components and core functions that are perceived to be essential to the transformational leadership role, such as idealized influence, inspirational motivation, intellectual stimulation, and individualized consideration (Bass & Avoleo, 1993). Hitt (1993) believes it is essential to possess knowledge related to self, the organization, and global society. In order to function at this level the core attributes one must possess are strong self-identity, independence, authentic behavior, responsibility to self and the profession, courage, and integrity (Tomey, 2000). Transformational leadership has also been defined as "the ability to articulate a vision of the future with a group of people and to work with them to transform that dream into a reality" (Woods, 2003, p. 255). Sofarelli & Brown (1998) emphasize the following competencies, which were identified by Bennis & Nanus (1985) as important requirements for the transformational leader: management of attention, meaning, trust, and self. These four components underscore the leader's ability to empower, communicate a vision, establish trust, and achieve self-actualization. Transformational leaders, as noted by Trofino ". . . will be the catalyst for expanding a holistic perspective, empowering nursing at all levels and maximizing use of technology in the movement beyond patient-centered health care to patient-directed health outcomes" (Trofino, 1995, p. 12).

The Leadership Effectiveness Checklist

	Very Much	Somewhat	Not At All
A. Knowledge			
1. Do you have as much or more knowledge as the rest of your group?	☐	☐	☐
2. Do you feel confident of your knowledge in this situation?	☐	☐	☐
3. Are you able to speak to the group on their level?	☐	☐	☐
4. Have you identified the needs and motives of the people in the group?	☐	☐	☐
5. Have you identified the sources of power and authority in the situation?	☐	☐	☐
6. Have you critically analyzed the situation, including the leader, co-actor(s), and environment?	☐	☐	☐
7. Have you kept an open mind about the situation?	☐	☐	☐
B. Self-Awareness			
1. Do you know what your own needs are?	☐	☐	☐
Have you found ways to meet these needs?	☐	☐	☐
2. Do you know what you expect to gain from this situation?	☐	☐	☐
3. Are you able to empathize with the people in the group?	☐	☐	☐
4. Do you think of yourself as a leader?	☐	☐	☐
C. Communication			
1. Do you know what channels of communication are usually used?	☐	☐	☐
Are you using them?	☐	☐	☐
2. Is there an adequate flow of information?	☐	☐	☐
3. Have you created any new channels of communication?	☐	☐	☐
4. Are your communications open and direct?	☐	☐	☐
5. Do you attend and respond (listen actively) to what others are saying?	☐	☐	☐
6. Do you check out your perceptions of the situation with other people?	☐	☐	☐
7. Do you see and point out connections (links) between the statements of different people?	☐	☐	☐
8. Have you deliberately increased and strengthened your network(s)?	☐	☐	☐
9. Do you have a vision for the group?	☐	☐	☐
Have you shared it with the group?	☐	☐	☐
D. Energy			
1. Are you interested in the work of the group?	☐	☐	☐
2. Have you shared your interest and enthusiasm with the group?	☐	☐	☐
3. Do you monitor your energy level?	☐	☐	☐
4. Do you monitor the energy level of the group?	☐	☐	☐
5. Do you have enough energy for the task?	☐	☐	☐

Figure 25–1 Test your leadership effectiveness.

During these times of rapid change within the healthcare system, expanding knowledge as a result of technological advances, informatics, threats of bioterrorism, health disparities, and lack of resources, the characteristics of transformational leadership become essential. Some of the specific attributes that have been identified in

E. Goals	**Very Much**	**Somewhat**	**Not At All**
1. Have you identified:	☐	☐	☐
Your personal goals?	☐	☐	☐
Group members' personal goals?	☐	☐	☐
The organization's goals?	☐	☐	☐
The larger system's goals?	☐	☐	☐
2. Are your goals congruent with the group's goals?	☐	☐	☐
3. Do you identify with the group?	☐	☐	☐
Do you use "we" instead of "I" and "you"?	☐	☐	☐
4. Do members of the group see you as identifying with the group?	☐	☐	☐
5. Have you clearly and specifically stated the group's goals, including:	☐	☐	☐
The people involved?	☐	☐	☐
The target?	☐	☐	☐
The expected outcomes?	☐	☐	☐
F. Action			
1. Have you defined your nursing role and communicated this to the group?	☐	☐	☐
2. Have you developed a plan for getting the work done?	☐	☐	☐
3. Have you organized the work efficiently?	☐	☐	☐
4. Do you share your ideas with the others?	☐	☐	☐
5. Do you call the group together often enough?	☐	☐	☐
6. Do you use the authority you have?	☐	☐	☐
Do you delegate it?	☐	☐	☐
Have you tried to increase it?	☐	☐	☐
Have you tried to empower your group?	☐	☐	☐
7. Have you mobilized support systems?	☐	☐	☐
8. Are you willing to take risks?	☐	☐	☐
Have you taken any risks?	☐	☐	☐
9. Do you confront when it is needed?	☐	☐	☐
10. Do you initiate action when it is needed?	☐	☐	☐
Without delay?	☐	☐	☐
11. Do you seek feedback?	☐	☐	☐
Informally?	☐	☐	☐
Formally?	☐	☐	☐
12. Do you provide feedback?	☐	☐	☐
Informally?	☐	☐	☐
Formally?	☐	☐	☐
13. Have you tried to improve your leadership effectiveness?	☐	☐	☐

the literature review are the ability to provide a vision and direction and the willingness to be flexible and adapt to change (Sofarelli & Brown, 1998); empowering and inspirational communication (Carney, 1999); and the ability to focus on relationships and build partnerships.

What will practice be like in 2020? The transformational leader will be expected to develop trusting relationships and demonstrate a high level of ethical behavior in the clinical setting. He or she will be called on to create and design working environments that support the organization's mission and philosophy without compromising the professional employees. The leader of the next millennium will use self effectively to accomplish the vision and mission of the organization and maintain the employee's respect (Barker, 1990).

The transformational leader is viewed as "charismatic." The effectiveness of a leader is influenced by their insights into personal behavior, attitudes, and beliefs. A good leader needs to be able to examine his or her own behavior and its effect on the environment and personnel. According to Barker, "Transformational leadership is a relationship in which the purposes of the leaders and followers become fused, creating unity, wholeness, and a collective purpose. Collective purpose is crucial to this concept and success is measured on the realization of the intended social change. The change must have a positive impact on all those involved and be consistent with their values" (Barker, 1990, p. 42).

The transformational nursing leader will be very valuable in providing direction and support to members of the new specialty area, forensic nursing, which requires all of these competencies and a collective action that focuses on social change.

The profession recognizes that leadership in the clinical setting across all disciplines will be essential to safe, quality practice in the decades to come. The forensic nurse is a clinical leader in a challenging environment and works collaboratively across multiple settings. The competencies recommended for this specialty will facilitate role development that fosters beneficial partnerships in leadership and policy.

It is essential that nursing leadership recognizes and addresses the personal and professional needs of the changing workforce. The newest members of the workforce will come from the group born in the late 1970s and early 1980s. This group is referred to as Generation X, and responds to the concepts related to transformational leadership. Generation X expects to be "led," not managed. They want respect, trust, and empowerment. They are integrated with technology, creative, and independent. Generation X is not a group of joiners; they prefer to work individually with goals, deadlines, and action. They work best with transformational leaders who are secure in their own role and ready to facilitate self-empowerment of the individual with whom they work (Barker, 1990).

The issues that face the forensic nursing specialist are local, national, and international. "We live in an increasingly violent society that is affected by violence all around the globe" (Ferrell, quoted in Benn, 2001). The forensic leader must be a transformational leader who exhibits the behaviors and core competencies necessary to lead the workforce of the future.

Leadership in Policy

Many questions about policy and issues related to policy development need to be addressed by the nursing community. Nursing has the potential to significantly influence policy formation and health policy. Nursing has been involved in the policy arena since its inception; however, it has not been until the last decade that this participation has influenced policy.

As a profession, nursing has a charge to be involved in social policy formation by virtue of the *Code of Ethics* for nursing and the *Social Policy Statement.* The *Social Policy Statement* (Figure 25–2) recognizes the need for professional self-regulation. Nurses should be active participants in the development of policies and the review mechanisms designed to promote patient safety, reduce errors, and address environmental and human factors that present increased risk to patients. It is part of the social responsibility of nurses to report adverse events. Nursing is self-regulating, defines practice, supports practice with evidence-based research, directs education, establishes healthcare delivery structures, provides for quality review, maintains standards of practice, conducts peer reviews, and maintains a system for credentialing.

Nursing's role in social policy is well defined by the profession via its *Social Policy Statement,* a contract between society and the profession of nursing. Nursing, like other professions, is an essential part of the society from which it evolves. Nursing is dynamic, always changing to reflect societal needs. Societies determine their socioeconomic, political, and cultural conditions and values and what professional skills and knowledge are essential to their populations. Therefore, professions are the property of society. The practice of nursing is based on a social contract with society. The social contract acknowledges professional rights and responsibilities as well as mechanisms for social responsibilities. Society grants the profession authority over its functions and permits them autonomy in the conduct of their affairs. However, the profession must be accountable to society and act responsibly, always mindful of public trust. Self-regulation to assure quality of performance is the authentic hallmark of the profession.

The *Social Policy Statement* makes clear the definition of nursing and the core concepts and knowledge that is essential to nursing practice in the new millennium. It clearly defined decision making and the ability to make choices and social policies and their effect on the health of individuals, families, and communities. The advanced roles of nurses, as stated in the *Social Policy Statement,* recognizes the need for nurses educated and involved in the policy arena, as social policy analysts.

Source: American Nurses Association, 2003.

Figure 25–2   Social policy statement for nursing.

The profession of nursing, as represented by associations and their members, is responsible for "articulating nursing values, for maintaining the integrity of the profession and its practice, and for shaping social policy" (ANA, 2003).

Historically, nursing practice has focused on the nurse–patient relationship, which is inadequate today to meet the needs of client populations. Ballou (2000) addressed professional nursing's obligation to participate in sociopolitical activities. She poses the question: Does the scope of professional nursing practice include an obligation to participate in sociopolitical activity? After careful review and analysis of the *Social Policy Statement* and *Code of Ethics,* and establishing a clear definition of what constitutes sociopolitical action, she concluded "that professional nursing has a social responsibility and a moral and professional obligation to political activism as a client advocate." She further concludes that the *Code of Ethics* is a clear, unequivocal mandate for sociopolitical activity. Nursing is the greatest potential resource for the health of the public; however, nursing must find its own value and worth and empower itself as a profession (Ballou, 2000, p. 180). In order to achieve autonomy, nurses must be able to view themselves as key players in the healthcare arena. Many writers believe that it is nursing's lack of or inadequate participation in professional organizations that indirectly affects political participation. It should be noted that political activity is the strongest influence on policy at the national level. The professional organizations of nursing must maintain a vibrant presence at the state and federal levels in order to influence policy outcomes. The *Code of Ethics* for nurses (ANA, 2001), shown in Figure 25–3, outlines the responsibilities to the public.

The *Social Policy Statement* and *Code of Ethics* direct our professional responsibility. We have given ourselves the charge. The questions now are how do we proactively engage the next generation of nurses to participate in the sociopolitical arena? How do we prepare them to be lead-

---

Nurses, individually and collectively, have a responsibility to be knowledgeable about the health status of the community and existing threats to health and safety. Through support of and participation in community organizations and groups, the nurse assists in efforts to educate the public, facilitates informed choice, identifies conditions and circumstances that contribute to illness, injury and disease, fosters healthy life styles and participates in institutional and legislative efforts to promote health and meet national health objectives. In addition, the nurse supports initiatives to address barriers to health, such as poverty, homelessness, unsafe living conditions, abuse and violence, and lack of access to health services.

Source: American Nurses Association, 2001.

Figure 25–3   Code of ethics for nurses.

ers in policy development? What skills do they need? What skills do they possess? What experiences do they need to make them leaders in the policy arena?

Twenty years ago, Senator Edward Kennedy noted, "Nurses are America's largest group of health professionals, but they have never played their proportionate role in helping to shape health policy, even though that policy profoundly affects them as both health providers and consumers" (cited in Cramer, 2002, p. 98). Cramer suggests, "with over 2.2 million active registered nurses in the United States, the profession's participation in politics and policy is far less than their potential strength in numbers warrant" (p. 98). One needs to ask: Has our collective influence increased in the policy arena? If the answer is no, we must examine the roots of this problem and its related variables. The answer may be related to nursing's difficulty in developing as a profession and in identifying the fundamental responsibilities that professionalism mandates. Professional membership is a key component of the professional role. We must review the educational process and its role in the growth and development of professionalism.

Policy Defined

Policy "encompasses the choices that a society or an organization makes regarding its goals and priorities and how resources will be allocated" (Mason & Leavitt, 2002, p. 8). Public policies are formulated by local, state, or federal governments (Mason & Leavitt). Policy is made on behalf of the public, developed or initiated by government, and interpreted and implemented by public and private bodies (Birkland, 2001, cited in Mason & Leavitt, p. 55). Social policies "pertain to policy decisions that promote the welfare of the public" (Mason & Leavitt, p. 8).

Health policy "includes the decisions made to promote the health of individual citizens" (Mason & Leavitt, 2002, p. 8). Health policy encompasses issues related to economics, housing, environment, budget, and health services policy. Most people see health policy as focusing on the finance, organization, and delivery of personal health services. Longest (2002) defines health policies as "authoritative decisions that pertain to health or influence the pursuit of health. Health policies are established at the federal, state and local levels and usually influence individuals, communities and organizations" (p. 11). For example, a state may legislate against smoking in public places, including restaurants and bars. The intent of the health policy legislation is to protect the staff and patrons from second-hand smoke. Any public policy that has the potential to affect the health of the public should be of interest to nurses.

Points to Ponder During Leadership Development

Political acumen is the result of a learning process and experience in a broad range of healthcare-related activities, culminating in identifying the mechanisms of change. (Refer to Figure 25–6, the Political Self-assessment Tool on page 757.) The forensic nurse must consider several questions when assessing leadership needs and effectiveness. Among those questions are:

- In your state, what health policy has been legislated during the past 2 years?
- What effect has this legislation had on the public's health potential?
- What effect has this legislation had on nursing practice and/or education?
- What factors will motivate and influence the policy participation of nurses?
- Are professional nurses in your work setting involved in the development of policy? What types of policy are they developing?
- How do you define leadership?
- What attributes do you possess that compliment the leadership role?

Nurses, at the minimum, need to be involved in the voting process. Nurses who vote are making their voices heard and understand the power of that voice. Voting allows nurses to use their education, experience, and expertise to select candidates who support issues of concern related to patient safety (Wilding & Zimmerman, 2000).

Gebbie, Wakefield, & Kerfoot (2000) found that nurses' involvement in policy was a natural evolution in some career paths. Nurses interviewed for their research were able to articulate what they believed were key competencies related to becoming leaders in the policy arena. These included communication skills, the ability to multitask, decision making, collaboration, conflict resolution, analysis, and viewing the big picture (Gebbie et al.). These competencies are now being developed in the educational sector. The ability to utilize these competencies comes after reinforcement across the continuum of professional education. It is the educator's responsibility to foster development of these leadership competencies in nursing through theory, experience, mentoring, and role modeling.

Gebbie et al.'s (2000) research illustrates that most nurses enter the policy arena accidentally. Their career in nursing practice evolves to policy, which then becomes their practice arena. Personal experience, such as role modeling through participation in activist events; educational activities that fostered student participation in programs focused on politics and social change; and mentors and educators who provided encouragement and challenged students toward continued growth in the policy arena influenced nurses to become active in promoting public policy.

EMPLOYMENT

Employment can also be viewed as a catalyst for involvement in health policy activities, particularly when the issues are related to organizational policy that directly affects one's specialty area. "Can the future be sculpted to enhance nursing's voice and visibility in forums related to health care quality as well as in the policy arena? Nursing lost much of its influence in decision making a decade ago, when nursing leadership was dismantled" (Lang & Jennings, 2002, p. 60). Nurses must regain their influence in health delivery systems in order to participate in decision-making processes affecting institutions and broader areas of healthcare policy. Such influence is essential if nursing leaders hope to guarantee the provision of safe, quality care and act as key designers of organizational policy.

Lang (2002) believes it is difficult for nurses to be spokespersons for nursing and related healthcare issues without sounding self-serving. When dealing with universal health concerns, the nursing-relevant healthcare issues lose significance. A major challenge is to connect nursing's legitimate workforce issues to the larger public health concern of improving care access. Nurses need to articulate how improvement in employment conditions relate to quality health care and affect client outcomes. Professionals must, with their breadth and depth of knowledge, be involved in all aspects of policy development, implementation, and evaluation (Fawcett & Russell, 2001).

Fawcett & Russell (2001) present a model for policy development and analysis (see Figure 25–4). In order to be effective in the policy arena, nurses must develop their skills in the political process and they must understand relationships. Nurses must also learn to examine political issues from a global perspective to evaluate these issues and the benefits of proposed legislation at the state and federal level.

Nurses, however, ultimately serve the public. Indeed, the mission of the National League for Nursing (NLN) is to improve the quality of people's health care. The knowledge that nurses bring to the policy arena affords the profession the opportunity to develop policy related to specific professional issues. However, the scope of knowledge that nurses utilize in their professional roles may also facilitate a broader involvement in health policy at the local, state, and federal levels. Nurses are providers

The problem
　What problem is to be solved by policy?
　What is the magnitude of the problem?

The solutions
　What are the possible solutions to the problem?
　What has worked in the past?
　What innovative solutions have been proposed?

The stakeholders
　Who supports each solution?
　Who opposes each solution?

The costs–benefit analysis
　What is the cost of each solution?
　What are the principal sources of funding?
　What are the benefits of each solution?
　What are the benefits of the status quo?
　What are the intended effects of the policy on society as a whole?
　What basic social and political values are to be promoted by the policy?

The recipients
　To whom or what is the policy directed? What is their political power base?
　How will the policy affect them?
　What other people might indirectly benefit from this policy?
　Will any group suffer as a result of this policy? What is their political power base?

What is the proposed policy?
　Does it focus on healthcare services, personnel, expenditures, or some combination of the three?
　To which level is the policy directed?
　Who is to be involved in the formulation and evaluation of the policy?
　Who and what are needed to implement the policy?
　How will the policy be administered?

(*Source:* Fawcett & Russell, 2001, p. 114).

Figure 25–4   Guidelines for policy analysis.

who impart care 24 hours a day, 7 days a week, and work in a variety of settings. This knowledge and experience are key to the development of a healthcare delivery system that will guarantee quality care and access for all.

Nursing's Agenda for Health Care Reform (ANA, 2002a) proposes to support our nation's efforts to create a healthcare system that assures access, quality, and affordable services. This nursing agenda supports immediate reform of the healthcare delivery system, requiring a paradigm shift from an illness model to a prevention model. The healthcare system must be realigned toward prevention and wellness care (ANA, 2002a), which is consistent with the leadership role of the forensic nurse.

Cramer's (2002) research noted that individual activity in the policy arena is important. Some specific strategies discussed are: joining the professional organizations, mentoring novices, becoming knowledgeable about policy issues, capitalizing on the positive image that the public has of nursing, volunteering in the community, and participating in intern programs at the capital. The role of the professional organization in policy is often invisible to the practicing nurse; however, at the state and national levels, the professional organizations set an agenda in collaboration with the constituent state organizations. The state organizations also set policy agendas via their policy subcommittees. The state organizations are involved in reviewing all proposed legislation for its potential impact on the public health and the nursing disciplines. Nursing representation in the policy arena at the state level is essential to the provision of safe, quality care. It is through the state legislature that the law regulating nursing practice is negotiated. In the past decade, many academic programs and professional and specialty organizations have begun to focus on developing nurses for roles in the policy arena. Nurses at the legislative level have effectively utilized their knowledge to effect policy change that directly influences practice. An example of advancing policy through collaboration was seen when the Connecticut Nurses Association in conjunction with the Connecticut Nurse Practitioners Group, Inc.; the Connecticut Association of Nurse Anesthetists; the Connecticut Nurse Psychotherapists; and the Connecticut Medical Society collaboratively influenced statutory changes in the Connecticut Nurse Practice Act that were implemented during the 1998–1999 legislative sessions.

NURSES IN GOVERNMENT

The following questions should be answered as informed citizens: How many national nurse legislators currently hold office? What is their party affiliation? What is their policy agenda? Who are your legislators at the state level? Are there any nurses in the state legislature from your district? What is their policy agenda?

State Representative Lenny Winkler, a nurse legislator from Groton, Connecticut's 41st District, is an example of an effective nurse leader in the forensic policy arena in the Connecticut Legislature. In 2001, she was the primary sponsor of Public Act 01-124, which has been hailed as landmark legislation by medical authorities throughout the United States. This legislation (found at http://www.housegop.state.ct.us), the first in the nation to address the overuse of psychotropic drugs by children, merited national and international attention. It was unanimously passed by the Connecticut State House of Representatives and Senate in April, and signed by the governor the following month. The law requires each local board of education to develop and implement a policy that prohibits school personnel from recommending to parents or guardians the use of psychotropic drugs for children under their care. It does not restrict school personnel from encouraging physician evaluation or from consulting with a medical practitioner with the consent of the child's guardians. The law protects parents' rights to refuse such treatment unless that refusal results in abuse or neglect as defined by Connecticut statutes. Representative Winkler is the author of several major initiatives to prevent child abuse and neglect, and a key sponsor of "Megan's Law," which requires convicted sex offenders to register with the police in the community where they live for 10 years after completing their sentences. In addition, Megan's Law allows authorities to inform the public under certain circumstances when a convicted sex offender moves into the community. Representative Winkler also played an instrumental role working with the state judicial branch to establish an intensive supervision program for sexual offenders released from prison. The program is now operating on a pilot basis in New London County, Connecticut.

Proactive legislation related to child abuse and neglect has been another focus of forensic nurse activists. In Connecticut, Representative Winkler sponsored legislation in 2003 to protect Connecticut children against abuse. An amendment to House Bill 6118, An Act Concerning Placement of Children Committed to the Department of Children and Families, would require the Department of Children and Families (DCF) to remove *all* children from a home when one child is removed for suspected child abuse. House Amendment D specifies, "If the child is removed from the home due to suspected child abuse, all children shall be removed from such home and taken into the custody of the Department of Children and Families" (http://www.housegop.state.ct.us).

On the national level, forensic leaders have worked closely with Senator Joseph Biden of Delaware to raise awareness in Congress about the needs within the forensic nursing profession that will enable practioners to enhance victim care and perpetrator identification and apprehension. (See the Foreword of this text.)

POLICY INSTITUTES

Many nursing specialty organizations offer policy internships; these internships are geared toward knowledge building and developing skills in policy development through guided programs. More recently, academic institutions are developing educational degree programs that focus on policy.

At the organizational level, it is important to foster institutes for policy and leadership that support the social policy statement. Nurses should utilize the public trust to develop policy that addresses health concerns. In the educational sector, the curriculum in every program should include a course on policy and encourage collaborative relationships. Students at all levels in nursing education should be well informed about government at the state and national levels.

PROACTIVE LEADERSHIP AND POLICY INITIATIVES

At the state and federal levels, endeavors are already underway that serve as a model for proactive policy development. In Connecticut, under the auspices of the Connecticut Hospital Association, an initiative to address the future of nursing commenced in June 2003. The Future of Nursing in Connecticut Project is a broad-ranging initiative designed to prepare, increase, and strengthen the nursing workforce to play a vital role in meeting people's healthcare needs. This proactive model is dedicated to addressing workforce issues for the next decade.

A core group of nurses from education, service, and government discussed healthcare issues and the future of the profession using the guiding question, "What will it take for the nursing workforce to address healthcare needs in the state over the next 10 years?" The group identified eight major focus areas, outlined priorities for four of them, and agreed to develop workgroups to concentrate on these areas, as shown in Figure 25–5. The charge of the leadership and policy group involves engaging nurses in Connecticut to lead change for the profession of nursing and for the health of the public, through the use of partnerships and the political process.

At the national level, *Nursing's Agenda for the Future* offers direction for leadership and policy-making activities through the year 2010.

The future of forensic nursing, and nursing in general, is directly related to the need to develop well-prepared nurse leaders who are capable of assuming positions of power and influence, affecting key decision-making bodies throughout the profession, and acting as policy makers at the local, state, national, and international levels. In order to accomplish these goals, we as a profession must mobilize the necessary resources and develop leaders in policy who are involved at every level of government. Some of our members are already leading on forensic issues, but we must utilize the strength of our numbers to develop more leadership momentum. Therefore, the nursing community must foster the development of educated, articulate leaders in the policy arena through education and assessment. Figure 25–6 is an example of an assessment tool, which can be used in various clinical and educational settings, to raise awareness of nurses' political acumen.

Nursing as a Profession
Educating the public about nursing and supporting the career development of nurses.
- Consumer focus groups to collaborate in defining nursing
- The "practicing out loud" initiative
- Programs that reward and recognize nurses, as well as provide forums for nurses to share support, such as "Nurses Healing Nurses"
- Requirements for internship post-graduation
- White paper on public and professional accountability to mentor current and next-generation nurses
- Referrals to Nursing Career Center program for provision of career guidance for nurses
- Development of a position paper on definition of nursing, and the career growth process to include educational and experiential paths

Leadership and Policy
Engaging nurses in Connecticut to lead change for the profession of nursing, and for the health of the public, through use of the political process and partnerships.
- Information database on the nursing workforce
- Strengthening the nursing board of examiners
- Education of key legislators about nursing issues via various forums
- Examination of political vacancies and identification of potential candidates
- Establishment of a leadership and policy institute
- Education of the grassroots level on the political process

Identify Healthcare Needs
Illuminating the current and projected healthcare needs of the population of Connecticut, and the capacity of the nursing workforce to meet them.
- Develop information base regarding nursing preparation in gerontology and expertise within the state
- Examine nursing school curricula relative to end-of-life care
- Gather information from hospitals on current nursing practice in pain management, palliative care, and hospice
- Develop exemplars of nursing leadership in health promotion and illness prevention, including support of various legislative initiatives
- Conduct document review for identified and perceived healthcare needs and create a compendium

Research
Create a center to support improved nursing practice, through research and evaluation.
- Identify problems in nursing practice that call for improvements
- Create alliances across Connecticut's 31 hospitals and other care facilities
- Collect data across institutions to evaluate proposed solutions
- Disseminate the results of these projects to Connecticut's practicing nurses as "Best Practices"
- Develop an online "library" of research discoveries and evidence-based practice initiatives
- Support the development of proposals for research and evaluation through the establishment of core resources
- Pursue support of the center through grants and gifts

Source: American Nurses Association, 2002a.

Fig. 25–5 Future of Nursing in Connecticut Project work group plan highlights.

Place a check next to those items for which the answer is "yes." Then give yourself one point for each "yes." After completing the inventory, compare your total score with the scoring criteria.

_____ 1. I am registered to vote.
_____ 2. I know where my voting precinct is located.
_____ 3. I voted in the last general election.
_____ 4. I voted in the past two elections.
_____ 5. I recognized the names of the majority of candidates on the ballot and was acquainted with the majority of issues in the last election.
_____ 6. I stay abreast of current health issues.
_____ 7. I belong to the state professional or student organization.
_____ 8. I participate (as a committee member, officer, etc.) in this organization.
_____ 9. I attended the most recent meeting of my district nurses' association.
_____ 10. I attended the last state or national convention held by my organization.
_____ 11. I am aware of at least two issues discussed and stands taken at this convention.
_____ 12. I read literature published by my state's nurses' association, a professional magazine, or other literature on a regular basis to stay abreast of current health issues.
_____ 13. I know the names of my senators in Washington, DC.
_____ 14. I know the names of my representatives in Washington, DC.
_____ 15. I know the name of the state senator from my district.
_____ 16. I know the name of the representative from my district.
_____ 17. I am acquainted with the voting record of at least one of the above in relation to a specific health issue.
_____ 18. I am aware of the stand taken by at least one of the above in relation to a specific health issue.
_____ 19. I know whom to contact for information about health-related issues at the state or federal level.
_____ 20. I know whether my professional organization employs lobbyists at the state or federal level.
_____ 21. I know how to contact these lobbyists.
_____ 22. I contribute financially to my state and national professional organization's political action committee (PAC).
_____ 23. I give information about effectiveness of elected officials to assist the PAC's endorsement process.
_____ 24. I actively supported a senator or representative during the last election.
_____ 25. I have written to one of my state or national representatives in the past year regarding a health issue.
_____ 26. I am personally acquainted with a senator or representative or a member of his/her staff.
_____ 27. I serve as a resource person for one of my representatives or his/her aide.
_____ 28. I know the process by which a bill is introduced in my state legislature.
_____ 29. I know which senators or representatives are supportive of nursing.
_____ 30. I know which House and Senate committees usually deal with health-related issues.
_____ 31. I know the committees of which my representatives are members.
_____ 32. I know of at least two issues related to my profession that are currently under discussion.
_____ 33. I know of at least two health-related issues that are currently under discussion at the state or national level.
_____ 34. I am aware of the composition of the state board, which regulates the practice of my profession.
_____ 35. I know the process whereby one becomes a member of the state board, which regulates my profession.
_____ 36. I know what DHHS stands for.
_____ 37. I have at least a vague notion of the purpose of DHHS.
_____ 38. I am a member of a health board or an advisory group to a health organization or agency.
_____ 39. I attend public hearings related to health issues.
_____ 40. I find myself more interested in political issues now than in the past.

Scoring

0–9	Totally unaware politically
10–19	Slightly aware of the implications of politics on nursing
20–29	Beginning political astuteness
30–40	Politically astute...Asset to nursing

Source: Goldwater, M., Zusy, M. J. (1990). *Prescription for nurses: Effective political action.* St Louis: Mosby. Reprinted with the permission of Marilyn Goldwater.

Figure 25–6   Political self-assessment tool.

Fawcett & Russell (2001) proposed an evolving "conceptual model of nursing health policy." Fawcett states that there is: "a need to articulate Nursing's distinctive role in the multidisciplinary field of health policy as a catalyst for the development of this conceptual model of nursing and health policy" (2001, p. 108). Fawcett & Russell's model reflects philosophic assumptions about nursing and participation in the field of health policy. The model examines individual practice, nursing practice delivery systems, subsystems of healthcare delivery, the healthcare system (geopolitical system), and the broadest category—world health. The model focuses on process and outcome within existing and emerging models of nursing practice and theories, with which the proposed model can be linked to support nursing discipline health policy research.

The forensic nurse leader is charged by the social policy statement to alleviate, protect, and promote health for the public they serve. "Forensic nurses investigate real and potential causes of morbidity and mortality in a variety of settings. Responsibilities range from collecting evidence to testifying in court as expert witnesses. Forensic nurses are the bridge between the criminal justice system and the health care system" (Burgess, Burger, & Boersma, 2004).

Violence is not a new problem. It is, however, a growing issue and a major public health problem, nationally and internationally. Nurses in community/public health, school nurses, and emergency room nurses are first observers. However, the forensic nurse has the education and applied training to perform careful, detailed assessment and the skill to bring forward evidence to support legal action. The forensic nurse has a mandate by virtue of education in the specialty to develop appropriate protocols related to this area of expertise. An initial area of practice for the forensic nurse was in cases of sexual assault. The first national meeting of sexual assault practitioners led to the development of the specialty and the formation of the International Association of Forensic Nurses. This politically proactive organization moved to a recognized specialty status within four years. This move led to the development of standards of practice and a definition of scope of practice (Lundy & Jones, 2001).

The International Association of Forensic Nurses (IAFN) recently published sexual assault nurse examiner (SANE) educational guidelines and is working with the Department of Justice, Office on Violence against Women (OVW) to develop a national forensic assault protocol. The OVW will develop educational standards to accompany the protocol (cited in Burgess et al., 2004, p. 62). Evidence to date suggests that the SANE publication has made a profound difference in the care provided to sexual assault victims and in outcomes of prosecutions. The standards of forensic practice vary from state to state (see www.sane-sart.com) and practice is defined under each state's Nurse Practice Act. The Nurse Practice Act includes a definition of nursing practice, regulation of educational programs for nursing, rights of nurse licensure, and licensure requirements (ANA, 2001).

In order to deal with this new body of knowledge and practice, providers must develop organizational policies based on the standards of practice and legal mandates. At the specialty level, the forensic nurse needs to redefine the scope and standards of practice as his or her role evolves and expands to new settings. The forensic nurse must have a sound knowledge base related to the law and the criminal justice system.

SUMMARY

The charge inherent in professional nursing practice via the social policy statement and code of ethics for nursing mandates involvement in policy process across all levels. The preparation of leaders in nursing enhances the potential to involve a group of well-prepared, competent, articulate individuals in the policy sector at the state, national, and international levels. The issue that is paramount is the understanding of the moral mandate of professional nurses to participate in the sociopolitical arena.

QUESTIONS FOR DISCUSSION

1. What is leadership, and how is it defined for the forensic nurse?
2. What are the leadership challenges for the 21st century?
3. What are the special leadership challenges of the new generation of nursing professionals?
4. What are the core competencies of leadership related to forensic nursing?
5. How does effective leadership impact the profession?
6. Define health policy.
7. Describe healthcare policy development.
8. What influences the formulation of policy at the local, state, and national levels?
9. What is the role of the professional organization related to development of policy?
10. What are the responsibilities of the nurse to the professional organization in the policy arena?
11. What is the role of the forensic nurse in the policy arena?
12. How can the individual nurse shape health and public policy for forensic practice?

REFERENCES

Aiken L. H., Clarke, S. P., Cheung, R. B., Sloane, D. M., & Silbr, J. H. (2003). Educational levels of hospital nurses and surgical patient mortality. *JAMA, 290*(12), 1617–1623.

American Association of Colleges of Nursing. (2003). *Working paper on the role of the clinical nurse leader.* Retrieved September 22, 2004, from http://www.aacn.nche.edu/Publications/WhitePapers/CNL.htm.

American Nurses Association. (2001). *Code of ethics.* Washington, DC: American Nurses Publishing.

American Nurses Association. (2002a). *Nursing's agenda for health care reform.* Retrieved September 22, 2004, from http://www.nursingworld.org/readroom/rnagenda.htm.

American Nurses Association. (2002b). *Nursing's agenda for the future, a call to the nation.* Washington, DC: American Nurses Publishing.

American Nurses Association. (2003). *Nursing's social policy statement* (2nd ed.). Washington, DC: American Nurses Publishing.

Ballou, K. A. (2000). A historical-philosophical analysis of the professional nurse obligation to participate in sociopolitical activities. *Policy, Politics, and Nursing, 1*(3), 172–184.

Barker, A. M. (1990). *Transformational nursing leadership: A vision for the future.* Baltimore: Williams and Wilkins.

Bass, B. M. & Avoleo, B. J. (1993). Transformational leadership and organizational culture. *Public Administration Quarterly, 17,* 112–121.

Beaudin, L. & Berger-Spirack, L. (2004). *Leadership and policy: A summary.* Futures of Nursing Project Connecticut. Unpublished manuscript.

Beaudin, L. & Gillis, C. (2003). *Futures of nursing project Connecticut.* Unpublished manuscript.

Benn, J. (2001). Spotlight on nurses; professional chats: On the edge of forensic nursing with Lynda Benak. Retrieved September 22, 2004, from http://www.nursezone.com/stories/SpotlightOnNurses.asp?articleID=7834.

Bennis, W. & Goldsmith, J. (1997). *Learning to lead: A workbook on becoming a leader* (rev. ed.). Reading, MA: Addison-Wesley.

Bennis, W. & Nanus B. (1985). *Leaders: The strategies for taking charge.* New York: Harper & Row.

Brown, B. S. (2001). The multigenerational workforce: mixing it up at the coffee station. *Review 7–11* 3, 19. Glen Allen, VA: Virginia Hospital and Healthcare Association.

Buerhaus, P. I., Staiger, D., & Auerbach, D. I. (2000). Implications of an aging registered nurse workforce. *JAMA, 283*(22), 2948–2954.

Buerhaus, P. I. (2001). Expected near- and long-term changes in the registered nurse workforce. *Policy, Politics, and Nursing Practice, 2*(4), 264–270.

Burgess, A. W., Berger, A. D., & Boersma, R. R. (2004). Forensic: Investigating the career potential in this emerging graduate specialty. *American Journal of Nursing, 104*(3), 58–64.

Burns, J. M. (1978). *Leadership.* New York: Harper & Row.

Carney, M. (1999). Leadership in nursing: Where do we go from here? The ward sisters' challenge for the future. *Nursing Review 17*(2), 13–18.

Cramer, M. E. (2002). Factors influencing organized political participation in nursing. *Policy, Politics, and Nursing Practice, 3*(2), 97–107.

DePree, M. (1989). *Leadership is an art.* New York: Doubleday.

Fawcett, J. & Russell, G. (2001). A conceptual model of nursing and health policy. *Policy, Politics, and Nursing Practice, 2*(2), 108–116.

Gallup Organization. (2001). *Honesty and ethics poll.* Princeton, NJ: Author.

Gebbie, K. M., Wakefield, M., & Kerfoot, K. (2000). Nursing and health policy. *Journal of Nursing Scholarship, 32*(3), 307–315.

Goldwater, M. & Zusy, M. J. (1990). *Prescription for nurses: Effective political action.* St. Louis: Mosby.

Hall-Long, B. A. (1995). Nursing's past, present, and future political experiences. *N&HC: Perspectives on Community, 16*(1), 24–28.

Hitt, W. D. (1993). The model leader is a fully functioning person. *Leadership and Organization Development Journal, 14*(7), 4–11.

Lang, N. & Jennings, B. (2002). Nurses and nursing in health care quality policy arena. *Journal of Professional Nursing, 18*(2), 60–112.

Longest, B. B. (2002). *Health policymakers in the United States* (3rd ed.). Foundation of the American College of Healthcare Executives, Chicago: Health Administration Press.

Lundy, K. S. & Jones, S. (2001). *Community health nursing: Caring for the public's health.* Sudbury, MA: Jones & Bartlett.

Mason, D. J. & Leavitt, J. K. (2002). *Policy and politics in nursing and health care* (4th ed.). St. Louis: Saunders.

Oakley, E. & Krug, D. (1994). *Enlightened leadership.* In Yoder-Wise, P. S. (2003). *Leading and managing in nursing* (3rd ed.). St. Louis: Mosby.

O'Neil, E. & Morjikian, R. (2003). Nursing leadership: Challenges and opportunities. *Policy, Politics, and Nursing Practice, 4*(3), 173–179.

Robert Wood Johnson Foundation. (2002). *Health care's human crisis: The American nursing shortage.* Princeton, NJ: Author.

Sexual Assault Resource Service. (1994). Sexual Assault Nurse Examiner Development and operation Guide. Retrieved from http://www.sane-sart.com.

Sofarelli, D. & Brown, D. (1998). The need for nursing leadership in uncertain times. *Journal of Nursing Management, 6*(4), 201–207.

Stewart, I. M. (1953). *The education of nurses.* New York: Macmillan.

Tappen, R. M. (2001). *Nursing leadership and management: Concepts and practice* (4th ed.). Philadelphia: F.A. Davis.

Tomey, A. M. (2000). *Guide to nursing management and leadership* (6th ed.). St. Louis: Mosby.

Trofino, J. (1995). Transformational leadership in healthcare. *Nursing Management, 26*(8), 42–47.

U.S. Department of Health and Human Services, Division of Nursing, Nursing Data and Analysis Staff. (2000). *National sample survey of registered nurses.* Raw Data on CD-ROM.

Wilding, M. & Zimmerman, K. (2000). *Don't underestimate the nursing vote.* Retrieved from http://www.nursingcenter.com.

Woods, N. F. (2003). Leadership—not for just a few! *Policy, Politics & Nursing Practice, 4*(4), 255–256.

World Health Organization. (n.d.) Retrieved from http://www.who.int.

Yoder-Wise, P. S. (2003). *Leading and managing in nursing* (3rd ed.). St. Louis: Mosby.

What Forensic Nurses Should Know about Public Policy and How to Influence It

Michael E. Moynihan
Tracy A. Swan

This chapter will review, define, and describe public policy and the ways in which policy decisions influence nursing practice. Nurses historically have not been very involved in either developing policies or lobbying for or against policies that impact nursing practice. This chapter will enhance current knowledge and assist in developing new knowledge that can be applied to addressing the development of forensic nursing practice in the 21st century.

CHAPTER FOCUS

Definition of public policy
Categories of public policy
Types of public policy
Public policy-making process/cycle
Administrative agencies
Policy makers
Policy influencers
Specific policy areas of interest to forensic nurses
Advocacy role of forensic nurses and associations

KEY TERMS

administrative agencies
advocacy
agenda setting
authoritative technique
capacity technique
distributive policy
economic policy
executive department
government corporation
hortatory technique
incentive technique
independent agency
independent regulatory commission
interest groups
legislature
policy adoption/decision making
policy formulation
policy implementation/administration
problem recognition/identification
professional associations
programs
public policy
redistributive policy
regulatory policy
rule making/regulations
social policy

WHAT IS PUBLIC POLICY?

Public policy is a relatively stable, purposeful course of action followed by a government in addressing some problem or matter of concern that is shared by a substantial number of individuals, corporations, or organizations (Anderson, 2003, p. 2). Public policies are government policies based on law and are authoritative and binding (O'Connor & Sabato, 2002, p. 430).

There are several categories of public policies: substantive, procedural, material, symbolic, distributive, regulatory, self-regulatory, redistributive, and those policies involving public or private goods. The types of public policies that affect the field of forensic nursing and that would be of most interest are distributive, regulatory, and redistributive. These kinds of policies differ from other types by their effect on society and the relationship among those involved in the formation of the policy (Anderson, 2003, p. 7).

Distributive policies involve allocation of services or benefits to particular segments of the population—individuals, groups, corporations, or communities. Some distributive policies may provide benefits to just one or a few beneficiaries, whereas other distributive policies, like health aid for the elderly, tax deductions for home mortgage interest payments, free public school education, and job training programs, provide benefits to a vast number of individuals. Distributive policies typically involve using public funds—taxes—to assist particular groups, communities, or industries (Anderson, 2003, p. 7).

Redistributive policies involve deliberate acts by the government to shift the allocation of wealth, income, property, or rights among a broader class in society or to specific groups, like from the wealthy to the poor. This type of policy is usually heatedly debated in the media, among elected officials, and between political parties because redistributive policies transfer some power, rights, or money from one group to another. Examples of some successful redistributive policies are the graduated income tax, Medicare and Medicaid, the Voting Rights Act, and the Civil Rights Act (Anderson, 2003, p. 10).

Regulatory policies impose restrictions or limitations on the behavior of individuals, groups, and industries. This type of policy reduces the freedom or discretion to act of those regulated, whether they are bankers, utility companies, liquor stores, physicians, or engineers. The most extensive variety of regulatory policies deals with criminal behavior against individuals and property. The formulation of regulatory policies usually occurs because of conflict between two groups or coalitions of groups, with one side seeking to impose some sort of control on the other side. Typically, the other side views the proposed control as unnecessary or inappropriate for the desired result and, thus, opposes the regulation.

Regulatory policies take several forms. Some set general rules of behavior, directing that certain actions be taken or not taken. Others set standards for quality—quality of goods, services, or information—as with the Food and Drug Act, Consumer Credit Protection Act, or the hundreds of professions that require licensing in order to practice (Anderson, 2003, pp. 8–9).

The previously discussed categories of public policies can be further classified into two areas—*social* and *economic* (both fiscal and monetary). Social policies are those addressing individuals' overall well-being, in particular dealing with health care, education, employment, poverty, crime, and housing. Social regulatory policies deal with issues that regulate personal behavior, such as affirmative action, school prayer, gun control, pornography, and abortion (Anderson, 2003, p. 8). Economic policies address the well-being of our economy with regard to employment, interest rates, labor, agriculture, and taxes.

WHEN DOES A PROBLEM COME TO THE ATTENTION OF THE PUBLIC?

The extent to which an issue is perceived to be a problem and is shared by many is the catalyst for generating interest in addressing/solving the issue. Four factors can influence the perception of an issue as a problem that must be addressed:

1. *Image of the problem:* Is the problem one that is truly shared by many and worthy of being addressed? Can the problem be solved or impacted in a meaningful way?
2. *Influence and number of constituents affected by the issue or interested in the issue:* The greater the number of individuals affected by the issue and the greater their political "clout"—voting power or financial influence—the more likely the issue will be considered.
3. *Political acceptability of the issue:* Can policies be developed that would have an impact on the issue? Do voters care about this issue?
4. *The issue's point in history:* Must the issue be dealt with now? Can it be put off until later?

Some problems will never rise to the level of public concern because they are accepted as trivial, appropriate, inevitable, or beyond the control of government (O'Connor & Sabato, 2002, p. 432). Figure 26–1 depicts the relationship between the political environment and the policy-making process.

Public policies are created out of a need, which can be social or economic, as already discussed. The need usually requires some kind of change, such as greater access to health care for the retired, more employment opportunities for those on welfare, lower interest rates in order to spur buying and borrowing, or stronger restrictions on pollution in order to enjoy cleaner air and water. When the government steps in to create a policy, regardless of whether the proposed policy is social or economic, it is usually to promote efficiency in situations where the market (our economy—the exchange of goods and services) is believed to have failed, or to foster a more desirable distribution of goods, services, and rewards among individuals in society (Starling, 2002, p. 31).

The Environment

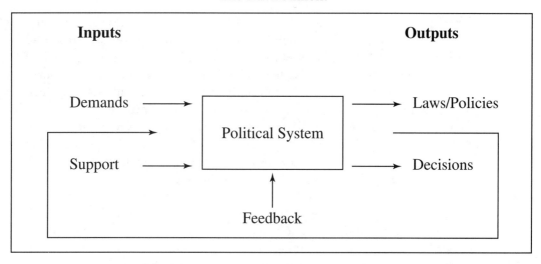

Figure 26–1　A model of the political environment where policy is created. *Source:* Anderson, 2003, p. 15.

Markets fail in four distinct ways:

1. They organize themselves such that there is little or no competition, which can cause prices to skyrocket (e.g., a monopoly).
2. They release a byproduct that is harmful to the public/environment, such as pollution, when manufacturing their goods.
3. They tend not to produce or underproduce a needed/wanted public good (e.g., public roads, parks, defense, judicial system) because they find it difficult to make a profit selling the public good.
4. They withhold vital consumer information such as drug side effects or qualifications of professionals, like physicians, that could lead to consumer harm.

Besides market failures, some other situations in which private issues can rise to the level of public concern and warrant attention as part of the public agenda include:

- Breakdowns of systems, such as family relationships
- Low living standards that result from well-functioning markets that do not reward individuals very generously if they lack marketable assets and skills
- Discrimination against racial and other minorities
- Areas where government is expected to function effectively, but in fact is not, such as providing excellent public education (Bardach, 2000, pp. 3–4).

THE POLICY PROCESS/CYCLE

Political scientists and other social scientists have developed many theories and models to explain the public policy process. Presented here is a widely used model that outlines the process as a sequence of stages or functional activities. Models of the public policy process usually do not explain *why* the policy was created, outside of identifying and addressing a shared problem, or *who* initiated the process or dominates the formulation of the policy. As you review the model presented in this chapter (see Figure 26–2), please keep in mind that sometimes in the policy process some of the stages may merge, such as the policy formulation and adoption stages, or the adoption and budgeting stages. As well, it is important to recognize that what happens at one stage in the policy-making process affects action(s) at later stages, and sometimes such action is done deliberately with these effects in mind. For instance, how does the content of legislation (policy formulation) ease or complicate its implementation? Or, how does implementation affect its impact (evaluation)? As well, the policy cycle is flexible and open to change and refinement as the policy progresses through the stages. The cycle also highlights the relationships, or interactions, among the participants in the policy-making process. Political parties, interest groups, legislative procedures, presidential commitments, public opinion, and the media can be tied together as they drive and explain the formulation of the policy (Anderson, 2003, p. 30).

Problem Recognition and Definition

A problem is identified as some condition or situation that causes distress or dissatisfaction or generates needs for which some kind of relief or corrective action is sought—often from the government (national, state, or local) (O'Connor & Sabato, 2002, p. 432). Often there is not a single agreed-on definition of the problem. This can lead to political struggle because how the problem is defined helps determine what sort of action is appropriate to adopt.

Agenda Setting

Once a problem is recognized and defined, it must be brought to the attention of public officials and it must secure a place on the government's agenda—a set of problems to which policy makers believe they should be attentive (O'Connor & Sabato, 2002, p. 433). Not all the problems that attract the attention of public officials have been widely discussed by the general public; as well, not all the problems widely discussed by the general public attract the attention from public officials. The two most pressing factors for a shared problem to receive

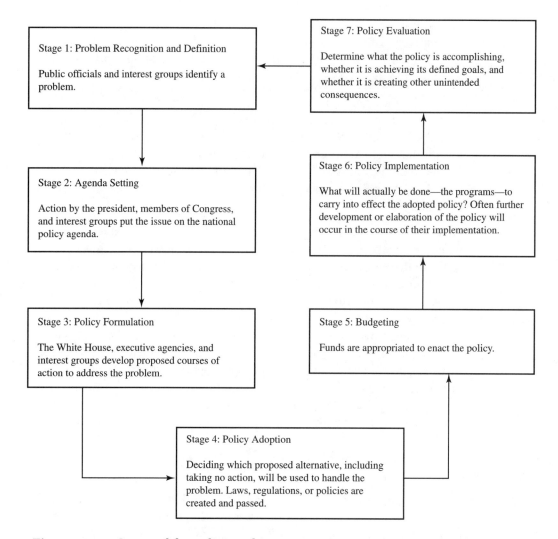

Figure 26–2 Stages of the policy-making process. *Source:* O'Connor & Sabato, 2002, p. 431.

attention from public officials is the influence and number of constituents affected by or interested in the problem, and the political acceptability of the problem and its solution.

Policy Formulation

This stage involves the crafting of appropriate and acceptable proposed courses of action, or policy alternatives, to ameliorate or resolve the public problem. Policy formulation may be undertaken by various players in the political environment—from the president and his aides to agency officials, from appointed task forces and commissions to interest groups, from think tanks to legislators and their staffs. In developing the policy alternatives, often a preliminary analysis of their success, which includes costs and practicability for implementation and political acceptability, occurs.

Many different methods for analysis can be used here or as part of the next stage. The most commonly used method is a cost–benefit analysis. This method compares the costs of creating and implementing each policy alternative (usually in terms of expense, but also political feasibility) against that alternative's benefits. The analysts need to determine if the benefits outweigh the costs, or if the benefits justify the costs regardless of how high they are.

To evaluate an alternative's political feasibility, an analyst looks at whether elected officials would vote for the proposal and make it law *and* whether appointed officials will support the law and implement the policy in a way that makes its success possible (Munger, 2000, p. 15). There is only one way to ensure that politicians and bureaucrats will be likely to support a policy, or at least not to oppose it: Get them involved from the beginning of the cycle. The two most important stages in which to get these officials involved are in the problem recognition and definition stage and the policy formulation stage. Because politicians and bureaucrats have different kinds of veto power over many policies, it is especially important to get their views on each policy alternative before you move on to the next stage in the policy-making cycle (Munger, p. 15).

Policy Adoption

In this stage, also referred to as *decision making,* the different policy alternatives are compared to determine which alternative is the most appropriate, and usually cost-effective, to address the defined problem. The adoption of one alternative must be approved by the people with the requisite authority to do so, such as the legislature or chief executive. This approval gives the policy legal force. Successful policy adoption requires the building of majority coalitions like interest groups, labor organizations, political parties, or general citizenry. Policy adoption is "political" in that it usually includes conflict, negotiation, the exercise of power, bargaining and compromise, and sometimes even deception and bribery (Anderson, 2003, p. 29). It is crucial that the policy adopters correctly state in specific language what the policy is to accomplish, and by whose authority, so as to adequately guide the implementation of the policy and to prevent distortion of legislative intent (O'Connor & Sabato, 2002, p. 434).

Not all policy adoption requires the formation of majority coalitions. Presidential decision making, such as on foreign affairs and military actions, is often unilateral. Although inundated with information and advice from many aides and advisors, the final decision rests with the president. As well, the president also has the power to veto a bill—a piece of legislation that would address a public, shared problem— passed by the legislature.

Budgeting

As with most things, a crucial stage in the policy-making cycle is funding. Most public policies require financial support in order to be carried out successfully. Many of the distributive and redistributive types of policies involve the transfer of money from taxpayers to the government and back to those individuals that the policy was created to benefit. Whether a policy is well funded or not has a significant effect on its scope, impact, and effectiveness. An absence of funding or a refusal to fund can virtually nullify a policy. As well, other plans or programs developed to meet the objectives of the policy can suffer from inadequate funding, such as the No Child Left Behind Act (O'Connor & Sabato, 2002, p. 435).

The budgetary stage also gives the president and Congress an opportunity to review the hundreds of government policies and programs, to inquire into their administration, to appraise their value and effectiveness, and to exercise some influence on their conduct (O'Connor & Sabato, 2002, p. 435).

Policy Implementation

This stage (also referred to as *administration*) defines *how* policies are carried out. Most public policies are implemented primarily by administrative agencies. These administrative agencies are given a mandate by Congress to create the necessary programs that will meet the objectives of the policy passed by the legislature. While creating the programs, administrative agencies often engage in elaboration of the policy and even creation of policy through enactment of the programs' rules and standards. Figure 26–3 shows how a public policy is implemented through agency plans, which are administered through various programs that reflect policy goals.

There are four different types of administrative organizations, which encompass roughly 1,150 agencies. The first is the *executive departments* of the executive branch of government. These are the fourteen cabinets of the president that have the responsibility for conducting a broad area of government operations (examples are the Departments of Justice, Defense, Commerce, Agriculture, Education, Health and Human Services, and Housing and Urban Development) and are led by presidentially appointed secretaries with Senate approval. Most of these

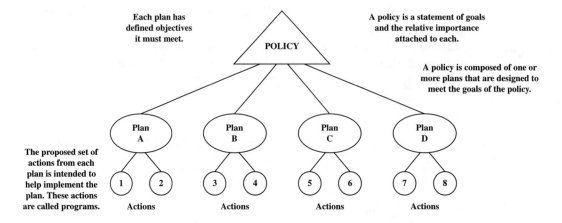

Figure 26–3   The structure of a public policy. *Source:* Starling, 2002, p. 187.

departments are further organized into bureaus, divisions, sections, and other smaller units, such as the Department of Justice's Office on Violence Against Women. It is here that much of the day-to-day policy and program implementation work is handled.

The second type is *independent regulatory commissions,* which are agencies created by Congress that engage in the regulation of private economic activities, such as the stock market, banks, and labor–management relations. These agencies are headed by presidentially appointed regulatory commissioners who serve fixed, staggered terms and can be removed only because of malfeasance, inefficiency, or neglect of duties. An example of an independent regulatory commission is the Joint Commission on Accreditation of Healthcare Organizations.

The third type is *government corporations*, such as Amtrak and the United States Postal Service. These agencies handle business-like or commercial activities of the government. They are created by Congress when the government decides to engage in commercial activities. They produce revenue and require greater flexibility than Congress generally allows regular departments. They are wholly owned by the federal government and have greater financial and personnel flexibility than other governmental agencies. Government corporations usually charge a fee for the goods and services they produce.

Lastly, *independent agencies* make up the largest number of agencies and employees of the four types. Although these agencies are organized outside of the executive branch of government for symbolic and practical reasons, the federal government and the political party in charge still largely influence them. Agencies are headed by an appointed director, and thus most likely hold the same views on policies and programs as the elected official who made the appointment. These agencies resemble the cabinet departments; however, they have a narrower area of responsibility and often have a watchdog or review capacity (Anderson, 2003, pp. 202–204; O'Connor & Sabato, 2002, pp. 242–245). An example of an independent agency is the Centers for Disease Control and Prevention.

Administrative agencies may be enabled to use a number of techniques to implement policies in their jurisdictions. These techniques can be categorized as authority, incentive, capacity, and hortatory techniques. *Authoritative techniques* are based on the assumption that people's actions must be directed or restrained by government in order to prevent or eliminate activities or products that are unsafe, unfair, evil, or immoral. Examples of these actions are driving while intoxicated, unsafe consumer products like poorly designed baby cribs, or broadcasting obscenities over the radio. Agencies enforce policies by issuing rules and standards that individuals and corporations must follow. Compliance with these rules and standards is determined through inspections and monitoring. Penalties may be imposed if individuals or corporations are in violation of the rules and standards that are set forth in a particular policy.

Incentive techniques are based on the assumption that individuals are maximizers of goods and services and act in their own best interest, and thus must be provided with payoffs or financial inducements to get them to comply with the policy. Examples of financial inducements to create certain desired behaviors are tax deductions for charitable donations or grants awarded to companies for installing pollution control equipment. As well, sanctions such as high taxes imposed on luxury goods (such as furs and diamonds) and sin goods (such as gasoline, tobacco, and liquor) are intended to discourage consumption of these products.

Capacity techniques are based on the assumption that society has the incentive or the desire to do what is right but lacks the capacity to act accordingly. This technique provides individuals with information, education, training, and resources that will enable them to undertake the desired activities. Examples of this are job training for the unemployed and accurate information about interest rates for consumers.

Hortatory techniques are based on the assumption that people decide to act on the basis of their personal beliefs and values, such as equality, justice, and what is right and wrong. These techniques encourage individuals to comply with a policy by appealing to their better instincts, such as the Smokey the Bear "Only You Can Prevent Forest Fires," "Don't Be a Litterbug," and "Just Say No" publicity campaigns (Anderson, 2003, pp. 220–221).

The effectiveness of public policies depends largely on the ability of the agencies to promote understanding and consent, thereby reducing violations and minimizing the use of sanctions (Anderson, 2003, p. 236).

Policy Evaluation

This stage determines whether the course of action—the program—is achieving its intended goals and objectives. Policy evaluation may be conducted by a variety of players from congressional committees to presidential committees, from administrative agencies to university researchers, and from private research organizations or think tanks to the General Accounting Office of the federal government. Evaluations may lead to amendments that would hopefully correct problems or shortcomings in the policy.

WHO CREATES POLICY?

Official policy makers are those who have the legal authority to engage in the formation of public policies. These policy makers include legislators (federal, state, and local), executives (president, governor, county executive, and mayor), administrative agencies, and judges. They each perform somewhat functionally different policy-making tasks from one another (Anderson, 2003, p. 46).

Policy makers can be broken up into two distinct categories: primary and supplementary. *Primary policy makers* have direct constitutional authority/power to create policy. These include legislators and executives. The main function of our legislature is to engage in the central political tasks of lawmaking and policy formation in our political system (Anderson, 2003, p. 47). Our president's authority to exercise legislative leadership is clearly established by the U.S. Constitution and legislation, and is an accepted practical function and political necessity of the executive branch. Presidents are generally more interested in policy initiation and adoption than in policy administration (Anderson, 2003, p. 52).

Supplementary policy makers, such as administrative agencies and judges, operate from the power granted to them by primary policy makers. Due to our increasingly complex society and its social, technical, and economic needs, as well as a lack of time for legislators to become experts in the vast number of policy areas, our political system created administrative agencies for the specific purpose of adequate control of public policies. This creation caused the delegation of much discretionary authority, which often includes extensive rule-making power, from legislatures to administrative agencies. Consequently, administrative agencies make many decisions and issue many rules that have far-reaching political and policy consequences (Anderson, 2003, p. 53).

Rule making by administrative agencies is the creation of agency statements of general applicability and future effect that concern the rights of private parties. These guidelines have the force and effect of law. Under the requirements of the federal Administrative Procedures Act, general notice of a proposed rule must be published in the *Federal Register* so interested parties can have the opportunity to present their opinions on it through a presentation of written data. The *Register*, published five days a week, also lists the latest presidential orders and rules adopted by agencies and a great variety of other official notices (Starling, 2002, p. 58). In addition to adopting new policies, rule making also involves modifying existing policies.

As administrative agencies implement policy, conflicts can and do arise between the agencies and individual citizens. *Adjudication* is a quasi-judicial process conducted by agencies to determine if their decision on some matter involving an individual or corporation was within their scope of jurisdiction (for example, denial of a permit).

The courts, specifically the national and state appellate courts, have often greatly affected the nature and content of public policies through their powers of judicial review and statutory interpretation. Judicial review is the power of courts to determine the constitutionality of actions by the legislative and executive branches of our government. Courts can declare actions null and void if they find them in conflict with the U.S. Constitution. Courts also interpret and decide the meaning of statutory provisions that are ambiguous or unclearly stated and open to conflicting interpretations. When the court accepts one interpretation over another, it in effect gives preference to the winning party's explanation of the policy (Anderson, 2003, pp. 54–55).

WHO INFLUENCES POLICY?

In addition to the primary and supplementary policy makers, several other entities influence policies through their opinions, specialization and expertise, and ability to influence others. Some of these entities are individual citizens, labor unions, professional organizations, research organizations, media, nonprofit groups, public corporations, lobbyists, political parties, legislative staff, and interest groups.

A pictorial representation of these influences on the policy-making process is shown in Figure 26–4.

Individual citizens—constituents—can influence policy in three distinct ways: voting, party affiliation, and political activism. Some policies are

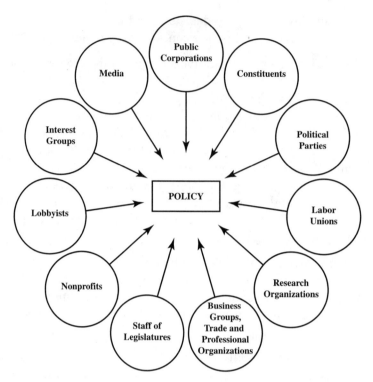

FIGURE 26–4   Influences on policy making.

taken to the public for a vote (for example, referendums and proposi-tions), whereas other policies are actually proposed by the people—initiatives. As well, constituents unhappy with elected officials and the officials' policy decisions and adoptions can always exercise their right to vote against them in the next election. Individuals can also influence policy by their support of certain policies or elected officials through volunteerism, contributing financial resources, and advocating in the political environment for or against a public policy, such as staging protests.

Legislators are targets of a wide variety of lobbying activities from both *professional lobbyists* and *interest groups*. These activities consist of congressional testimony from experts in policy areas, letters of interest from group members, campaign contributions, and sometimes even the outright payment of money for votes (O'Connor & Sabato, 2002, p. 371). Interest groups try to work closely with agency administrators in an effort to influence policy formulation and, more importantly, policy implementation. Lobbyists and interest groups are often seen as experts on a particular issue (for example, the environment, the elderly, or gun control), and thus are consulted by policy makers. Interest groups are especially poised to help policy makers form coalitions in order to suc-cessfully adopt a particular policy alternative.

Political parties greatly influence policy through their endorsements of specific candidates and domination of elected seats in government. Parties endorse candidates by raising and donating money for their campaigns, and recruit and organize volunteers for campaign efforts and other group efforts like "get out the vote" campaigns. As well, by creating a new political party, like the Green Party, a candidate can help to spotlight an issue of concern.

Keep in mind that the president appoints most high-level positions in the administrative area of our government (executive departments, regulatory commissions, and independent agencies), with approval from the Senate. As well, elected officials' staffs are handpicked by the elected official. It stands to reason that the president, and thus the president's political party, will appoint leaders who share the same political views and ideals as they do. In general terms, the Republican Party tends to be more conservative on issues and the Democratic Party tends to be more liberal. Whichever party controls the presidency and the majority in Congress tends to advance more of its own views on public issues during its term.

Research organizations are composed of policy analysts and researchers. They exist to provide policy makers with information and data on policy alternatives and even on proposals for new policy alternatives. As well, they provide the public with their opinions on the effectiveness of public policies. These organizations usually have a policy bias and distinct ideological leanings—conservative or liberal.

Other entities that may lobby policy makers or contribute financially to elected officials' campaigns in exchange for favorable votes on policies are corporations, labor unions, nonprofits, business groups, and trade and professional associations.

One of the most influential entities regarding policy, at least on the evaluation of public policies, is the media. Again, different media outlets usually have political biases and specific ideologies that affect their evaluations of elected officials and their policies.

KEY TECHNIQUES FOR INFLUENCING POLICY

There are several techniques forensic nurses can employ to influence policies that are of interest and impact their occupations:

- *Join a professional organization* such as the American Nurses Association, the International Association of Forensic Nurses, or your state's nurses association.
- *Determine the specific public and health issues of interest* that impact the field of forensic nursing.

- *Become informed* about the public policies and health policies currently under consideration at the federal level of government.
- *Study the federal rule-making process* and learn how to present your opinions for consideration by an administrative agency.
- *Become familiar and comfortable with the Federal Register.* It will publish directions on where to send comments and the deadline for the public comment period.
- *Offer your expertise* to your state's nurses association in assisting with the development of new regulations or modifying existing regulations. Also, offer your expertise to help the association prepare comments on proposed regulations (American Nurses Association, 2005).

POLICY ISSUES AND FORENSIC NURSING

Some specific issues that may be of interest to those in the field of forensic nursing are DNA analysis; sexual assault forensic examiner (SAFE), forensic nurse examiner (FNE), and sexual assault nurse examiner (SANE) certification; prevention of violence and abuse; specifically sex-based crimes; prisoner rights; healthcare services in prisons; bioterrorism; forensic examination protocol; patient education programs for at-risk populations; Web-based crimes; and, of course, the adequate funding and support to address these issues.

SUMMARY

Governmental policy, whether federal, state, or local in origin, develops through the many stages discussed in this chapter. These stages provide numerous opportunities for the forensic nurse to help shape policy and its implementation in programs that will serve clients in diverse populations. However, the forensic nurse often has little experience with governmental agencies or policy administration. Therefore, forensic nurses should familiarize themselves with the policy making process by taking advantage of opportunities to participate at the local and state levels in grassroots organizations, to raise local awareness of issues of interest, and to network with individuals from other professions who have similar interests and concerns.

One way to network with groups and forensic nurses in other jurisdictions is through the use of the Internet. Most national, international, or advisory groups have websites that are readily accessed. Forensic nurses can use the information provided by these groups to supplement their own experiences and understanding of an issue as they work to shape public policy. In addition, the forensic nurse should access all appropriate federal executive and legislative branch websites. This will help when evaluating local and national trends in policy making. These same websites are used by administrators and legislators themselves to research policies and programs and to develop ideas for legislation. Thus, one can anticipate statutory trends and responses by legislators by studying the same materials they rely on. The forensic practitioner can develop the skills necessary to further public policy in areas of interest by utilizing all available resources and working with legislators and administrators to respond to client's needs.

QUESTIONS FOR DISCUSSION

1. What is public policy?
2. When does a problem rise to the attention of the public?
3. What are the steps in the policy-making process?
4. Who creates policy?
5. Who influences policy?
6. What strategies might the forensic nurse employ to influence policy and assist in its implementation?

REFERENCES

Anderson, J. E. (2003). *Public policymaking*, (5th ed.). Boston, MA: Houghton Mifflin.

American Nurses Association, Government Affairs—"ANA in Action" located at www.ana.org/gova. Retrieved February 02, 2005.

Bardach, E. (2000). *A practical guide for policy analysis.* New York: Seven Bridges.

Munger, M. C. (2000). *Analyzing policy.* New York: Norton.

O'Connor, K. & Sabato, L. J. (2002). *Essentials of American government. Continuity and change.* New York: Addison Wesley Longman.

Starling, G. (2002). *Managing the public sector* (6th ed.). Belmont, CA: Wadsworth/Thomson Learning.

Forensic Nursing Education: Developments, Theoretical Conceptualizations, and Practical Applications for Curriculum

Arlene Kent-Wilkinson

Forensic nursing's time has come: Events covered in the media have contributed to public awareness of how the applied sciences are used to help solve crimes, to determine psychiatric assessment of those accused, and to educate professionals in the identification, treatment, and prevention of trauma and catastrophic injuries. Now students from all over the world are inquiring about how they can become forensic nurses, and where and how they can take forensic nursing courses. To meet these requests, forensic nursing education programs are rapidly appearing in curriculums of leading colleges and universities. This chapter provides practical applications for developing forensic nursing and multidisciplinary curriculums using classroom, distance, and online delivery modalities. Images detailing many facets of course development are included, showing frameworks for content structure and content concepts, as well as teaching and learning strategies for forensic interactivities. Visual learning objects include the use of animation, Macromedia Shockwave, and Internet resources in combination with an international perspective to the fascinating forensic field.

CHAPTER FOCUS_____

Systems and services where forensic nurses work
How do I become a forensic nurse?
Educational levels of forensic nursing courses
Policies and standards guiding forensic nursing education
Responsibilities of forensic nurse educators
Methods (modes) of course delivery (on site/online)
Forensic nursing curriculum content
Effective teaching and learning strategies
Research in online forensic nursing courses
The future of forensic nursing education
Forensic nursing programs globally

KEY TERMS_____

asynchronous
forensic historical time lines
learning objects
international perspective
synchronous
WebCT and Blackboard

INTRODUCTION

"How can I become a forensic nurse?" "What education do I need?" Students all over the world are inquiring about where they can take forensic nursing courses and where to find jobs that employ forensic nurses.

Although forensic nursing courses have been rapidly appearing in curriculums of many leading colleges and universities, forensic nurse educators themselves also have questions: "How do we best organize and disseminate this unique body of knowledge?" "What content should be included in each course or program of study?" Perhaps the most important questions educators have is this: "Are we conceptualizing forensic nursing consistently with other programs locally, nationally, and internationally?"

This final chapter will attempt to address these practical inquiries for educators. In addition, it will answer common student questions, such as: "Where can I work as a forensic nurse?" "What content can I expect in a forensic nursing course?" and "Is classroom better than distance education?" The different on-site and online choices in delivery modalities will be described with content outlines that have been used in specific forensic nursing programs. Samples of learning objects for student interactivities will be included. Finally, to answer the universally asked question "Where are the programs?" a list of the known forensic nursing programs available globally will conclude this chapter.

SYSTEMS AND SERVICES WHERE FORENSIC NURSES WORK

Forensic nurses practice not only in the complex organization of hospitals within the healthcare system, but also in facilities of many interfacing systems: the criminal justice system, the mental healthcare system, the medical examiner/coroner system, the child welfare system, and in government-approved facilities. Forensic nurses have adapted to practices within many systems and with many disciplines on interdisciplinary teams, but their practice remains within the scope of nursing. Figure 27–1 illustrates where forensic nurses work within the many systems and services that have forensic nursing roles.

HOW DO I BECOME A FORENSIC NURSE?

The generic undergraduate baccalaureate degree in nursing is first required, as forensic nursing is a specialty that requires additional skills and knowledge in a specific area. Several graduate programs are available in forensic nursing, and more are in the planning stages. However, it is possible to attain additional skills in particular areas of forensic nursing, such as sexual assault nurse examiner (SANE) or legal nurse consultant, through programs of continuing education rather than through formal graduate study. Students enrolled in undergraduate nursing programs who have an interest in forensic nursing could inquire into the possibilities of forensic placements for a clinical practicum, and could focus written assignments on a forensic nursing role, or a forensic health issue.

Because forensic nursing education is relatively new, the programs of study are in the early development stages at colleges and universities scattered around the world. The courses for the most part have been and are being written by forensic nurse clinicians and nurse educators with a passionate interest in the area. Because educational programs were not previously available, nurse educators developing the programs are drawing from their own forensic clinical experiences and/or from what has been published in the forensic nursing literature.

Many nurses identified themselves as forensic nurses and practiced with forensic populations long before education was available in this specific field. This is similar historically to many nursing specialty areas, including emergency, critical care, and nurse midwifery. Nurses who worked in the area and learned on the job saw the value of having

SYSTEMS	SERVICES/FACILITIES	ROLES
• Health care system	• Hospitals • Communities • Emergency departments, • Sexual assault clinics • Women's shelters • Medical clinics	• Sexual assault nurse examiners (SANE) • Forensic clinical emergency specialists • Interpersonal violence nurse specialists • Forensic pediatric nurses • Forensic geriatric nurses
• Criminal justice system	• Penitentiaries • Correctional centers • Remand or pretrial centers • Half way houses	• Prison nurses • correctional nurses • Forensic mental health nurses • Nurse attorneys • Forensic nurse consultants
• Medical examiner • Coroner's system	• Medical examiner's offices • Coroner's offices • Morgues	• Forensic nurse death investigators
• Mental health care system	• Special hospitals • State or provincial hospitals • Regional psychiatric units • Medium, high & low security units • Forensic community services • Forensic psychiatric inpatient units • Forensic psychiatric outpatient units • Forensic psychiatric services	• Forensic psychiatric nurses • Forensic mental health nurses • Forensic nurse consultants • Forensic community mental health nurses (FCMHN)
• Child welfare system • Government systems	• Social services • Long term care services • Geriatric services	• Forensic nurse consultants • Forensic geriatric nurses
• Legal firms • Insurance companies • Private practice • Government services	• Legal services	• Legal nurse consultants • Forensic nurse consultants • Nurse attorneys
• Education system	• Colleges and universities	• Forensic nurse educators

Source: © Kent-Wilkinson, 1999a

Figure 27–1   Forensic systems, services, and forensic nursing roles.

additional education to learn the unique aspects of certain specialty areas, and thus developed educational programs.

EDUCATIONAL LEVELS OF FORENSIC NURSING COURSES

By the end of the twentieth century, it was evident that an exciting movement toward forensic nursing was taking place internationally in every method of educational delivery possible: traditional classroom, distance, and Internet delivery with varying levels of certificate, diploma, baccalaureate, and graduate credit. With many different levels of forensic nursing courses and programs becoming available, it is difficult for student nurses and anyone interested in the forensic area to sort out what level of program is best to take for their individual situation. The following sections discuss the main levels of nursing education in general, and specify whether programs or courses of study exist in forensic nursing at that level.

Certification

Certification is an examination process that verifies whether a professional has a sufficient amount of current knowledge in a selected specialty area. Usually the professional organization in the field of study determines the criteria for certification and the length of time for which the certification is valid. Certification is separate and different from a formal academic diploma or degree, neither of which guarantees qualifying for employment in the area of practice. In some countries, and for some specialties of nursing, students are expected to achieve advanced practice certification appropriate to their specialty after graduation with a diploma or baccalaureate degree in nursing. For example, in the United States, the American Nursing Credentialing Center offers certification exams for some nursing specialty areas; in Canada, the Canadian Nurses Association (CNA) offers certification exams for some nursing specialties, such as mental health nursing.

With regards to forensic nursing, certification already exists for some of its subspecialties: correctional nursing has certification examinations offered by the National Commission on Correctional Healthcare; the American Association of Legal Nurse Consultants provides legal nurse consultants with certification examinations; and the International Association of Forensic Nurses began offering SANE certification in 2001. Only some areas of nursing practice require certification to obtain employment; thus far it is not a requirement for most areas of forensic nursing. However, New Jersey has made SANE programs mandatory in its counties in an effort to improve the care and treatment of sexual assault survivors (Naught, 2002).

A certification exam currently is under development by the IAFN that will cover a broad range of forensic nursing in general. In 2003–2004, international forensic nurse specialists and educators, through the IAFN, collaborated to develop the core curriculum to provide the foundational concepts for certification exams and a guideline for formal forensic nursing educational programs at the graduate level for the advanced practice forensic nurse.

Certification examinations are often developed by a professional interest group or association, which determines whether the level of certification is at the advanced practice graduate level or at the diploma/baccalaureate level. Although certification for the subspecialties of forensic nursing (correctional nursing, legal nurse consulting, and SANE) is at the diploma/baccalaureate level, those who wish to sit the certification examination for forensic nursing in general, when it is available, will be required to have a graduate degree in nursing.

Certificate Program

A certificate program is a series of courses in a selected specialty of professional practice (e.g., mental health, emergency, critical care, neonatology, gerontology). After completion, the student has a certificate in a specific area of practice. A certification program is required in some areas of practice to obtain employment. A certificate forensic nursing program is a series of courses in the specialty of forensic nursing (e.g., forensic heath studies certificate). After completion, the nurse has a certificate in specific areas of forensic nursing.

Graduate Degree Nursing Program

A master's of nursing degree requires advanced practice nursing studies, which are beyond a baccalaureate degree in nursing and include graduate nursing courses. "Advanced Practice Nursing is the application of an expanded range of practical theoretical and research based therapeutics to phenomenon experienced by patients within a specialized clinical area of the larger discipline of nursing" (Hamric, 2000; Hanson & Hamric, 2003, p. 205).

When studying for a master's in nursing, students may want to choose to focus on the specialty area of forensic nursing or forensic healthcare issues for their articles or thesis. A graduate degree forensic nursing program provides a master's degree in the specialized area of forensic nursing study.

Doctoral Degree Nursing Program

A PhD nursing program of study (which culminates in a doctoral degree in nursing) requires studies beyond a graduate degree in nursing. When pursuing a doctoral degree in nursing, students may want to focus on the specialty area of forensic nursing or forensic healthcare issues for their research or dissertation. A forensic nursing PhD program requires studies beyond a graduate degree in nursing where the special focus of the program is advanced practice forensic nursing at the doctoral level.

None of the previously mentioned levels of education guarantees obtaining employment in the area of forensic nursing practice. Currently, certification in forensic nursing is not required in most forensic nursing subspecialties to obtain employment, but due to the laws of supply and demand, as with many other nursing specialties, certification may be required in the future. Nurses, like most other healthcare professionals, may choose to take educational programs outside of their discipline. Many forensic nursing courses could easily be designed or already are designed for multidisciplinary study, and most are recognized within other disciplines. Mason (2002) notes that nursing does not have absolute rights to the forensic specialty of study. Many other disciplines have a forensic specialty of practice, such as forensic medicine, forensic psychiatry, forensic psychology, and forensic social work, to name only a few, each of which follows the standards of practice and codes of conduct of its specific discipline.

POLICIES AND STANDARDS GUIDING FORENSIC NURSING EDUCATION

Nurses, as the largest group of healthcare professionals, have advantages when marketing, developing, and delivering programs for forensic nursing and multidisciplinary educational programs at all levels. The discipline of nursing has a strong and clear metaparadigm with a professional scope as well as standards of practice, a code of ethics, and ideologies that provide a framework for the development of forensic nursing educational programs.

IAFN Educational Policies and Standards of Practice

Clearly delineated standards of nursing practice inform professional nursing care and provide a framework for responsibility and accountability. The IAFN has begun to make a significant contribution to global policies for forensic nursing education. The *Sexual Assault Nurse*

Examiner Standards of Practice (IAFN, 1996) and the *Forensic Nursing Standards and Scope of Practice* were both developed by the IAFN membership (ANA, 1997). Forensic nursing certification became available in 2001 for the subspecialty of sexual assault nurses. On October 1, 2001, an IAFN resolution on terrorism called for worldwide support of nursing education that includes mass disaster preparedness (IAFN, 2001a). At the same time, an IAFN resolution on forensic nursing education called for the development and implementation of comprehensive forensic nursing content at all levels of formal nursing education (IAFN, 2001b).

The IAFN policies encourage forensic nurses to acquire and maintain current knowledge in forensic practice (ANA, 1997). The forensic nurse may seek additional knowledge and skills appropriate to the practice setting by participating in educational programs and activities, conferences, workshops, interdisciplinary professional meetings, and self-directed learning, thereby embracing a lifelong learning policy. The IAFN has taken a leadership role in the health policy arena to champion positions on national and international issues. IAFN nursing leaders have had the opportunity to participate in meetings about national policy regarding sexual assault victims and interpersonal violence.

RESPONSIBILITIES OF FORENSIC NURSE EDUCATORS

Although it is a privilege for forensic nurse educators to develop some of the first forensic nursing and forensic multidisciplinary academic programs, it is also a responsibility. The media, through magazines, movies, and television, have played a role in enhancing awareness of the forensic area, but forensic nurse leaders in the field are responsible for communicating their unique knowledge of the specialty. These forensic nurse specialists have to take responsibility for making both themselves and their specialty understood. Articulating the specialization in any discipline is serious, rigorous, and demanding. It requires the members of each area of specialization, beginning with the leaders and scholars in each field, to take on the hard work of defining what they do. To date, forensic nurses globally have authored an impressive body of knowledge. Discourse is alive in the important debates of the specialty in forensic nursing's current years of early development.

Forensic nurse educators also have a responsibility to mentor and advise those interested in a forensic nursing career. Forensic nurse educators need to be knowledgeable and up front that some areas of forensic nursing, particularly in certain locations, have very few available jobs. Advising newcomers to the forensic specialty as to where forensic nurses have pioneered their own jobs and how they made these inroads provides insight as to current and future career opportunities within the forensic arena. Forensic areas can exist anywhere healthcare professionals deal with victims or perpetrators of catastrophic accidents, physical or emotional trauma, violence, and crime.

Nursing professional bodies in North America and around the world have mandated that nurses become more culturally aware and sensitive to the diversity of their patients. Cultural components are required to be included in nursing educational curriculums and registration examinations (ANA, 1997, 2000; CNA, 2000, 2004). Students learn to understand and appreciate diverse perspectives through a dialogue with their peers, facilitated by a dialogue with the instructor, who helps students learn the unique knowledge content of forensic nursing. Many subspecialties of forensic nursing are exposed to the dilemma of "crime or culture" when caring for culturally diverse groups. Health-related issues of female genital mutilation raise many ethical concerns for nurses who care for these female clients. Nurses must interact in a culturally sensitive manner and know when and to whom to voice their concerns about cultural practices.

METHODS (MODES) OF COURSE DELIVERY (ON SITE AND ONLINE)

Whenever a new teaching method comes along in education, educators and students debate which teaching and learning modalities (i.e., classroom, distance, and most recently online distance education) are the most efficient and effective models. Arguments about the role of technology in education go back at least 2,500 years. For the ancient Greeks, oratory was the means by which people learned and passed on learning (Bates & Poole, 2003). Oratory was soon challenged by the advent of reading and writing, and the debate then turned to a concern for which of the two was more effective for learning.

Today, one of the prominent educational debates concerns the efficacy of on-site education versus online or distance education. We are beginning to realize that "virtual" or online education is not necessarily better or worse than face-to-face education. The old distinction between on site versus distance technology blurs rapidly as the increasing availability of network resources and collaborative software stimulates a convergence of the two.

The Classroom/On Site/Lecture Method

For hundreds of years, the lecture format was traditional for classroom delivery. The word *lecture* stems from the Latin word for *reading* because it was mainly based on readings in Latin from ancient handwritten manuscripts. The philosophical position that informs this teaching method is scholasticism, which trains students to consider a text according to certain pre-established, officially approved criteria, which are painstakingly and painfully drilled into them (Bates & Poole, 2003). The traditional classroom teaching method has evolved to include numerous delivery methods for the exchange of information. The lecture, the seminar, group discussion methods, and elaborate multimedia technology enhancements make this an effective and more enjoyable learning mode than the original lecture format.

Classroom forensic nursing courses can be multidisciplinary in nature, overviewing the emerging forensic specialty. During a classroom forensic nursing course, experts in the unique forensic practice areas can be brought in as guest lecturers. Complementing the classroom instruction are field trips or clinical practicums organized to include local forensic facilities, such as secured facilities (jails or penitentiaries), young offender centers, forensic psychiatric units, homeless shelters, courts of law, women's shelters, or the medical examiner's or coroner's offices. These on-site experiences introduce students to the actual clinical settings where roles for forensic health professionals are clearly visible in practice. Classroom forensic courses, including a variety of teaching approaches, can be duplicated in any educational institution teaching forensic nursing.

Distance Education

Distance education is learning that takes place when the instructor and student are not in the same room, but are separated by physical distance. It is therefore a solution for those who require a creative and flexible way to learn. Many associate distance learning with correspondence learning, the original form of distance learning. This type of education provides course materials through the mail. Ahern and Repman (1994) noted that because correspondence courses relied on the mail, the pace of the course was slow, and reciprocal interaction between teacher and students was difficult. Eventually, the correspondence course overcame the constraints of place through a mechanical process of course design and distribution involving the Internet; this became known as distributed or online learning.

When first introduced, distance education was considered a prepackaged text or audiovisual course, with little or no interaction between the student and the instructor. Today's evolving interactive communication technology allows learning experiences to occur at any time between instructor and student, student and student, and student and expert. When developing a course online many elements of the classroom can be incorporated (Figure 27–2). Internet technology has gone beyond the

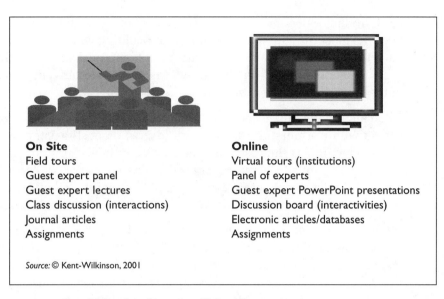

On Site	Online
Field tours	Virtual tours (institutions)
Guest expert panel	Panel of experts
Guest expert lectures	Guest expert PowerPoint presentations
Class discussion (interactions)	Discussion board (interactivities)
Journal articles	Electronic articles/databases
Assignments	Assignments

Source: © Kent-Wilkinson, 2001

Figure 27–2   On-site and online parallels of course content.

issues of distance to honor the interactive, communal character of learning and the emerging capabilities of the Internet (Kent-Wilkinson, Mckeown, Mercer, McCann, & Mason, 2000).

The use of computer technology in healthcare education has proliferated. Technology now is a part of patient care in many settings, thus requiring its instruction in undergraduate educational programs; its use also continues to grow in graduate and continuing education programs (Hawley & Desborough, 1998). Hybrid courses that combine the traditional classroom with online methods are commonly being used, and evaluations suggest that this combination provides for more resources, and more efficient communication.

FORENSIC NURSING CURRICULUM CONTENT

The most difficult aspect of course development for nurse educators is how to best organize and structure the forensic course content. This task is magnified for forensic nursing content because there are many subspecialties of forensic nursing; many concepts are similar among all the specialties, but some content is unique to each subspecialty. In addition, the courses are often written for a multidisciplinary audience with an international perspective to the forensic issues. Forensic nursing content can be organized and disseminated in many different ways. The challenge of turning the content of a successful classroom-delivered forensic nursing course into content delivered online is an onerous undertaking.

An introductory course on all subspecialties of forensic nursing is perhaps the most difficult course to develop. Deciding what to include and what to leave out from a massive amount of theoretical and clinical concepts is overwhelming. The job at hand is to include only an overview of the key roles and concepts.

Often an undergraduate course on forensic nursing may be only a single course within a nursing baccalaureate degree or post-registration program. When this is the case, there is not a continuous series of courses, each focusing on a different subspecialty. Therefore, the challenge is to organize a single course that provides a student with the best overview possible of this umbrella specialty.

When the concepts to include have been decided, then decisions must be made as to how to organize the content. The author has included a navigation framework unit or module outline that she developed (Figure 27–3). This framework serves equally as well for forensic nursing courses as for example a cultural diversity and Aboriginal health course. The content of many different courses can be inserted into the categories of this framework.

Section/Unit Outline

Forensic history/laws

Forensic theories/philosophy

Forensic specialties/roles

Forensic systems/services

Forensic practice/prevention

Forensic populations (at risk)

Forensic concepts

Forensic issues

Forensic education

Forensic research

Forensic career opportunities

Source: Kent-Wilkinson 1997; 1999; 2002

Figure 27–3 Section/Unit outline for forensic nursing content.

Although forensic nursing course content may be structured or organized into many different overall sections/units, one of the challenging points to sort out is the hierarchical structure of the terms for the course—index, topics, sections, units, and modules. Terms differ when developing courses with different instructional design teams, at different universities, and in different countries. The term *topics* in Australia seems to correspond to the term *sections* in North America, and within these are units and modules.

Two methods of organizing content for an introductory course are included here. The first method is to divide the forensic nursing content into two main focuses of study for all subspecialties of forensic nursing: 1) those who care for the victim, and 2) those who care for the offender. This division could also be called *forensic science* and *forensic behavioral science* (Figure 27–4).

Forensic nursing and a multidisciplinary forensic content could also be divided into the five topics of forensic nursing, forensic psychiatric, forensic medicine, forensic corrections/prison health, and forensic clinical emergency. If the semester is short, students can be given the choice to select just three of the five topics. The student would be required to do the topic of their discipline (e.g., if they are in the nursing program they are required to do forensic nursing, and if they are in psychology they are required to do forensic psychiatry), but only have to complete the modules for two other areas of most interest to them. Students given these criteria have appreciated this choice to reduce the workload, but they also have access to all the resources and content of the other topics, so they can learn by reading the postings on the discussion board from students doing the topics they did not select (Figure 27–5).

Course Management Systems and Templates

There are also many different ways in which a course can be delivered. The choice of model will depend on the scale and complexity of the course, and the centrality of the use of technology (Bates & Poole, 2003). Since the late 1990s the two most popular course management systems for online course templates have been WebCT and Courseware Blackboard. Within the online educational community, there is a debate: Is the software version of Blackboard better than WebCT? Both support excellence in online teaching and learning with course tool software, resources, and academic expertise.

Prior to the development of course management systems like WebCT and Blackboard, most colleges and universities that delivered online courses developed their own template. For example, Mount Royal College, in Calgary, Alberta, Canada, developed a template in 1996 that proved to be an effective tool for its online courses (Figure 27–6).

I.

Forensic Nursing (Forensic Science) (Forensic Medicine/Forensic Clinical Medicine)	Forensic Nursing (Forensic/Behavioral Sciences) Forensic Psychiatric/Correctional Prison Health
History & Theory Historical & legal timelines Laws & acts & reporting policies Theories & philosophies	**History & Theory** Historical & legal timelines Laws & acts & reporting policies Theories & philosophies
Forensic Nursing Specialties & Roles Forensic nurse Clinical forensic ER nurse Forensic nurse investigator (death) Forensic nurse consultant (legal) Forensic educator/researcher Forensic nurse examiner Sexual assault nurse examiner Sexual assault resource team Sexual assault forensic examiner Forensic geriatric nurse Forensic pediatric nurse Interpersonal violence forensic nurse Multidisciplinary Team Medical examiner Coroner Crime scene investigator Criminal profiler/police Forensic scientists Police surgeon ER physician Sexual assault nurse examiner Sexual assault resource team EMT/paramedic Police	**Forensic Nursing Specialties & Roles** Forensic nurse Forensic correctional nurse Forensic psychiatric nurse Forensic nurse consultant (legal) Forensic educator/researcher Forensic psychiatrist Forensic psychologist Forensic occupational/recreational therapist Forensic psychiatric nurse Forensic social worker Court/judge/police Forensic psychomotrist Prison medical officer Correctional nurse Institutional psychologist Correctional officer Parole/probation/police
Systems & Services Health Care system Mental health system Medical examiner system Coroner system Government-approved facilities Child welfare system Emergency medical services Judicial legal system Police services Sexual assault nurse examiner Sexual assault resource team	**Systems & Services** Health Care system Mental health system Criminal justice system Forensic psychiatric services Correctional services Judicial legal system Solicitor general services
Practice & Prevention Standards of practice Professional associations Assessment (risk)/identification/screening Documentation Evidence collection Therapeutics/intervention/treatment/evaluation Medication management Health prevention/promotion Wound care/ballistics Custody of body procedures sudden/accidental/unexplained death	**Practice & Prevention** Standards of practice Professional associations Assessment (risk)/identification/screening Documentation Evidence collection Therapeutics/intervention/ treatment/evaluation Medication management Health prevention/promotion Fitness/insanity/assessments/evaluations Pretrial/presentence/assessment

Figure 27–4 Forensic nursing—course content index: two topics.

2. **Forensic Nursing (Forensic Science) (Forensic Medicine/Forensic Clinical Medicine)**

Practice & Prevention (continued)
Examinations
Addictions/suicide
Toxicology
Fingerprinting
Crime scene investigation

Populations at Risk
Accidental death victim
Culturally diverse victim
Child abuse/neglect victim
Child sexual abuse victim
Child prostitution victim
Drowning victim
Elder/senior abuse victim
Female circumcision victim
Families of victims
Homicidal victim
Munchausen syndrome by proxy victim
Nurse abuse victim
Sexual abuse victim
Shaken baby syndrome victim
Spouse abuse victim
Sudden Infant Death Syndrome Victim
Suicidal

Concepts
Abuse/neglect
International
Stigma
Suicide
Violence

Issues
Confidentiality issues
DNA issues
Euthanasia/mercy killing
Media/technology issues
Organ donation issues
Rights (human/patient/victim/deceased)
Violence/terrorism/ school/workplace/bullying

Future
Education (international)
Research (international)
Careers (international)

Forensic Nursing (Forensic/Behavioral Sciences) Forensic Psychiatric/Correctional Prison Health

Practice & Prevention (continued)
Not criminally responsible/dangerous/risk
Assessment/mental status/addictions/suicide

Populations at Risk
Aboriginal/multicultural offender
Addicted offender
Aging offender
Chronically ill offender/HIV offender
Culturally diverse offender
Dangerous offenders
Disabled/mentally challenged offender
Families of offenders
Female offender
Homicidal filicidal offenders
Mentally ill offender
Nurse abuse
Sex offender
Suicidal/self harm offender
Young offender

Concepts
Abuse/neglect
Anger/aggression
Capital punishment
Caring/custody/control
Deinstitutionalization
Homicide/filicide
International
Recidivism
Restraint/seclusion
Stigma
Suicide
Violence

Issues
Confidentiality issues
Deinstitutionalization
Homicide/filicide
Media/technology issues
Pornography (Internet)
Recidivism
Restraint/seclusion
Rights (offender)
Tx vs. Warehousing

Future
Education (international)
Research (international)
Careers (international)

Source: Kent-Wilkinson 2000

FORENSIC NURSING (RN)

History & theory
Specialties & roles
Systems & services
Practice & prevention
Populations at risk
Concepts & issues
Future/education/research/career opportunities

Forensic Nursing History & theory
Historical & legal time lines
Theories & philosophies

Forensic Nursing Specialties & Roles
Forensic nurse
Clinical forensic
ER nurse
Correctional nurse
Forensic nurse consultant (legal)
Forensic nurse examiner (sexual assault)
Forensic nurse investigator (death)
Forensic geriatric nurse
Forensic pediatric nurse
Forensic psychiatric nurse
Forensic educator/researcher

Forensic Nursing Systems & Services
Healthcare System
Mental health system
Criminal justice system
ME/coroner system
Gov't approved services

Forensic Nursing Practice & Prevention
Standards of practice
Professional associations
Assessment/identification/screening/treatment
Documentation/evidence collection
Therapeutics/intervention/treatment/evaluation
Medication management
Health prevention/promotion

FORENSIC PSYCHIATRIC

History & theory
Specialties & roles
Systems & services
Practice & prevention
Populations at risk
Concepts & issues
Future/education/research/career opportunities

Forensic Psychiatric History & Theory
Historical & legal time lines
Theories & philosophies

Forensic Psychiatric Specialties & Roles
Forensic psychiatrist
Forensic psychologist
Forensic OT/RT
Forensic psychiatric nurse
Forensic social worker
Court/judge/police
Forensic psychometrist

Forensic Psychiatric Systems & Services
Mental health system
Criminal justice system
Forensic psychiatric services
Forensic community & private services
Judicial legal system

Forensic Psychiatric Practice & Prevention
Standards of practice
Professional associations
Assessment/pretrial/presentence/NCR/dangerous/risk fitness/insanity
Documentation/evidence collection
Therapeutics/intervention/treatment/evaluation
Medication management (psychotropic)
Health prevention/promotion

FORENSIC MEDICINE

History & theory
Specialties & roles
Systems & services
Practice & prevention
Populations at risk
Concepts & issues
Future/education/research/career opportunities

Forensic Medicine History & Theory
Historical & legal time lines
Theories & philosophies

Forensic Medicine Specialties & Roles
Medical examiner
Coroner
Forensic nurse investigator (death)
Crime scene investigator
Criminal profiler/police

Forensic Medicine Systems & Services
Coroner system
Medical examiner system
Healthcare system
Solicitor general services
Police services

Forensic Medicine Practice & Prevention
Standards of practice
Professional associations
Assessment sudden/accidental/unexplained
Documentation/evidence collection
Therapeutics/intervention/treatment/evaluation
Custody of body procedures
Health prevention/promotion

FORENSIC CORRECTIONS

History & theory
Specialties & roles
Systems & services
Practice & prevention
Populations at risk
Concepts & issues
Future/education/research/career opportunities

Forensic Corrections History & Theory
Historical & legal time lines
Theories & philosophies

Forensic Corrections Specialties & Roles
Prison medical officer
Correctional nurse
Institutional psychologist
Correctional officer
parole/probation/police

Forensic Corrections Systems & Services
Criminal justice system
Mental health system
Forensic psychiatric services
Correctional services
Judicial legal system

Forensic Corrections Practice & Prevention
Standards of practice
Professional associations
Assessment/mental status/addictions/suicide
Documentation/evidence collection
Therapeutics/intervention/treatment/evaluation
Medication management (prison health)
Health prevention/promotion

FORENSIC CLINICAL (ER)

History & theory
Specialties & roles
Systems & services
Practice & prevention
Populations at risk
Concepts & issues
Future/education/research/career opportunities

Forensic Clinical ER History & Theory
Historical & legal time lines
Theories & philosophies

Forensic Clinical ER Specialties & Roles
Police surgeon
ER physician
Clinical forensic
ER nurse
Interpersonal violence nurse
SANE/SART nurse
EMT/paramedic
Police

Forensic Clinical ER Systems & Services
Healthcare system
Child welfare system
Emergency medical services
Judicial legal system
Police services
SANE/SART services

Forensic Clinical ER Practice & Prevention
Standards of practice
Professional associations
Assessment/identification/screening/examinations/wound care/ballistics
Documentation/evidence collection
Therapeutics/intervention/treatment/evaluation
Medication management
Health prevention/promotion

Forensic Nursing Populations at Risk
(Victim/offender/family)
Child prostitution
Child pornography
Families of deceased
Nurse abuse

Forensic Nursing Concepts & Issues
Rights (human/patient)
Media/technology issues
Violence/terrorism/rage
school/workplace/bullying
Confidentiality/stigma

Forensic Nursing Future
Education (international)
Research (international)
Careers (international)

Source: Kent-Wilkinson, 2002

Forensic Psychiatric Populations at Risk
(Mentally ill offender)
Aboriginal/multicultural offender
Addicted offender
Aging offender
Chronically ill offender/HIV offender
Dangerous offender
Disabled/mentally challenged offender
Families of offenders
Female offender
Mentally ill offender
Nurse abuse
Sex offender
Suicidal/self harm offender
Young offender

Forensic Psychiatric Concepts & Issues
Rights (mentally ill offender)
Media/technology issues
Violence/anger/aggression
Homicide
Filicide

Forensic Psychiatric Future
Education (international)
Research (international)
Careers (international)

Forensic Medicine Populations at Risk
(Deceased)
SIDS
Homicide
Drowning
Accidental
Suicidal
Families of patients/victims

Forensic Medicine Concepts & Issues
Rights (deceased)
Media/technology issues
Violence/intentional death
DNA
Organ donation
Toxicology

Forensic Medicine Future
Education (international)
Research (international)
Careers (international)

Forensic Corrections Populations at Risk
(Offender)
Aboriginal/multicultural offender
Addicted offender
Aging offender
Chronically ill offender/HIV offender
Dangerous offender
Disabled/mentally challenged offender
Families of offenders
Female offender
Homicidal/filicidal offenders
Mentally ill offender
Nurse abuse
Sex offender
Suicidal/self harm offender
Young offender

Forensic Corrections Concepts & Issues
Rights (offender)
Media/technology tssues
Violence anger/aggression/
Caring/custody
Capital punishment
Deinstitutionalization
Recidivism
Restraint/seclusion
Suicide
Tx vs. Warehousing

Forensic Corrections Future
(Prison) Education (international)
(Prison) Research (international)
(Prison) Careers (international)

Forensic Clinical ER Populations at Risk
(Victims)
Child abuse/neglect
Child sexual abuse
Child prostitution
Female circumcision
Munchausen Syndrome by Proxy
Shaken Baby Syndrome
Families of victims
Elder/senior abuse
Sexual abuse
Spouse abuse
Nurse abuse

Forensic Clinical ER Concepts & Issues
Rights (victim)
Media/technology issues
Violence/catastrophic/
biochemical/terrorism
Confidentiality/control
Organ donation

Forensic Clinical ER Future
Education (international)
Research (international)
Careers (international)

Figure 27–5 Forensic nursing—course content index: five topics.

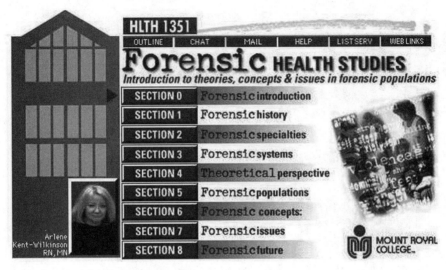

Figure 27–6   Forensic template for home page. *Source:* Kent-Wilkinson, 1997.

EFFECTIVE TEACHING AND LEARNING STRATEGIES

Forensic nurse educators and instructional designers can use the educational software now available to develop a variety of instructional methods, often in combination, to promote active student participation. Information is exchanged through various methods, such as animation/simulation, streaming audio interviews, expert panels, and slide presentations of case studies. Interactions then are facilitated through e-mail, the course listserv, and the course discussion board.

Forensic Interactivities

Interaction can occur between not only the student and the instructor and the student and other students, but also between the student and the content of the course. Thus, the key to success in an online class rests not only with the content that is being presented, but also with the method by which the course is delivered. The effective use of interactivity deepens the learning experience and creates a more satisfying outcome for everyone. When content is delivered in multiple ways, it also addresses different student learning styles and creates a more interesting course overall. It is pedagogy, not technology, that is critical to the success of an online course (Kent-Wilkinson & Hanson, 2002). The following are examples of some of the interactivities used in online forensic nursing courses developed by this author and a team of instructional designers and technicians.

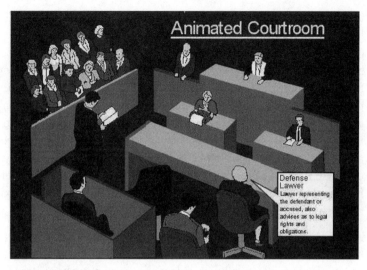

Figure 27–7   Animated courtroom. *Source:* Kent-Wilkinson, 1997.

Animation

A courtroom animation can provide students the layout of a typical courtroom. As a unit activity, students can be asked to research online what the differences are between this and a courtroom in other countries. They can also be asked to identify the different terms globally for the roles of the courtroom players; a simple rollover provides a definition for each person in the courtroom (Figure 27–7).

Field Trips and Clinical Practicums

Teachers of classroom courses at a college or university can arrange field trips to various forensic facilities in the area. Online students can also participate in the field trips if they live nearby. The forensic facilities of interest for forensic nursing and multidisciplinary courses can be any of the following: medical examiner's or coroner's office, local jails, young offender centers, provincial or state penitentiaries, forensic psychiatric units, sexual assault centers, and women's shelters. Students appreciate the opportunity to tour these facilities, and the staff at the institutions look forward to talking about their area of work to students who may in the future work at the institutions as volunteers or employees. Following the tours, students often state they would never have considered working in the area had they not had the opportunity to actually go to the facility.

In a formal program of forensic study, nursing students are required to accumulate a certain number of hours in actual hands-on experience with forensic clients. The same venues that students visit in introductory course field trips may be used for these clinical practicums. Students are assigned for specific intervals to a variety of settings, and based on their program of study they may be allowed to choose an area for further concentration. Students studying forensic nursing in a distance education model must be more innovative in their approach to clinical experience than those in an on-site program. In some cases, they may be asked to seek out their own clinical experience or even to secure a mentor who must be approved and prepared for the role by the faculty of the college or university. In other situations, the students may be required to come to the campus for an intensive clinical experience in one or more venues.

Alternatively, the college or university may have agreements with forensic institutions in various geographic areas that the students may use if convenient. Some students enjoy the opportunity to travel to institutions that are known to have outstanding educational opportunities, regardless of the distance. The parameters and requirements for the clinical practicum must be clearly articulated and understood by the student before a commitment to a formal program leading to a credential in forensic nursing is undertaken.

Virtual Tours

Online students can participate in live field trips if they live nearby; however, most students live at great distances. For them, a virtual tour is the next best thing. A virtual tour has the advantage of not requiring the trip to be scheduled with the facility or the clearance of security checks to enter the building. A virtual tour can be facilitated by using photographs of the inside of forensic facilities (with the consent of management) in a PowerPoint presentation that is then added to the content of the WebCT or Blackboard online forensic courses. For example, a series of pictures can walk the student through many aspects of a forensic psychiatric unit—the security doors on entering, the nurses' station, the offender admission and visiting area, the bedrooms, the community and recreation areas and the security or time-out room. The security room of the forensic psychiatric unit has many elements worth pointing out in an online picture, such as the cameras, the special bathroom facilities, and the fiberglass bed frame.

Innovative teachers and students can take full advantage of the Internet to move from a paradigm of delivery to one of interactivity (Brown & Duguid, 1996). As our technologic society increases its rate of change, education will become increasingly important, and we will need to make our existing methods of instruction more effective, efficient, and appealing in a wide variety of contexts.

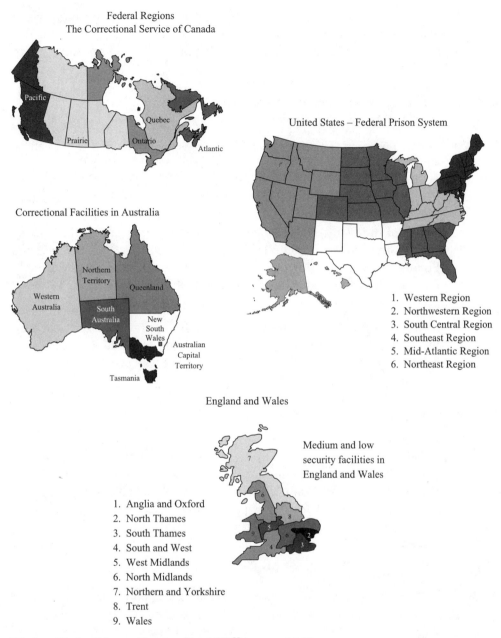

Federal Regions
The Correctional Service of Canada

United States – Federal Prison System

Correctional Facilities in Australia

1. Western Region
2. Northwestern Region
3. South Central Region
4. Southeast Region
5. Mid-Atlantic Region
6. Northeast Region

England and Wales

Medium and low
security facilities in
England and Wales

1. Anglia and Oxford
2. North Thames
3. South Thames
4. South and West
5. West Midlands
6. North Midlands
7. Northern and Yorkshire
8. Trent
9. Wales

Figure 27–8   Maps. *Source:* Kent-Wilkinson, 1997.

Using Maps to Highlight Forensic Systems and Services

Maps are another visual tool that is effective in forensic courses to provide
a broader understanding of the structure of the systems and services in
which forensic nurses practice. Many maps are now available online at
federal and local Web sites, including maps of forensic/correctional services by region in four different countries (Figure 27–8). Forensic nursing

educational programs, now available globally, could be put on a world map; however, like the written list included later in this chapter, it is difficult to keep updated, as forensic nursing programs are beginning to proliferate.

Using Flags to Provide an International Perspective

An international perspective is critical to teaching and learning about forensic nursing. The use of countries' flags is an effective way to show students what country each author is from when listing the required readings. In addition to putting a flag beside the required reading article, the author's name can be linked to a database containing that particular forensic expert's picture and biography. The article itself may be linked to any of the many electronic article database services that the university library may have contracted with (e.g., Ovid, Proquest, Academic Premier, Medline), allowing the student to access the article directly from any location in the world (Figure 27–9).

Flags can also be used to delineate the country-by-country time lines for historical events, laws and acts, and statistics or prevalence rates of each unit of study. As an interactivity, the question to students could be to speculate on reasons why the statistics or rates vary so much from country to country (Figure 27–10).

Multidisciplinary Expert Panels

Expert panels can be as effective online as in the classroom. Macromedia Shockwave can be used to facilitate the online functioning of the expert panel. When the picture of the panel member is selected online, his or her biography appears, and the student can select that expert's response to the questions asked of the panel. Involving the local community

---

Required Online Articles

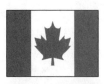

Kent-Wilkinson, A. (1999). Forensic family genogram: An assessment and intervention tool. *Journal of Psychosocial Nursing and Mental Health Services, 37*(9), 52-56. Retrieved May 22, 2004, from ProQuest database http://search.proquest direct.asp

Martin, T. (2001). Something special: Forensic psychiatric nursing. *Journal of Psychiatric & Mental Health Nursing, 8*(1), 25-32. Retrieved December 12, 2002, from Academic Search Premier database http://search.epnet.com/direct.asp

Figure 27–9   Required readings.

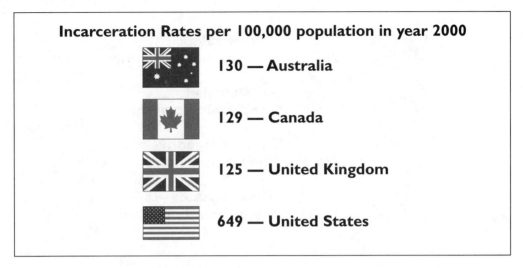

Figure 27–10   Incarceration rates, 2000. *Source:* Kent-Wilkinson, 1999a.

forensic experts in the course also serves to promote awareness of the course at the college or university.

Because the multidisciplinary team is integral to every subspecialty of forensic nursing, an expert panel could represent many members of the team. Local experts representing each discipline can be solicited for their picture and answers to interview questions regarding specific topics. Example questions could include the following: What drew you to your forensic profession? What makes you want to stay in this career? What are the specific roles of your practice? What are the current health-related issues of your practice? What research is needed? These provide the student with an understanding of the career paths taken by the multidisciplinary team.

International Ethical Discussions

For sensitive issues such as capital punishment, abortion, and euthanasia, it is often better for the students to view the excerpts online and read pro and con responses to the issues rather than having a debate among the students themselves. The point is not to present what is "right" or "wrong" in a debate, but rather to present "how it is" in a discussion. The reasons why countries have adopted certain laws and what the ethical issues are for forensic nurses in their practice are what the student needs to discover.

International Policies

Unique to forensic nursing are many laws, acts and policies of many countries that relate to the forensic populations of offenders and victims—living and deceased—that forensic nurses care for in their prac-

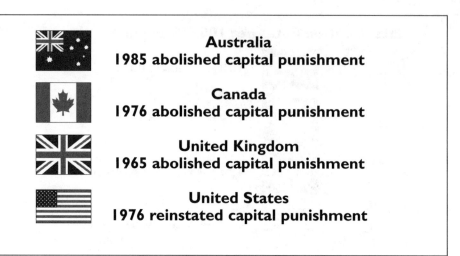

Australia
1985 abolished capital punishment

Canada
1976 abolished capital punishment

United Kingdom
1965 abolished capital punishment

United States
1976 reinstated capital punishment

Figure 27–11   Capital punishment policies. *Source:* Kent-Wilkinson, 1999a.

tice. Exposing the students to international policies, laws, and acts provides far more information for the student to question when the differences and similarities between countries are so visually evident. As an example, a policy such as capital punishment that is the law in some states or countries is a human rights violation in others. The years that certain policies were abolished or reinstated are interesting when comparing them to other countries in the world (first world and third world) (Figure 27–11).

Firsts and Facts

Forensic nursing, forensic science, and criminal justice science have had many historical advancements over the years. The many firsts and facts events should be included in time lines where achievements can be appreciated from country to country (Figure 27–12).

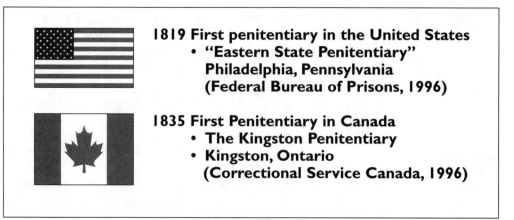

1819 First penitentiary in the United States
  • **"Eastern State Penitentiary"**
    Philadelphia, Pennsylvania
    (Federal Bureau of Prisons, 1996)

1835 First Penitentiary in Canada
  • **The Kingston Penitentiary**
  • **Kingston, Ontario**
    (Correctional Service Canada, 1996)

Figure 27–12   Firsts and facts. *Source:* Kent-Wilkinson, 1997.

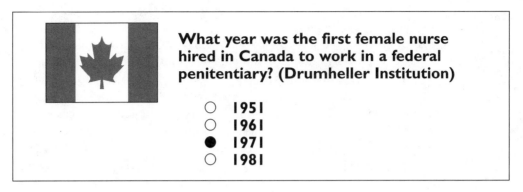

What year was the first female nurse hired in Canada to work in a federal penitentiary? (Drumheller Institution)

- ○ 1951
- ○ 1961
- ● 1971
- ○ 1981

Figure 27–13 Interactive quiz. *Source:* Kent-Wilkinson, 1999a.

Interactive Quizzes

"Forensic firsts" provide good content for interactive quizzes online. Most management systems for online courses contain quiz software. The unit quizzes can be used for self-assessment or for grading. The answers are tabulated and a mark for each quiz is recorded electronically. The software permits the students to see the marks they receive immediately and also to view the correct answers (Figure 27–13).

Online Glossaries

A glossary is often developed with a forensic course. The advantage of an *online* glossary is in the ease of use for the students and educators. A hypertext link can be created between specific forensic terms and the online glossary, which means as a student is reading online and comes across a term they may not be familiar with they can simply click on the word and be connected directly to its definition within the online glossary. For the educator the glossary can be utilized as a tool, for example: Terms from different units can be easily pulled together in an interactive quiz. (A forensic online glossary developed by the author of this chapter is accessible to students and educators worldwide at http://forensiceducation.com.)

Learning Objects

Learning objects, according to the Learning Object Metadata working group, are defined as "any entity, digital or non-digital, which can be used, or reused or referenced during technology supported learning" (Beck, 2003; Wiley, 2000, p. 4). Some of the popular learning objects for forensic nursing courses were created using Macromedia Shockwave. These templates can be reused, and the content can be changed for different units in the course. For example, a forensic puzzle can be reused as a new interactivity in a different unit, and an expert panel Shockwave template can be used in many different ways as well.

Case Studies

High-profile forensic cases are now often played out in the media. An inter-activity or an assignment for the student could be to identify as many forensic issues as possible in specific forensic cases, and to determine which forensic healthcare professionals have a role in the event and what their responsibilities are. For example, many child abduction cases have been discussed in the media. These cases often involve many of the foren-sic nursing subspecialties: victims, offenders, and forensic science. New laws may have resulted from the cases (e.g., Amber Alert, Megan's law, and Brian's law). Before, during and after the media event transpires, there would be points where the various forensic nursing subspecialties could be involved.

International Experts as Guest Lecturers Online

Students involved in an online forensic nursing course at the University of Calgary in Canada have had the opportunity to learn about and inter-act with forensic expert nurses from around the world (such as Singapore, Australia, and England). In a unit on terrorism, Lydia Lanxner, disaster preparedness nursing manager responsible for the readiness of the Laniado Medical Center in Netanya, Israel, in case of conventional terrorist attacks, unconventional use of biochemical agents, and global chemical warfare, explained to the students how she and her staff prepared for mass disasters during the 2003 Iraq war. As a guest expert, she responded to students' questions about mass terrorism and posted pictures of preparations that they had made in their emer-gency department in Israel (Figure 27–14). That winter semester, while the Iraq war was in progress, the students experienced a personal con-nection with a nurse whose department had experienced 11 terrorism attacks in the previous 12 months. They also heard of her personal fears for her own family's evacuation, as the possibility of terrorist attacks occurring near their own residence was also a constant reality.

Online Discussion Board

Students can respond to questions about all of the preceding interactivities on an online discussion board. Online discussion boards can be either *syn-chronous,* which is real time (similar to instant messenger services like ICQ), or asynchronous, where the questions are preposted and students can respond at a time convenient for them within the time frame of the course. Advantages and disadvantages to each exist. The disadvantage of synchro-nous discussion is that a time has to be arranged for all of the students and the instructor to be online. In many ways, this defeats one of the major advantages of online learning, which is flexibility. Also, it is difficult to arrange a time that is feasible for all when some students may live in dif-ferent time zones across the country or around the world. The asynchro-

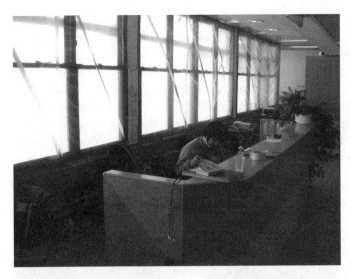

Figure 27–14
This three-part figure illustrates how an Israeli Medical Center prepared for mass disasters during the 2003 Iraq war. *Source:* Kent-Wilkinson, 2002. Photos from online lecturer Lydia Lanxner, Disaster Preparedness Nursing Manager for Laniado Medical Center in Netanya, Israel.

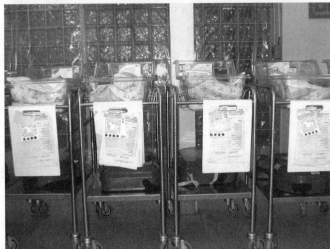

(Top) Lanxner sits at the nurses' station in front of windows taped and bagged in an effort to prevent glass from spreading in the event of a bombing.

(Middle) The Laniado Medical Center nursery prepares for the possibility of evacuation by equipping bassinets with respiratory packs.

(Bottom) Patient units fully secured and equipped in preparation for possible terrorist bombings.

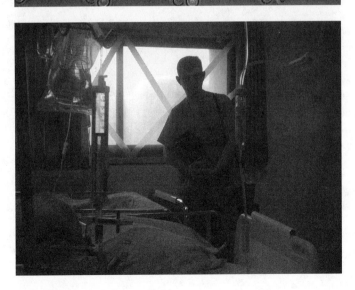

nous discussion board method is most popular for online courses, though since communication is not in real-time, the response is delayed. The interactive questions can be posted by the instructor each week or at the beginning of the semester. A *loaded discussion board* is a method in which all of the course questions for each unit interactivity are preloaded before the course starts. When the students begin the course, they can immediately see all of the questions to be answered in the time frame of the course semester and gauge for themselves how quickly they want to proceed (Figure 27–15).

Research suggests that online discussion groups can contribute to the development of competence. Students enjoy more *think time* in asynchronous online discussions. Higher-level thinking and independence are fostered in threaded discussion groups, as students collect, evaluate, and create in this unique learning environment. Individuals who tend to be timid or reserved in face-to-face discussions sometimes see online discussions as a lower risk environment and will thus contribute more.

RESEARCH IN ONLINE FORENSIC NURSING COURSES

An exploratory study done in 1998 may have been the first research done on forensic nursing online courses. Mount Royal College conducted a study of its first forensic nursing Internet course. Data from the

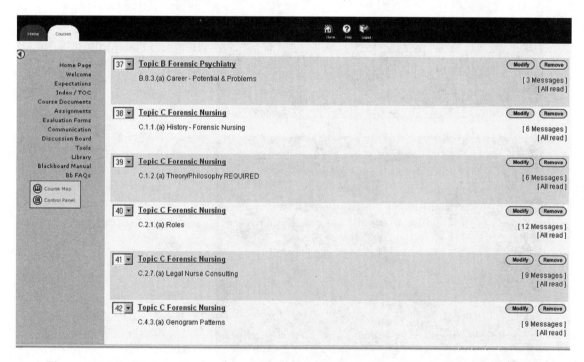

Figure 27–15   Discussion board: asynchronous interaction. *Source:* Kent-Wilkinson, 2002.

student evaluations were analyzed to determine what technical and content design characteristics affected student learning outcomes when instructional technologies were used online in the delivery of distance education in forensic nursing. An independent researcher contracted by the college conducted the research to determine the efficiency and effectiveness of Mount Royal College's first forensic online course.

The findings revealed that students valued time and place flexibility, access to course topics that they could not otherwise access, and interaction with instructor, students, and special guests globally. Students also valued the course delivery and development of new technical knowledge. Students also provided commentary on how their experience would be different without online course delivery. The immediacy of communication, access to online resources, and an ability to take the course despite geographic location/prior family and professional commitments were seen as areas that would have been compromised or absent in a traditional modality delivery (Harvey, 1998).

The 1998 study found that most participants in the forensic online course surveyed chose to participate in the course because of their interest in the subject matter. Over half of the participants chose the course because of the way it was delivered. Personal enrichment and reasons related to career opportunities or enhancing current career status were most often cited as reasons for taking a forensic course at that time. Close to 70% of participants involved in the distance-delivery studies were new to technology, most having used a computer for less than 1 year or not at all. Only 10% of students were experienced users who had computer experience of 6 to 10 years. Participants in the study agreed or strongly agreed that courses that used technology resources for distance delivery worked as well as those offered in a more traditional setting (Harvey, 1998).

Quantitative feedback supported findings that because of the online resources students had increased access to materials, could work at their own pace, and acquired relevant skills and abilities that they will extend beyond the course in studies, career, and in some cases everyday life. Graphics in the course were highly valued also. Finally, quantitative data supported the findings that the discussion board allowed students to consider the comments they made and to participate in discussions which explored issues related to the course material and that access to the instructor was enhanced (Harvey, 1998).

For many students, in 1997, threaded discussion groups, listservs, and chat resources were new. Significant increases in ability ratings of computer skills were reported by students by the end of the course. The listservs provided opportunities for interesting discussions that broadened the scope of the knowledge offered. Students also appreciated the humor involved in these exchanges (Harvey, 1998). The full study can be viewed online at the Web site provided in the references.

THE FUTURE OF FORENSIC NURSING EDUCATION

Significant changes are occurring in nursing education around the world as institutions restructure to address financial constraints and the changing needs of the profession. Many universities are implementing specialized forensic programs and developing an educational niche for themselves driven by the passion of forensic nurse experts, many of whom have pioneered forensic nursing roles in their clinical practice and/or published early works on forensic nursing concepts. Specialization in forensic nursing is a popular focus area that many universities are embracing. In addition, forensic areas of research with regard to prevention and marginalized populations are gaining attention as important areas of funding.

Not only is there a need for more forensic nursing programs, but there is also a need for a forensic nursing educational framework to promote standardization and program structure. This framework should emphasize international concepts within the forensic nursing curriculum.

Because forensic nursing is a relatively new specialty, there has been limited research regarding development of models specifically designed for forensic nursing education. The use of educational models would provide the needed framework not only for theoretical education, but also for practical applications in the clinical areas.

Changes are occurring in education and technology at the same time that interest has increased internationally in the emerging specialty of forensic behavioral science. Media exposure has brought a recent fascination about and heightened interest in the understanding of the mind of infamous perpetrators, and the social/legal issues of how to deal with offenders and care for their victims are in the forefront. Because of this recent interest in the study of forensic health practices there is increasing demand for forensic courses internationally. Although the media, by inadvertently propagating the term *forensics,* may have brought forensic areas and working with stigmatized marginalized groups to prominence and acceptability in society today, the responsibility to transmit the unique knowledge and philosophical underpinnings of the forensic nursing specialty falls to forensic nursing leaders.

Not only have forensic nurses become the most common providers of primary care for many of society's vulnerable and stigmatized populations, but forensic nursing has also gained prominent recognition and specialty status as the nursing profession's response to the preclusion and repercussions of criminal and interpersonal violence in society. With the number of forensic nursing publications mounting and with the media's publicity bringing awareness to this dynamic field, the future looks promising for forensic nursing education.

ACKNOWLEDGMENT

The author acknowledges the international experts, the instructional designer teams, and the computer technicians who participated in the panels and interactivities, globally, for their clerical and administrative support that make the content of forensic nursing courses a virtual reality: Mount Royal College and University in Calgary in Calgary, Alberta and the University of Saskatchewan in Saskatoon, Canada. Also, a special thank you to Lydia Lanxner for her contributions.

QUESTIONS FOR DISCUSSION

1. Where can I work as a forensic nurse?
2. How are on site and online forensic nursing courses similar and different?
3. What content can I expect in forensic nursing courses?
4. What teaching and learning strategies have been effective in forensic nursing courses?
5. Where can I take forensic nursing courses?

REFERENCES

Ahern, T. C., & Repman, J. (1994). The effects of technology on online education. *Journal of Research on Computing in Education, 26*(4), 537–546.

American Nurses Association (1997–2000). *Ethics and human rights position statements: Cultural diversity in nursing practice.* Washington, DC: Author. Retrieved May 16, 2004, from http://www.nursingworld.org/readroom/position/ethics/etcldv.htm.

Bates, A. W., & Poole, G. (2003). *Effective teaching with technology in higher education: Foundations for success.* New York: Jossey-Bass/Wiley. Retrieved December 21, 2003, from http://www.batesandpoole.ubc.ca

Beck, R. J. (2003). *Learning objects.* Milwaukee, WI: Centre for International Education: University of Wisconsin. Retrieved July 5, 2004, from http://www.uwm.edu/Dept/CIE/AOP/learningobjects.html

Berg, B. L. (2001). *An introduction to content analysis: Qualitative research methods for the social sciences* (4th ed., pp. 238–267). Toronto, Ontario, Canada: Allyn & Bacon.

Brown, J., & Duguid, P. (1996, July/August). Universities in the digital age. *Change: The Magazine of Higher Learning,* 11–19.

Canadian Nurses Association. (2000, February). Cultural diversity: Changes and challenges. *Nursing Now—Issues and Trends in Canadian Nursing, 7.* Ottawa: Author. Retrieved April 14, 2003, from http://www.cnanurses.ca/_frames/search/searchframe.htm.

Canadian Nurses Association. (2004). *Promoting culturally competent care* [Position Statement]. Retrieved January 31, 2005, from http://canaiic.ca/

CNA/documents/pdf/publications/PS73_Promoting_Culturally_Competent_Care_March_2004_e.pdf.

Hamric, A. B. (2000). *Advanced Nursing Practice.* Philadelphia, PA: W.B. Saunders.

Hanson, C. M. & Hamric, A. B. (2003). Reflections of the continuing evolution of advanced practice nursing. *Nursing Outlook,* 51(5), 203–211.

Harvey, P. (1998). *On-line distance learning in acute critical care nursing and forensic health studies: Preliminary case-study report.* Calgary, Alberta, Canada: Mount Royal College. Retrieved November 13, 2003, from http://www.mtroyal.ab.ca/olt/main2a.htm

Hawley, P., & Desborough, K. (1998). The computer as tutor. *The Canadian Nurse/L'infirmiere canadienne, 94*(4), 31–35.

International Association of Forensic Nurses. (1996). *Sexual assault nurse examiner standards of practice.* Thorofare, NJ: Slack. (Available online at: http://www.forensicnurse.org/ShopIAFN).

International Association of Forensic Nurses. (2001a, October 1). *Resolution I: Terror on September 11.* IAFN 9th Annual Scientific Assembly, Orlando, FL: Author.

International Association of Forensic Nurses. (2001b, October 1). *Resolution II: Forensic nursing education.* IAFN 9th Annual Scientific Assembly, Orlando, FL: Author.

Kent-Wilkinson, A. (1997). *FORE 4401 - Forensic history, risk population and issues. Forensic Studies.* Calgary, AB, Canada: Mount Royal College. Retrieved February 9, 2005, from http://www.mtroyal.ca/healthcomm/ashs/FOREcoursedesc.php?textfile=FORE4401.txt

Kent-Wilkinson, A. (1999a). *FORE 4403 - Forensic history, risk population and issues. Forensic Studies.* Calgary, AB, Canada: Mount Royal College. Retrieved February 9, 2005, from http://www.mtroyal.ca/healthcomm/ashs/FOREcoursedesc.php?textfile=FORE4403.txt

Kent-Wilkinson, A. (1999b). *Forensic icons.* Forensic education website. Retrieved December 7, 2004, from http://www.forensiceducation.com

Kent-Wilkinson, A. (2000). Forensic nursing course proposal [Course content index]. Graduate Certificate in Health - Correctional Nursing. Flinders University of South Australia, School of Nursing and Midwifery, Adelaide, Australia.

Kent-Wilkinson, A. (2001, October 17). *Forensic nursing: International educational technologies.* [Invited Plenary Address] Psychiatric Nurses Association (FPNA), Blackpool, England, UK.

Kent-Wilkinson, A. (2002). *NURS.503.08. Focus on forensic: Forensic nursing and health care in forensic populations* [Course content index]. Post Registration BN Program, Calgary, AB, Canada: University of Calgary.

Kent-Wilkinson, A. & Hanson, L. (2002). *Collaboration in the development of multimedia interactivities within the development of a Forensic WebCT Course.* Retrieved May 27, 2004, from http://www.forensiceducation.com/forensic_edu/proposal677.html

Kent-Wilkinson, A., Mckeown, M., Mercer, D., McCann, G., & Mason, T. (2000). Practitioner training, future directions, and challenges for practice. In

D. Mercer, T. Mason, M. Mckeown & G. McCann (Eds.), *Forensic mental health care: A case study approach* (pp. 349–357). Edinburgh: Churchill Livingstone.

Mason, T. (2002). Forensic psychiatric nursing: A literature review and thematic analysis of role tensions. *Journal of Psychiatric and Mental Health Nursing, 9,* 511–520.

Naught, P. (2002). Compassionate care: Flight nurse heads program to assist sexual assault victims. *Forensic Nurse Magazine.* Retrieved June 7, 2004, from http://www.forensicnursemag.com/articles/281feat2.html.

Wiley, D. A. (2000). Connecting learning objects to instructional design theory: A definition, a metaphor, and a taxonomy. In D. A. Wiley, (Ed.), *The instructional use of learning objects: Online version.* Retrieved May 18, 2001, from http://reusability.org/read/chapters/wiley.doc

APPENDIX A: FORENSIC NURSING PROGRAMS GLOBALLY

Included here is a list of all known existing forensic nursing educational programs to-date. Compiled by Arlene Kent-Wilkinson 2003.

Africa

South Africa, Africa
University of the Free State, South Africa
http://www.uovs.ac.za
Faculty of Health Sciences School of Nursing
Qualification in Forensic Nursing
http://www.uovs.ac.za/fac/health/registerednursing/ForensicNursing.doc

Australia

North Queensland, AU
Townsville and Cairns,
James Cook University in Australia
http://www.jcu.edu.au/theuni/
MSc in Forensic Mental Health
NS5360:03 Issues in Forensic Mental Health 1
NS5362:03 Issues in Forensic Mental Health 2
http://www.jcu.edu.au/courses/handbooks/2004/subjects/ns5360.html

South Australia
The Flinders University of South Australia
Adelaide, SA
http://www.flinders.edu.au/
Graduate Certificate in Health (Clinical Forensic Nursing)
http://www.flinders.edu.au/courses/postgrad/clin_forensic.htm
Graduate Certificate in Health (Correctional Nursing)
http://adminwww.flinders.edu.au/courses/postgrad/correct_nurse.htm

Western Australia
Edith Cowan University (flexible delivery)
School of Nursing and Public Health
Perth, WA
http://www.cowan.edu.au/
Postgraduate Certificate in Forensic Mental Health Nursing
http://www.ecu.edu.au/acserv/hb2002/pg/chs/school_of_nursing_and_
public_health/post_graduate_certificate_in/forensic_mental_health_
nursing.html

Western Australia
University of Notre Dame
Fremantle, WA
http://web.nd.edu.au
Postgraduate unit in clinical forensic nursing
http://web.nd.edu.au/news/media/2003/forensic_nursing.shtml

Canada

Alberta
Mount Royal College
Calgary, AB
http://www.mtroyal.ca
Forensic Studies
http://www.mtroyal.ca/forensic

Alberta
University of Calgary
Calgary, AB
http://www.ucalgary.ca
NURS 503.08 Introduction to health care and forensic populations
http://www.forensiceducation.com/forensic_edu/503.08description.htm

British Columbia
British Columbia Institute of Technology
http://www.bcct.ca
Forensic Science Technology: Advanced Specialty Certificate Program

British Columbia
Douglas College
Vancouver, BC
http://www.douglas.bc.ca/
Forensic Nursing Certificate
"Intro" to nursing in the justice system
http://www.douglas.bc.ca/calhtm/courses/cnurs.htm

Saskatchewan
University of Saskatchewan, College of Nursing
Saskatoon, SK
http://www.usask.ca
NURS 486.3 Forensic nursing in secure environments
http://www.usask.ca/nursing/postreg/index.htm
MN with forensic focus
http://www.usask.ca/nursing/masters/index.html

Ireland
Royal College of Surgeons
St. Stephens Green
Dublin, Ireland
Psychiatric Nursing in Forensic and Secured Environments
(1 year) certificate course
http://www.rcsi.ie

New Zealand

Wellington
Whitireia Community Polytechnic
Porirua, NZ
http://www.whitireia.ac.nz
Postgraduate Certificate in Forensic Psychiatric Care
http://www.whitireia.ac.nz/programme.php?key=67&career_id=
Forensic%20Psychiatric%20Carer

United Kingdom

England
University of Liverpool
Liverpool, England
http://www.liv.ac.uk
Post-graduate Diploma in Forensic Behavioral Science
leading to 2 yr Masters degree MSc
in forensic behavioral science (thesis)

England
University of Teesside
Middlesbrough, UK
http://mental-health.tees.ac.uk/
Forensic Health and Social Care
Forensic Multidisciplinary Practice
24 credits
Mental Disorder and Crime
http://www.tees.ac.uk/schools/soh/subjects/modspec.cfm?ID=
271&SubAreaID=14

Scotland
University of Dundee
Dundee, Scotland
http://www.dundee.ac.uk
Forensic Medicine, School of Nursing
BN Forensic Nursing Module
http://www.dundee.ac.uk/forensicmedicine/nurse/nurseindex.htm

England
King's College London, University of London
Institute of Psychiatry at the Maudsley
http://forensic.iop.kcl.ac.uk/msc/downloads/Forensic-Mental-Health-Science.pdf
MSc in Forensic Mental Health Science.
http://www.iop.kcl.ac.uk/iopweb/departments/home/default.aspx?locator=431

United States

California
American Forensic Nurses
Palm Springs, CA,
http://www.amrn.com
Forensictrak
http://www.forensictrak.com

California
University of California
Riverside Extension
Riverside, CA
Forensic nursing certificate program (online)
http://www.ucrextension.net/certificates/forensic-nurse.html

Colorado
Beth-El College of Nursing
University of Colorado
Colorado Springs, CO
http://web.uccs.edu/bethel/
Graduate Certificate in Forensic Nursing
http://web.uccs.edu/bethel/grad_cert_programs.htm

Connecticut
Quinnipiac University
Hamden, CT
http://www.quinnipiac.edu
Master of Science in Forensic Nursing
http://www.quinnipiac.edu/x1338.xml

Idaho
Canyon College
Caldwell, ID
Online Forensic Nursing Certificate Program
http://www.canyoncollege.edu/forensicnur.htm

Louisiana
Louisiana State University Health Sciences Center (LSUHSC)
New Orleans, LA
http://www.lsuhsc.edu
Introduction to Forensic Nursing
http://www.nursingsport.lsuhsc.edu/
http://nursing.lsuhsc.edu/ContinuingEducation/Programs/Spring/
Forensics2.cfm

Maryland
Johns Hopkins University School of Nursing
Baltimore, MD
http://www.jhu.edu
Masters of Science in Nursing; clinical nurse specialist, forensic nursing
http://www.son.jhmi.edu/academic_programs/masters/hlthsys/
forensics.asp

Massachusetts
Fitchburg State College
Fitchburg, MA
http://www.fsc.edu
Masters of Science in Forensic Nursing
http://www.fsc.edu/nursing/grad/index.html
Forensic Nursing Certificate Program
http://www.fsc.edu/catalog/Grad/forensicnursing.html

New Jersey
Monmouth University
West Long Branch, NJ
http://www.monmouth.edu
Forensic Nursing Certificate
http://www.monmouth.edu/academics/schools/graduate/programs/
fngc.asp
Masters of Science in Forensic Nursing
http://www.monmouth.edu/academics/registrar/msnforensic02.asp

New Jersey
Seton Hall University, College of Nursing
South Orange, NJ
http://www.shu.edu

Graduate Nursing
Dimensions of Violence: Individual course
Assessment of sexual assault survivors

New York
Kaplan College
New York, NY
http://www.kaplancollege.edu
Forensic Nursing Certificate Program online
http://www.elearners.com/program/4038.htm

Ohio
University of Cleveland State
Cleveland, OH
http://www.csuohio.edu/nursing
Masters of Science in Nursing: Population Forensics
http://www.csuohio.edu/nursing/Forensic%20graduate%20bulletin.pdf

Ohio
University of Cincinnati
College of Nursing
http://nursing.uc.educ
Cincinnati, OH
Advanced Concepts in Forensic Nursing
http://nursing.uc.edu/ProfessionDevelop/ForensicNursing.html

Ohio
Xavier University
Cincinnati, OH
http://www.xu.edu
Masters of Science in Nursing with Forensics Concentration
http://www.xu.edu/MSN/forensics/forensics.html

Oklahoma
University of Central Oklahoma
Edmond, OK
http://www.ucok.edu
Department of Nursing
Masters of Science in Forensic Sciences (Forensic Nursing)
http://204.154.117.68/nursing/msin.htm
http://nurse.ucok.edu:8080/MSForensic.jsp

Pennsylvania
Duquesne University
Pittsburgh, PA
http://www.nursing.duq.edu
Forensic Nursing (MSN, Post MSN, PhD) online
http://www.nursing.duq.edu/gradMsnForen.html

Pennsylvania
La Roche College
Pittsburgh, PA
http://www.laroche.edu/home.asp
Forensic Nursing Certificate Program
http://www.laroche.edu/schools/professions/DisciplineDetail.asp?
DisciplineID=596

Pennsylvania
University of Scranton
Scranton, PA
http://matrix.scranton.edu
Nursing 444 Forensic Health Care of Victims

Pennsylvania
University of Pennsylvania, School of Nursing
Philadelphia, PA
http://www.nursing.upenn.edu/
MSN Minor in forensic nursing
Forensic science, forensic mental health nursing, victimology

Tennessee
Vanderbilt University, School of Nursing
Nashville, TN
http://www.vanderbilt.edu/
Masters of Science in Nursing Program, Forensic Nursing
http://www.mc.vanderbilt.edu/nursing/msn/forensic.html

Tennessee
University of Tennessee
Health Science Centre
http://www.utmem.edu/
Memphis, TN
MSD, PhD Forensic Focus, DNSc
The Integrated Model of Forensic Nursing
http://www.utmem.edu/nursing/

Washington State
Gonzaga University
Spokane, WA
http://www.gonzaga.edu
Masters of Science in Nursing, with option of forensic/corrections

Washington
University of Washington
Seattle, WA
Advanced Practice Forensic Nurse Specialist
APFNS program leading to MN
38-credit course of study leading to a Masters of Nursing (MN) degree
http://www.son.washington.edu/eo/apfns/

West Virginia
Carilion Health System
Forensic Nurse Examiner Program
http://www.carilion.com/sane

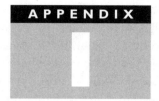
Legal Issues in Forensic Nursing: Search and Seizure of Evidence

Mary M. Galvin

Forensic nurses by definition are required to navigate the areas where law and medicine intersect. Some of these areas include sexual assault examinations where medical treatment is administered and evidence is collected for use in court; medical examiner autopsies and investigations; child sexual abuse interviews and examinations; treatment for physical assaults and domestic violence; and forensic mental health assessments and examinations.

This appendix is intended to provide an overview of certain areas of the law that will frequently arise in the forensic context. Forensic nurses should be aware of the basics of search and seizure law, the requirements for chain of custody of evidence, the admissibility of statements made by defendants and others, and legal foundations for expert opinion testimony.

FOURTH AMENDMENT

The Fourth Amendment to the U. S. Constitution commands that:

> The right of the people to be secure in their persons, houses, papers, and effects, against unreasonable searches and seizures shall not be violated, and no warrants shall issue, but upon probable cause, supported by oath or affirmation, and particularly describing the place to be searched, and the persons or things to be seized.

The U.S. Supreme Court has ruled that the Fourth Amendment protects any person who has a "reasonable expectation of privacy" (*Katz v. U.S.*, 389 U.S. 347, 88 S.Ct. 507 [1967]). This means that if police search a person or his or her property for which there is a reasonable expectation of privacy, then either the officer must have a search warrant issued by a judge or there must be an exception to this warrant requirement. When a defendant in a criminal case claims that the Fourth Amendment has been violated, he does so by moving to suppress the evidence. The court's suppression of improperly seized evidence is done pursuant to what is called "the exclusionary rule." In addition, a defendant must have standing to claim a violation of Fourth Amendment rights. The doctrine of standing requires that the police must have violated the *defendant's* individual right to privacy, not someone else's. In other words, the defendant cannot use the exclusionary rule to exclude evidence based on a violation of a victim's or third party's Fourth Amendment rights. The defendant can only use this right to claim a violation of her *own* privacy rights. As a result, a motion to suppress evidence from the medical examination of the victim based on a claim of an improper search or seizure would not be available to a defendant in a criminal case.

The forensic nurse should recognize that the use of a criminal search warrant is one proper way that the police comply with the U.S. Constitution. There are also exceptions to the warrant requirement, and these also comply with the U.S. Constitution. It is perfectly proper for the police to use one of the following exceptions to seize evidence:

- Plain view
- Exigency
- Consent
- Inventory
- Caretaker
- Stop and frisk
- The car doctrine
- Search incident to a lawful custodial arrest

There are also three areas where it has been held that the Fourth Amendment does not apply and does not provide its protection:

- Open fields
- Private party searches
- Abandonment

Of these various warrantless searches, a forensic nurse is most likely to encounter the exceptions of exigency, plain view, consent, caretaker, or search incident to a lawful custodial arrest. The other exceptions to the warrant requirement are usually found in contexts that do not involve a forensic nurse.

The exigency exception applies to situations in which the police must act hastily to enter a location in order to prevent the loss of evidence, to alleviate danger to life, or to prevent the escape of a wanted felon. Furthermore, when police come upon the scene of a homicide or serious assault, they may perform certain legitimate emergency activities without a warrant. At such a scene, the police may make a search for other victims or for suspects and may seize any evidence that they find in plain view during these legitimate emergency activities (*Mincey v. Arizona,* 437 U.S. 385, 98 S.Ct. 2408 [1978]).

The plain view doctrine allows law enforcement officers who are in a place where they have a legal right to be to seize any item that they have probable cause to believe is evidence of a crime.

A properly executed consent to search constitutes another exception to the warrant requirement of the Fourth Amendment. A valid consent to search must be freely and voluntarily given by a person who is capable of giving that consent. A reviewing court will examine various factors including age, education, intelligence, and physical condition to decide if the person is capable of giving a valid consent. As a result, police may inquire of a nurse as to whether an individual is competent to give consent. Police officers often will prefer a written consent because it is usually easier to establish in court than a verbal consent. Although the person giving consent is not required to have direct physical control over the item that is the object of the consent, that person must have mutual authority over the property or must have joint use of the item if it is shared property. Sometimes this means that a parent may legally consent to a search of their child's belongings.

Caretaker searches occur when law enforcement officials seize property as part of their caretaking function. The courts rarely utilize this exception; some of the few situations in which it has come up involve the seizure of clothing cut off of a patient by a nurse or EMT. Such removal of clothing has been held to constitute abandonment of neither the clothing nor any possessions contained within the clothing. Nevertheless, the seizure of such property may be upheld under the caretaker exception, because the items were taken into custody to protect them and take care of them. In some jurisdictions a warrant or consent will be required before any further examination or testing can be performed on items seized under the caretaker exception.

When an arrestee is taken into lawful custody, the police may seize his or her clothing as an incident of that arrest. This is often referred to as a station house seizure of clothing, and is done to preserve the clothing for evidence and for forensic examination and testing. An arrestee's clothing can be a valuable source of evidence including bodily fluids, hair, and trace evidence.

In conclusion, the Fourth Amendment protects citizens from unreasonable searches and seizures. These rights are individual and must be asserted by the person whose privacy interests have been impacted. Therefore, when a victim is examined, and evidence is seized from the victim, the offender cannot claim a Fourth Amendment violation because the offender's reasonable expectation of privacy is not involved. Only the victim's expectation of privacy is involved in such an examination. A defendant's Fourth Amendment rights are personal and must arise from his or her own reasonable expectation of privacy.

CHAIN OF CUSTODY

When clothing or evidence is seized from a victim of a crime, some common legal challenges to the admission of that evidence are based upon improper chain of custody, contamination of the evidence, or spoliation of the evidence.

The law requires that a proper chain of custody be kept on seized evidence to the extent necessary to provide a reasonable assurance to the court that the evidence to be introduced is the same evidence that was seized by the police and that its condition is substantially unchanged. Therefore, unique or individualized items will generally require a less strict chain of custody than generic or fungible items. When evidence is seized during a medical examination of a victim, it is very important to properly document who has obtained the evidence, who packaged the evidence, and the police officer to whom any evidence was given. All of these steps are necessary to ensure a proper chain of custody. Claims that evidence was contaminated can involve situations where samples are mixed or improperly packaged. Spoliation of evidence can occur when an item is not properly preserved, when it is discarded, or when relevant evidence is not seized and is therefore lost.

EXPERT OPINION

Pursuant to Rule 702 of the Federal Rules of Evidence, an expert may render opinion testimony:

> If scientific, technical, or other specialized knowledge will assist the trier of fact to understand the evidence or to determine a fact in issue, a witness

qualified as an expert by knowledge, skill, experience, training, or education, may testify thereto in the form of an opinion or otherwise, if

(1)   the testimony is based upon sufficient facts or data
(2)   the testimony is the product of reliable principles and methods
(3)   the witness has applied the principles and methods reliably to the facts of the case

Before allowing such expert testimony, the court may examine the expert's credentials and qualifications to make sure that the witness is qualified to render an expert opinion. Nurses have been qualified to render relevant opinions in courts in the United States. The specific science that an expert like a nurse is testifying about may also be reviewed by the court and must be found to be reliable. The case of *Daubert v. Merrill Dow Pharmaceuticals* (509 U.S. 579, 113 S.Ct. 2786 [1993]) controls the admission of expert testimony and requires that before an expert is allowed to testify, their science must pass through the following gatekeeper test for expert testimony:

1. The scientific theory or technique can be and has been tested.
2. The theory or technique has been subjected to peer review and publication.
3. The scientific technique has a known or potential rate of error or follows set standards.
4. The theory or technique has general acceptance in the relevant scientific community.

Essentially the *Daubert* gatekeeper test guarantees that any expert testimony given by a nurse be about a scientific theory or technique that has been established as valid and reliable. The thrust of the *Daubert* case was to make sure that courts don't admit "junk" science or untested theories.

STATEMENTS

Questions frequently arise about the admissibility of statements that are obtained in a hospital. Such statements may be obtained from defendants who are receiving treatment and are being questioned by the police. Sometimes statements from victims or other witnesses are given while seeking treatment and become part of the hospital record. The law makes provisions concerning the admissibility or inadmissibility of these various statements.

When a defendant makes a statement in a hospital or in the presence of a nurse, that statement may be admissible as evidence against the offender at trial. Some important legal requirements must be met before the defendant's statement will be admitted into evidence. If the defendant was in police custody at the time of questioning, then he must be advised of his rights pursuant to *Miranda v. Arizona* (384 U.S. 436, 86 S.Ct. 1602 [1966]) before questioning begins. The defendant must waive these rights and agree to talk to the police. Another constitutional requirement that must be met in order for an offender's confession to be admitted is voluntariness. In order for a statement by a defendant to be admitted in court, the statement must have been "the product of his free and rational choice" (*Mincey v. Arizona, supra*). If the defendant's physical condition is impaired to the degree that she cannot exercise her free and rational choice, then her statement will not be admitted in court. As a result of this rule, police will frequently check with the nurse or head nurse in a hospital before questioning a suspect. The fact of hospitalization does not preclude a finding of voluntariness of a confession. The court will review each situation on a case-by-case basis to assess whether a defendant was capable of giving a voluntary statement. It is not uncommon for police to request the presence of medical personnel when they take a statement or confession from a hospitalized person. This is done to ensure that the police officer will not be accused of overriding the suspect's free will, and so that medical personnel will be available to testify accurately concerning the suspect's condition and ability to speak with the police.

Although many out-of-court statements are excluded from evidence by the hearsay rule, the statement of a victim or witness made for the purpose of medical diagnosis or treatment is admissible under an exception to the hearsay rule. The following reflect Rule 803 (4) of the Federal Rules of Evidence concerning hearsay exceptions:

> Statements made for purposes of medical diagnosis or treatment and describing medical history, or past or present symptoms, pain, or sensations, or the inception or general character of the cause or external source thereof in so far as reasonably pertinent to diagnosis or treatment.

This hearsay exception is carved out to specifically address the situation of an individual presenting himself to a hospital for diagnosis or treatment. Statements made to a doctor or nurse can fall under this exception to the hearsay rule, and if so, will be admissible into evidence. This exception is relevant when a sexual assault victim presents at the hospital, and allows such hearsay statements to be presented in court. Therefore, the importance of accurately recording statements made by victims and witnesses in the medical record is obvious for both medical and legal purposes.

In addition, some states have a doctrine called "constancy of accusation," wherein certain statements made by rape victims within a short time after the crime are admissible as evidence. It is not unusual for a nurse to be a "constancy of accusation" witness, specifically in the context of a prompt report and presentation for treatment by the victim. Again, the laws of each state apply, and there is wide variation in the existence and application of this hearsay doctrine.

VICTIMS' RIGHTS

All states have some form of assistance for victims of crime, and every state has passed some type of statute to provide assistance to victims. In fact, some states have enacted constitutional amendments to their state constitutions that can afford substantial rights to victims of crime. Some of the statutory provisions that have been passed to assist victims include notification requirements, compensation for various types of economic loss, rape shield laws, protection of personal information, and the right to be heard in court. Because significant differences exist among the states on the rights that are afforded to victims, it is necessary to review each state's statutes in order to ascertain which rights are provided to a victim in a specific state.

Potential victims also have a right to be notified of certain dangers. If a person seeing a therapist, which can include a psychiatric nurse, gives reasonable cause to believe the patient is dangerous to a third person, then the therapist has a duty to warn that potential victim (*Tarasoff v. The Regents of the University of California,* 17 Cal. 3d. 425; 551 P.2d 334 [Ca.1976]).

Individual states may afford their citizens, including victims and wrong-doers, greater rights than the U.S. Constitution provides (in other areas of constitutional and statutory law that are discussed in this appendix). In other words, the U.S. Constitution sets the minimal level of constitutional rights that must be afforded to every citizen. The states may give their citizens greater, but never less, protection than the federal constitution.

SUMMARY

Forensic nurses practice at the crossroads of law and medicine. They are in a field where knowledge of both medicine and law is essential. Although their emphasis is on the science of nursing, to be "forensic," they must also learn the law.

OTHER RELEVANT LEGAL CITATIONS

Exclusionary rule	*Mapp v. Ohio,* 367 U.S. 643, 81 S.Ct. 1684 (1961).
Standing	*Rawlings v. Kentucky,* 448 U.S. 98, 100 S.Ct. 2565 (1980).
Plain view	*Horton v. California,* 496 U.S. 128, 110 S.Ct. 2301 (1990).
Consent	*Schneckloth v. Bustamonte,* 412 U.S. 218, 193 S.Ct. 2041 (1973).
Third-party consent	*United States v. Matlock,* 415 U.S. 164, 94 S.Ct. 988 (1974).
Caretaker	*Cady v. Dombrowski,* 413 U.S. 433, 93 S.Ct. 2523 (1973); *State v. Joyce,* 229 Conn. 10 (1994).
Search incident	*United States v. Edwards,* 415 U.S. 800, 94 S.Ct. 1234 (1974).
Accusation constancy/consistency	*State v. Roldan,* 257 Conn. 156 (2001).

Evidence Collection Guidelines

SPECIMEN TYPE	IDENTIFICATION INFORMATION	PACKAGING	PRESERVATION	COMMENTS
Fingerprints				
Porous surface	Outside container	Box, paper	Package to prevent contact with other surfaces.	
Smooth surface	On lift	Individual labels on lifts in sealed envelope, number in sequence	Process with contrasting powder & lift print.	Only trained persons should attempt to dust and lift fingerprints.
Visible print (blood, oil, etc.)	On container	Entire item/relevant portion for lab processing	Prevent contact and chemical exposure.	Chemical enhancement may be necessary.
Postmortem prints	On collected prints	Envelope, once set	If finger tissue is removed, preserve in glycerol or other nondrying fluid.	Dry hands of cadaver thoroughly; take both finger and palm prints. Call laboratory for assistance if decomposition is advanced.
Imprints				
Smooth surface	Nonimprint area	Box original surface or lift.	Prevent contact with imprint.	Lift only if residue. Photograph appropriately prior to collection.
3D impression	Nonimprint area	Paper wrap or box	Make casting.	Photograph prior to cast.
On moveable item	Nonimprint area	Wrap flat in paper.	Avoid contact with imprint.	Submit entire item.
Hairs				
Individual hairs	On packet	Paper chemist fold/packet	Packet into outer envelope.	Individual hairs may be picked up with forceps. Vacuuming is not recommended.
On moveable item	On item	Wrap in paper.	Place in paper bag.	Avoid unnecessary activity and movement of item.
Known hair standards	On packet	Place in paper with chemist fold/ packet.	Packet into outer envelope.	Pulled hairs are best, 15–20 per area. If cut, place scissors against skin to get entire length of exposed hair.

SPECIMEN TYPE	IDENTIFICATION INFORMATION	PACKAGING	PRESERVATION	COMMENTS
Hairs (continued)				
Pubic/head hair combings	On packet	Comb over paper. Fold paper into chemist fold/ packet.	Place in an envelope and seal.	
Fibers				
Individual fibers	On packet	Paper chemist fold/packet	Packet into outer envelope.	Individual fibers may be picked up with forceps. Vacuuming is not recommended.
On moveable item	On item	Wrap in paper.	Place in paper bag.	Avoid unnecessary activity and move-ment of item.
Known fibers	On packet	Paper chemist fold/packet	Packet into outer envelope.	Sufficient sample should be collected to obtain all fiber types, weave, etc. in the fabric.
Rope, Twine, Cordage				
Any cord type	Tag or mark container	Entire length	Wrap securely in clean paper. If small strands, place in folds as fibers.	If cut during collection, clearly label ends as cut by you and their association.
Soil/Minerals/ Drugs/Other Powders				
Trace amounts	On container	Plastic or paper sealed container with no seams	If moist, be sure to use sturdy container.	Submit as soon as possible to avoid mold growth or deterioration. If on moveable item, collect entire item.
Standard samples	On container	At least 2 Tbsp in a sealed plastic or paper container	If moist, be sure to use sturdy container.	
Glass/Paint				
Fragments	On container	Individual fragments in paper fold	Place folds in an envelope or sealed container.	Maintain separate packets for individual samples.
Standards	On container	Individual paper fold/sample	Place each fold in an envelope or sealed container.	Collect known stan-dards as close to damaged area as possible.
Firearms/ Weapons				
Entire weapon	On weapon away from other evidence	Secured to prevent motion and abrasion	Avoid excessive con-tact with the object.	Handle for safety. May contain trace materials & body fluids. Do not place anything in the barrel of a gun.
Bullet, cartridge	On package	In paper packet or box	Avoid cotton in package. Do not wash. Handle to avoid loss of trace materials.	Do not place multiple projectiles or car-tridges together.

SPECIMEN TYPE	IDENTIFICATION INFORMATION	PACKAGING	PRESERVATION	COMMENTS
Unknown Material				
Powder	On package	Place in paper chemist fold before secondary package.	Chemist fold into envelope; avoid plastic bags to prevent loss by static.	Handle all unknown powders as potential infectious or hazardous material.
Liquid	On container	Up to 5 ml if homogeneous appearance in glass or inert plastic container	Seal around container opening. Place in plastic zipper bag to protect against loss.	
Body Fluids				
Urine/other liquid body fluid	On container, identifying type or appearance of material	Use a clean bottle or test tube with leak-proof stopper.	Keep samples separate. Refrigerate, if possible.	Entire liquid sample should be collected. At least 30 ml if voided urine. If diluted, collect a representative sample.
Stains on clothing	Tag or mark clothing item.	Fold entire item in paper. Place in paper bags. *Never* use plastic.	Avoid marking or folding in area of staining.	Handle carefully to protect stain patterns and to prevent loss of other trace materials. Do not roll item.
Organs/Tissue				
Tissue sample, product of conception, excised injury area, etc.	On container	Sterile glass jar or plastic container *without* additional liquid or preservative	Keep cool or refrigerate. Freeze for longer storage.	*Never* use chemical preservative or alcohol with tissues if DNA or other testing may be required.
Blood				
Liquid—draw	On container	Sterile tube with EDTA or no preservative; package to prevent damage or breakage.	Refrigerate; do not freeze.	Handle as biohazardous material.
Liquid—small quantity	On container	Sterile tube with EDTA or no preservative; package to prevent damage or breakage.	Refrigerate; do not freeze.	Collect entire sample, up to 5 ml.
Dry stain	On packet and outer container	Use a sterile swab wet with a small amount of dH_2O. Place dried swab in envelope.	Air dry swab under natural conditions or in swab dryer.	Maintain in cool, dry place. Do not lick envelope to seal.
Stained clothing, fabric, etc.	Label tag or mark directly on clothes.	Fold in paper, each item separately packaged. Place in paper bag.	If wet when collected, air dry under natural conditions.	Do not use heat to dry. Do not place bloody clothing in plastic bags.
Volatile Liquids				
Accelerants, alcohols, etc.	On container	Collect debris in clean paint cans. Place liquid samples in airtight glass containers.	Maintain in a cool, dry place or refrigerate.	

Selected Assessment Tools

The assessment tools included in this appendix may be useful in the evaluation of the forensic client. Forensic nursing practice involves treating or interfacing with clients from various age groups, ethnic groups, and socio-economic levels and in a variety of settings. The reason for the client/nurse interaction may vary, ranging from treatment to risk assessment to preparation for trial. In order to provide the most effective intervention as well as establish needs and predictors for further interventions, various assessment tools have been created. It is essential that these tools be utilized by those who have the skills to administer, interpret, and draw conclusions from the data obtained. In order to develop a level of comfort and self-confidence in administering these tools, the nurse should review the action to be undertaken once the assessment has been completed.

Nurses must consider HIPAA and ethical guidelines and have informed consent prior to undertaking any assessment procedures. We have listed only a sample of the many varied assessment tools available to the forensic nurse—the large number of possibilities exceeds the scope of this appendix. The resources identified in this appendix represent a sampling of guidelines currently available, and at times represent "works in progress" to be further developed by those practicing in the field. The forensic nurse should research the various assessment tools available for specific purposes. The Internet is an invaluable source of information, as are peer review, networking, and the exchange of information among colleagues. Any screening tool or scale must be culturally sensitive and age appropriate, and utilize language that the client can understand. Assessment tools may not exist for certain forensic client populations. The role of the forensic nurse as researcher and collaborator becomes even more important in those situations.

ASSESSMENT TOOLS

Children & Adolescents

Screening for Pregnant and Nonpregnant Clients by Her Gynecologist/ Obstetrician.
www.acog.org

Dienemann, J., Campbell, J., Landenborrer, K., & Curry, M. A. (March 2002). The domestic violence survivor assessment: A tool for counseling women in intimate partner violence relationships. *Patient Education and Counseling, 46*, 221–228.

Sherdan, D. J. (1988). *The Harassment Instrument.* Available from Dshen.dan@son.jhml.edu.

Council on Scientific Affairs. (1992). Violence against women relevance for medical practitioners. *Journal of the American Medical Association, 267*(23), 3184–3189.

Elder Abuse

Wolf, R. (2003). *Risk assessment instruments.* Available from www.elderabusecenter.org/default.cfm?p=riskassessment.cfm.

Reis, M. & Nahmiash, D. (1998). Indicators of abuse screen. *The Gerontologist, 38*(4), 471–480.

Post-traumatic Stress Disorder

National Center for Post-Traumatic Stress Disorder: www.ncptsd.org.

This resource provides clinicians and researchers with descriptive, reference, and contact information about child and adult measures of trauma exposure and response. This is a very valuable site for the forensic nurse; however, there are strict ethical guidelines related to administration of assessment tools.

American Psychiatric Association. (2000). *Diagnostic and statistical manual IV.* Washington, DC: Author.

Teen/Adolescence

Center for Disease Control and Prevention Youth Risk Behavior Surveillance System. Washington, DC: Department of Health and Human Services. Retrieved from www.cdc.gov/mccdphp/dash/yrbs/2001 on June 19, 2003.

Merell, K. W. (1999). *Behavioral, social, and emotional assessment of children and adolescents.* Mahwah, NJ: Lawrence Erlbaum Associates.

Domestic Violence/Intimate Partner Abuse

Centers for Disease Control and Prevention: Division of Violence Prevention
www.cdc.gov/ncipc/dvp/dvp.htm

Chalk, R. (2000). Assessing family violence interventions. Linking programs to research based strategies. *Journal of Aggression Maltreatment and Trauma, 4*(1), 29–53.

Knopp, P., Hart, S., Webster, C., & Evans, D. (1995). *Manual for the spousal risk assessment guide.* Vancouver, Canada: British Columbia Institute on Family Violence.

McFarlane, J., & Parker, B. (1994). *Abuse during pregnancy—A protocol for prevention and intervention.* New York: National March of Dimes, Birth Defects Foundation.

McFarlane, J., Hughes, R. B., Nosek, M. A., Groff, J. Y., Swedland, N., & Mullen, P. D. (2001). Measuring frequency, type and perpetrator of abuse toward women with physical difficulties. *Journal of Women's Health and Gender-Based Medicine, 10*(9), 861–866.

McFarlane, J., Parker, B., Soeken, K., & Bullock, L. (1992). Assessing for abuse during pregnancy. *Journal of the American Medical Association, 267*(3), 3176–3178.

National Domestic Violence Hotline
1-800-799-SAFE(7233)
1-800-787-3224 (TTY)

Rape, Abuse & Incest National Network/New Haven Sexual Assault Hotline
1-800-656-HOPE
1-800-656-4673
www.rainn.org

Civil Rights

American Civil Liberties Union
132 W. 43rd Street
New York, NY 10036-6599
(212) 944-9800

Collective Violence

Centre for the Study of Violence and Reconciliation
www.wits.ac.za/csvr

Global Internally Displaced Persons Project
www.idpproject.org

Elder Abuse

Action on Elder Abuse
www.elderabuse.org.uk

International Network for the Prevention of Elder Abuse
www.inpea.net

National Center on Elder Abuse
www.elderabusecenter.org

National Committee for the Prevention of Elder Abuse
www.preventelderabuse.org/index.html

Mental Health

National Alliance for the Mentally Ill (NAMI)
www.nami.org

National Institute of Mental Health (NIMH)
www.nimh.nih.gov

Prevention Institute
www.preventioninstitute.org/mental.html

Migrant Workers

Association of Occupational and Environmental
Clinics
www.aoec.org

Migrant Clinicians Network
www.migrantclinician.org

National Alliance for Migrant Health
www.hispanichealth.org

National Center for Farmworkers Health
www.ncfh.org

Suicide

American Association of Suicidology
www.suicidology.org

Suicide Prevention Advocacy network
www.spanuss.org

Teens/Adolescence
www.preventioninstitute.org/schoolvio/4html

Violence Against Women

Global Alliance Against Traffic in Women
www.inet.co.en/org/gaatw

National Sexual Violence Resource Center
www.nsvrc.org

Office of Violence vs. Women
www.osp.usdos.gov/vawo/

Research, Action and Information Network for the Bodily Integrity of
Women
www.rainbo.org

Women Against Violence Europe
www.wave-network.org

Youth Violence

Center for the Prevention of School Violence
www.ncsu.edu/cpsv

National Center for Injury Prevention and Control
www.cdc.gov/ncipc

National Criminal Justice Reference Source
www.ncjrs.org/intlwww.html

United Nations Crime and Justice Information Network
www.uncjin.org/Statistics/statistics/html

Organizations

Amnesty International
www.amnesty.org

Centers for Disease Control and Prevention: National Center for Injury
Prevention and Control
www.cdc.gov/ncipc/pub_res/intimate.htm

Centro Latino-Americano de Estudos sobre Violencia e Saude
www.ensp.fiocruz.br/claves.html

Human Rights Watch
www.hrw.org

Inter-American Coalition for the Prevention of Violence
www.iacpv.org

International Center for the Prevention of Crime
www.crime-prevention-intl.org

Trauma.org
www.trauma.org/trauma/html

United Nations Research Institute for Social Development
www.unrisd.org

World Health Organization
www.who.int/

www.who.int/violence_injury_prevention/pdf/injuryguidelines.pdf
(injury surveillance guidelines)

Internet Resources

AMERICAN BAR ASSOCIATION

This is the site of the professional organization that represents the nation's attorneys. In addition to its role in providing member services, it sponsors many initiatives designed to improve the public's use of the legal system. It has many useful links located in a section on specialized resources, including Children & the Law, Domestic Violence, Homelessness and Poverty, Human Rights, and Senior Citizens.

http://www.abanet.org

AMERICAN MEDICAL ASSOCIATION (AMA)

This is the site of the professional organization that represents the nation's physicians. The AMA offers consumer health information, a doctor finder, journals and research information for physicians, and policy and advocacy information. It contains many links to topics of interest to forensic nursing.

www.ama-assn.org

AMERICAN NURSES ASSOCIATION (ANA)

The is the site of the professional organization that represents the nation's 2.6 million registered nurses. Its stated mission is to "foster high standards of nursing practice, promote the economic and general welfare of nurses in the workplace, project a positive and realistic view of nursing, and to lobby the Congress and regulatory agencies on healthcare issues affecting nurses and the public." It contains many useful links including up-to-date news and press releases, an online journal, career opportunities, and a bioterrorism site. There are also links to the organization's other entities, the credentialing center, and the American Nurses Foundation. Other organizational specialty affiliates as well as constituent members can be accessed as well.

http://nursingworld.org

AMERICAN PSYCHOLOGICAL ASSOCIATION

This is the website of the professional organization that represents psychologists. It provides a great deal of information relative to all aspects of violence and suicide.

http://www.apa.org

ANA DEFINITION OF ADVANCED PRACTICE NURSING

This is a good site for a quick review of the state of advanced practice nursing in the United States including definitions, statistics, and commentary on nurses' roles.

http://www.nursingworld.org/readroom/fsadvprc.htm

ANTHRAX AND SMALLPOX—BEING PREPARED FOR BIOTERRORISM

The National Network for Immunization Information (NNII) has compiled resources with information on bioterrorism agents (anthrax and smallpox) and vaccine need/supply. The NNII's partner organizations in this effort include the Infectious Diseases Society of America, American Academy of Pediatrics, American Nurses Association, American Academy of Family Physicians, and American College of Obstetricians and Gynecologists.

http://www.immunization.org/

BIOTERRORISM AND DISASTER PLANNING

This site, linked from the ANA website, provides information on how to plan for a bioterrorist attack, and contains links to the American Hospital Association planning site, the American Red Cross, the Johns Hopkins Center for civilian biodefense strategies, and information regarding the volunteer medical reserve corps.

http://nursingworld.org/news/disaster/bioprep.htm

BROOKINGS INSTITUTION (PUBLIC POLICY)

The Brookings Institution describes itself as "an independent, nonpartisan organization devoted to research, analysis, education, and publication focused on public policy issues in the areas of economics, foreign policy, and governance. The goal of Brookings activities is to improve the performance of American institutions and the quality of public policy by using social science to analyze emerging issues and to offer practical approaches to those issues in language aimed at the general public." There are many useful links on this site including listings of events and forums, research topics, and publications. There is also a search engine and a link to the three study programs—economic, foreign policy, and governance.

http://www.brookings.org

CENTERS FOR DISEASE CONTROL AND PREVENTION (CDC)

The CDC serves as the national center for developing and applying disease prevention and control, environmental health, and health promotion and education activities designed to improve the health of the people of the United States. As such, it is the clearinghouse for up-to-date public health emergency response and preparedness information.

http://www.bt.cdc.gov

CHILDREN, BIOTERRORISM, AND DISASTERS

This American Academy of Pediatrics (AAP) site is a compilation of AAP resources and materials on disasters, bioterrorism, and psychological support of children. It also provides links to other sites with resources on bioterrorism and to directories of health departments.

http://www.aap.org/advocacy/releases/cad.htm

COMPETENCIES FOR MASS CASUALTY RESPONSE

This site, provided by the American Association of Critical Care Nurses, includes, among other things, a report of the International Nursing Coalition for Mass Casualty Education's competencies, entitled "Educational Competencies for Registered Nurses Responding to Mass Casualty Incidents." The premise of developing these competencies is that every nurse must have sufficient knowledge and skill to recognize the potential for a mass casualty incident, identify when such an event may have occurred, know how to protect oneself, know how to provide immediate care for those individuals involved, recognize his or her own role and limitations, and know where to seek additional information and resources. Other links provided at this site include the American Red Cross, the National Nurse Response Team, Public Health Security and Bioterrorism Preparedness and Response Act of 2001, and federal legislation related to the September 11 attacks.

http://www.aacn.org/AACN/pubpolcy.nsf/vwdoc/Sept11

CREDENTIALING

This site provides information on certification and recertification through the American Nurses Credentialing Center (ANCC), a division of the American Nurses Association. In addition to credentialing information, this site provides links to conferences, workshops and seminars, educational research, magnet programs, and consultation services.

http://nursingworld.org/ancc/

DEPARTMENT OF JUSTICE

This site describes the department's mission to ensure the enforcement of the laws of the nation fairly and effectively and to defend the interests of the United States according to the law. It contains many subsections including Publications, Press Releases, Civil Rights & Liberties Violations, Disabilities, Dispute Resolution, Domestic Violence, Faith-Based & Community Initiatives, Fraud, Immigration Information, Prison & Parole Information, Safe Communities, Trafficking in Persons, Youth Violence, Victims of Crime, Fugitives, Grants, and Bioterrorism. It also contains many useful links to other federal sites pertaining to law, including a separate site for children and youth.

http://www.usdoj.gov

DEPARTMENT OF HOMELAND SECURITY

This site describes the mission of the department as being first and foremost the protection against terrorist attack and also to protect the rights of American citizens and to enhance public services, such as natural disaster assistance and citizenship services, by dedicating offices to these important missions. Features on this site include Emergencies and Disasters, Travel and Transportation, Immigration and Borders, Research and Technologies, Threats and Protection, and Press Releases. It contains useful links to other agencies such as Immigration and Naturalization Services, the FBI, U.S. Customs Services, the Federal Emergency

Management Agency (FEMA), Strategic National Stockpile and the National Disaster Medical System (HHS), Nuclear Incident Response Team (Energy), and Domestic Emergency Support Teams (Justice).

http://www.dhs.gov/dhspublic

ELEMENTS OF EFFECTIVE BIOTERRORISM PREPAREDNESS— A PLANNING PRIMER FOR LOCAL PUBLIC HEALTH AGENCIES

This 28-page document was developed by the National Association of County and City Health Officials (NACCHO) to help local public health officials and their partners to identify their public health and safety roles when responding to bioterrorism.

http://www.naccho.org/files/documents/Final_Effective_Bioterrism.pdf

FEDERAL BUREAU OF INVESTIGATION

The Uniform Crime Reports and other statistical reports of interest are published here, at the site of the Federal Bureau of Investigation. Analyses of trends in violent crime can also be found here.

http://www.fbi.gov

FOOD AND DRUG ADMINISTRATION

This site describes the role of the government in protecting the public health by assuring the safety, efficacy, and security of human and veterinary drugs, biological products, medical devices, our nation's food supply, cosmetics, and products that emit radiation. Among the many links contained on this site are several for bioterrorism and counterterrorism. There is also an extensive A–Z index providing information on a vast array of topics of interest to forensic nurses.

http://www.fda.gov/

GROUP VIOLENCE

This website offers a series of mini-lectures and discussions that address the origins and prevention of group violence. The activities described are intended to serve as a model for healing through connection and understanding, particularly in the area of group violence and genocide. There are many interesting links to related sites as well as to publications. It is a joint project of the Trauma Research Education and Training Institute and the University of Massachusetts at Amherst.

http://www.heal-reconcile-rwanda.org/

AN INTRODUCTION TO FIREARMS IDENTIFICATION

This site focuses on one of the disciplines of forensic science, firearms identification. Firearms identification concerns identifying fired bullets, cartridge cases, or other ammunition components as having been fired from a specific firearm. This site serves strictly as an educational resource, and is not affiliated with any government agency, professional organization, or commercial entity. It has a number of helpful features including an archive of previously published articles and a message board.

http://www.firearmsid.com

JOHNS HOPKINS UNIVERSITY CENTER FOR GUN POLICY AND RESEARCH

This site provides information and statistics on firearm injuries. It also serves as a resource for those interested in policy related to firearms and provides links to research in this area.

http://www.jhsph.edu/gunpolicy

MANAGING RADIATION EMERGENCIES: GUIDANCE FOR HOSPITAL MEDICAL MANAGEMENT

This site provides information that not only addresses basic explanations and definitions related to radiation, but also offers guidance to those responding both at the scene of an accident (prehospital) and at the hospital. The Radiation Emergency Assistance Center/Training Site is a 24-hour emergency response program at the Oak Ridge Institute for Science and Education (ORISE) that trains, consults, or assists in the response to all types of radiation accidents or incidents.

http://www.orau.gov/reacts/care.htm

MEN STOPPING VIOLENCE

Provides links and information on the prevalence and effects of men's violence against women in intimate relationships.

www.menstoppingviolence.org

NATIONAL ASSOCIATION OF CLINICAL NURSE SPECIALISTS

This is the official site of the National Association of Clinical Nurse Specialists (NACNS), which was founded in 1995. The mission of the NACNS states that it exists to enhance and promote the unique, high-value contribution of the clinical nurse specialist to the health and well-being of individuals, families, groups, and communities, and to promote and advance the practice of nursing. Members of NACNS benefit from national, regional, and local efforts of the association to make the contributions of CNSs more visible. The mission statements, core competencies, and a plan for graduate education of CNSs are available, although still in draft form at this time. There are links to all major professional nursing organizations, a discussion forum, and a student page.

http://www.nacns.org

NATIONAL CENTER ON ELDER ABUSE

This site provides information and statistical reports in addition to resources for prevention and intervention. Links to various publications are provided.

http://www.elderabusecenter.org

NATIONAL CENTER FOR POLICY ANALYSIS (NCPA)

According to its mission statement this organization is "a nonprofit, nonpartisan public policy research organization" whose goal is to "develop and promote private alternatives to government regulation and control, solving problems by relying on the strength of the competitive, entrepreneurial private sector. Topics include reforms in health care, taxes, Social Security, welfare, criminal justice, education and environmental regulation."

http://www.ncpa.org

NATIONAL COMMITTEE TO PREVENT CHILD ABUSE

This site provides data relative to the incidence and characteristics of child abuse, including fatalities.

http://www.childabuse.org

NATIONAL CRIMINAL JUSTICE REFERENCE SERVICE

A division of the U.S. Department of Justice, this site contains a large database of statistics, policy statements, and other communication related to violence and the criminal justice system.

http://www.ncjrs.org

NATIONAL INSTITUTES OF HEALTH

This is the site of the biomedical research arm of the federal government. Links provided at the site include that for the National Institute of Child Health and Human Development, which supports research on child health, including the risk for violence.

http://www.nih.gov

NATIONAL LEAGUE FOR NURSING

The stated mission of the organization is to advance quality nursing education that prepares the nursing workforce and to support nurse educators. The organization has an affiliate that serves as a credentialing body for academic programs in nursing. There are several useful links including a career site, a site for information and involvement in issues of public policy, and various position papers issued by the organization.

http://www.nln.org

NURSE ADVOCATE: NURSES AND WORKPLACE VIOLENCE

This website is dedicated to the recognition and resolution of workplace violence experienced by nurses, in support of those who have experienced violence and in memory of those who have died.

http://www.nurseadvocate.org

NURSING NETWORK ON VIOLENCE AGAINST WOMEN, INTERNATIONAL

The Nursing Network on Violence Against Women, International's mission is to eliminate violence by advancing nursing education, practice, research, and public policy. Their website includes pertinent links and legislative and conference information.

http://www.nnvawi.org

NURSING'S AGENDA FOR THE FUTURE

This site contains a strategic plan for addressing current issues facing the profession. Excerpts can be read at this site, or the entire document can be downloaded.

http://www.nursingworld.org/naf

PHYSICIANS FOR A VIOLENCE-FREE SOCIETY

This is a national nonprofit organization of physicians, other members of the healthcare community, and concerned citizens who are committed to reducing violence in the United States. This website includes educational resources, links to other sites, and information about conference and training opportunities.

http://www.pvs.org

PHYSICIANS FOR SOCIAL RESPONSIBILITY (PSR)

PSR has a violence prevention program that is building a national violence prevention network of physicians, public health professionals, PSR staff, and supporters working to reduce the number of firearms in the United States and eliminate domestic violence.

http://www.psr.org

PUBLIC HEALTH FOUNDATION (PHF)

This site states that it is a national, nonprofit organization dedicated to supporting, convening, and advancing efforts of local, state, and federal public health agencies and systems to promote and protect the health of people living within their respective jurisdictions. PHF is dedicated to improving the public's health by helping strengthen and build capacity and infrastructure of the public health system, including agencies, organizations, workforce, and communities. They do so by conducting applied research, sharing knowledge, providing training and technical assistance, anticipating future needs, and leading constructive change. The foundation has established core competencies for practice in the arena of public health that can be accessed through a link on the site's home page. Other links provide access to current project initiatives and research, public health training and resource materials, and a calendar of events.

http://www.phf.org

PUBLIC HEALTH—AMERICAN PUBLIC HEALTH ASSOCIATION (APHA)

APHA is an association of individuals and organizations working to improve the public's health and to achieve equity in health status for all. Its mission is to promote the scientific and professional foundation of public health practice and policy, advocate the conditions for a healthy global society, emphasize prevention, and enhance the ability of members to promote and protect environmental and community health. The APHA is the oldest and largest organization of public health professionals in the world, representing more than 50,000 members from over 50 occupations of public health. The organization states as its concerns a broad set of issues affecting personal and environmental health, including federal and state funding for health programs, pollution control, programs and policies related to chronic and infectious diseases, a smoke-free society, and professional education in public health. Many links to specific programs and initiatives, state and local public health agencies, continuing education programs, and other resources are provided.

http://www.apha.org

REGIONAL HEALTHY PEOPLE 2010 EVENTS AND PRIORITIES

Use resource listings, event information, and contacts on this site to get information relative to regional Healthy People 2010 activities and priority area(s), as determined by the U.S. Department of Health and Human Services. There are links to maps or state listings with information specific to all of the priority regions. For each region's priority area(s), one can download, print, or search listings of action resources in Acrobat Reader. Two-page resource listings describe Healthy People 2010 companion resources, sites with evidence-based strategies, and other tools to achieve and promote relevant objectives.

www.phf.org/HPtools/regions.htm

SEXUAL ASSAULT NURSE EXAMINER-SEXUAL ASSAULT RESPONSE TEAM

The SANE guide is designed for nursing professionals involved in providing evaluations of sexually abused victims. It can be found on this website, which provides information and technical assistance to individuals and institutions interested in developing new SANE-SART programs or improving existing ones.

http://www.sane-sart.com

SMALLPOX, BIG PROBLEM?

This article from *Nature* reports on a new model that suggests that if smallpox were to return, the disease would spread as fast as it did before vaccination. Swift detection and rapid intervention would be essential to control an outbreak. The results of the new model give a gloomier prognosis than another recent smallpox model by researchers at the Centers for Disease Control and Prevention (CDC), which concluded that the United States has enough vaccine to control a smallpox outbreak.

http://www.nature.com/nsu/011213/011213-15.html

TERRORISM AND SECURITY COLLECTION

This National Academies Press site provides free access to 26 recent publications from the National Academies about the science and policy issues surrounding terrorism and security. Included among the titles is a 2001 publication, *Firepower in the Lab: Automation in the Fight Against Infectious Diseases and Bioterrorism* and a 1999 report, *Chemical and Biological Terrorism: Research and Development to Improve Civilian Medical Response.*

http://www.nap.edu/terror/

THOMAS

This website provides information about federal legislation. Databases available include bill text, the *Congressional Record* text, Bill Summary & Status, and the *Congressional Record Index*. Links are provided to Frequently Asked Questions; House and Senate Directories, including member committee assignments and additional member information; and Congressional Internet Services, as well as to the websites of other legislative agencies, including the House, Senate, Library of Congress, Government Printing Office (GPO), General Accounting Office (GAO), Congressional Budget Office (CBO), and the Library of Congress.

http://thomas.loc.org

U.S. AGENCY FOR HEALTHCARE RESEARCH AND QUALITY (AHRQ)

The stated mission of this federally funded organization is "to support research designed to improve the outcomes and quality of health care, reduce its costs, address patient safety and medical errors, and broaden access to effective services." AHRQ funds research and demonstrations to translate the knowledge and tools acquired into measurable improvements in health care. In addition, AHRQ develops partnerships with public and private-sector organizations to disseminate the knowledge and tools for use in the health care system.

http://www.ahrq.gov

U.S. CENSUS BUREAU

The Census Bureau serves as the leading source of data about the nation's people and economy. In addition to providing information from demographic and economic surveys, the bureau also conducts surveys for various other organizations including the Bureau of Justice Statistics and the National Center for Health Statistics. Links to detailed information by state are provided.

http://www.census.gov

U.S. INSTITUTE OF PEACE

This is the website of an independent, nonpartisan federal institution created by Congress to promote the prevention, management, and peaceful resolution of international conflicts. Established in 1984, the Institute meets its congressional mandate through an array of programs, including research grants, fellowships, professional training, education programs from high school through graduate school, conferences and workshops, library services, and publications. The site contains links to all of these programs as well as to press releases and current news.

http://www.usip.org

WORKPLACE VIOLENCE

This site is sponsored by the ANA and contains information and documents related to workplace violence, including a list of legislative initiatives pertaining to workplace violence and their status, OSHA guidelines for preventing workplace violence for healthcare workers, and highlights of the Bureau of Justice Statistics special report on violence in the workplace.

http://nursingworld.org/dlwa/osh/violence.htm

Index